Jane Hiscock

Elaine Stoddart

Jeanine Connor

BEAUTY THERAPY

2nd edition

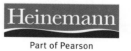

Part of Pearson

D1330285

Heinemann is an imprint of Pearson Education Limited, a company incorporated in England and Wales, having its registered office at Edinburgh Gate, Harlow, Essex, CM20 2JE. Registered company number: 872828

www.pearsonschoolsandfecolleges.co.uk

Heinemann is a registered trademark of Pearson Education Limited

Text © Jane Hiscock, Elaine Stoddart, Jeanine Connor, 2010

First published 2010

12 11 10
10 9 8 7 6 5 4 3 2 1

British Library Cataloguing in Publication Data
A catalogue record for this book is available from the British Library

ISBN 978 0 435 02701 8

Edited by Helen Atkinson

Designed by Wooden Ark

Typeset by Oxford Designers & Illustrators Ltd

Original illustrations © Pearson Education 2010

Illustrated by Hardlines and Oxford Designers & Illustrators Ltd

Cover design by Wooden Ark

Picture research by Susi Paz

Cover photo/illustration © Image Source

Printed in Italy by Rotolito Lombarda S.p.A

Websites
The websites used in this book were correct and up-to-date at the time of publication. It is essential for tutors to preview each website before using it in class so as to ensure that the URL is still accurate, relevant and appropriate. We suggest that tutors bookmark useful websites and consider enabling students to access them through the school/college intranet.

Acknowledgements

The author and publisher would like to thank the following individuals and organisations for permission to reproduce photographs:

Shutterstock/tonobalaguerf pp3, 348; Nigel Riches www.imagesource.com p9; Felix Mizioznikov/Shutterstock p18; Cut2White pp20, 119, 418, 517, 552; Jason Stitt/Shutterstock p41; Science Photo Library (boil) pp45, (wart) 46, (ringworm) 47, (chloasma) 238, (strawberry naevus) 239; Dr P. Marazzi/Science Photo Library (impetigo) pp45, (measles) 46, (blepharitis, conjunctivitis) 47, (bruise, scar tissue, eczema, psoriasis) 236/377, (acne rosacea) 237, (lentigo, haemangioma) 238, (spider naevus) 239; Western Ophthalmic Hospital/Science Photo Library (stye) p45; St Bartholomew's Hospital/Science Photo Library (cold sore) pp46, (dermatitis) 236, (acne vulgaris) 237; Biophoto Associates/Science Photo Library (chickenpox) pp46, (thrush) 47; Alain Dex Publiphoto Diffusion/Science Photo Library (cold) p46; Lorraine Kourafas/Shutterstock p54; Carlton Professional pp56, 60, 279, 286, 299, (percussion vibrator) 359, 360, 425, (top) 538; John Warburton-Lee Photography/Alamy p59; BeautyExpress pp63, (make-up) 298; Shutterstock/Apollofoto p88; Shutterstock/coka pp118, 173; Martin Barraud/Stone/GettyImages (young men) p122; Ariel Skelley/Stone/GettyImages (40+ ladies) p122; Trinette Reed/BlendImages/Photolibrary (young girls) p122; Yellow Dog Productions/Riser/GettyImages p126; Dima Kalinin/Shutterstock p127; Imagesource pp135, 153, 383; Jeffrey Blackler/Alamy p136; Dermalogica p138; CNRI/Science Photo Library p170; Flashon Studio/Shutterstock (black skin) p174; Sam Dcruz/Shutterstock (Asian skin) p174; AVAVA/Shutterstock (Oriental skin) p175; nolie/Shutterstock (mixed race skin) p175; Patrick Renice/Photononstop

Photolibrary p176; Steve Gschmeissner/Science Photo Library p179, 535; Stefano Ginella/Shutterstock p194; Shutterstock/Yuri Arcurs pp222, 421; Diego Cervo/Shutterstock p225; Bliznetsov/Shutterstock p228; Lucian Coman/Shutterstock p231; Dr Harout Tanielian/Science Photo Library p234; Jane Shemilt/Science Photo Library (cut) p236; Scott Camazine/Phototake/Alamy (skin tag) p237; Dr H.C.Robinson/Science Photo Library (milia) p237; B. Boissonnet/Science Photo Library (melanoderma) p238; James Stevenson/Science Photo Library (vitiligo) p238; moodboard/Alamy (freckles) p238; Medical-on-Line/Alamy (dilated/split capillaries) p239; John Radcliffe Hospital/Science Photo (port wine stain) p239; Skinlogic.co.uk (skin scanner) p241; Andrey Sukhachev/Shutterstock (Woods lamp) p241; SkinLogic p242; Julian Winslow/Photolibrary (normal skin) p243; Pinon Pinon/Photolibrary (dry skin) p243; Olga Sapegina/Shutterstock (oily skin) p243; Kirill Mikhirev/Shutterstock (sensitive skin) p244; Monkey Business Images/Shutterstock (mature skin) p244, 344, 510; Roxana Gonzalez/Shutterstock p245; Laurent Lucuix/Shutterstock (teens) p248; Lev Olkha/Shutterstock (20s) pp248, 494; iofoto/Shutterstock (30s) p248; Zsolt Nyulaszi/Shutterstock (40s) p248; Yuri Arcurs/Shutterstock (50s) p248; Dmitrijs Dmitrijevs/Shutterstock p249; Hans Neleman/Stone+/GettyImages p251; Brenda Carson/Shutterstock p252; Shutterstock/Alena Ozerova p256; Shutterstock/VladGavriloff p275; Ambrosia/www.lonie.com (pre-treatment cleanser) p277; Elemis p290; Guinot pp297, 298; Serg64/Shutterstock (fruit and veg) p298; www.familychiroandskincare.com p312; www.equipmedical.com p318; Andresr/Shutterstock p320; Shutterstock/eyedear p324; Stock Connection Blue/Alamy pp337, 355; Humbert/Severine/Photolibrary p338; Medicimage Medicimage/Photolibrary p339; vario images GmbH & Co.KG/Alamy p342; Kokhanchikov/Shutterstock p343; Solid Web Designs Ltd/Shutterstock p345–6; Cassiede Alain/Shutterstock p349; Imagemore Co. Ltd./Alamy (pool) p354; Dale Saunas (sauna) pp354, (shower) 355; Jerko Grubisic/Shutterstock (spa pool) p355; Shutterstock/Tatjana Strelkova p362; Christopher Futcher/Shutterstock p381; www.massagetablestore.com (stool) p387; Weleda p432; Shutterstock/Phase4Photography p434; Shutterstock/Valua Vitaly p456; Reda/Shutterstock p476; Hive (heater) pp487, (marble stones) 488, 499, 500; Diane Macdonald/Alamy (marine stones) p488; Stuart Pearce/Photolibrary p492; David Scharf/Science Photo Library p535; BalletNeedles/HofBeauty.com (bottom) p538; Vasiliy Koval/Shutterstock p542; Thorsten Rust/Shutterstock p553.

All other photos: Pearson Education Ltd/MindStudio; Pearson Education Ltd/Stuart Cox; Pearson Education Ltd/Lord and Leverett; Pearson Education Ltd/Studio 8 Clark Wiseman; Pearson Education Ltd/Gareth Boden; Pearson Education Ltd/Rob Judges.

With thanks to the following for their permission to reproduce realia: Health and Safety Executive p69; Federation of Holistic Therapists; www.fht.org.uk p84; Pictures supplied by Carlton Professional, leading UK manufacturers of Electrotherapy Equipment p313; Courtesy of Hive of Beauty Ltd www.hiveofbeauty.com p470, Sterex Electrolysis International Ltd pp527, 554.

Grateful thanks for their help in sourcing photographs to Trudy Sawyer at the Carlton Group, Joanne Etherson and Joyce Chan from Beauty Express, Amy Rowe from Hive of Beauty and Terry at HOF Beauty.

Every effort has been made to contact copyright holders of material reproduced in this book. Any omissions will be rectified in subsequent printings if notice is given to the publishers.

Crown copyright material reproduced with permission of the Controller of Her Majesty's Stationery Office and the Queen's Printer for Scotland.

Author acknowledgements
Whilst writing the Level 3 Beauty Therapy student book, Elaine and I have been fortunate to have been helped, advised and inspired by our colleagues, as well as guided by the wonderful team at Pearson who shaped our text into such a great finished product! Our heartfelt thanks go to all the support given by suppliers, copy editor Julia Naughton for her eagle eye and Faye Cheeseman and Caitlin Swain for their expertise and knowledge. My personal thanks must go to my husband Stephen, who took over all other aspects of our lives whilst I was immersed in writing, and my two beautiful daughters Victoria and Venetia – both beauty therapists – who shared their own experiences and training knowledge. Huge thanks also to Peter Symonds College: Alex Day my Director, the tutors, all the students and centre staff who were just fantastic when roped in to model or take part in the photos. Many, many thanks.

**Jane Hiscock; Head of Hairdressing,
Holistic and Beauty Therapy; Peter Symonds College**

Contents

Units B26/B27 Provide female and male intimate waxing services, B21 Provide UV tanning services and B25 Provide self tanning services are available on the Pearson Education website at www.pearsonfe.co.uk/BeautyTherapyLevel3units

Answers to the Check your knowledge quizzes are available on the Level 3 Tutor Resource Disk.

Introduction

Welcome to your Level 3 (NVQ/SVQ) Diploma in Beauty Therapy! This professional handbook has been written in an accessible format to provide all the underpinning knowledge and practical skills you need to succeed in your Level 3 course. The book is designed to guide you through the 2010 Level 3 National Occupational Standards (NOS) and is tailor-made for the Level 3 Beauty Therapy General and Massage Routes.

The treatments and specific skills that you will learn during this Level 3 course build on the knowledge and techniques you learned and practised in your Level 2, or equivalent, course. By enhancing your expertise, this Level 3 course extends your career options. With a Level 3 qualification, the world is literally your oyster and your career will take off in all sorts of directions – consider this book a good investment for your future!

What is a Diploma (NVQ/SVQ)?

NVQ stands for National Vocational Qualification and SVQ for Scottish Vocational Qualification (for those studying in Scotland). These qualifications are based on the National Occupational Standards (NOS) for Beauty Therapy which are written by HABIA – the organisation that represents the industry. NVQs/SVQs are assessment-based qualifications.

How do I gain a Certificate/Diploma (NVQ/SVQ)?

The qualification is gained by collecting a variety of **evidence** within each unit. It is practically based and will give you a good grounding for working with clients in a salon.

How do I get my evidence?

Many forms of evidence are acceptable. These will be recorded on **evidence sheets** provided and will form a **portfolio** – a collection of evidence. The following types of evidence are valid:

- observed work
- witness statements
- assessment of prior learning and experience (APL)
- oral questions
- written questions and/or assignments
- other (for example, photographs, videotape or client record cards).

What evidence do I need?

You should ask your assessor about the most suitable method for the work you are doing. Most of your evidence will be derived from direct observation of your work by your assessor; however you should also include a variety of evidence. All of the evidence needs to be recorded in your candidate logbook and collected together over a period of time in your portfolio to demonstrate your competence.

If you have previous experience (APL) – perhaps gained whilst working – or recent qualifications, they can also be counted. For example, if you work in a shop, part-time, and have experience using the till, dealing with customers and handling complaints, then a witness statement from your employer that is current, valid, signed and dated is very acceptable evidence.

What do I have to achieve?

First, your training establishment will register you with its awarding body. The awarding body will then issue you with your assessment book. Take care of it; it is very precious. It will become your only source of evidence for all your hard work.

Within your assessment book your will be given guidance on how to achieve each unit. Each unit is divided into Outcomes.

How is the qualification structured?

The new Level 3 (NVQ/SVQ) Diploma in Beauty Therapy qualification has been designed to enhance the career path of those wishing to have an all-round qualification, or provide routes for those wishing to specialise in massage or make-up. To complete the full award you must achieve eight units.

The mandatory units (which *must* be completed) are:

- G22 Monitor procedures to safely control work operations
- H32 Contribute to the planning and implementation of promotional activities

These are compulsory to all students, and cover all aspects of health and safety, product promotion and how to become a good team worker for your salon. You must take these two, and then choose one of the following routes:

- Beauty Therapy General Route
- Beauty Therapy Massage Route
- Beauty Therapy Make-up Route

This book provides all the mandatory units for both the General and the Massage Routes. Whichever route you decide to follow you must complete the following units:

Beauty Therapy General (Mandatory units)	Beauty Therapy Massage (Mandatory units)
B13 Provide body electrical treatments	B20 Provide body massage treatments
B14 Provide facial electrical treatments	B23 Provide Indian head massage
B20 Provide body massage treatments	B24 Carry out massage using pre-blended aromatherapy oils
B29 Provide electrical epilation treatments	B28 Provide stone therapy treatments

You will then be required to complete *two* further optional units. These include units such as G11 Contribute to the financial effectiveness of the business, B26/B27 Provide female and male intimate waxing services, and so on.

There are also two units available on the Pearson website at the following link: www.pearsonfe.co.uk/BeautyThearapyLevel3units. They are B21 Provide UV tanning services and B25 Provide self tanning services.

How to use this book

This book has been designed with you in mind to:

1. lead you through the Level 3 (NVQ/SVQ) Diploma in Beauty Therapy, providing background, technical guidance with suggested evidence collection and key skills

2. provide a reference book that you will find useful to dip into, long after you have gained your qualification. Comprehensive cross-referencing within the individual chapters will guide you through the NVQ units and indicate where the information applies.

Each of the practical units contains the same essentials — the **Professional basics**. This has been presented as a separate section that should be worked through and adapted to the unit you are taking at the time. The **anatomy and physiology** required for each unit has also been separated so that it can be accessed and referred to easily.

Features to help your learning

To reinforce your learning process and get you thinking, this book contains several features to help you.

Key terms — highlight terms that are central to your understanding of the topic, that you may not have come across before.

Think about it — activities to get you to think about applying theory to a practical situation. They will give you an opportunity to think about what you are doing when you are carrying out treatments, to ensure that you are striving for and achieving best practice.

Salon life — a full-page feature designed to look like the page of a magazine, covering a key issue or problem, including an account of a therapist's experience in the salon and expert guidance on the issue or problem covered.

My story — short, real-life accounts from people working within the industry with tips and suggestions. They are designed to get you to think about the different things you may need to think about in your day-to-day life as a beauty therapist.

Frequently asked questions — expert advice and answers to some of the most commonly asked questions — questions that may come up as you work through the practical units.

Check your knowledge — a list of multiple-choice and/or short-answer questions provided at the end of each unit to help you check your knowledge and understanding. Answers are provided on the Level 3 Beauty Therapy Teacher Resource Disk.

For your portfolio — tasks or activities which encourage learning through research and investigation. They are designed to help you to gather and generate evidence for your portfolio and key skills.

Getting ready for assessment — helpful information and advice about how each unit is assessed and guidance on what you will need to be able to demonstrate to your assessor in terms of skills and competencies.

Saks

We are pleased that this book has been endorsed by Saks. Saks Education is officially acknowledged as the UK's Best Training Provider, having been awarded Beacon Status by the Quality Improvement Agency and all grade ones by the Adult Learning Inspectorate for providing outstanding training. It is the only hair and beauty work-based learning provider to have been awarded both accolades.

Saks recognise that Education is the key to success! A good sound education can lead to numerous career opportunities within the beauty industry and the basis for that is NVQ Level 3.

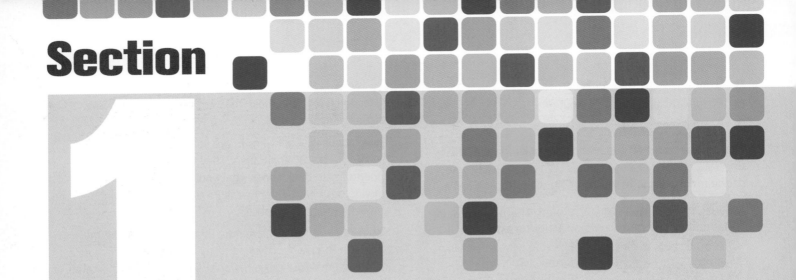

Section

1

Professional basics

Professional basics

What you will learn

- You – the therapist
- You and your client
- You and your working environment
- You, your client and the law

Introduction

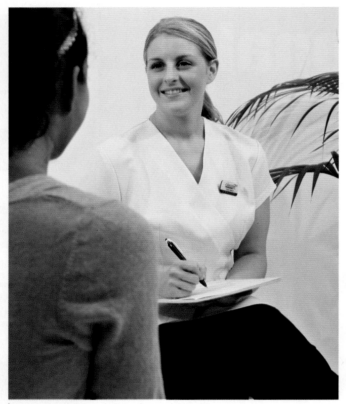

A thorough consultation before treatment is important for developing a good relationship with your client

The professional basics are literally everything that underpins the skills you will require to become a qualified beauty therapist.

Before you can decide upon the most suitable treatment for your client, or prepare **treatment plans**, you need to have a clear understanding of the basic underlying principles of what you are doing. Understanding the basics is very important to your development within the role of a professional beauty therapist and will help you to achieve your NVQ qualification.

It sets the highest of standards, which you should always aspire to. This is your transition from student to employee, and your employer will have a very high expectation of the new Level 3 recruit!

This section covers the basic knowledge you will need before you start working through any practical unit. You will need to refer back to this section each time you start a new practical unit.

You – the therapist

In this section you will learn about:

- personal appearance
- personal presentation
- personal safety and security
- personal risk assessment
- managing resources within the limits of your authority
- becoming an holistic therapist.

Before beginning any new training or learning new skills, you will need to go back to the fundamental basics of beauty therapy and start by looking at yourself – the beauty therapist. While not a novice at beauty therapy – you already have qualifications – it is very important that you assess yourself in a slightly different light and re-evaluate yourself in all aspects of professional life.

At this level, clients will also have a greater expectation from their treatments. A mental 'spring clean' and re-think will eliminate any bad habits which you may have and encourage you to develop the good practices you have adopted. Sometimes senior students become complacent – you should be setting an example to new students, as they really do look up and aspire to be like you, and not fall into careless habits, which can be hard to break.

Key terms

Treatment plan – a personal guide for each client, outlining the most suitable course of treatments to offer the client. It includes a comprehensive consultation, analysis of needs, suitable treatments, aftercare and homecare with retail suggestions. This is then written on a record card for both client and therapist to follow, depending upon time and cost considerations.

Think about it

It is not just about the skills you will learn, it is about developing an intuitive approach to your clients, having patience and a calm attitude, and wanting to help your client and putting them first. The outside troubles and stresses of normal life should be left behind by the client, and it is up to you to create the right sort of atmosphere in your treatment room to enable that to happen. This is true whether you are taking the beauty route or the massage route.

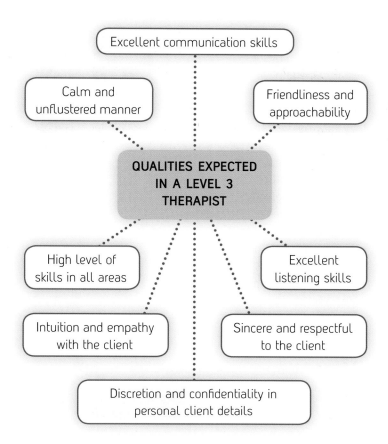

Excellent communication skills

Calm and unflustered manner

Friendliness and approachability

QUALITIES EXPECTED IN A LEVEL 3 THERAPIST

High level of skills in all areas

Excellent listening skills

Intuition and empathy with the client

Sincere and respectful to the client

Discretion and confidentiality in personal client details

NVQ Level 3 work requires a thorough approach as the electrical equipment used, if handled incorrectly, could cause your clients harm and you will need to be fully aware of **health and safety** implications.

Key terms

Health and safety – literally to be free from risk of injury, illness, disease or danger. Health and safety policies in the workplace are a set of rules to be followed by everyone to ensure risk and hazards and any potential problems to health are minimised.

Personal appearance

How you look not only represents you as an individual and your skill levels; you represent your college and your profession – all of us in the Beauty and Spa industry. We nearly all make snap judgements about people within the first ten seconds of meeting them. You want your first impression to be a good one, to encourage your clients to have faith in you, to inspire confidence and to encourage them to become a regular client.

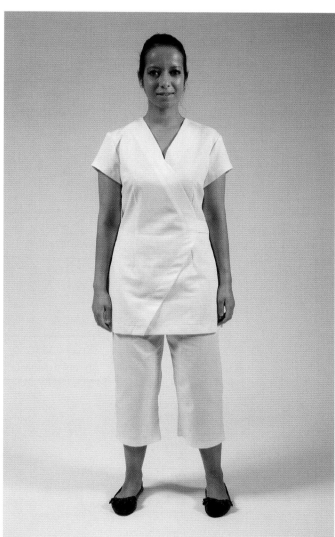

A professional appearance will give clients confidence in you

Your professional appearance says so much about you, your business and your abilities. All this is reflected in your personal appearance, body language and attitude. So you have just ten seconds to make the right impression, and convince the client that you are the therapist for his or her needs, while giving a caring and competent reflection of your abilities!

Think about it

Appearance is combined with spoken language and non-verbal communication to convey a variety of messages – an important thing to remember when greeting and dealing with clients.

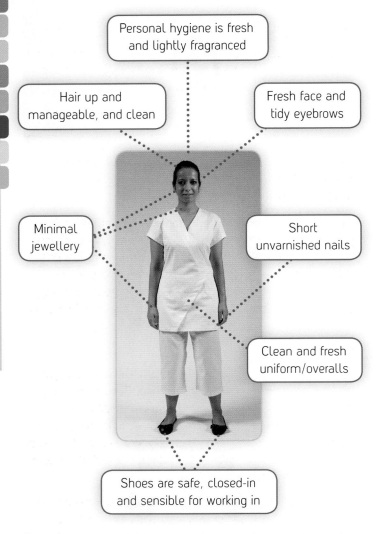

Personal hygiene is fresh and lightly fragranced

Hair up and manageable, and clean

Fresh face and tidy eyebrows

Minimal jewellery

Short unvarnished nails

Clean and fresh uniform/overalls

Shoes are safe, closed-in and sensible for working in

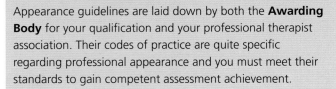

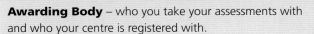

You have just ten seconds to make the right impression!

Think about it

Appearance guidelines are laid down by both the **Awarding Body** for your qualification and your professional therapist association. Their codes of practice are quite specific regarding professional appearance and you must meet their standards to gain competent assessment achievement.

Key terms

Awarding Body – who you take your assessments with and who your centre is registered with.

Uniform

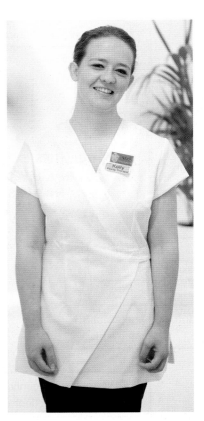

Be critical about your overalls. If you have had them since you first started training, they may not be as immaculate as they once were. Level 2 treatments can take their toll on your uniform. Do you have tint splashes or wax stains which never seem to quite fade away, or has the whiteness of your uniform simply faded after so many hot washes? Your college or training establishment may have a different colour of uniform to show you are a Level 3 therapist, and it certainly instils a sense of professionalism (and shows your capability) to have a pristine clean uniform, whichever level you are.

Salons vary in uniform codes and the expected dress for work, so you must always check exactly what is expected of you within your own training establishment. Different dress codes are acceptable, and you should try to be flexible, as long they are safe, comfortable and easy to maintain. Some fabrics are totally unsuited for uniforms, such as silk, which is not hard wearing and requires dry cleaning. Polyester and cotton mixtures wear and wash well, and many companies are incorporating linen blends in their fabrics, which look very professional.

Many training establishments encourage a different look for the more senior students, and it is possible to invest in some professional work wear, which is a little more reflective of your new status. Trousers and tunic tops are encouraged by lots of salons as uniforms, and are both comfortable and very practical – you may change tops more than trousers.

Overalls for large groups need to suit all figure types. The most important function of any uniform is to allow the wearer a free range of movement. It is advisable to go up a size to allow free movement, or at least try it on with arm movements tested! Looking trim in a fitted overall to look the part may be nice but is highly impractical!

Think about it

The dress code for your assessments is set by your Awarding Body and they will stipulate how you should look – not only for professional appearance but for health and safety. You will also have some guidance from your college or your training provider – this may be in a salon, college or private school – and the dress code will be in line with both the Awarding Body and the college policies. This may vary. Some colleges do not allow students to wear cropped trousers, others will not mind. Others do not like trousers and a full overall will be expected. As long as you take your assessments in the salon under full assessment conditions and your Awarding Body criteria and your External Verifier are satisfied, you will be competent!

Hair style

Whatever length your hair is, it should always be clean, tidy and presentable. If it keeps dropping in your eyes and irritates you, you can be sure it is going to distract you from your treatment. For hygiene reasons you must also make sure it does not come into contact with the client. Hair up in a professional style is both attractive and practical, so go back to the good habits of your initial training. Fresh, clean hair also enhances the overall hygiene of a person. If it is short, have regular trims and keep it well-groomed, and also remember that a re-growth of colour near the scalp makes the hair look dirty, even when it isn't, so keep the colour up if you tint, bleach or highlight your natural hair colour.

Footwear

Feet need the protection of safe shoes – with toes covered and no high heels – for your own safety and to maintain a good posture. Work shoes should meet industry standards and your college regulations, but students often forget to change from outdoor shoes into appropriate salon footwear. It is quite easy to get into bad habits and wear footwear with little or no support. When slipper/ballet pump styles of shoe are older, they lose all firmness and support; this is very bad for you and will make your feet ache. Also, it is annoying and will detract from your treatment if you have heels that make a noise when working or have shoes that do not stay on your feet, causing you to shuffle when you walk .

Some work-wear companies advertise clothing with the models wearing an open toe or flip-flop style shoe. This is not suitable salon wear, and will probably not be approved by either your Awarding Body or the insurance company for your training centre.

Think about it

Leather shoes allow the feet to breathe and are more hygienic as they prevent a build-up of bacteria which may cause odour problems and lead to athlete's foot.

Skin

While you do not need to wear full make-up to look professional, you should remember that Level 3 treatments are all about skin improvement and that your face can be used to advertise your abilities.

Your skin should reflect your therapist skills and be fresh, glowing and healthy looking. The advice you give to clients also applies to you – enough sleep, a sensible diet, a little exercise, reduced coffee and alcohol intake and plenty of water, will pay dividends with a clear skin, plenty of energy and a positive glow. You can help inspire clients to look after their skin by setting the example, and looking good.

Oral hygiene

Regular dental care will prevent tooth decay and keep gums healthy, so stopping bad breath forming. Regular brushing, mouth sprays, sugar-free mints and breath fresheners are also advisable to prevent stale breath being passed over the client. Remember that bad breath can be a sign of illness, so it may be worthwhile getting a dental or medical check-up if you think you may have a problem.

It is courteous to your client to avoid strongly flavoured foods, such as curry, garlic and onions, especially at lunchtime. Smoking can also cause odours that cling to the breath – a good excuse to give up smoking, even if only at work.

Think about it

It's not only on the breath that smoke lingers – it clings to clothing and the hair, which can be really off-putting if you are delivering a treatment, because you are in very close contact with your client. A mint cannot hide all of that! Smoking in public places has been banned since the law came into effect on July 1st 2007. If you are caught smoking in your workplace you will be liable to a heavy fine – £50 up to a maximum of £200 if prosecuted. See 'You, your client and the law', page 74, for more detail .

Hands and nails

Your hands are your most important tool of all, and nails reflect both your hygiene standards and your profession. Short, unvarnished nails are essential to giving an intuitive massage, without fear of stabbing clients' skin, and for maintaining a clean appearance. Always wash your hands after a toilet visit, handling food or stock, and after handling money – the worst offender for spreading dirt and germs! If you accompany the client to the till and handle money, just check and see how dirty your hands have become.

Always wash your hands at the beginning and the end of a treatment – the client will expect to see you do this. You will also need to wash your hands during a treatment, for example if you have blown your nose or touched your face. Certain procedures such as extraction will also require a mid-treatment hand wash. Remember to thoroughly dry your hands to prevent dermatitis. If you train to become a nail technician, then your clients will expect to see beautifully manicured nails, but it would be impractical to take any form of massage assessment wearing nail extensions.

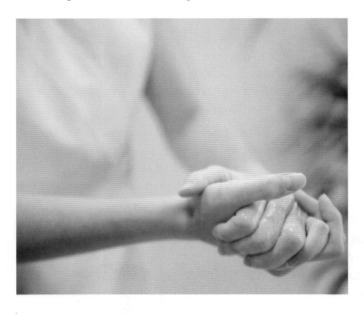

Use antibacterial handwash and wash your hands regularly

Jewellery

Jewellery is neither safe nor practical within Level 3 treatments. Rings can scratch clients' skin, ruining the relaxation of the treatment. They are also dangerous to wear when carrying out electrical procedures, as metal is a good conductor of electricity. A minimal amount of jewellery is recommended by all Awarding Bodies – a wedding band, small earrings and nothing else. It is not safe to have necklaces and earrings dangling when working and it may affect any insurance entitlement if negligence is claimed. There is also the risk of your best jewellery getting lost at work, or ruined by products and wear and tear.

Personal presentation

Presentation is about the whole package – not just the uniform or face, make-up and nails, but your entire image, facial expressions, body language and attitude.

Preparing for the day ahead

It takes organisation, care and dedication to be ready to work effectively. You should aim to be calm, relaxed and to ignore any personal problems and focus your whole attention on the client.

It is not just the décor of a salon that creates atmosphere; it is the ambience created by the people within it. How the therapist mentally prepares for work goes a long way to producing the calm, relaxed atmosphere of a salon which allows the client to gain maximum benefit from the treatment.

The right mindset

Your attitude and your approach to your job and to your clients is a reflection of your personal self. Part of feeling calm, relaxed and unhurried is your preparation for work, both at home and when you get into the salon. Preparation is the key to feeling composed, unruffled and serene – which is what you want your client to feel and pick up on, as he/she enters your treatment room. You need to centre yourself and achieve a stillness of mind, which allows you to totally immerse yourself in your clients' needs. This is virtually impossible if you are disorganised, agitated because you are late, or do not feel professional because your overall is still at home. This is not acceptable at Level 3: you may still be a student, but you must now also demonstrate that you are a serious professional.

Think about it

The beauty therapy industry is a service industry. The general public are your clients and they pay for your service and expertise. Therefore, they should also be entitled to your full attention and care.

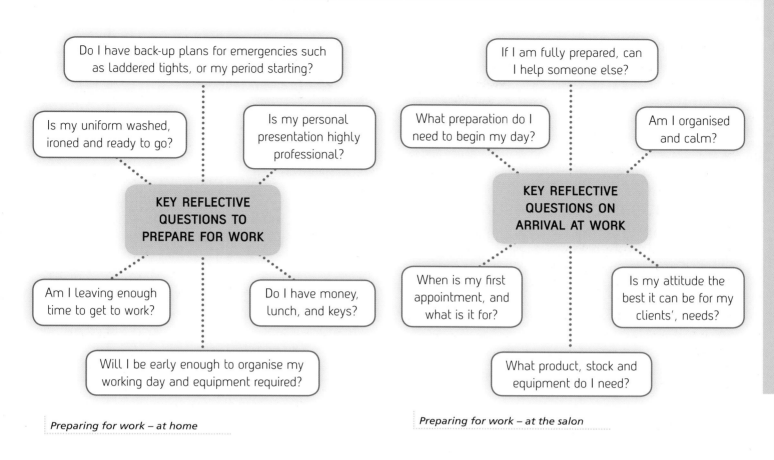

Do I have back-up plans for emergencies such as laddered tights, or my period starting?

Is my uniform washed, ironed and ready to go?

Is my personal presentation highly professional?

KEY REFLECTIVE QUESTIONS TO PREPARE FOR WORK

Am I leaving enough time to get to work?

Do I have money, lunch, and keys?

Will I be early enough to organise my working day and equipment required?

Preparing for work – at home

If I am fully prepared, can I help someone else?

What preparation do I need to begin my day?

Am I organised and calm?

KEY REFLECTIVE QUESTIONS ON ARRIVAL AT WORK

When is my first appointment, and what is it for?

Is my attitude the best it can be for my clients', needs?

What product, stock and equipment do I need?

Preparing for work – at the salon

You – the therapist

My story

Getting enthusiastic about products

Hi, my name is Sarai. I am originally from Thailand but now work in England running a top spa in a well-known hotel chain. I am enjoying the management aspects of my job, but one of my jobs is personnel and making sure we have the right staff for our clients. I have just had to ask a new therapist to leave us, as she had not passed her probation period of three months. I took her on straight from her college training and I think she treated our salon a bit like a day at college. She was often late, quite disorganised, not professional with her treatments and not very flexible if I asked her to work late or cover an unexpected treatment. Twice she had to borrow a uniform from the laundry, as she had forgotten hers, and I know the more senior spa staff were concerned about her casual attitude. She did have a lovely manner with clients when she settled to do a treatment and she made friends easily, but she was just not consistent or reliable. I didn't enjoy our last review or telling her we would not be offering her a permanent contract. I just hope she learns her lessons and gives more to her next job role.

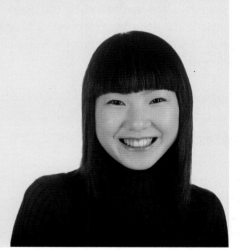

Professional practice

Be totally attentive to the client and his or her needs. If you do not show interest in the client, then he or she may not return to the salon for other treatments. As you prepare your working area, clear your mind of all angry thoughts. The client does *not* want to hear about *your* problems. Centre yourself with a few deep breaths and visualise peace and harmony surrounding you.

Personal safety and security

This section is about you taking responsibility for yourself, for your actions and for others. There is **legislation** that you must adhere to and you will always be expected to act in a sensible and professional manner. The Health and Safety at Work etc. (HASAW) Act 1974 states: 'Employees have responsibilities to take reasonable care of themselves and other people affected by their work and to co-operate with their employers in the discharge of their obligations' (see page 69). It is absolutely essential that you remember this when dealing with electrical equipment, the wet area and body treatments. You must never jeopardise the safety of your client (or yourself), as the consequences are serious.

Each piece of equipment used in the practical units has its own risk assessment and safety regulation, safe use and storage guidelines, and so on. This Professional basics section is more about you as a therapist, rather than the specifics of individual equipment, which are dealt with in each specialist chapter. This section refers to you and your attitude to work, and how you can keep yourself and everyone around you safe.

Beauty therapists often work very long hours and may be on the go all day. They are usually in a busy salon environment, with people present all the time — clients, other beauty therapists, sales representatives, managers, receptionists, cleaners, etc. If the therapist does not have a sense of personal safety and respect for the safety of others, accidents will occur.

Key terms

Legislation – laws created by government.

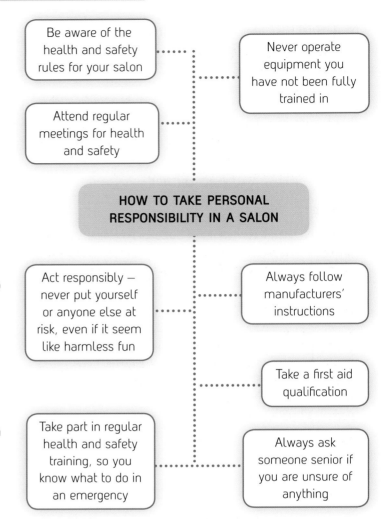

Be aware of the health and safety rules for your salon

Never operate equipment you have not been fully trained in

Attend regular meetings for health and safety

HOW TO TAKE PERSONAL RESPONSIBILITY IN A SALON

Act responsibly — never put yourself or anyone else at risk, even if it seem like harmless fun

Always follow manufacturers' instructions

Take a first aid qualification

Take part in regular health and safety training, so you know what to do in an emergency

Always ask someone senior if you are unsure of anything

Think about it

It is the employer's responsibility to provide health and safety frameworks and procedures, but it is the responsibility of each employee to follow the rules. You may be found personally negligent if you do not.

Informing others of your whereabouts

Ensure that someone in the salon knows where you are or what you are doing, regardless of how simple the task may appear. If you stand on some steps to change the light bulb, then make sure that another member of staff is with you, to prevent you being knocked off, and to take the old bulb from you. Do not be tempted to stand on a chair, or an old delivery box, or anything else remotely unstable.

Think about it

There are many types of potential harm – verbal, mental or physical – and they can come from many sources, often unexpected ones.

If you go to the local shop for lunch, pop to the bank or run an errand, tell someone when you will be back, and where you are going. You may wish to carry a personal alarm but make sure that you keep it handy, in a pocket of your coat for example (not at the bottom of your bag), ready to be activated in an emergency.

The salon should have a list of telephone numbers by the phone in case of emergency, such as the local police station or security guard room. This will save time when it really counts.

Do not be unprotected. For example, do not leave outside doors open when working in a treatment room, do not leave the till draw open, etc. Do not be naive enough to think that it could not happen to you! If unsure, seek professional advice from the local crime prevention officer or local police station, both for building security advice and also for personal safety hints for staff and clients.

As a professional therapist, always follow your professional guidelines.

- Do not treat a male client alone in the salon late at night.
- There should be a minimum of two people working in the salon on winter evenings when it gets dark early.
- Always lock up the premises together.
- If you drive a car to work, think about the best place to park it. Always choose an area that will be well-lit after dark.
- Do not park in a multi-storey car park if you know that you will be going home late and in the dark.
- Do not travel home after work alone in the dark — phone a taxi, family member or friend.
- Do not put yourself at risk in any way.

Think about it

If the therapist does not have a sense of personal safety and respect for the safety of others, accidents will occur.

Personal security for staff

The salon should provide lockable staff storage cabinets or similar so that personal belongings can be locked away. Handbags and purses are always vulnerable to the opportunist thief, who may slip in and out of the salon undetected. Staff should be discouraged from bringing large amounts of cash into work and should avoid wearing expensive jewellery, which has to be removed during treatments and is therefore vulnerable to loss or theft.

The salon's takings should be transferred to a bank or night deposit daily. Avoid taking the same route to the bank at the same time of day. Someone may be watching!

Be very aware of clients' jewellery. Let them see that this is placed in a bowl on the trolley, do not forget to return it when finishing the treatment and do not put yourself in danger of being called a thief by slipping it into your overall pocket!

Be aware of suspicious packages left unattended. Inform a supervisor and if necessary, call the emergency services.

Your posture

Good posture can protect you from aches and pains, as well as the development of more permanent back problems, repetitive strain injury (RSI) and time off work due to illness. Try to avoid stooping and slouching, to prevent back problems occurring.

Maintain a good posture and evenly distribute body weight by standing correctly with the feet slightly apart. This will prevent accidents and injury. A full body massage is a very demanding treatment to give, and you may treat several clients on the same day, so good posture is essential to avoid muscular problems in the shoulders and lower back. Poor posture may lead to discomfort and, in the worst cases, can cause permanent problems with vertebrae. It is common for therapists to suffer from RSI in both the wrists and the lower back, especially if the therapist specialises in massage, and does five or six treatments in a day. Prevention is so much better than cure — and often there is no cure for a bad back, just rest and avoidance of the activity.

For this reason, try to work with a couch or bed which is set at the correct height for you. It should be at a comfortable height so that you do not have to bend at the waist or bend your arms at the elbow. When trying out a couch you will need to take into account the added height of the client's body, so when purchasing, ask a colleague or friend to lie on the couch to allow you to judge the correct height.

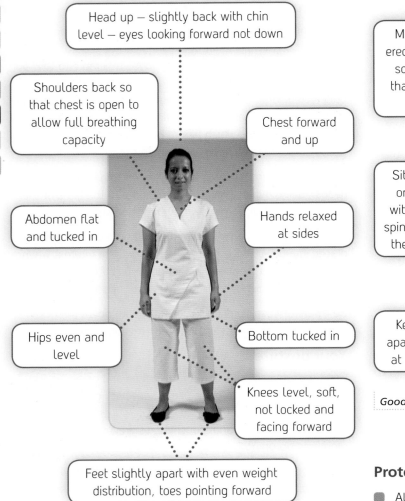

Head up – slightly back with chin level – eyes looking forward not down

Shoulders back so that chest is open to allow full breathing capacity

Chest forward and up

Abdomen flat and tucked in

Hands relaxed at sides

Hips even and level

Bottom tucked in

Knees level, soft, not locked and facing forward

Feet slightly apart with even weight distribution, toes pointing forward

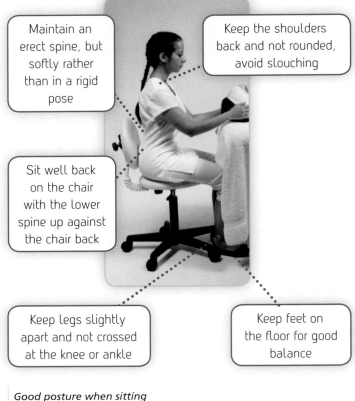

Maintain an erect spine, but softly rather than in a rigid pose

Keep the shoulders back and not rounded, avoid slouching

Sit well back on the chair with the lower spine up against the chair back

Keep legs slightly apart and not crossed at the knee or ankle

Keep feet on the floor for good balance

Good posture when sitting

Hydraulic adjustable couches are ideal, but are expensive to purchase. It may be possible to raise the couch by using wooden blocks under the legs, but these must be approved by your health and safety officer, put under the couch before the client is on it, and of a suitable size and material to support the weight of the client. If the block is not solid, or the couch leg is perched on the edge of the block, an accident could happen.

You will also need to ensure that your equipment is posture friendly. Do not position your trolley or machine so far away from you that you are continually leaning over to reach it. This would mean that you are over-extending, and you will not be in full control of the machine for safety and client comfort.

Protection and personal cleanliness

- Always wear the correct protective clothing provided to shield a uniform.
- Always wear gloves when using chemicals or if there is a possibility of coming into contact with body fluids.
- Always follow the correct disposal regulations for gloves and waste materials.
- If an establishment provides a uniform as part of a corporate image, then wear it!
- Hair should be tidy. Clip back loose hair. Avoid long hair styles as these are considered unhygienic and may be unsafe (see the table on the next page).

Think about it

For your personal protection it is always wise to keep immunisations (such as tetanus, hepatitis and flu) up to date if you are considered vulnerable, for example asthmatic.

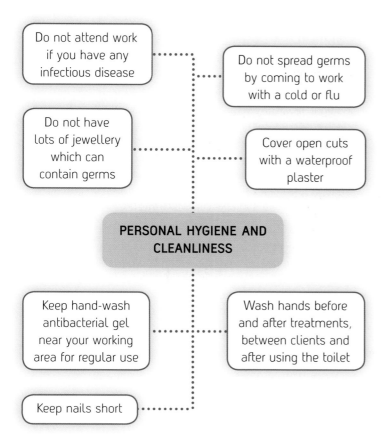

Do not attend work if you have any infectious disease

Do not spread germs by coming to work with a cold or flu

Do not have lots of jewellery which can contain germs

Cover open cuts with a waterproof plaster

PERSONAL HYGIENE AND CLEANLINESS

Keep hand-wash antibacterial gel near your working area for regular use

Wash hands before and after treatments, between clients and after using the toilet

Keep nails short

A high standard of cleanliness will ensure no cross-infection can occur

Personal risk assessment

Worker health and safety competence

In Unit G22 Monitor procedures to safely control work operations, you are asked to confirm that worker health and safety competence is up to date. This means being safe and responsible throughout your working day, and you will be referring back to that unit for all your practical treatment applications. You will also need to carry out a personal risk assessment which involves considering your dress code and presentation, how you handle electrical equipment, and the way you deal with clients and carry out your duties. This means that personal risks can be controlled safely and effectively.

Dress code and presentation

The table below looks at some of the reasons why it is essential to view your salon uniform and presentation as a safety issue and some of the possible consequences for the therapist if she fails to do so.

Key terms

Hazard – something that could cause harm, such as an electrical cable trailing across the floor.

Risk – the likelihood of the hazard actually causing harm, for example the therapist tripping over the cable and injuring herself.

Uniform / Presentation issue	Potential risk	Control of risk
Shoes	High heels may cause you to be unstable on your feet. They may cause you to trip over or fall sideways off the heel. If you trip while carrying equipment, you could injure yourself and damage the equipment. Open-toed shoes provide no protection if equipment or products should fall on your toes.	Adhere to your salon dress code and the code of your professional body. Buy a safe, sensible pair of shoes with closed-in toes. Try on the shoes before purchase and walk around in them. Are they comfortable and safe? Do you feel unstable or as if you are tottering around? Keep sling-backs, high heels and open-toed shoes for evening wear and non-work occasions.
Overalls	Baggy sleeves may catch on handles, products and equipment. Overalls that are too tight will restrict movement, which will inhibit safe conduct. Trousers which are too long may cause you to trip.	Adhere to your salon dress code and the code of your professional body. Try on overalls before purchase and stretch and move as in treatments. Are they comfortable and safe? Stop wearing a tightly fitting overall and purchase a larger size. If your overall is far too large, either alter it yourself or ask a professional seamstress to alter it for you.

Continued

Uniform / Presentation issue	Potential risk	Control of risk
Hair style	Long hair dangling in the eyes may distract you or prevent you seeing clearly and may cause eye irritation. Hair is a conductor of electricity, and if you make contact with a client via your hair while he or she is having a galvanic facial, you may cause the current to short circuit, causing sparking and pain for the client. Not regarded as hygienic.	Does your hairstyle feel comfortable? If it is scraped back and too tight, it will give you a headache and may make you feel irritable. Make sure that your choice of style does not cause you to constantly fiddle with your hair, which is distracting and unhygienic. Check your hair from all angles using a mirror. Seek advice. Your manager will tell you what is acceptable and what isn't. Go to a hairdresser and ask for a lesson on putting hair up. Invest in a good haircut, which will provide you with a professional look.
Nails	Long nails or jagged nail edges will inhibit massage movements and can cause skin damage to clients if you scratch or jab them. If not kept scrupulously clean, nails may harbour germs and pass on infections.	Keep nails very clean by scrubbing with a suitable antibacterial cleanser. Keep nails at a workable length to prevent damage to clients' skin. Look at your fingers with the palm towards you – if you can see the free edge of the nail plate, over the fingertip, then they are too long! If you cannot work safely with longer nails, then file or cut them to a suitable length.

Risk control: who could be harmed? Everyone you come in contact with!

Handling all your tools – electrical equipment, oils and products

How you handle your tools of the trade can have consequences for health and safety. The table below gives an overview of the risk analysis you should carry out before working with any item that you use on your clients. Individual equipment will have specific hazards, and these are explained within each practical unit.

Tools – Electrical equipment

Potential risk

- serious injury – electric shock, burns
- damage to the equipment
- fire
- scarring as a result of negligence – the client may seek damages from the therapist, which could cost you your business, or your salon owner a hefty fine
- loss of earnings
- trailing leads – which may cause an accident if someone trips over them
- not putting all dials back to zero to avoid the next person accidently switching onto a high setting.

Control of risk

- Never abuse the equipment.
- Never operate equipment you have not been trained to use.
- Follow manufacturers' guidelines.
- Arrange regular maintenance checks – these should be carried out by a qualified electrician (refer to Electricity at Work Regulations 1989).
- Report faulty equipment.
- Never use equipment which you think may be defective.
- Attend regular updates for training and safety.
- Follow salon safety guidelines – e.g. never use equipment with wet hands.
- Always complete a full consultation and check for **contra-indications**.
- Always test the equipment on yourself before the client.
- Always explain the treatment to the client.
- Always follow manufacturers' instructions.
- Always turn all dials back to zero when finished with them.
- Never overload the plug socket.
- Remove the defective equipment from use.
- Clearly label the equipment as unusable.
- Make sure all staff are aware of the problem.
- Have the equipment repaired by an authorised repairer.
- Return new equipment that is found to be faulty to the manufacturer.

Continued

Tools – Essential oils

Potential risk

- Overdose, or oils and toxicity occurring causing headache, nausea and sickness
- Sensitivity to a particular oil causing skin irritation
- Incorrect dilutions
- Putting undiluted oils directly onto the skin
- Using prohibited oils during pregnancy which can cross over the placenta
- Spillage and slipping on an oily patch
- Flammability of oils

Control of risk

- Undertake full training and a qualification in how to use the oils.
- Correctly dilute in a carrier oil.
- Carry out a full consultation with client, including medical history.
- Store oils safely and correctly.
- Correctly dilute oils using a dropper system for easy measuring.
- Learn how to deal with spillage through training.
- Undertake fire training as part of health and safety.

Tools – Products

Potential risk

- Contact sensitisation – irritation of skin in applied area, burning or heat rash (all **contra-actions**)
- Eye irritation if accidently used in eye area
- Wrong products used for skin type with electrical appliances, causing skin reactions
- Spillage

Control of risk

- Make sure you are fully trained in how to use products.
- Do not use products you are not trained to use.
- Make sure your first aid training includes eye irrigation.
- Follow manufacturers' instructions.
- Always carry out a full consultation with client, including medical history.

Risk assessment: controlling personal risks as a therapist

Key terms

Contra-indication – a condition that will prevent a treatment from taking place or that will require a treatment to be adapted.

Contra-action – a reaction that occurs as result of a treatment or service.

Your conduct in the salon

When you work in a salon you may have a manager who supervises what you do, or you may have junior staff who are your responsibility throughout the working day.

When working under a manager:

- you will need to accept that he or she is in charge
- you should be able to take instructions and act upon them
- you will need to communicate effectively
- you will need to take responsibility for your job role and do it to the best of your ability
- you will need to accept their judgement and experience and be respectful
- you should always show professional courtesy to others.

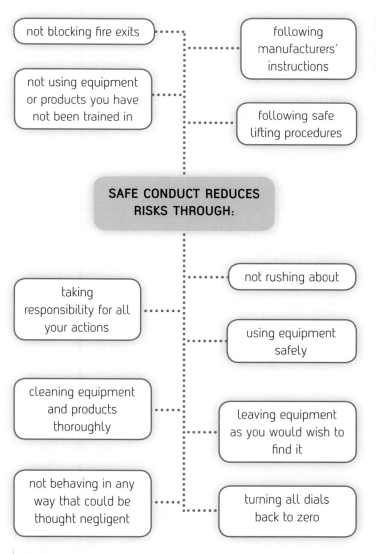

The importance of safe conduct in the salon

Working together as a team:

- means supporting each other, not being in conflict with one another or just looking out for yourself
- requires good communication
- gives the salon a good atmosphere which the client senses
- provides a reliable service
- gives excellent results.

Unacceptable behaviour

Whatever your position within the salon, there is a certain etiquette which must be followed, and respect for colleagues is top of the list. There may be a certain rivalry between staff if treatments and product sales are organised on a commission basis and the therapists are in competition with one another, but if the therapists are made to feel part of a team and the division of labour allows everyone to succeed, then serious rivalry can be avoided.

A sense of pride should be instilled in all staff, with regular training and positive feedback. A strong management structure will ensure that minor problems never get out of hand, and that staff morale is good. This can be encouraged in the salon by showing the staff that they are valued and treated with respect, for example through shared tips, rewards of products or treatments and through social events such as Christmas lunches and charity events.

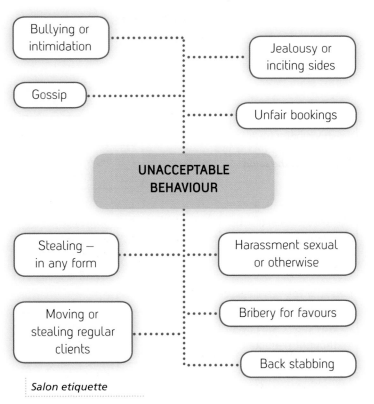

Salon etiquette

Think about it

As an employee, you are expected to be responsible about your work, reliable and dependable. You are accountable for all your actions and the possible consequences of irresponsible action.

Dealing with conflict

If you find yourself in a situation, in the salon, at college or at work, where you feel victimised or undermined in some way, then you should deal with it quickly. It is important to maintain a sense of proportion, and to be mature in your reaction.

Ask the person involved for a private talk, and avoid spreading rumours or innuendo among other members of staff. There is a danger that if the issue gets blown out of proportion, it will become a bigger conflict than it needs to be, so act quickly and sensibly to sort out the problem. Often, a one-to-one discussion will clear the air if it is handled correctly. If it is a conflict with another student, go to your tutor and ask for a meeting with your tutor present.

Avoid apportioning blame, and try not to be either aggressive or defensive — tears are not appropriate in this type of meeting and they make the atmosphere very emotional. It is better to begin with something like 'I don't know if you are aware of it, but I feel very undermined when you question me in front of clients', or whatever the problem is. This then allows the offender to say that he or she was not aware of this and to apologise, and gives you the opportunity to clear the air and move on. Your aim always is to build a better working relationship.

Before the meeting, practise what you are going to say, and be clear and as factual as you can. The problem may not be something that the other person has recognised, and if an apology is offered, then be gracious and accept it.

Think about it

This is not school, and you should not be bullied — you are an adult and you can have your grievances stated quite openly, with good, clear communication. However, you also have to be grown up and accept that you may be partly to blame for the situation. Do not resort to emotional blackmail, tears and harsh words or dramatically run out — it will not help solve the issues. Try and remain calm and objective, and try to sort out the issues in a responsible manner.

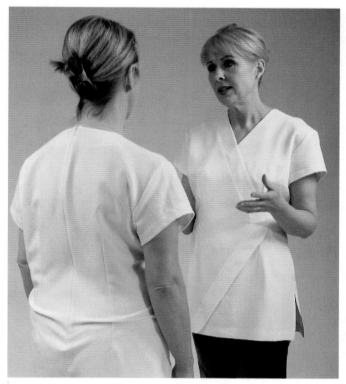

A private talk is a positive way of resolving conflict

At the meeting, remember to keep calm and follow these guidelines.

● *State your feelings clearly.* The other person cannot dispute that you may feel undermined or devalued. Your feelings are personal to you; it is the other person's behaviour which is making you feel a certain way, and this needs to be looked at. You may want to prepare for the meeting by jotting down a few notes, just key points that you want mentioned, and are likely to forget in the pressure of the meeting.

● *Avoid blackmail, emotional or otherwise.* Being negative and stating that you will have to seek employment elsewhere is a risky strategy. Your bluff may be called, and you may find yourself job hunting. Only use the threat of resignation as the very last resort, if this and subsequent meetings fail to resolve the problem. And, only if you really mean it — if the job has become unworkable.

● *Be receptive.* The person may understand your side of the problem and realise his or her behaviour is unacceptable to you, but he or she may also want you to understand that your own behaviour may have contributed to the situation. It could be that if you have not said anything before, it was assumed that you accept the situation. For example, if a manager regularly teases you, he or she will not know that you find it irritating unless you say so.

● *Be clear* in what you are asking for. State firmly that you wish the behaviour to stop. If you do not say this, then the meeting will be a waste of time.

● *Be positive and upbeat.* You all have to work together, so be encouraging. State clearly that you are pleased to be able to clear the air and move forward.

● *Have closure.* This American phrase sums up how to end the conflict. Do not drag it up at every available opportunity. Forgive and forget, and respect others as you wish to be respected.

Managing resources within the limits of your authority

When managing your resources there are three main areas to consider:

● what you are responsible for, and expected to do

● what you are not responsible for, and should not attempt to do

● who you should go to — reporting to the right authority.

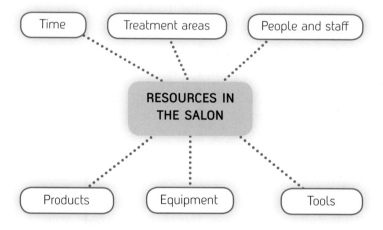

Resources in the salon

Knowledge and good management are essential in working within your job limits and not exceeding your own authority. Knowing what you are not allowed to do is as important as knowing what is expected. (See also Unit G11 Contribute to the financial effectiveness of the business, for guidance on financial resource management.)

Tools

The tools of your trade are precious resources and should be kept in pristine condition — not only for hygiene reasons and to reduce the possibility of cross-infection but also because they are expensive to replace. Your tools reflect your

My story

Matthew's story

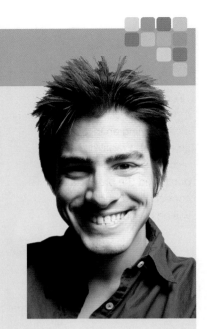

I am the stock controller for a very large beauty studio in London, with ten beauty rooms and six massage areas, as well as a wet room and a large retail section in our reception. Our turnover is very large and I spend a lot of my time counting stock and reordering when we reach minimum levels. I am also in charge of small pieces of equipment and tools required – any larger items get ordered via purchase order from our sales director.

Last year, I noticed that a lot of our small tools seemed to go missing – nothing major but the therapists always seemed to be asking for brushes, tweezers and cuticle nippers, and even some leads for a galvanic machine went astray. So, I went on the hunt, and watched everyone working. It soon became apparent that one of the junior therapists was helping herself to equipment and other people's stock. It wasn't as if she was taking them home and using them, she was just accumulating them in her workstation. I had to report it to the personnel manager and I didn't want to accuse her of stealing without fair grounds.

When we did get the issue out in the open, I think the girl was just a bit scatty, and it was not done in any deliberate sense. Every time she needed a small piece of equipment, she would take someone else's from their work station, and use it, sterilise it, and put it in her trolley. We found eight cuticle nippers in her drawer! It wasn't stealing, as the articles were not being taken off the premises, but she was genuinely sorry and we were able to support her with a lot more training in stock control and management. The moral is, never borrow from someone else, just because it's easier!

professionalism. Whose job is it to see that they are clean, sterile and ready for use after each client? Yours. Abuse and mistreat them, and not only will you lose customers, but you will also be replacing expensive tools more often than you would wish. Replace small items such as sponges and mask brushes before they disintegrate on the client's skin! By having a number of sponges and mask brushes, you will be able to rotate their use and prolong their life. It will also allow you to have some in the autoclave, while using others.

Products

Products are the profit base of any therapy business – no therapist can work without them. They are one of the most expensive ongoing outlays for the salon (especially if they are just sitting on a shelf gathering dust) but, used wisely, they can also bring in a good return.

- Always treat products as if you have personally paid for them.
- Do not be wasteful. For example, when decanting a product into a small bowl prior to application, only use what you need – you must not reuse or pour back the product into the container because of the contamination risk.

- Do not use too little of the product – you should always use the correct amount or the product will not perform its function. With experience, you will find that you can judge exactly how much you need. However, you cannot, for example, always estimate how much oil a very dry back will soak up during massage. If you pour only a small amount into a bowl, you can always add more, but if you start off with too much, you cannot pour it back.

- Do not substitute one product for another if you have run out, on the assumption that 'it will do': it may not be suitable for the client's needs and may actually cause harm.

- Accidents will happen, and you may find that your salon runs a policy of breakage being paid for by the member of staff responsible for the accident. Be informed and find out beforehand!

- Avoid having expensive products on show or on display near the reception area and doorway, where they are easy to steal. Displays and stock for sale should be kept under lock and key, and dummies used for open display areas.

Giving clients good aftercare advice and recommending the correct products to use at home will reinforce the benefits of salon treatments and continue your good work. For example, if the client is not cleansing her face properly at home, or if she is using an incorrect product, then all improvements an electrical facial gives will be lost. However, if you have recommended the correct skin care routine, she has purchased the products and you have instructed her on the correct usage, then her skin will improve enormously, and she will be delighted.

To get the best from a product, clients should be fully aware of:

- when to apply it
- how to apply it
- what it works well with
- how often to use it — daily, weekly, monthly
- its benefits and advantages
- storage
- shelf life.

You should also check that they have understood all you have said. When talking an application through with clients, or demonstrating, look for lots of eye contact and nodding, which you will see if clients have understood your instructions. If clients look confused, bored or distant, you have lost their interest, they are unlikely to use the product and may even return it.

Ask clients to repeat back to you what you have said. Check understanding by asking questions such as:

- When do you apply it?
- How is it put on?
- How regularly?
- How much do you need?

This will confirm that clients have full knowledge of how and when to use the product. Write any product purchases in clients' record cards and the next time you treat them remember to ask them how they got on and if they are pleased with the results. Be interested in clients' efforts and comment on the effects of their product use, as this will confirm your recommendations were correct. If there is a brochure/pamphlet or product leaflet for further reading, then put in into the bag with the client's goods and they can refer to it later, to read at leisure.

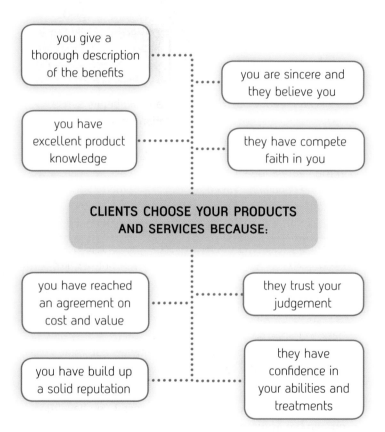

you give a thorough description of the benefits

you are sincere and they believe you

you have excellent product knowledge

they have compete faith in you

CLIENTS CHOOSE YOUR PRODUCTS AND SERVICES BECAUSE:

you have reached an agreement on cost and value

they trust your judgement

you have build up a solid reputation

they have confidence in your abilities and treatments

Factors which influence clients to use your products or services

Do you speak with confidence, enthusiasm and knowledge about your products? Do you know them inside out, the benefits, advantages, costs and sizes? You must have a full knowledge of products to pass on to your clients to meet their individual needs.

Client understanding of product use

(See also the information on clients' rights in 'You, your client and the law', beginning on page 68.)

Product displays

Product displays are generally included in the job role of the receptionist. However, if you have a spare hour and wish to promote your own range of products, say for electrical treatments, then you may be asked to be 'hands on' with displaying and promotion of products. Have a fresh look at products in your display cabinet and ask yourself the following:

- Are they clean and smart looking?
- Do they represent what you want to say about your business and treatments (smart, hygienic, professional)?
- How long have they been in the cabinet?

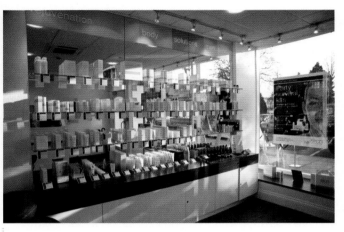

Product displays may be organised by product type

- Are the products still in stock, in date and in fashion?
- Have they deteriorated through sunshine or heat exposure? (Nail varnishes and creams split and become watery, which does not look professional.)

Retail sales will always boost a salon's profits and are a key factor in enhancing the benefits of the clients' salon treatments by encouraging use of the correct products at home. Therefore, running out of a popular line of stock or having poor displays of products neither makes good business sense nor gives the reception area a professional look. Nothing looks more off-putting than empty shelves!

By taking regular stock checks, the salon can see exactly what is required, which products are the most popular and sell well and which are slow moving and may require a promotion to boost sales. Keep product displays simple, clean and neat. No one is going to be tempted to buy a dusty pot of cream, or one which looks as if it is past its sell-by date.

Product displays may be organised in two ways:
- by product type
- by design.

Think about it

If your salon uses a particular product line, they will have specific ways of setting out their stock. For example, Dermalogica favours straight lines and boxes of all the same height, in rows, rather than flowers or other decorative enhancements being used. Always check with your representative how they would like to see the displays. Large corporations such as John Lewis have windows dressers who all do the same displays in the same manner, so no matter where you are in the country the windows will be identical. This is called a corporate image.

Think about it

Whichever display type is used, the products need to be locked up to avoid shoplifting of stock — security should be an important factor.

If there are many products in the range, then use the display cabinets to double up as storage and display the products in a logical order, that is by size or by product type: for example all cleansers together, toners together, and so on. Display by height and size so that clients can easily compare the value of buying the larger economical size (always a good selling point — the larger the product, the better the saving).

Products can also be displayed to look attractive — usually using 'dummy' (empty) boxes, and organising them in an artistic display, with flowers or ribbons to complement the colouring of the display cabinet. The boxes are usually clustered to form a small display within a glass case, and stock is held in a cupboard below for easy access.

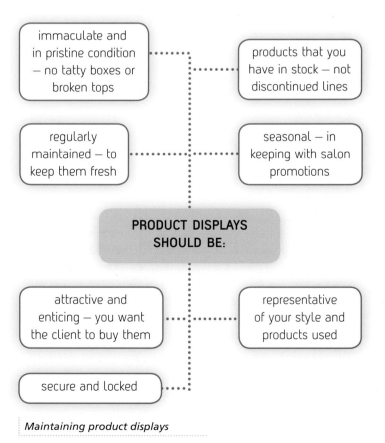

Maintaining product displays

PRODUCT DISPLAYS SHOULD BE:
- immaculate and in pristine condition — no tatty boxes or broken tops
- products that you have in stock — not discontinued lines
- regularly maintained — to keep them fresh
- seasonal — in keeping with salon promotions
- attractive and enticing — you want the client to buy them
- representative of your style and products used
- secure and locked

Prompt delivery of goods

If, following your advice, clients wish to purchase either a product or treatments, you will need to ensure they understand the time constraints or delivery expectations. When you order stock the time taken to deliver it will vary between suppliers, depending on their resources and stock levels, and whether the supplier is based in your area. It may be a next-day delivery if the company is local, or it might mean a wait of several weeks if the suppliers are themselves awaiting a shipment. The client may be enthusiastic about the product, but if it needs to be ordered, make sure that you keep the client fully informed about delivery dates, to avoid misunderstandings. Be honest with your client and you will keep your integrity!

When ordering products ensure you know how to order the correct goods, or refer to the staff member who is responsible for the salon's purchasing. Take responsibility for your actions — if you make an effort to get it right, the client will appreciate this.

Refer clients to alternative sources

There are times when you cannot recommend or offer clients want they need. This could be because you are not yet trained in the particular treatment or it may be that your salon does not offer the recommended treatment. For example, should a client require a sunbed session and the salon does not have one, or the client would like a specialist epilation (hair removal) treatment and the salon does not offer it, then you may recommend a *reputable* therapist who can provide the treatment required.

There is the possibility that you will lose the client altogether, but he or she may approve of your professionalism and remain loyal to you for other treatments. At the same time, you could take the opportunity to recommend to the manager or owner that the salon should investigate the possibility of offering the required treatment to expand business opportunities, if there is sufficient demand and the salon is losing clientele by not offering it.

Try to do your own research on costing of equipment and training needs, profit margins and expected returns, and then make a short presentation to the staff — you will learn a lot and so will they, as well as being impressed by your initiative!

Time

Time management is crucial to any business. You cannot afford to rush your clients, as they are paying for your attention, but you need to manage all clients within a busy working day so they all feel happy with the services they have paid for. You must:

- organise your own working day
- organise your work space
- organise appointments
- manage your responsibility so that jobs get done
- delegate tasks to others so that time management is shared
- avoid being stressed and irritable with clients because of poor time management
- avoid giving client dissatisfaction through poor time management
- meet deadlines and times for stock deliveries and products.

Client time management

Time management is easy to grasp in theory but often very hard to put into practice! Your time as a therapist is expensive: you give one-to-one treatments and this should be reflected in the treatment price. For example, a full hour's body massage is labour intensive. You stay with clients throughout the treatment and they receive a full hour of your time. A one-off treatment is very easy to time-manage, and if the client takes his or her time getting undressed, falls asleep on the couch, and takes time getting dressed, then that is fine. But you do not give one-off treatments. Your working column is full for the whole day, and you are probably going to give a variety of treatments, say three body massages, a galvanic facial and a couple of tanning treatments, along with epilation and a sauna and body treatment.

Good time management involves working out the amount of time each treatment needs. There are a number of things that you will need to take into account.

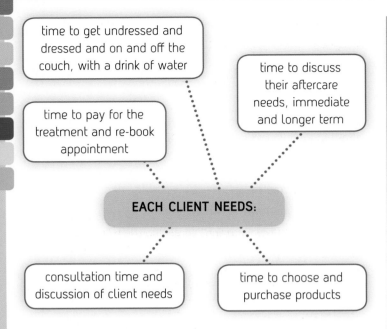

EACH CLIENT NEEDS:

- time to get undressed and dressed and on and off the couch, with a drink of water
- time to pay for the treatment and re-book appointment
- time to discuss their aftercare needs, immediate and longer term
- consultation time and discussion of client needs
- time to choose and purchase products

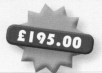

HEALTH & BEAUTY PACKAGES

Total Bliss salon Top-to-Toe Day £195.00

Full Body Massage (60 mins)
Clarins Personal Blend Facial (70 mins)
Jessica Manicure (40 mins)
Jessica Pedicure (40 mins)
Clarins Professional Make-up
Two-course lunch and a glass of wine in the Spa
Full use of the Spa facilities

Thalgo Top-to-Toe Day £175.00

Detoxifying Exfoliation (30 mins)
Marine Algae Body Wrap (75 mins)
Thalgo Marine Facial to suit your skin type (60 mins)
Full Body Massage (60 mins)
Two-course lunch and a glass of wine in the Spa
Full use of Spa facilities

A sample price list showing treatment times

The following table will also give you some idea of the amount of time you should allow for individual treatments. You should add on the time you need to consult and prepare.

Service (excluding consultation and preparation time)	Maximum time in minutes
Facial treatments	Approximately 60
Full body massage including head	75
Full body massage excluding head	60
Back massage	30
Aromatherapy body massage	60
Indian head massage	45
Hot stone treatment	As for body massage
Epilation	15 mins per session/area
Spa treatments (wet areas only – add other treatments on top, e.g. body massage)	60

Calculating how much time is needed for individual treatments

Each client deserves the same professional attention, and they may also like to chat and extend the treatment time because he or she has enjoyed it so much. So the problem is that, although you think you are responsible for your own time management, you really are not — the client structure dictates how long you have for the whole day.

A good receptionist (or the person who books in the appointments) will understand this, and make allowances for the consultation and dressing and undressing, but you still cannot afford to go over time. If each booking runs over by just ten minutes, by the end of the day your last client is likely to be waiting for up to an hour for his or her appointment, as the time lost has accumulated through the day.

How to prevent the client being dissatisfied with the treatment

Good service is expected — and clients are very aware of their legal rights and expectations — so all salons want to avoid the bad publicity which follows a client being unhappy with the service or treatment. Word of mouth advertising is very effective — the client is very happy and tells everyone who will listen how great the salon is. Unfortunately the opposite is also true — negative feedback is also very powerful. You really do not want clients telling friends and family how bad your treatments are! Always consider the following:

- *Give the client your full attention.* For the time they are with you, they are all that matters. To avoid projecting your troubles and problems onto your client, read the section 'Centre yourself as a therapist' on page 27. This gives advice on how to focus and earth yourself, so that you do not keep or pass negative energy onto your clients, or hold onto theirs.

- *Keep communication open.* If an unexpected occurrence happens, tell the client and explain the situation. No one really minds waiting a few minutes if they know why, but being kept waiting and not knowing anything is very frustrating for anyone.

- *Dealing with disturbances.* Apologise if you are interrupted, keep it brief and then give the client a few extra minutes of treatment if you can. Better still, try not to be disturbed when you are with a client.

- *Check client satisfaction.* Always give clients an opportunity to say if they are unhappy. If necessary, offer compensation. For example, if you know you have cut corners with time and the treatment has not gone smoothly, it is worth giving a free small treatment to keep the client happy. Everyone likes something for nothing!

- *Client comfort.* At intervals during your treatment, always check your client is comfortable, positioned correctly, well-supported, warm enough and enjoying the treatment.

- *Give proper consultations.* Make sure the treatment is suitable for the client in the first place — give a full consultation, explain all aspects of the treatment and check they understand everything.

- *Treat your client as you would like to be treated.*

Organising your time

As well as organising client time management, you will need to allow time to:

- prepare the working area
- clean tools
- dispose of waste products
- sterilise necessary equipment
- gather new equipment, if required
- leave the working area as you would wish to find it.

For the newly qualified therapist, this can be quite a daunting task. Experience will help with spreading the workload. Remember to ask for help if you need it — there may be a spare pair of hands willing to help, and you can return the favour. This is all part of good teamwork.

Poor time management leads to stress, the feeling that there are not enough hours in the day, and job dissatisfaction, as you feel you cannot cope well, and seem to do nothing right. Ask for help before you get to that stage, and at an **appraisal** with your line manager you should be able to put into place a routine that will save you time. It often takes someone else to observe your working routine to be able to spot time-saving remedies.

Managing your work stress is important. The key is to be organised and prepared. Work at least one client ahead:

- What will I need next?
- Where is the galvanic unit — who is using it?
- How long have I got?
- Could a junior member of staff help me prepare something?

Also, expect the unexpected and give yourself a little 'wiggle room' to manoeuvre. There are many factors which could affect your plans for a stress-free day. Be prepared for the following:

- walk-in clients — without appointments
- clients arriving late

Think about it

Remember you will need written consent to enter into a treatment plan with all clients and especially those who require parental permission for a treatment, if they are minors. You must check with your Awarding Body for their policy on the treatment of minors and the age restrictions for treatment – this applies to all your Level 3 treatments .Some Awarding Bodies do allow treatment of minors if the parent or guardians are present in the treatment room – but always check, never assume.

Key terms

Appraisal – a one-to-one meeting with a line manger to discuss how the job role is going, identify further training required or give a considered opinion, estimation or judgement of an individual or an estimate of value.

Self appraisal – to evaluate one's own work performance and recognise one's strengths, weaknesses and training requirements.

- client treatment times overrunning
- clients wanting additional treatments — you must be realistic about the extra time given to one client, if it comes off the treatment time of the next. You may need to say no, and rebook the additions at a later date
- clients not wanting to leave the salon, as they are having a nice chat.

Good communication really helps. No client will be offended if you say politely 'I'd love to stay and chat, Mrs Brown, but my next client is due in soon, and I need to prepare for her. Why don't you go into the sun lounge and have a drink to help you relax after your treatment?' Be calm but firm with the client who hovers and does not seem to want to go. The client may have time to spare, whereas you have several more clients to see.

Resources

Ensuring that you have enough resources will also help to improve your time management. For example, getting a fresh face mask brush from the autoclave saves time, as do spare sponges, spare turbans and fresh towels. Having only one set of everything is really hard work and it is virtually impossible to keep up a safe level of hygiene.

Keep up standards

No matter how stressed you get, do remember you must always deliver quality, otherwise the client is entitled to feel cheated! Do not be tempted to cut corners in order to save time. You cannot afford to compromise either the safety or hygiene of the client and this could be a very expensive problem in the long run, should negligence be proven.

Unforeseen problems

The other main problem with time management is the unforeseen event, which you cannot be prepared for, such as:

- a sick member of staff
- a piece of equipment becoming faulty and needing to be removed from service
- the client who turns up late and still expects to be treated
- the staff member who cuts herself badly and has to go to hospital for treatment.

Solutions

One or any combination of these problems and your time management collapses as easily as a pack of cards! Here are some possible solutions:

- Hold regular planning meetings and ensure that strategies, or contingency plans, are in place to cope with the unforeseen event. Staff will then know what to do in the case of cover being required and what is expected.
- Implement salon policies and staff training on time management.
- Make late arrivals and no-show clients aware of the salon's policy. Some salons state that charges will be made if an appointment is not attended.
- Give training on covering staff who are absent due to illness, detailing who is the flexible stand-in, or who has the necessary skills to cover, and who would be able to cancel clients if needed.
- Give support from above. A good manager will fully support all staff decisions because he or she has put procedures in place, and the therapist will be acting in the knowledge that her decisions are the views of the management.

If the problem is a faulty piece of equipment, and there is no other available, then honesty is the best policy, and perhaps an alternative could be suggested, or the appointment rescheduled.

Think about it

Teamwork and good communication throughout the day with the front-of-house team who deal with appointments and bookings is essential. This will mean providing updates and progress reports for the therapists working in their therapy rooms. Good team players make all the difference to time management.

Equipment

Managing your own equipment is not so easy when you are sharing the bigger electrical machines with others — this equipment is not then solely for your use, and professional teamwork is needed here, too.

Again, it is largely a matter of having enough of the right equipment to go around. Some smaller salons, for example, have three or four facial steaming units as this is a popular

Think about it

Where possible, avoid lending or borrowing small items of equipment. Try to be self-sufficient as this will make you independent and you will then not need to reply on others to provide for you. It will also prevent your precious (and expensive to replace) equipment getting lost!

treatment, but they may have only one galvanic unit as this is an expensive piece of equipment to purchase.

Planning the day is essential, and a morning staff meeting, with the booking-in sheet for the day, should allow the team to stagger the use of equipment so that all client needs are accommodated. Very soon it will become apparent which equipment is most in demand and will therefore require further investment by the salon.

Think about it

You must manage your resources within the limits of your own authority – it may not be your decision to purchase new stock or equipment, change the staff rota or alter the running of the salon. Know your place, and stay there! There may be reasons unknown to you as to why certain things do or do not happen. Follow the management hierarchy within the salon and observe the correct protocol. If you have suggestions to make and recommendations which you think may help, then use the correct procedure for suggesting them – perhaps at a staff meeting. Try not to jump up the ranks, and go over people's heads: it is not professional and can be very undermining.

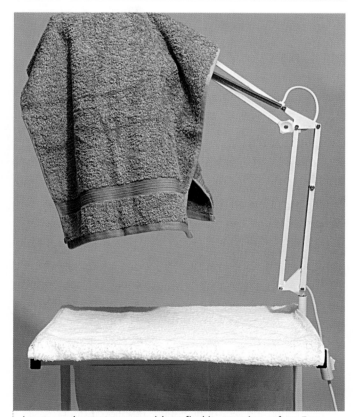

Leave equipment as you wish to find it, ensuring safety. For example, placing a towel over a hot infrared lamp safeguards the therapist from getting burnt

Sharing equipment with other staff

When sharing equipment remember the following:

- Leave the equipment as you would wish to find it – clean and ready for use.
- Set dials and settings to the '0' position – what is suitable for one client may not suit the next person.
- Unplug the equipment from the wall socket, so the therapist moving the equipment does not accidentally pull the lead out of the socket.
- Remove any heads or tubes which you have used but are as yet unable to clean or sterilise – the next client should not make contact with these.
- Ensure the equipment is placed safely on the trolley, and not balanced precariously.
- Do not clutter the equipment trolley with waste materials, used brushes or sponges – the next client does not need to see your rubbish!

Becoming an holistic therapist

You are embarking on a very exciting journey: your training and gaining your Level 3 qualification will equip you to apply for premium jobs and you should be confident in your abilities.

It is important that you see yourself as an **holistic** therapist, treating a client's mind, body and spirit. This means treating the client as a whole being rather than just a set of symptoms or a treatment list. You need to see the client in the context of social, economic, physical, psychological and spiritual aspects of their conditions. External and internal environmental influences have a huge impact on all of us, and you need to develop your intuition about the bigger picture, rather than seeing the client in the narrow confines of just a symptom or problem. For example, shoulder tension and muscular aches may be the physical symptom, but the root cause may be emotional – the client may have suffered a bereavement and the symptoms manifest into pain and tension.

Key terms

Holistic – from the Greek word *holos* meaning whole, this can refer to a style of treatment or a type of therapist. It means treating the person completely, altogether and in context, rather than just as one symptom or problem. It means you are treating the client on many levels: physically, psychologically and spiritually.

You will learn to probe a little deeper into underlying causes. This takes time to develop and a certain maturity on your part, but it can be highly rewarding for both you and the client. You can use the holistic approach for all treatments from massage and hot stones to facials and body treatments — in fact the more you use this approach with clients, the more insight you automatically gain: your perception is heightened into a client's needs and you will treat them instinctively.

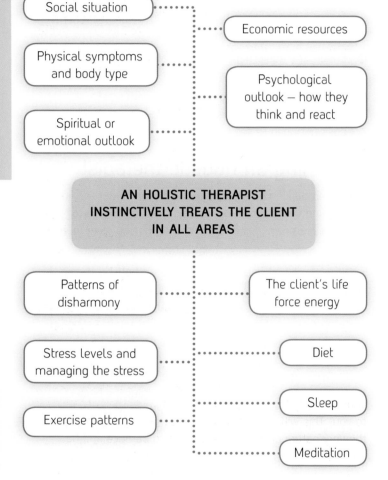

Social situation

Economic resources

Physical symptoms and body type

Psychological outlook — how they think and react

Spiritual or emotional outlook

AN HOLISTIC THERAPIST INSTINCTIVELY TREATS THE CLIENT IN ALL AREAS

Patterns of disharmony

The client's life force energy

Stress levels and managing the stress

Diet

Exercise patterns

Sleep

Meditation

Origins of holistic treatment

Holistic treatments have a very long history with eastern cultures; here in the west we are really only beginning to incorporate the holistic approach with beauty treatments, massage, medicine and nursing care.

The treatments you provide as a Level 3 therapist will be carried out with a thorough knowledge of the physical processes, but it is equally important to understand the eastern principles and practices which have shaped and informed those treatments. This is part of your holistic care of your clients, and you will be expected to demonstrate a basic understanding of the following principles and ideas.

Traditional Chinese Medicine (TCM)

This is the basis for the harmony and balance of the body or **Qi** (life energy). TCM uses meridians, tongue analysis, and pulses within the body for an holistic diagnosis of a problem with the *yin and yang* balance of the body. Holistic medicine and treatments is all about restoring balance and harmony, as imbalance leads to dis-harmony and eventually dis-ease.

Key terms

Qi, Ki or Chi – this means *life force energy*. *Chi* in Chinese, *Ki* in Japan, *Prana* in Indian (Sanskrit) and *Mana* in Hawaiian. Everything has a universal energy or life force within it which is constantly flowing and needs balancing to maintain maximum health. Holistic treatments are all designed to restore and rebalance the life force, as well as asking the client to re-evaluate their work/life balance and actively help in the balancing process.

Ayurveda

This refers to a treatment or therapist. In Sanskrit the word *ayur* means 'life' and *veda* means 'knowledge'. So, it is literally 'life knowledge' or the science of life. An ancient Hindu word for healing and promoting health through the use of herbs, good nutrition, oils, massage, meditation and yoga, diet and exercise to create a balance of mind, body and spirit for optimum heath. Ayurveda is based upon the five great elements from Mother Earth — *ether, air, fire, water and earth* — which underlie all things, and constantly ebb and flow and interact.

Integral biology/integral health

This is the study of our wellbeing in relation to our external pressures: all the small things which become an essential part of our environment and our mental health — our work/life balance and stress levels, everything which affects our bodies.

- *Negative factors*: for example, lack of sleep, lack of fresh air, poor diet with too much processed food, too much alcohol, smoking, stress, bereavement or serious illness, too many stimulants such as recreational drugs, caffeine or alcohol and lack of hydration. Emotional troubles, such as worrying, being alone or feeling isolated, not making time for recreation such as sport and socialising.

- *Positive factors*: for example, good sleeping patterns, a diet rich in fresh foods and variety of coloured vegetables, lots of water, moderate but regular exercise, fresh air, managing stress through exercise and meditation, with a good work/life balance, support of family and friends.

- *Homeostasis*: the state of relative stability or equilibrium of the internal body to maintain good health, such as blood pressure, temperature, heart rate, chemical reactions in the body, which are all disturbed by stress. By giving relaxing treatments the therapist is returning the body back to a good position of homeostasis.

- *Yin and yang*: in East Asian thought, yin and yang are the two complementary forces or principles that make up all aspects and phenomena of life.

- *Meridians*: over 5000 years ago, the ancient Chinese discovered a subtle energy in the body that can't be seen, but flows in channels called meridians. With much practice they can be felt or found with the senses. Meridians form the basis of acupuncture.

- *Chakras*: an important element of holistic treatments and Ayurvedic medicine is balancing the flow of energy in the body. The body is seen as having seven energy centres called chakras. The chakras also help make up an energy field around the physical body.

- *The aura*: this is the electromagnetic field that surrounds the human body (often referred to as Human Energy Field – HEF) and every organism and object in the universe.

Think about it

All touch and forms of massage have an effect on the meridian channels, chakras and auric fields – as we massage, we can clear and balance these and restore emotional balance, as well as helping any physical problems such as muscular tensions and dry skin.

The healing crisis

Often, these powerful holistic treatments produce mixed reactions within the client and this is called a healing crisis. The client may have unexpectedly strong physical and emotional responses, because they have had a rebalance and blockages have been cleared.

Physically, this may show up as the need to visit the toilet more frequently or diarrhoea. The skin may break out in spots or a rash, and/or the client may feel really tired, often with flu-like symptoms. This is quite common, and the body's way of ordering rest and relaxation to promote healing. Emotionally, the client may cry and feel quite sensitive and weak for a few days — especially if they have been holding on to something for a long time and 'coping' with it.

This is common with clients who have suffered bereavement or shock, car accidents, surgery or other major trauma, which has had a big impact on their lives and inner equilibrium. This should be seen as a good, positive thing and do warn the client this may happen — tears can be very healing and a release, and the client should be made to feel comfortable with this reaction. Recommend a light diet, lots of water and plenty of sleep, avoiding stimulating foods and alcohol, to help the client recover and move on.

Centre yourself as a therapist

Taking care of the therapist

When we as therapists take care to preserve our vital energy and work in a clear energy space, both we and our clients will receive the full potential of the treatment. This positive experience will speed up the natural healing process and build a successful practice. A therapist cannot give a relaxing and meaningful treatment if they are not themselves relaxed and centred, and any emotional irritation the therapist has may be passed on to the client.

Take time before the treatment to clear your thoughts, breathe deeply and block out all outer influences — forget the shopping list, parking ticket or your row with your boyfriend; in the treatment room, these problems do not exist.

It is also important that you protect yourself from the clients who will drain your energy levels and subconsciously draw your positivity from you, whilst passing over their negativity to you. This will always happen to some degree, as it is in the very nature of holistic treatments to balance and heal the client. Think of this as the client being the drain — and you being a radiator, giving off good energy vibrations. Some clients can become very needy and if you treat them on a regular basis, you must be careful to block their depressing or low energy. You cannot afford to absorb all of your client's problems as this would certainly make you ill.

Creating a sacred space

Whenever we give any treatment, the environment we perform the treatment in is vital to the outcome. After we have practically prepared the tools we need for treatment (such as hot stones, essential oils, towels and so on) it is also important to create a clear energy space. This will help

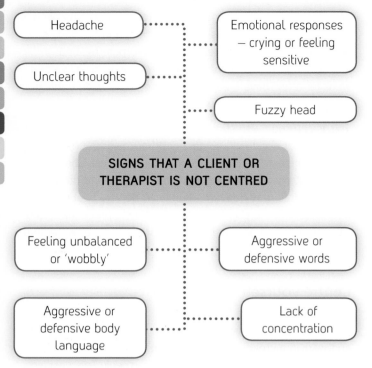

Headache

Emotional responses — crying or feeling sensitive

Unclear thoughts

Fuzzy head

SIGNS THAT A CLIENT OR THERAPIST IS NOT CENTRED

Feeling unbalanced or 'wobbly'

Aggressive or defensive words

Aggressive or defensive body language

Lack of concentration

to increase the power of the treatment and enable you to work without depleting your energy.

Here are some techniques you can incorporate into your practice. You may already have certain steps you follow and may wish to add or amend them.

Visualisation:

- Before and after every treatment, centre yourself in the room and take some slow deep breaths. Use your powerful imagination to visualise that fire is eating and burning away any lower energy, or imagine that warm water is raining down into the room, cleansing and clearing. You can also use a golden or pure white light to clear the space. When washing your hands visualise your own worries going down the plughole with the soapy water and leaving your body.

- Plant your feet apart and visualise roots growing out from your soles and connecting to the earth (the connection is even stronger if you can do this outside). You are then grounding yourself to Mother Earth and tapping into her energies and nature. Breathe deeply and imagine your roots draining any negativity away, whilst drawing positivity from the earth. White and purple are very healing colours so visualise this positivity as a white and purple ray coming from your feet until it reaches your head and surrounds you.

- Visualise a white egg of glowing light and step into the egg, which will cover you from head to toe. This is your personal space capsule and all negative energy will not be able to break through the outer shell, it will just bounce off.

Light:

- Candles are a fantastic way to invite purity and cleansing into a space. Prepare the room with candles and keep burning during the treatment. (Always uphold the health and safety precautions associated with naked flames.)

Aroma:

- All natural aromas have an unseen energy that interacts with all our energy bodies. Diffusing aromas creates atmosphere and clears the space. To cleanse the room choose one of the following: lavender, juniper berry, lemon, sage, thyme, pine or camphor. To create an uplifting atmosphere, use lemongrass, grapefruit, sweet orange or bergamot. For relaxation, ylang ylang, sandalwood, frankincense or jasmine. Use in a burner to infuse the whole room; it makes a fantastic atmosphere to the client to walk into and immediately sets the scene for relaxation.

Sound:

- The vibration of sound has a very profound effect on the energy of a space. You can play uplifting classical music such as Bach or Mozart, or nature music or light choral/chanting sounds. Tibetan singing bowls and chimes are also very effective.

How to centre a client

When you are centred and focused on the client and treatment, spend a few minutes centring your client, prior to treatment. Place your hands just above your client's body, at the nape of the neck and the small of the back. Ask your client to breathe deeply with you to the count of three in through the nose and five slowly out through the mouth. Repeat this several times. Silently offer a message that you give this treatment in a positive loving way, and mean the client no harm. Visualise a colourful rainbow in a beautiful clear blue sky and imagine you are melting into the colours of the rainbow, and being bathed in its warmth and light. The colours match the seven main chakras and you are helping both your own and the client's aura to become strong and positive. If you lose concentration at any time during your treatment, repeat the rainbow vision and reinforce the colour connections.

With practice this will become second nature and you will leave the client energised and refreshed. You, too, should feel bright and energetic after your day's work — if you feel washed out and drained, you are not protecting your own aura enough and have been drained by your clients. The use of stones and crystals will also help with your protection, and will give out positive energy vibrations. At the end of each treatment and at the end of your working day, renew and refresh both your working space and your body, with the sacred space suggestions from page 27.

You and your client

In this section you will learn about:

- communication
- body language
- the consultation
- hygiene and avoiding cross-infection.

This part of the unit considers the client, the all-important consultation and how to get the best out of the consultation to match your client's needs. This is a general introduction and is intended to refresh your consultation techniques.

The specific consultation details for either face or body treatments are covered within B14 Provide facial electrical treatments, page 275, and B13 Provide body electrical treatments, page 362, so please refer to those sections.

Think about it

You can also incorporate your Level 2 skills and treatments for the benefit of the client. In the normal working salon, and even under assessment conditions, if you are doing a body massage, for example, and you notice the client has very dry skin on the soles of the feet, then as part of your treatment package you can still recommend a paraffin wax pedicure. You could recommend the client has the treatment on another day, when you are not being assessed, or even be used as a model for assessment with another class — you will be creating revenue for your training salon, and the client is likely to be pleased to be treated.

Communication

Communication can be:

- verbal
- non-verbal
- written.

Think about it

People speak with their vocal cords, but communicate with the whole body.

Verbal communication

Verbal communication is what we say and is full of different expressions, which can be used to convey many emotions to suit the occasion. The words can be made to sound different by altering the pitch, tone and volume and the emotion behind the words — the same words can be said with kindness, harshness or sarcasm. Even a simple phrase like 'Thank you' can sound like a criticism.

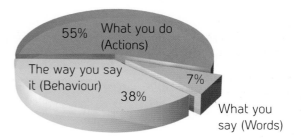

Speech is only 7 per cent of all communication; 38 per cent is the way you say something and 55 per cent is your actions, or what you do

Intonation	This is the tone of speech and it can significantly alter the meaning of words. 'Well done' can be made to sound sarcastic, or be genuine praise. The variation of tone enlivens speech, which would be very boring if it was all monotones, and the different speech patterns and accents add shades of meaning or emotion, and help retain the listener's attention. Flat boring tones will not engage listeners and will not help them understand what is being said. Intonation also helps distinguish people's home country, through their accent.

Continued

You and your client

You and your client

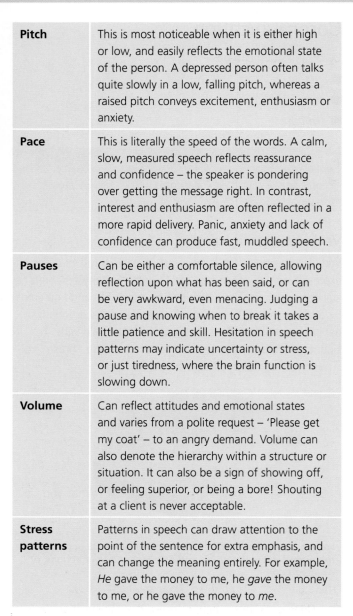

Pitch	This is most noticeable when it is either high or low, and easily reflects the emotional state of the person. A depressed person often talks quite slowly in a low, falling pitch, whereas a raised pitch conveys excitement, enthusiasm or anxiety.
Pace	This is literally the speed of the words. A calm, slow, measured speech reflects reassurance and confidence – the speaker is pondering over getting the message right. In contrast, interest and enthusiasm are often reflected in a more rapid delivery. Panic, anxiety and lack of confidence can produce fast, muddled speech.
Pauses	Can be either a comfortable silence, allowing reflection upon what has been said, or can be very awkward, even menacing. Judging a pause and knowing when to break it takes a little patience and skill. Hesitation in speech patterns may indicate uncertainty or stress, or just tiredness, where the brain function is slowing down.
Volume	Can reflect attitudes and emotional states and varies from a polite request – 'Please get my coat' – to an angry demand. Volume can also denote the hierarchy within a structure or situation. It can also be a sign of showing off, or feeling superior, or being a bore! Shouting at a client is never acceptable.
Stress patterns	Patterns in speech can draw attention to the point of the sentence for extra emphasis, and can change the meaning entirely. For example, *He* gave the money to me, he *gave* the money to me, or he gave the money to *me*.

Key terms of speech

All of the effects in speech (called prosodic effects) described above can influence the message the speech is to convey. So it is not just what you say, it is the way in which you say it, and emphasise it, which gets the right or wrong meaning across.

There is also some relationship to voice quality and personality types. Extroverts, for example, tend to speak more loudly and more rapidly than introverts, with fewer pauses and at a higher pitch. Confidence plays its part in making speech clear. If you wish to come across as competent in your job, then reflect that in your speech patterns.

Think about it

Listen carefully to people on television and judge their speech patterns. For example, do younger presenters talk more quickly than older presenters? How does the news delivery change with each topic? Who would you consider to be a very good public speaker, and why?

Speech pointers

● *Use straightforward language when talking to your client.* Use words that he or she will recognise and avoid jargon where possible. Jargon is verbal shorthand for the professional. It can seem as if you are showing off, and you will confuse the client if, for example, you talk about a galvanic facial. If you explain the treatment as a deep cleaning and rehydration of the skin, the client will be far more receptive to having the treatment.

● *Avoid slang, bad language and lazy speech.* Slang is acceptable in your own social circle, where everyone knows what is meant, but if you use slang with clients, they may not understand you! Bad language (swearing and cursing) is inappropriate in the salon. It is easy to fall into the habit of bad language, but remember that some clients may be offended. Lazy speech includes dropping Hs and missing Ts in the middle of words, which makes it hard to understand.

● *Always be respectful to clients.* Use titles and surnames where appropriate, for example Mrs Smith, Dr Patel, and so on. Do not view this as using language to give the client power; view it more as recognition of their importance to you and the salon.

● *Be aware of people's sensitivity and never be offensive.* Sexist, racist and ageist terms are not acceptable — your salon could find itself the subject of a lawsuit and a hefty fine if you use such terms. If you avoid all ethnic, age, gender and sexual orientation terms, then you cannot offend anyone!

Politeness in your job role

To build up a rapport with clients and establish a relationship, you will need to have respect for them, and this is shown in politeness, a broad term for the sensitivity that we should all show one another in conversation.

Examples of politeness include:

● using the appropriate forms of address

● speaking to others in a way that is fitting to the social relationship you have with them

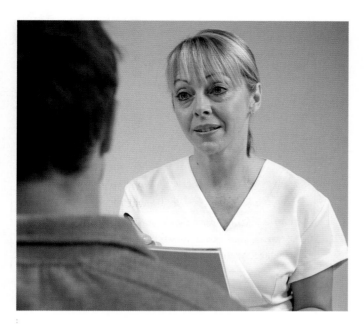

A supportive conversation involves good eye contact

- speaking with a degree of formality if required, especially for new clients
- showing an understanding of the conventions of speech — knowing when a conversation is beginning or ending
- listening carefully to what clients are saying — or not saying, which is often just as important.

Conversation support

It takes two to hold a conversation! To make sure that your conversation with a client is a two-way street, you will need to use supportive conversation techniques, otherwise the conversation may become stilted and may stop altogether. To support conversation, try some of the following techniques.

- Ask more questions — show interest in what the client thinks, and encourage him or her to participate.
- Give lots of supportive feedback when listening, for example through 'back channel' noises such as 'Mmm' and through expressions of agreement and understanding like 'Yes, I know'.
- Pay compliments where appropriate.
- Initiate more topics of conversation.
- Make an effort to bring others into the conversation — general family topics are usually safe, and pets and social activities are interesting to talk about (the client's — not yours!).
- Use 'you' and 'we' more often as it involves the client in the treatment and what is being said.

Think about it

Rapport + consultation = successful

Good rapport + consultation = very successful

Excellent rapport + good consultation = excellent success

Excellent rapport + excellent consultation = outstanding success

Try not to:
- interrupt
- express strong disagreement or criticise the client for expressing an opinion, such as 'You can't really like so-and-so's singing'
- ignore the client's utterances
- show reluctance to pursue the topic the client is initiating.

Questioning techniques

Asking questions is a skilled task. If you really want to find out what the client thinks and needs from you, you need to ask him or her. How you ask, what you ask and the type of question will dictate the reply you get. So, it is important that you give some care to your questioning technique.

If you ask the right questions and listen carefully to the answer, the treatment almost plans itself! All information should be included on the record card, which you will be filling out as you discuss details during the consultation. Use the record card as your guide. As already stated, verbal questioning will determine all the personal details — refresh your memory by looking at the record card on page 39. There are two types of questions, open and closed.

- *Open questions* — help to make the conversation flow, as they require a fuller response than a simple yes or no reply. For example, 'How did your skin feel after your facial last week?' would be a good question to break the ice. Open questions help you to build rapport with the client and put them at their ease.
- *Closed questions* — usually need only one-word answers. They do not allow conversation to flow, but they are good for confirming information, so they have their place. For example, 'Have you ever had high blood pressure?' will enable you to confirm or eliminate information when the client responds 'Yes, I have' or 'No, I have not'. Sometimes you have to use a closed question if you just require facts, but try to keep them to a minimum.

Non-verbal communication

Non-verbal communication (NVC) is a broad term, and refers to the way we all interact with one another, excluding the actual words. It includes not only body language (gestures, facial expressions and physical contact) but also appearance and non-verbal aspects of speech itself.

The functions of NVC include the following.

- Accompanying speech — to reinforce what you are saying, using gestures as you go along.
- Replacing speech — as in a sign, such as a thumbs up for OK, or a wave, or a horizontal shake of the hand to denote something uncertain.
- Betraying attitudes or feelings — unfortunately, when you tell a lie, your speech is saying one thing, but your unconscious body language is saying another! Expressions and closed gestures such as crossing the arms may give away your true thoughts, as will avoiding eye contact and touching the nose or ear when lying.
- Self-presentation — NVC contributes to the way you choose to present yourself, for example wearing a smart suit to an interview or the professional uniforms worn in the salon.
- Social rituals — people formally shake hands upon meeting, or the less formal European greeting among friends of kissing both cheeks.

Communication that is written down must be:

- clear and easy to understand
- concise — only information that is required should be given
- legible and easy to read
- well presented — handwritten or word processed
- correct — all the information should be included.

Avoid the shorthand that we now all use for texting on a mobile phone — not everyone understands this and it is a bad habit to get into. Write the words in full to avoid any confusion.

Clear written communication is important for many aspects of work within the busy salon environment, including health and safety, accident reports and record cards. For example, the client could be placed in danger if an allergic reaction warning on her record card is not readable. Messages for staff can also cause misunderstanding if appointments are cancelled or changed, but not fully understood by the person receiving the memo.

You and your client

INTERNAL MEMO

Date: 24th Feb 2010 Time: 10.30am	Taken by: Rasheda	For: Saskia – senior therapist

Message: Can Mrs Kaminski change her appointment from tomorrow to next week as she has just been signed off by her doctor with a nasty virus and is not going to work for the rest of the week. She doesn't want the girls in the salon to catch it and is too poorly to come in.

Action: If you agree can you just confirm by phone and leave a message on the answer machine. tel: 01234 56789012

Written communication must be clear and concise

Body language

Facial expressions

Orientation

Proximity

Eye contact

BODY LANGUAGE MAY BE BROKEN DOWN INTO THE FOLLOWING CATEGORIES:

Gestures

Posture

Touching

Head movements

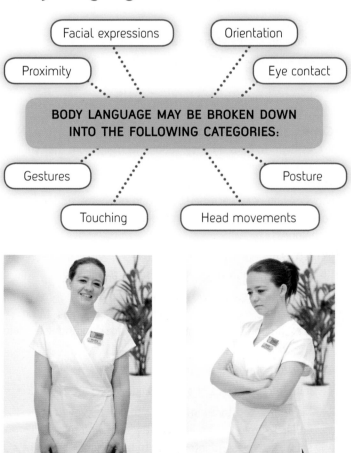

Be aware of your body language when working with clients and colleagues

Body language – what this means

For the therapist:

- Use open hand gestures and ensure you look approachable – crossed arms and legs, and/or a closed facial expression or a scowl on your face will discourage the client from coming over to you.
- Smile and make eye contact – body language that avoids eye contact with the other person gives the impression of being shifty or dishonest.
- Give the client her own personal space – avoid getting too close, which may make her feel uncomfortable.
- Read the signs from your client – she may be saying one thing with her voice, but her body language will give away her true feelings. Is the client nervous? Look for hair twiddling and agitation with the hands. Is the client looking confused? Watch for frowning and puzzled facial expressions. Adjust your body language to suit the client's and you will reassure her. Be calm and smooth in your actions – this shows confidence.

For the client:

- If the client sees you as open and friendly, she will feel able to approach you and will be less nervous or intimidated.
- The client will be more confident about you and your abilities if you look like you are an honest person.
- The client will be more likely to rebook and spend more money if you are a welcoming, responsive therapist – and she will probably ask for you again!

Whether your body language is good or bad, it will create a lasting impression on the client – so make sure it is good!

Proximity

This refers to the physical distance between people.

- The smallest is the *intimate zone* of about 50 centimetres, used only by close family members and partners.
- The *personal zone* is 0.5–1.5 metres, used when chatting at a party or with people whom you feel very comfortable with.
- The *social zone*, 1.5–4 metres, is used in a business setting, dealing with shop assistants and tradespeople.
- The *public zone*, 4+ metres, is used when delivering a speech or public address.

Think about it

In beauty therapy you are breaking into a person's most intimate space to deliver treatments, so the relationship between therapist and client has to be built upon trust, confidence and total rapport, otherwise the relaxation and benefit of the treatment is wasted. The client must feel comfortable with you for you to be able to touch them.

For your portfolio

Observe those around you and take time to study their communication skills – both in your learning environment and outside, especially if you have a part-time job.

Look at someone you admire and consider to have good communication skills – what do they do that makes it easy for you to get on with them and relate to them in a positive way?

Write a 150–200-word summary of how your boss communicates with you. How could you improve your own communication skills?

Orientation

This refers to the way you position yourself in relation to others. If you turn away from a person while in conversation, this shows either a lack of interest or that you wish to be separated or disassociated from that person. People who face towards each other, and even mirror each other's actions or position, signal interest and friendliness. This is very common when couples first fall in love!

Sitting on opposite sides of a desk, or couch, facing each other, may be interpreted as competitive or a sign of confrontation, whereas sitting side by side in a personal zone is much more harmonious and suggests empathy and co-operation. This is most useful to know when carrying out a consultation: you may think that being on the other side of the couch is fine – your client may perceive your signal differently!

Facial expressions

The face is a true reflection of what you are thinking and can convey all emotions, but remember to concentrate, as a look of boredom or tedium is very difficult to hide! In western cultures facial expressions tend to mean the same, and expressions are used to give feedback and show interest, with eye contact and smiling to offer encouragement. (However, conventions can differ around the world. In China, for example, sticking out the tongue shows surprise and delight at something.)

Eye contact

Eye contact is very important, not only at the beginning and end of a conversation, but to judge someone's level of self esteem, and to show confidence and interest. Lack of eye contact may just be shyness, but if it happens continually, it usually indicates the person is intimidated, frightened or lacks self-assurance.

Gestures

These can be used for clarification, to demonstrate or point to something, or to emphasise a point. Jabbing an index finger at a person, or invading their intimate space, during an argument would be a sign of aggression. Pointing can be a pre-signal to attack with a fist, and politicians are taught not to use such a bullying gesture during speeches. By contrast, shaking hands with someone originates from showing you have no concealed weapon in the palm of your hand and is a friendly gesture. Any gesture showing the palm is very good and can be used to show a client around, but flicking a thumb to show where the toilet is would be considered ill-mannered.

Posture

Posture can reflect the emotional state of a person. Sitting on the edge of a seat shows tension and anxiety. A dropped pair of shoulders and dragging feet will indicate that they are nervous, a bit low in self esteem or worried or anxious about something. A confident client will have more direct body language, more eye contact, with a spring in the step and an upright posture.

Head movements

The slightest inclination of the head can mean many things. Nodding forward and back shows both agreement and understanding, and side-to-side shaking can mean disbelief or disagreement. Tossing the head and shaking the hair usually accompany a bout of laughter, or can be part of the subtle mating ritual, showing interest, if aimed at an attractive partner! Tossing the head over the shoulder, if used to indicate where something is, can show lack of interest.

Think about it

There is a saying 'Fake it 'til you make it' and that is so true of posture. If you look confident and in control, people will believe your body language, even if you are quaking like a jelly inside! The more you practise being confident the better you become at it.

Touching

Touching is vital for human bonding, especially when we are babies. But as we grow up our personal space becomes more pronounced and we become more inhibited. This is, of course, a generalisation — some families are great huggers and kissers, both male and female, and the Continental Europeans are less inhibited than the British. Who we touch, how, and in what way, will depend upon the situation. Women tend to kiss more; men shake hands. We are more likely to touch in relationships familiar to us — you would not kiss your clients in the salon as it would not be appropriate, but if a family member came to visit you at work, you would be far more likely to.

Touching is, of course, the very basis of beauty therapy treatments, especially in all forms of massage, so it has to be appropriate, carried out professionally and in the correct context. Massage has been recognised as being very beneficial in the healing process, and is soothing and comforting for all ages.

Think about it

Only massage or treat a client who is undergoing medical treatment with the approval of his or her doctor. While beauty treatments can be very therapeutic, therapists are not medically trained and may be creating more problems for the client.

The consultation

A successful and profitable business will earn its reputation by providing an excellent personal service. It starts with a good consultation. The very first impression that you give to the client, the care and attention he or she gets, and the feeling of being comfortable and secure will last indefinitely, creating repeat business and expansion of clientele, as your excellent reputation will be spread through recommendation.

The consultation should be carried out in complete privacy, be complimentary (free of charge), and carried out when both parties have the time to be thorough and establish a good rapport with one another. Your manner should be polite, sensitive and supportive, encouraging the client to feel able to ask questions, especially if he or she is unsure of anything.

Often a consultation is used by a potential client to vet the staff and premises, before deciding to go ahead with a treatment or course of treatments, and therefore business can be lost or gained in an instant. The key words of professionalism, integrity and honesty sum up all the traits required during a consultation — any insincerity, talking about treatments of which you have no real knowledge, or general lack of interest will be detected and you will lose the client.

Position of the client

One of the key functions of the consultation is to determine if the client is suitable for treatment, as well as deciding upon the client's needs. Therefore, it makes sense to conduct the consultation with the client before he or she is prepared for the treatment, undressed and on the couch.

The client is normally taken into the working cubicle, which is quiet and private, and the record card and pen should already be prepared in anticipation. Make the client feel comfortable; ask him or her to remove outer clothing and to be seated. Some salons have a private room for consultation, which is separate from the working cubicles, off the main reception, in which case you must ensure the clients are given a conducted tour of all of the facilities, to familiarise themselves.

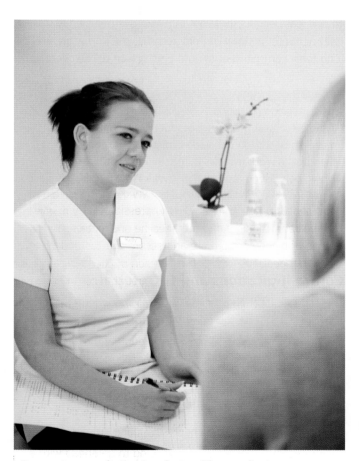

Carry out a consultation in private with your client

A client consultation

Some training establishments have the client on one side of the couch, and the therapist on the other. This may be to save space in a large training room, if the beds are quite close together. Ideally, there should be no barriers between you and the client. Seating side by side is ideal, and it allows you to touch the client should the need arise. Clients can feel very vulnerable in the initial consultation, and become emotional — it is nice to be able to reach out and hold the client's hand, to offer reassurance, if appropriate.

Not only is the 'how' of the consultation important, all the other skills required will make the process successful.

A good therapist will use a combination of all the skills to gain the information required for the consultation. However, it may take several visits before all the information is given freely; after all, a lot of the detail required is very personal, and the client may hold back about some things until the rapport has been built up.

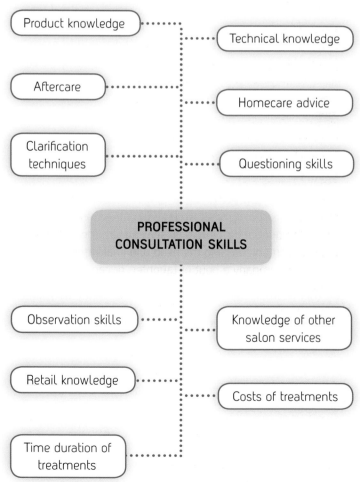

The consultation is the time for you and the client to agree on:

- the treatments
- the time span involved
- the total treatment costs
- the expected outcomes
- the client's contribution in the programme.

This treatment plan should be written, rather like a contract between you and the client, on the consultation form. If a treatment plan is not suitable for the client, for example because of time constraints and financial limitations, you will lose the client to a salon which can give a more realistic treatment plan.

Knowledge

In all parts of the consultation, it is very important that the therapist understands what she is talking about. If in doubt, ask a more senior therapist who has more experience, or who has the training in the treatment, to talk to the client. Do not make up benefits of a treatment, deliberately mislead the client in any way or give false information about the time or cost involved. Legally, the salon is not permitted to make untrue claims about treatments, and your salon would be liable to prosecution under the Trade Descriptions Act and the Supply of Goods and Services Act, if you did so (see 'You, your client and the law', page 68).

Think about it

Statements like 'Miracle anti-wrinkle cream removes all signs of the ageing process' or 'G5 treatment promises instant slimming results' or ' Lose ten pounds in the sauna' are just not true, and cannot be proven – and illegal, which could result in a hefty fine from your local Trading Standards office.

Be careful when using technical terms, or jargon, as your client may not understand them, and you could be perceived as showing off, or be thought patronising. Keep information straightforward and easy, and talk about benefits, rather than just how the equipment works.

Be honest with your product knowledge, too. Selling an unsuitable product, just because it happens to be the only one in stock, is very poor practice, and that all-important trust you have built up will be lost.

When giving advice, keep to the specific problem, rather than being too general, or giving too much advice. You are

the professional, but only in beauty therapy; your client may have previous or professional knowledge equal to or greater than your own, so never patronise.

The first few questions on a record card will be the personal details of name, address and so on. This is an ideal ice breaker, to build up a rapport with the client, leading into conversations about how easy it was to get to the salon and so on. It is also important to record details of the client's GP.

Price list

It is a very good idea to give the client your full brochure or price list. Treatment explanations and approximate timings should be included – clients do not retain all the verbal information you give them in the consultation, so it is useful to have something to take away to read at leisure. Again, be careful that the treatment explanation is correct and gives an accurate picture, with no hidden costs.

Working with the client

During the consultation, it is a good idea to emphasise the client's active participation in the chosen programme of treatments – the salon treatments are only half of the story. To see real benefits for facial skin improvement, body toning treatments, or a slimming programme, the homecare and long-term commitment should be stressed to the client.

Think about it

If the client uses the wrong products, fails to remove her make-up or eats an unbalanced diet, then expecting the therapist to work miracles in the salon is unrealistic. The client would be wasting money. This is where the holistic approach is needed. The consultation should view the wider picture of the client's lifestyle and nutrition, which play a large part in the body functioning efficiently, healing and repairing.

Contra-indications and GP referral

The contra-indication checklist will tell you whether the client is suitable for the treatment. Although you may be knowledgeable and able to recognise certain symptoms, the qualification you hold is not a medical one. As a beauty therapist, you are not permitted, nor should you attempt, to give an opinion about any symptoms the client divulges during the consultation.

A general contra-indication checklist is found on most record cards. Manufacturers often produce a specific contra-indications list to be used with individual items of equipment.

Contra-indications for treatments	Why you would avoid
Contagious skin diseases	There is a real risk that cross-contamination will occur and you pass the infection on.
Dysfunction of the nervous system	The client will be unable to respond or feel the current if sensory or motor nerves are impaired – you could cause damage to the underlying tissues.
Heart diseases or disorders	Circulation is stimulated during electrical treatments and if the heart is not functioning fully the treatment puts extra strain on it and may make the condition worse.
Ongoing medical treatment	Any electrical treatment may make the condition worse. You are not medically trained and therefore not in a position to say whether or not your treatment will be counterproductive to an existing medical condition.
Pacemaker	A pacemaker regulates the heart beat and is battery operated. The electrical current may be attracted to the metal and the function of the pacemaker may be impaired.
Recent scar tissue	The tissue is still healing and the blood-clotting process is still going on – there is a high moisture content within the blood and the current may be attracted to the scar, so there will be an intensity of current in the area, which is uncomfortable, and you may interfere with the healing process.
Undiagnosed lumps and bumps	Any swelling that is not yet medically checked has the potential to be a serious condition and no treatment should take place as you may make the condition worse.
Any medication which causes thinning of the skin (steroids, Accutane, retinols)	Electrical treatments are too stimulating for a thin skin, which may have a poor rate of healing or cellular repair. As the client is taking medication, the skin may already be injured or have an infection or condition such as acne, which you may exacerbate.

General conditions that would restrict treatment	Why you would adapt the treatment
Diabetes	Some diabetics (especially Type-2 older clients) tend to have thinner skin and poor healing qualities, so always seek GP approval before treatment and use minimal current, and/or lower settings.
Epilepsy	Some epileptics find that electrical current stimulates the nervous system too much and that may trigger a fit – the hazard is that the client is on the couch and at risk of falling off during a fit. Always seek GP approval.
High/low blood pressure	Circulation is stimulated during electrical treatments and high blood pressure may be aggravated. With low blood pressure the client may feel dizzy if they get off the couch too quickly; going from horizontal to vertical does not allow the blood flow to get to the brain and there is a risk of fainting.
Micro pigmentation	This is a semi-permanent make-up application using tattooing techniques – to colour in eyebrows, eyeliner or lip liner or any loss of natural pigment. If this has recently been carried out there is a risk that the electrical treatment will redistribute the pigmentation and disturb it – which would be very hard to correct.
History of embolism or thrombosis	If the client has a history of blood clots or impaired circulation it is best not to over-stimulate the veins with electrical current, as all treatments stimulate the circulation. You may aggravate an existing condition, so always seek GP approval.
Botox and dermal fillers	Any treatment carried out after an injectable treatment is at risk of disturbing the position of the product and redistributing it – it may be carried into neighbouring muscles, in the case of Botox, or moved, causing swelling in other areas, in the case of dermal fillers.

Continued

You and your client

You and your client

General conditions that would restrict treatment	Why you would adapt the treatment
Metal plates or pins, or piercings	Metal is a good conductor of electricity and the current will be drawn to the metal – especially if close to the surface or in the mouth, as is the case with some bridges. This needs to be discussed on an individual basis with the client.
Cuts, abrasions and bruising	See 'Recent scar tissue' in the Contra-indications for facial treatments table on page 37.
Chemical peels, IPL, laser or epilation	These are strong treatments and sufficient healing time should be factored in before any other treatments taking place.

Think about it

If a contra-indication is present, then it is important that you do not treat the client because:

- the disease or **infection** could be **contagious** and there is a risk of **cross-infection** to both therapist and other clients
- the condition may be made worse by a treatment
- there may be a reaction later, which puts the client's health at risk.

This is why it is essential to complete a thorough consultation, prior to any treatment being given.

Without causing any undue alarm or concern, the client should be referred to his or her GP and often, with a permission letter, the treatment can take place at a later date.

Key terms

Infection – the successful invasion, establishment and growth of micro-organisms to a sufficient degree to cause symptoms of disease in the host.

Contagious – term describing a disease which can be passed on to others through contact either with the sufferer or with articles which the sufferer has handled.

Cross infection, or contamination – the introduction of infectious material from one source to another, or transmission of different diseases or infection.

If the contra-indication is small and localised in one area, treatment may take place with some adaptation. For example, a minor cut would be covered with a plaster or avoided altogether. If the problem is on a part of the body which is not being treated, but there is current flowing through the body, then use some petroleum jelly to protect the damaged area.

If any clients are particularly nervous, you could ask them to read the contra-indications checklist, and tick any problems that relate to them, and then discuss these. This provides the client with something to focus on and he or she is actively participating. However, clients are notoriously forgetful — they may tick 'No' in all of the boxes to say there is nothing wrong with them, but then reach the 'Medication taken' section and you will find that they are on medication for all sorts of things! The card will then need to be amended.

Remember that all clients' personal details are confidential and should be kept with the client record card, locked away in a filing cabinet or a similar secure unit. You will need to check with the client that the personal details have not changed, but the reference on the consultation forms for both facials and body treatments should only have the client reference number on them. Therefore you will have only one personal detail card, but you may have hot stones, facials and massage consultation forms.

For your portfolio

For assessment purposes, it is best to talk through all of the contra-indications with your client, as your assessor will want to hear that as evidence!

Think about it

If you do your consultation with the client undressed and on the couch awaiting the treatment, and then discover a contra-indication which prevents treatment from taking place, your client will have to get dressed. You will have wasted time, and the client will be very disappointed to get so close to having a treatment, only to learn that it cannot take place.

Thermal and sensitivity testing

As well as going through the contra-indication checklist, it is important to check that the skin is receptive to electrical treatments, and that no nerve damage is present, causing a lack of sensitivity. This can cause injury, as the client can feel no depth of current or sensation.

Here is an example of a personal history card:

Client's full name:	Title: Mr ☐ Mrs ☐ Ms ☐ other, e.g. Doctor ☐
Address:	Contact details: Telephone home: Telephone work : Email address:
Postcode:	Name of doctor:
Date of birth: Under 21 ☐ 21–30 ☐ 31–40 ☐ 41–50 ☐ 51–60 ☐ 61–75 ☐ 75 + ☐	Surgery address:

Health details:		
Within the previous 12 months have you been under a doctor or dermatologist for treatment? Yes ☐ No ☐ If yes please specify:	Have you had any health problems in the past, surgery or procedures? Yes ☐ No ☐ If yes please specify:	Are you taking any regular medication? Yes ☐ No ☐ If yes please specify – this should include retinol and acne medication:

For female clients:

Could you be pregnant or are you trying to conceive?	Yes ☐	No ☐	Any other relevant details about your monthly cycle or related problems:
Are you taking oral contraception or HRT?	Yes ☐	No ☐	
Are your currently breastfeeding?	Yes ☐	No ☐	
Are you currently on a period or are you due one in a couple of days?	Yes ☐	No ☐	
Are you menopausal?	Yes ☐	No ☐	

Lifestyle details:

Do you smoke?	Yes ☐	No ☐	If yes please specify number and how often:
Do you regularly take exercise?	Yes ☐	No ☐	If yes, what exercise and how often:
Do you follow a restrictive diet or have medical dietary requirements?	Yes ☐	No ☐	If yes please specify:
Do you have metal implants, a pacemaker or body piercings?	Yes ☐	No ☐	If yes please specify:

Work/life balance:

Do you suffer with stress?	Yes ☐	No ☐	If yes please specify how it affects you, e.g. unable to relax, irritable bowel syndrome, poor sleeping:

Continued

How would you rate your stress levels?	1–10 1 being the lowest 10 being the highest	Please specify:
Do you generally enjoy the following? Good sleeping patterns A varied diet Healthy skin, hair and nails High energy levels A good level of health – no minor colds	Yes ☐ No ☐ Yes ☐ No ☐ Yes ☐ No ☐ Yes ☐ No ☐ Yes ☐ No ☐	If no, please specify.
Allergies: Do you suffer with any reactions to the following? Cosmetics or creams Any foods Any medication Animals Fragrance Metals Other	Yes ☐ No ☐ Yes ☐ No ☐ Yes ☐ No ☐ Yes ☐ No ☐ Yes ☐ No ☐ Yes ☐ No ☐ Yes ☐ No ☐	Please specify:
Occupation: What is your occupation/job or current situation?		Does this have any effects on your health, e.g. shift work? Please specify:
Any other details which are relevant to your treatments but have not been mentioned above:		

It is very important that tests are carried out in the area to be worked upon, not just a general test on an arm or leg. So, if a facial is being given, the tests must be carried out on a clean, grease-free face; if it is to be a cellulite treatment on the thighs, then the tests must be carried out on the legs.

The thermal test for the differentiation between hot and cold involves placing test tubes containing hot and cold water alternately on the skin, so that the client can tell you which is which. Ideally, the client should have his or her eyes closed, but if the test tubes are identical, it will not be possible to distinguish temperature just by looking.

The sensation test will enable you to tell whether the client can feel the difference between sharp and soft objects. The client will need to close his or her eyes for the test. For the soft test, stroke over different areas of the skin with a cotton wool pad. For the sharp, use the end of an orange stick, as this provides a sharp enough sensation for the client to tell the difference. Just put slight pressure on the skin; do not stab the client to cause pain (or draw blood!).

These tests are very important, as they inform the therapist that the nerve endings in the skin for temperature and sensation are working properly. Should the client be unable to distinguish hot/cold and soft/sharp, do not commence the treatment but refer the client to his or her GP.

Think about it

A thorough consultation protects both you and everyone else in the salon from possible cross-infection from any disease a client might have. It also protects your business should the client decide to sue for negligence or malpractice. If the client agrees with the treatment, declares any contra-indications present and then you both sign the treatment plan, this record would act as evidence of your client care and attention in the event of a court case. Be both vigilant and thorough with your consultation.

Think about it

You should find out about all contra-indications, even though they may not seem relevant to the treatment you are about to give. For example, your client may have come in for a facial treatment, but you discover a contra-indication in or on the body. A small bruise on the ankle will not affect the facial condition, but systemic problems will, such as fluid retention caused by kidney problems. Use your judgement and experience to decide whether to go ahead with the treatment. If in doubt, ask a more senior therapist for advice, or gain the client's GP approval before going ahead.

Analyse the client for treatment

Regardless of whether you are carrying out a consultation for a facial or body treatment, some of the consultation will have a common theme; other parts will not. For example, your questions will be similar, but your observations will differ — as the skin and its related problems differ on different areas of the body.

Your consultation techniques will include:

- questioning
- observing
- manual examination.

Questioning

Follow the questions within your record card as a guide to what you need to ask. Be polite, and clarify any points which you feel need further investigation. Be prepared to answer the questions clients have — they may (quite rightly) want to know why you need the information. You will need to reassure clients that the reasons are for their safety and health, not because you are being nosy! You should also understand the effect the treatment may have on particular conditions and why the treatment cannot go ahead. For example, if the client has epilepsy, then an electrical current may stimulate the brain into triggering a seizure, so cannot be offered as a treatment option. It is possible to offer non-electrical facials and body treatments, so alternatives are available. As long as the explanation offered is full, then clients should understand and be open to other options.

Client modesty

The client's modesty and privacy must be preserved; in a closed cubicle, ask the client to remove all outdoor and heavy clothing for the initial verbal consultation. Protecting the client's privacy is not only about personal modesty but is also about safeguarding personal information and maintaining client confidentiality. The topics you discuss with your client, and their possible medical nature, are private to them, and should not be discussed outside the cubicle, unless it is in a consulting, professional manner (should you need to seek clarification on something you are unsure of). Even then, ask the client's permission to consult with a more senior colleague or your lecturer.

Once the initial consultation has been completed and you are happy that no contra-indications are present, you are ready to begin a facial or body analysis, which means you can prepare the client for treatment and instruct him or her to lie on the couch or bed.

My story

Beenal's story

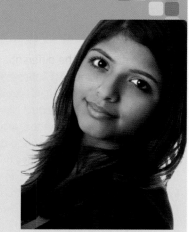

I had just qualified in electrical facials and was eager to introduce one of my clients, who regularly had manual facials, to the benefits of the galvanic current. The client was also enthusiastic to try something new. As I carried out the thermal and sensitivity testing, I became aware that the client had areas on her face and neck where she had no sensation at all.

I went over the areas twice but still the client could feel nothing. I stopped the testing and explained to her why the treatment could not go ahead. The client was a little confused and asked me my opinion on what was wrong, but I said that as I had no medical training I could not comment on why this was occurring. I suggested she visit her GP.

About a month later, the client came into the salon with a beautiful bunch of flowers for me. She wanted to thank me for the trouble I had taken. The client's GP had referred her to a neurologist who diagnosed a disease of the nervous system. Although serious, early diagnosis had allowed prompt treatment to take place.

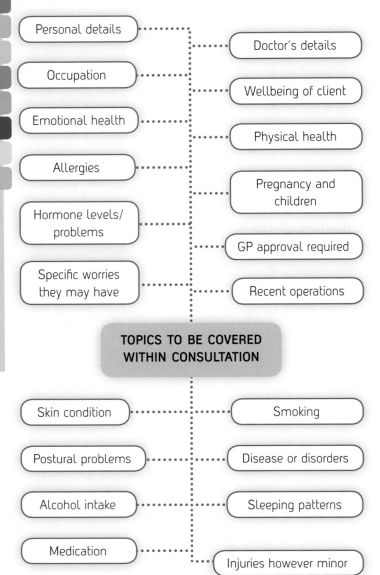

Personal details

Doctor's details

Occupation

Wellbeing of client

Emotional health

Physical health

Allergies

Pregnancy and children

Hormone levels/ problems

GP approval required

Specific worries they may have

Recent operations

TOPICS TO BE COVERED WITHIN CONSULTATION

Skin condition

Smoking

Postural problems

Disease or disorders

Alcohol intake

Sleeping patterns

Medication

Injuries however minor

Hygiene and avoiding cross-infection

Hygiene and avoiding cross-infection are of the utmost importance within beauty therapy, as treatments necessarily demand close human contact. However, many of the benefits of the treatments would be ruined if protective clothing and gloves were worn — imagine giving a full body massage with gloves on — so care must be taken to provide the maximum protection against cross-infection.

All professional bodies' codes of practice state clearly that all members are expected to abide by a standard of good practice in relation to hygiene. Special care must be taken to ensure that cross-infection does not occur and official guidelines are respected. You will be assessed on your hygiene practices during assessment, but they should be good habits that you carry out automatically, not just something you do because you are on assessment.

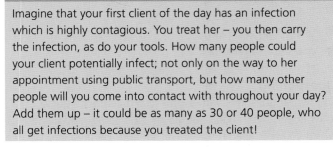

Think about it

Imagine that your first client of the day has an infection which is highly contagious. You treat her — you then carry the infection, as do your tools. How many people could your client potentially infect; not only on the way to her appointment using public transport, but how many other people will you come into contact with throughout your day? Add them up — it could be as many as 30 or 40 people, who all get infections because you treated the client!

Hygiene should be regarded as a protection against disease and illness. As a professional therapist, good hygiene practices will:

- maintain your own health
- maintain your clients' health
- maintain your colleagues' health
- protect your business reputation, and ultimately your business.

Good hygiene practices are also a legal requirement.

Expert advice on hygiene can be confusing. Conflicting reports have been seen in the media with regard to AIDS and hepatitis, and the resistance of some bacteria, such as MRSA, commonly found in hospitals, to antibiotic treatment. (MRSA is a drug-resistant strain of a very common bacterium called Staphylococcus aureus.) The most valuable up-to-date information can be gained from your Awarding Body's

Think about it

What *you* decide for individual clients may not necessarily be their goal — it is therefore their decision which treatments and homecare they opt for. Being too dictatorial and not working with clients may mean that they decide not to have any treatments with you. For example, putting the client on a very low carbohydrate diet to lose three stone (19 kilograms) in three months may not be what the client wants, and this will affect motivation, results and ultimately cost you the client's business. Talk to clients about what *they* want to achieve in their time with you — and allow that to happen, rather than being forceful and dogmatic in your treatment approach.

Think about it

Disposable gloves

There are a wide variety of disposable gloves on the market and all beauty therapists must ensure that all health and safety legislation is adhered to, to protect themselves and their clients from cross-contamination. Most Awarding Bodies also specify that gloves should be worn for some treatments in which there is a possibility of contact with bodily fluids and/or the skin is being pierced – especially epilation, use of micro lance, intimate waxing and microdermabrasion.

There are a few guidelines for gloves you need to be aware of for health and safety.

- Always buy medical-standard disposable gloves from a reputable manufacturer. This ensures that they comply with British Standards BS EN 455 which states that gloves must be thoroughly tested for holes, chemical penetration, tears, tension testing and are fit for purpose.
- The gloves should state that they are for single use only and can be disposed of safely – so check the box .
- Look on the box and check the symbols for the manufacturing and expiry dates. (because the gloves are treated with chlorine which cleanses the surface of the rubber, they are only guaranteed for a limited period).
- You can buy Nitrile (blue) gloves which are latex-free and powder-free, Vitrile (green) gloves which blend Nitrile rubber with vinyl components, and synthetic gloves which are also latex- and powder-free. Nitrile rubber is more resistant than natural rubber to oils, acids and punctures but they are less flexible.
- Gloves should be chosen to fit snugly on the hands; however both Nitrile and Vitrile gloves are close-fitting and you may need to purchase a bigger size to obtain a comfortable fit .
- Never reuse the gloves.
- Do not apply talc to the hands prior to use as this may cause an allergic reaction.
- Always wash and dry hands thoroughly before and after using gloves.
- If the hands dry out with constant use then apply a reconditioning hand cream to keep hands from cracking or breaking open.
- Do not substitute heavier cleaning or domestic rubber gloves for use on clients.
- Do not use the gloves if they are damaged, smell or have holes in them.

Note: latex gloves should be avoided as they may cause an allergic reaction.

code of ethics or practice (refer to it for more details). These guidelines have been established after a great deal of research on behalf of the beauty industry, and are most likely to be current.

It is important to understand the responsibilities we each have under the Health and Safety at Work Act 1974, and under the COSHH (Control of Substances Hazardous to Health) regulations. Refer to the legislation section on pages 68–82 for extra guidelines.

In order to maintain the highest hygiene standards, you will need to understand how infection can occur. An infectious disease is one which can be passed from one person to another. All germs need warmth and moisture to multiply so a therapy treatment area is an ideal breeding ground for germs.

Disease can be spread:

- by direct contact with a person who has a disease or infection
- by infection from droplets in the air, as when someone sneezes near you
- indirectly – when you touch an infected item such as a towel, tissues, cotton wool.

Infection is caused by three different groups of micro-organisms. A micro-organism is any organism that is too small to be seen by the naked eye. They are ever-present in the environment and include:

- bacteria
- viruses
- fungi.

Think about it

Tetanus

When was your last tetanus jab? They only last for ten years, and that soon goes by. Ask at your local surgery to look on your medical records – you are at risk if your immunisations are not up to date.

You can avoid the bacterial infection tetanus through an injection of antitoxin. Tetanus causes violent muscle spasms and, in extreme cases, may be fatal. The tetanus jab needs boosting every ten years, and should be given after a suspect injury such as a cut from a rusty blade. Cutting your hand while gardening and then getting the spores in the cut may lead to tetanus.

You and your client

Bacteria

Bacteria are classified according to their shape, as shown in the table below.

Shape	Description	What they look like	Disease they cause
Round – cocci	They can protect themselves by forming tough outer coats, and in this condition they are known as spores		Spores themselves cannot cause disease in this state: they are too immature. As spores they can survive for a long time without food or water. However, when conditions improve – when water, a suitable food source and temperature become available – the spores grow, mature and cause disease. Spores can enter the body through cuts, and may be present in pot-plant soil.
Round in couples – diplococci	Bonded together in pairs		**Parasitic** bacteria including pneumococcus causing pneumonia
Round in bunches – staphylococci	Cocci bunched together, forming clumps		Acne, boils, barber's rash
Round in chains – streptococci	Cocci linked together at the ends to form chains		Impetigo, sore throats
Rod-shaped – bacilli	Separate rod shapes		Scarlet fever
Spiral-shaped – spirochetes	Single threads that form in a spiral, lack a rigid cell wall and move by muscular flexions of the cell		Diphtheria and typhoid, tuberculosis, whooping cough
Comma-shaped – vibrios	They have thicker bodies and a tail-like structure		Venereal disease (such as syphilis), cholera

Classification of bacteria

Key terms

Parasitic – an organism which attaches to living tissue and feeds off it to survive.

Secondary infection – infection at a site on the body already vulnerable, for example a cut or open wound.

Saprophytes – bacteria which live on dead organic matter.

Pathogen – an organism capable of causing disease.

Pathogenic – general term for diseases found on humans and animals (living beings).

Sepsis – the presence of harmful micro-organisms or their toxins in the blood or other tissues.

Septicaemia – blood poisoning, the presence of pathogenic bacteria in the bloodstream.

Bacteria need a number of conditions to survive and thrive:

- food
- warmth
- alkalinity
- darkness
- oxygen
- moisture

Boils	This bacterial infection forms at the base of the hair follicle. Bacteria can spread through an open scratch in the skin. The area is raised, red and painful. **Pus** may be present.	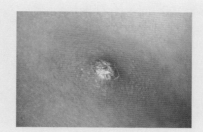
Impetigo	Highly infectious, this bacterial infection starts as small red spots, which then break open and form blisters. Most common around the corner of the mouth and if picked, will spread. It can be spread through use of **unsanitised** equipment.	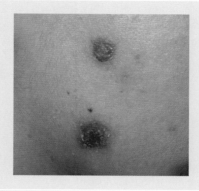
Stye	This is a small boil at the base of the eyelash follicle, which is caused by a bacterial infection. It is raised, sore and red, and there may be considerable swelling in the area.	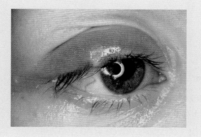

Examples of bacterial infections

Viral infections

A virus consists of a protein shell, within which are particles of genetic material, either DNA or RNA. The virus infects a cell and uses the host's genetic material to reproduce itself. Viruses can then leave the host cell and invade other cells.

Most viruses enter the body through the mouth or skin and then spread to cells throughout the body, via the bloodstream. Because the cells can multiply only in living cells, they cannot survive in the horney layer of the epidermis — they need to be deeper within the epidermis to find a living host cell.

Key terms

Pus – a product of inflammation consisting of fluid and white blood cells.

Inflammation – a common response to any infection. When cells are injured they release chemicals that allow blood cells and fluid to move into the tissues. This bloodflow results in four signs of inflammation: heat, pain, redness and swelling (the suffix –*itis* indicates inflammation, for example appendicitis and tonsillitis).

Unsanitised – unhygienic.

You and your client

Viruses cause:

- the common cold
- cold sores (herpes simplex)
- measles
- rubella (German measles)
- hepatitis A, B and C
- HIV.
- mumps
- warts
- flu
- chickenpox

Cold sores	The cold sore virus appears on the lips, cheeks and nose. Blisters form, the skin is broken and painful. The blisters are likely to spread when open and weepy and then crusts form.	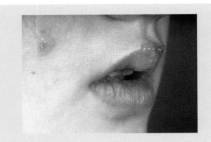
Warts	Warts are caused by a virus. They are small, compact raised growths of skin. They can be light or brown in colour.	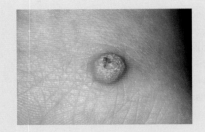
Measles	Measles is an acute, highly contagious viral disease causing fever and a blotchy rash. It can cause more serious complications.	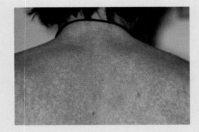
Chickenpox	Chickenpox is a mild, specific contagious disease of childhood, caused by a virus. It causes crops of spots which scab and are itchy, and may cause scarring.	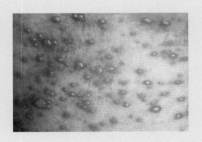
The common cold	The common cold is easily spread. Streaming eyes and nose, coughing and sneezing are its symptoms.	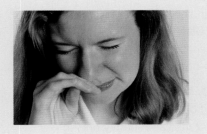

Examples of viruses

You and your client

Fungal infections

Fungal/yeast infections cause:

- ringworm of the foot, body, head and nail
- thrush
- infection to the heart and lungs, which may prove fatal.

Protozoa (large group of microscopic single-cell animals) cause:

- diarrhoea
- malaria
- **amoebic dysentery**.

Key terms

Amoebic dysentery – an inflammatory disorder of the intestine, especially of the colon, caused by an amoeba (a microscopic organism). It results in severe diarrhoea, containing mucus and/or blood. It can be fatal if untreated.

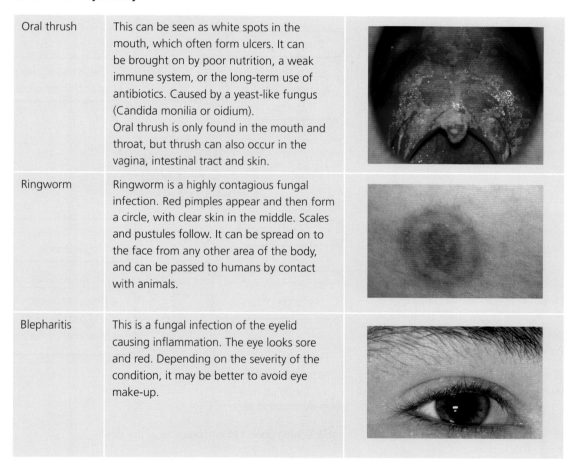

Oral thrush	This can be seen as white spots in the mouth, which often form ulcers. It can be brought on by poor nutrition, a weak immune system, or the long-term use of antibiotics. Caused by a yeast-like fungus (Candida monilia or oidium). Oral thrush is only found in the mouth and throat, but thrush can also occur in the vagina, intestinal tract and skin.	
Ringworm	Ringworm is a highly contagious fungal infection. Red pimples appear and then form a circle, with clear skin in the middle. Scales and pustules follow. It can be spread on to the face from any other area of the body, and can be passed to humans by contact with animals.	
Blepharitis	This is a fungal infection of the eyelid causing inflammation. The eye looks sore and red. Depending on the severity of the condition, it may be better to avoid eye make-up.	

Examples of fungal infection

A general infection – for example:

Conjunctivitis	Conjunctivitis is an inflammation of the conjunctiva in the eye; it may be bacterial, viral or allergic in origin. This is a nasty eye condition. The eyelids are red, sore and itchy .	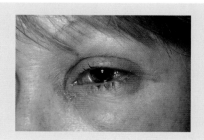

You and your client

47

Micro-organisms enter the body through any route they can:

- damaged, broken skin
- ears, nose, mouth and genitals
- hair follicles
- the bloodstream via a bite from blood-sucking insects, such as malaria-carrying mosquitoes.

Think about it

The symptoms and severity of the infection or disease will depend on the type of invasion, the strength of the person's immune system, whether it is able to defend the body, and their general health. If a person is run down, then the micro-organisms have more chance of multiplying rapidly. They also thrive in poor hygiene. The best ways of avoiding these are prevention – through good hygiene practices.

Obviously, some of these diseases are life threatening, but many are not and can be prevented by good hygiene. For example, protozoa can be transmitted from contaminated food and water, which grow and infect the bowel, causing diarrhoea and ill health.

For your portfolio

Many of these diseases are also radically reduced by vaccination. Precautions can be taken against both hepatitis B and tetanus; these precautions are recommended for beauty therapists. Most school children are given immunisation against measles, mumps and rubella, unless there are medical reasons not to have the injections. Whooping cough has been dramatically reduced by the same method of immunisation.

When you have completed your course, if vaccinated, put your medical certificate in with your portfolio.

If you go abroad to work, or work on cruise liners, you will need different injections to protect you against malaria, TB and diphtheria – always check with your doctor and your employer. You will not be able to work or travel without the required certificates.

Think about it

All good hygiene practices should be continuously carried out to ensure that no cross-infection takes place – starting with preparation of the work area, throughout the treatment itself, through to leaving the work area and equipment clean and tidy ready for the next treatment. The client will then have total confidence in the salon and it ensures you are following all the required health and safety regulations.

Hygiene practices in the salon

Risk Assessment for Hygiene

Refer also to Unit G22, Monitor procedures to safely control work operations.

The best way to prevent infection occurring in the salon is to look at the systems and procedures in place regarding personal hygiene, client safety and sterilisation methods. Prevention is always better than cure, and sterilisation is the only sure way to destroy organisms, so it is worth investing in some modern and efficient equipment.

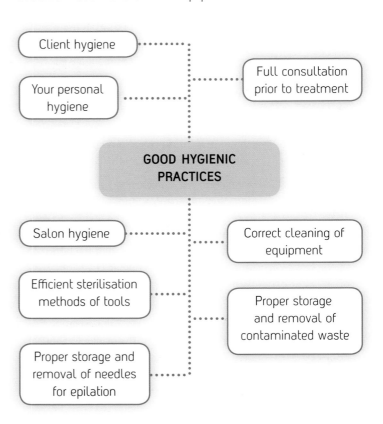

Maintaining good hygiene practices in the salon

Think about it

If you intend to set up your own business, either as a mobile therapist or in a salon, purchase the best sterilising equipment you can afford and which is practicable.

When going for an interview in a salon, check its hygiene standards by asking lots of questions and looking for the right equipment. If a salon has poor hygiene, is it really the type of place where you would want to work?

Poor hygiene practices

How it affects the therapist

Potentially the therapist could bring infection into the salon through infections spread from open wounds, harboured in jewellery, long nails or on clothing.

Prevention (Ask yourself – How can I prevent this?)

- Wash hands before and after every treatment – use bactericidal or antibacterial gel if possible.
- Wear disposable gloves for treatments if there is a possibility of an exchange of body fluids – when waxing, for example.
- Wear personal protective equipment (PPE).
- Cover cuts or broken skin with a waterproof plaster.
- Keep nails short and scrub under them with a nail brush.
- Do not come to work if you know you have an infection or disease likely to put anyone else at risk – impetigo, for example.
- Wash hands thoroughly after every visit to the toilet.
- Follow guidelines on personal presentation and clean overalls, etc. (see page 5).
- Attend training programmes for hygiene and use of sterilising equipment.
- Do not use equipment that is cracked or broken as germs will be present (this includes chipped cups, plates or glasses).

Corrective action (Ask yourself – What should I do if things are not right?)

- Take preventative measures – seek expert advice.
- Report unhygienic practices.
- Hold regular staff meetings to ensure all staff have the same procedures for hygiene and prevention of infection.
- Contact your local federation for advice and guidance on the latest information on hygiene and the latest legislation.

How it affects the client

Potentially the client could:

- bring infection into the salon
- have a treatment knowing a contra-indication is present
- not wash hands after using the toilet
- not use protective steps put in place by the salon, for example not treading upon the couch roll when getting out of the shower.

Corrective measures for the client (Ask yourself – What should I do if things are not right during the treatment?)

- Stop the treatment immediately and refer the client to their GP.
- Disinfect the area where the client has been.
- Sterilise the equipment which was being used.

Also:

- Constantly look and ask clients about possible infection.
- Carry out spot checks on clients' record cards.
- Keep up-to-date record cards.
- Insist clients follow your directives for maintaining hygiene standards.
- Seek GP approval for clients with any contra-indications or who may present a slight risk.

Think about it

You must explain to your client about the homecare hygiene practices to be carried out – especially after treatment such as extraction or epilation, when there may be blood spotting. This is also relevant if the skin is vulnerable, such as after microdermabrasion. There is a risk of infection occurring if the client does not follow simple hygiene rules such as keeping the area clean, covered with a plaster (if necessary) and avoiding picking at the skin.

General preventative steps

◉ Display a notice in the reception area asking clients to check that they are not knowingly suffering from any contagious diseases.

◉ Always carry out a full consultation to discover any contra-indications.

◉ Always perform a physical check of the area to be treated. Do not treat if any unrecognised problems are present.

◉ Ask the client to sign the declaration on the record card stating that all medical and other information is correct to date, to avoid possible repercussions later.

◉ Always wipe the area to be treated prior to commencement with appropriate lotion, for example surgical spirit, Hibitane or the recommended choice of your training establishment.

◉ Provide all possible protection for clients and insist they use the provided procedure, for example treading on the couch roll if their feet are bare to avoid touching the floor surface.

◉ Discourage clients from having a treatment if they have the beginnings of an illness — explain that you would not wish to infect other clients.

The salon environment

Possible risks include:

- infection from equipment
- towels/blankets/headbands/sheets/quilts
- products may cause multiple infections with a risk of cross-contamination
- work surfaces/couches/trolleys/sinks can harbour germs.

Prevention (Ask yourself — How can I prevent this?)

- Sanitise equipment used as fully as possible. This means following manufacturer's instructions for individual equipment, for example using the recommended cleaner.
- Tools should always be washed in hot, soapy water, rinsed well and dried thoroughly, before using a sterilising fluid or a UV box.
- Invest time and correct training in the use of sterilisation equipment such as an autoclave or sanitising unit.
- Clean the treatment area/room daily and wipe generally after each treatment has taken place.
- Clean all work surfaces regularly with hot water and detergent.
- Use couch roll and towels as a barrier between blankets and the clients — these can then be disposed of and fresh ones put on for each client.
- Tuck tissues into the headband or turban — these can be disposed of after use and keep the turban looking fresh.
- Wash towels after use — your training salon needs to invest in towels to ensure you do not run out!
- Wash towelling robes for clients.
- When carrying out a facial and wrapping the client up in blankets, use a cotton sheet as a barrier between the blanket and the client.
- Decant creams and oils, using a spatula, into a smaller bowl and throw away any excess.
- Never pour back into the original container any product that has been in contact with the hands and the client. To be cost effective, be careful not to pour out too much, which may be wasted.
- Use disposable spatulas for massage creams — that is, one use from pot to client, to avoid contamination.
- Do not accept products from the manufacturer which have been opened or where the seal is broken.
- Never use products past their shelf life.
- Conduct regular cleaning sessions.
- Sign a duty rota when the tasks have been completed.
- Carry out spot checks.
- Return faulty products to the manufacturer and seek their assurances for fresh products — or change suppliers, stop all treatments immediately.
- Close the salon for a whole cleaning day.
- Enrol professional help — employ professional cleaners to steam clean areas, if necessary.
- Buy new sterilising equipment — a new autoclave will be an excellent investment.
- Carry out a risk assessment: infections.

Sterilisation

The three main methods of sterilisation are:
1. heat   2. chemical   3. radiation.

The advantages and disadvantages of each method are shown in the table at the bottom of this page.

Key terms

Sterilisation – the total destruction of all living micro-organisms.

Disinfection – the destruction of some but not all micro-organisms.

Think about it

Most commercial washing powder manufacturers now make a washing powder which is antiseptic/bacterial at a 40 degree wash – use it for all linens and you will be safeguarding the client's hygiene.

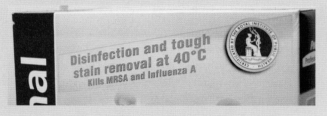

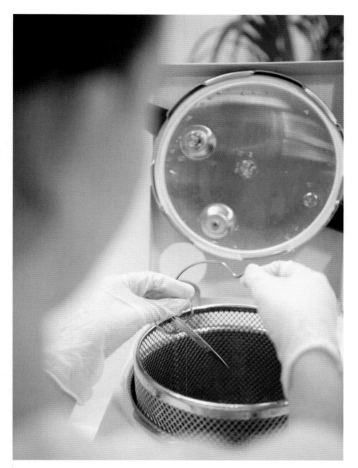

An autoclave in action

Method	Suitability	How it works
Oven	Not very practical in the salon, and only some items can go in an oven – plastic bowls, for example, would melt. The oven would need to be in constant use and be very large	An object needs to be the oven for one hour at 160°C – this will destroy even spores
Naked flame	Not practical – risk of fire, especially with so many inflammable chemicals in the salon Can only be used on metallic equipment Blunts the instrument, so cuticle nippers would be rendered unusable in a short time	Flame needs to be red hot to destroy all the germs – a small metallic object such as a needle will then be sterile
Burning	Not practical to burn salon's paper refuse in a bonfire – risk of fire getting out of control, pollution (environmentally unfriendly) May be illegal in some areas	Destroys germs and spores
Glass bead steriliser	Small electrically heated box with a cylinder full of small glass beads. Because of its size the steriliser can only hold small items – not practical. Items to be sterilised should be inserted deep into the glass beads and removed with a clean pair of forceps	Temperatures vary from 190–300°C. It takes from one to ten minutes to sterilise, but the steriliser takes up to one hour to reach the correct temperature (the unit cannot be used for at least 30 minutes after being switched on), so this method may have time constraints

Continued

Moist heat		
Boiling	Washing machine hot wash cycle will destroy germs in towels, robes, turbans, etc. Not suitable for items which rust or melt in hot water	Most germs destroyed at 100°C (boiling point of water) within 15 minutes; spores are more resistant and take longer
Autoclave	Similar to a pressure cooker; used to sterilise equipment. Most suitable for small metal equipment, e.g. eyebrow tweezers, manicure tools Refer to individual manufacturer's instructions for use Remove instruments with a clean pair of forceps and place in a kidney bowl with tissue soaked in isopropyl alcohol or similar	By heating water under pressure to a higher temperature than 100°C, creates an environment where germs cannot survive
Chemical vapour	Most useful for sterilising non-metallic tools as metal tools may develop pitting in the surface, and can also cause bluntness Unpleasant fumes Equipment must be washed with soap and water prior to sterilisation	A foam strip is soaked in 5 per cent formalin liquid, which is heated, releasing fumes, becoming formaldehyde. The fumes circulate in the sterilising box, which has open shelves for storage The formaldehyde destroys the germs
Radiation	Only suitable for sterilising equipment without body fluids on it, so tweezers need to be put into the autoclave As the ultraviolet waves travel in straight lines, the tools need to be turned over to allow both sides to be sterilised Equipment must be washed with soap and water prior to sterilisation Useful to store small items, but not very powerful	A mercury vapour lamp emits ultraviolet (UV) radiation inside a cabinet which has perforated wire shelves on which to lay the equipment. The process works by irradiating the equipment with UV light at a wavelength of 254 nanometres (1 nanometre = one-millionth of a millimetre). When a suitable dose has been delivered, bacteria are made inactive. (Refer to individual manufacturer's instructions, and see tanning unit for electro-magnetic spectrum in Unit B21 Provide UV Tanning Services on website.) The cabinet must be kept very clean as grease is a barrier to UV radiation The lamp must be changed after 2000 hours' use, the equivalent of one year's use at eight hours per day, five days per week

Advantages and disadvantages of methods of sterilisation

A guide to controlling micro-organisms

There are a great many commercial products on the market for cleaning and sterilisation — with lots of different trade names. This is merely a general guide. Please check the manufacturer's instructions for each individual piece of equipment. Most companies have their own particular favourites that they recommend.

Alcohol

Alcohol-based disinfectants are very good for soaking metal instruments such as small manicure equipment. The usual dilution is 70% isopropyl alcohol — or a surgical spirit base.

Once it has been used, the disinfectant should be thrown away and a fresh solution made up for every client. Isopropyl alcohol is an antibacterial solvent used in all sorts of products, from aftershave to hand lotions and cleaners. It is made from propylene which is obtained during the cracking of petroleum. It is a good cleaner but the fumes can be an irritant, so surgical spirit, commonly bought over the counter at a chemist or from a local wholesale supplier, can be used instead.

Ammonia

Ammonia is commonly used as a base for trade liquids that kill bacteria, for example barbicide, which is used to soak suitable instruments in salons. The drawback with using ammonia is its strong smell!

Antibiotics

An antibiotic is a chemical substance that destroys or inhibits the growth of micro-organisms. Antibiotics are usually used to treat infections that will respond well to them, such as fungal or bacterial infections, and are given to humans and some animals for treatment. They can be taken as tablets, or as a cream applied to the area, or in an injection. In hospitals, they can also be administered in a drip form straight into the bloodstream. They are not available over the counter to buy. They are only issued on prescription from a doctor.

Antiseptic

An antiseptic is a chemical agent which destroys or inhibits the growth of micro-organisms on living tissues, thus helping to prevent infection when placed onto open cuts and wounds.

Autoclave

An autoclave is a piece of equipment rather like a pressure cooker, used to sterilise equipment. It works by heating distilled water under pressure to a higher temperature than 100°C, therefore creating an environment where germs cannot survive. It is most suitable for small metal equipment, such as eyebrow tweezers and manicure items.

Ideally, the autoclave should heat up to 121°C for 15 minutes. There is a stacking system of baskets in the base so that lots of small tools can be put in together, but they should be washed and clean prior to sterilisation. If several therapists use the autoclave at one time, be sure that the equipment is easily identifiable — perhaps with a blob of nail varnish, otherwise you will not know which tools belong to whom! The autoclave is only good for stainless steel or glass equipment. Refer to individual manufacturer's instructions for use.

Bactericide

A bactericide is a chemical that will kill bacteria but not necessarily the spores, so reproduction may still take place. It can also be called biocide, fungicide, virucide or sporicide.

Chlorhexidine

Trade names for chlorhexidine include Savlon and Hibitane. Chlorhexidine is widely used for skin and surface cleaning and some sunbed canopies. Check individual manufacturer's instructions for cleaning.

Detergent

A detergent is a synthetic cleaning agent that removes all impurities from a surface by reacting with grease and suspended particles, including bacteria and other micro-organisms. Detergents need to be used with water but are ideal for cleansing large surface areas.

Disinfectant

This is a chemical that kills micro-organisms but not spores — most commonly used to wash surfaces and to clean drains. Disinfectants can only work against bacteria and fungi. They reduce the number of organisms, minimising the risk of infection. In medicine, disinfectants (such as Triclosan) are used to clean unbroken skin.

Hypochlorous acid is a weak unstable acid, occurring only in solution, which can be used as a bleach and disinfectant. Products containing sodium or calcium hypochlorite can be used on large surfaces, such as floors and walls, as they are relatively inexpensive to buy. They can however be corrosive and are not suitable for soaking metal instruments or applying directly onto the skin.

Phenol compounds

Phenol compounds are ideal for large areas that need cleaning, but phenol does have a chlorine base and should not be used on the skin. It is used in industrial cleaning preparations and the old-fashioned carbolic soap.

Sanitation

Sanitation (from the Latin *sanitas*, meaning health) is a generic term relating to health and the measures for the protection of health, i.e. to be free of dirt and germs, and to be hygienic. It is used to describe facilities and measures that are put into place to promote hygiene and prevent the spread of disease.

Sterilisation

Sterilisation is the complete destruction of all living micro-organisms and their spores.

Surgical spirit

Surgical spirit is widely used and easily available from chemists. It can be used for skin cleansing, and to remove grease on the skin. Surgical spirit comes in varying strengths of dilution. A 70% alcohol base concentration is acceptable for cleansing.

Ultraviolet boxes

Some salons use an ultraviolet (UV) light box to destroy bacteria. UV rays are generated from a quartz mercury vapour lamp (similar to a mini sunbed) with a low rate of penetration. The tools have to be thoroughly clean and dry before they go into the box, otherwise germs will cling to the dirt or dead skin cells on the surface and form a barrier preventing sterilisation from fully taking place. The tools also need to be turned around after 15 minutes because the rays only clean the surfaces of the tools. Only metal tools such as cuticle nippers are suitable for UV sterilisation and, of course, once you touch them, taking them out of the box, they are no longer sterile.

UV rays are harmful to the eyes, so the box should be switched off before you open it. UV bulbs have a limited life, so a log of usage should be kept and the bulbs replaced when recommended by the manufacturer. Always follow manufacturers' instructions .

You and your working environment

In this section you will learn about:

- hygiene in the treatment area
- setting up the resources you require
- environmental conditions
- fire precautions and evacuation procedures
- first aid
- accident reporting procedures.

This part of the unit looks at where you work, whether it's a cubicle, a room or a large salon space, and how you manage it. This includes health and safety within the area, managing your resources, and using your surroundings to create the right setting for a pampering and relaxing treatment.

Hygiene in the treatment area

When preparing and managing your treatment area, you will need to ensure that your working environment meets the legal, hygiene and treatment requirements, as set by both your Awarding Body and government guidelines.

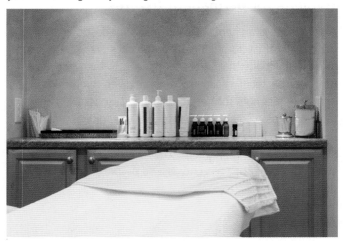

Your treatment area must be immaculately clean

Hygiene is important for:
the permanent fixtures in the salon, such as:

- walls
- doors
- flooring
- windows.

The portable equipment you use, including:

- the couch
- small equipment
- machines
- products.

You will need to refer to the Health and Safety at Work etc. (HASAW) Act 1974 for full guidance (see page 69) and also to work to the specifications of the Workplace (Health, Safety and Welfare) Regulations 1992, which require all premises used as workplaces to have effective means of:

- lighting
- ventilation
- temperature control
- providing adequate work space
- maintaining cleanliness
- arranging safe salon layout (see page 95).

Think about it

Dust and dirt in the salon are made up of particles of old skin cells, fluff from towels and clothing, ash and dirt brought in from outside and floating particles of products. In a busy salon, dust and dirt can build up very quickly.

You will need to refer to the 'You, your client and the law' section of this unit for a full list of treatment and working regulations (from page 68). Below is the information you need on environmental conditions for creating the right atmosphere.

Hygiene for permanent fixtures

The salon should be regularly cleaned to prevent the spread of infection, and to make it welcoming for the client. A dirty salon will be judged on its appearance rather than on the treatments carried out.

Most colleges and training establishments employ a cleaning firm, usually on a fixed contract, which provides staff to do the daily chores for hygiene maintenance: floor cleaning, emptying of general waste bins, sweeping the stairs, and so on. More staff may be employed to carry out longer-term spring cleaning of windows, paintwork and re-sealing of the floors.

Small salons do not normally subcontract their cleaning duties – it tends to be done on a rota system, with junior staff doing most of the jobs. Any idle pair of hands will be asked to get on with some cleaning duties, and all staff can expect to share the workload – it is almost part of the job description. It would be unrealistic to expect otherwise.

For your portfolio

Who does your company/training establishment employ to do the cleaning, if anyone? How much does the service cost? Who is responsible for checking the job is well done? What happens if it isn't?

Salon décor needs to be attractive yet practical, with suitable surfaces. There is a fine line between the clinical décor of a hospital and a welcoming salon which is easy to keep clean.

Flooring	Should be made of non-slip material, such as vinyl tiles or a softwood finish, which is easy to sweep or vacuum everyday. Carpet or carpet tiles may look good to start with, but can be high maintenance when getting old, and are not practical for spillage or keeping in pristine condition. A good disinfectant and mop will lift most dirt and grease from a floor, which should be cleaned nightly.
Walls and doors	Should be painted for two reasons: they are easier to wipe with a disinfectant or abrasive cleaner such as sugar soap, and it is easy to maintain a high standard of décor, as redecorating just involves a quick coat of paint! Any household preparation or spray cleaner will clean finger marks or dirt from paintwork, using a damp cloth. Sugar soap (granules which dissolve in hot water) will cut through long-term grease and make a good preparation of the surface for the new coat of paint.
Light switches	Along with dado rails, light switches tend to collect finger marks and general dirt, so they also need a spray with a household cleanser – but spray the cloth, rather than the light switch, and wipe over, to avoid getting the electric cable behind the switch wet.
Ceilings	These can get very grubby, Ceilings are actually quite a focus for clients as they often lie in the supine position (facing upwards) and a dirty ceiling will certainly catch the eye, and be very off-putting – especially the old swirl-effect Artex ceilings, where dirt can accumulate in the grooves. Washing ceilings should only be done when the salon is empty, and by using the correct ladder, or wide steps, for health and safety reasons. If the salon has subcontracted its cleaning, the contractor would normally have carried out the correct risk assessments and training for this task. Always remember to look up when vacuuming the carpet, so that you can vacuum up those long cobweb formations, which accumulate in corners, with the nozzle of the vacuum cleaner.
Windows	These are as hazardous as ceilings to clean, and should be left to an outside contractor, especially the high, external ones. When cleaning the insides of windows the old-fashioned recipe of vinegar diluted in hot water and rubbed with newspaper is highly effective. Never open a big window which is high up to try and clean the outside, or lean out to clean – that is an accident waiting to happen. Vinegar works equally well on mirrors, and modern window cleaning sprays have vinegar additives in them, as it cuts through greasy smears, leaving windows and mirrors streak-free.

Continued

You and your working environment

Shelving and worktops	These can collect dust very easily and need regularly stripping and wiping with disinfectant – a flick with a feather duster will remove the dust particles but, should the dust mix with grease or moisture, dirt forms and cannot be just waved away. If you use a scouring powder on some surfaces, then tiny scratches will be engrained onto the surface and bacteria will soon breed in them. Some salons have worktops over their units, which is very practical as these are hardwearing and easy to clean.
Basins, sinks and toilets	These need to be kept extra clean, as they are a place where germs and bacteria may breed and flourish. The ideal conditions of heat and moisture make sinks and toilets very appealing to bacteria. Any household bleach containing chlorine is ideal for work surfaces, toilets and sinks. Be careful not to mix bleach with other toilet cleansers as a reaction will occur and poisonous fumes can be given off. Having bins for paper towels and providing covered waste bins for sanitary items is essential. Pump-action soap dispensers in the showers and hand basins stop contamination, with multiple users, as do disposable paper towels rather than a shared towel on a roll.

Think about it

Many women judge the cleanliness of a toilet as a good indicator of the standard of hygiene in an establishment, whether it is a restaurant, hotel or a salon. Unsatisfied customers will leave and take their business elsewhere, rather than be somewhere they consider to be unclean. Always make sure that your toilet/washroom facilities pass the hygiene test.

Hygiene for portable equipment

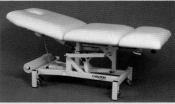

Couches need to be cleaned at the beginning and end of the working day. Remove the fitted couch cover or towelling material and wash the vinyl covering with a disinfectant solution. When dry, the couch cover should be placed over the top, and the couch set up for the next treatment. The cover can stay on all day, as it tends to be covered by bath-sized towels and couch roll, and does not attract a lot of dirt because of this. However, if there is a spillage, the couch will need to be stripped, cleaned and a fresh cover fitted. Most salons buy fitted couch covers to match the towels and general décor, which gives a calming and soft effect.

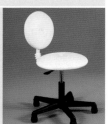

Chairs should be covered with a washable vinyl, which can be wiped. Cloth covers look lovely until they get dirty and then they will need to be cleaned with a special upholstery cleaner. Clients' outdoor clothing may bring in dirt and grease from outside (they might have brushed against a dirty car), with the likelihood that the dirt may transfer onto the salon chairs. Tell the client, as he or she will probably not be aware of it, and remove the offending mark as soon as possible. If the therapist's chair is an adjustable one, be careful of the accumulation of grease around the two pistons underneath, used for height adjustment – that can get on clothing, too.

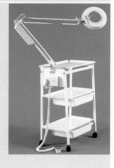

Trolleys should be made of metal or strong moulded plastic and have removable trays for easy access and cleaning. Avoid purchasing glass-topped trolleys as these are unsafe – if the glass gets hot from equipment on it, it may shatter. Covering trolley tops with towels and couch roll prevents them getting too dirty, and you can change the couch roll after every client, which looks smart and hygienic. Like couches, trolleys only need a cleaning morning and night if they are covered all day – except in the case of spillage. Trolleys seem to gather dust in their corners every day, from the cotton wool fibres and tissues used, so they do need emptying and thoroughly cleaning at the end of every day.

Towels, turbans and couch covers can be washed in a hot wash cycle in the washing machine, and tumble-dried. The salon should have a plentiful supply of these, so there is no shortage while dirty ones are being washed and dried. Always check washing instructions to avoid shrinkage and avoid mixing dark and light colours together to prevent colour runs. Ideally, whites should be washed separately – one dark item in a white wash can turn the whole load 'grey'. When changing the décor in the salon, some salons will invest in a clothes dye, which can be used in a washing machine, and then all towels, turbans and gowns can be dyed the same shade – it can be very effective, and may give tired towels a new lease of life.

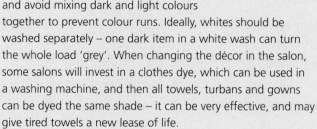

Machinery should always be cleaned following manufacturers' instructions, to prevent damage and avoid accidents. Never immerse a machine in water to clean it or scrub the surface, as you could rub off the dial markings which show heat intensity or strength of current. If that happens, you cannot be in control of the machine and it should be removed from service. Rubber will perish if cleaned with strong products, such as alcohol-based cleaner, and glass will develop scratches and not work well if an abrasive cleaner is used. If in doubt, ask, and if necessary, contact the manufacturer for advice.

Think about it

Equipment needs to be sterilised according to manufacturers' instructions as not all small equipment is suitable for immersion or the autoclave. (See 'Hygiene and avoiding cross-infection', page 51, for more details on sterilisation methods.)

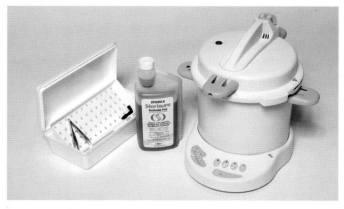

Methods of sterilisation

Keys to good practice

Here are some golden rules to managing your treatment area.

- Be hygienic by wiping down all surfaces and equipment with your chosen antibacterial cleaner, and then use couch roll on trolley tops and on the floor to keep the area clean.

- Inspect the area both before and after treatment – would you like to have a treatment there?

- Be tidy. Tidy as you go, use a bin for waste products, tissues, and so on – never accumulate them in a heap on your trolley.

- Wash up as you go. If the working area has a sink and you can wash out your applicator brush, for example while the client has a facemask on, then do so. But do not leave the client unattended, and if the client is disturbed by the noise, then wash up later.

- Be organised. Have one trolley for products and small equipment, which is separate from the equipment trolley, and return them to the place where they came from.

- Keep it simple. If all the product labels are facing you, then there can be no mistake in product application and you are safeguarding the client.

- Be methodical. Replace lids immediately after you have decanted the product to prevent spillage. Be economical with products – only put out what you will need. This also stops products and gels drying out in the hot salon atmosphere.

- Leave the room or area as you would wish to find it. Another therapist may be using the treatment area after you, and the client would be most put off by your mess not being cleared up!

Think about it

The same rules you learned in your Level 2 assessments apply to Level 3 assessments. Good working practices will ensure that your treatment area is fit for every client, every time!

Setting up the resources you require

When setting up your treatment area for the day, you may have an indication from the booking-in page about the treatments you will be carrying out, but you do not yet know if the client is suitable for them. You may have new clients, without known treatment requirements/expectations, and you may have the unexpected client who appears without an appointment. So – preparation is the key, both for assessment criteria and so that you do not leave the client unattended, or waste time setting up because you were not organised.

Think about it

If you have to leave the client unattended while you go off to seek a turban which you lent to a colleague, it may cost you your assessment, because you were not fully prepared in the first place.

Below is a suggested bed and trolley layout which will allow you to complete a facial electrical treatment, body massage or a body electrical treatment. However, because some of the equipment, such as the body testing equipment, is likely to be shared between several therapists it is up to you to manage your resources well. In the case of assessments taking place in the salon, inform your salon manager of your need for the equipment and, with good communication and teamwork, all students should have access to suit their needs.

Suggested treatment area equipment

Couch or massage plinth/stool
Stool or chair
Trolleys (x 2)
Magnifying lamp
Towels, large and small
Towelling robe/gown and disposable footwear
Headband/turban
Cotton wool rounds or squares
Sponges
Tissues
Couch roll
Containers for client's jewellery and spatulas
Spatulas
Mask brushes
Waste bin with liner
Record card and pen
Test tubes (for thermal testing)
Sharp and smooth objects (for sensitive testing)
Gloves
Talcum powder
Petroleum jelly
Products – depending upon treatment
Eye goggles and shower products if giving a tanning treatment
Tape measure, fat callipers, peak flow and blood-pressure machine (sphygmomanometer)

Environmental conditions

Most treatment objectives are primarily for relaxation and a sense of wellbeing for the client, regardless of whether the treatment is on the face or body. In order to relax and enjoy the treatment, clients need to feel safe and confident in your capabilities and be in an environment conducive to relaxation.

Many factors influence the relaxation dynamics in the salon, including:

- lighting
- heating
- ventilation
- general comfort
- suitable music and sound
- atmosphere.

Lighting

Lighting is one of the most instant mood enhancers – get it right and the client is encouraged to relax tense muscles, the eyes are soothed and the stress begins to melt away. Get it wrong and the facial muscles contract – harsh, strong lighting makes the client wince and the atmosphere is spoilt.

Natural daylight is very good for mood enhancement, as everyone loves sunshine streaming through the window, but on winter days there is not enough natural light to illuminate the salon all through the working day. Big windows, such as a shop front, will allow natural light in, but are impractical for treatment areas as they would allow the client little privacy. There needs to be enough light to work by, but at the same time ensure that the client is not distracted by too much light. It is important to be able to see what you are doing, and inadequate lighting over a period of time can cause eyestrain, so you certainly need enough light to write out the consultation card comfortably. It is important to get the salon lighting just right, so the client can relax and you can see to work.

For health and safety reasons, sufficient lighting is essential in some areas, for example the stairwell, and when using electrical equipment, mixing chemicals or during epilation. In the treatment area, avoid direct lighting where possible. A ceiling light or strip fluorescent lighting is quite harsh, and shines into the eyes when the client is in supine position (face up) on the couch. Soft wall lights spread the light and are soft and relaxing. Up-lighter shades, which allow the light to be arched towards the ceiling, are ideal, and are relatively inexpensive to purchase. Corner lighting from tall standard lamps, or modern wrought-iron stands, has the same effect – although there is always the danger of knocking them over. Ideally, a corner position means that they are not in the way of traffic flow through the room.

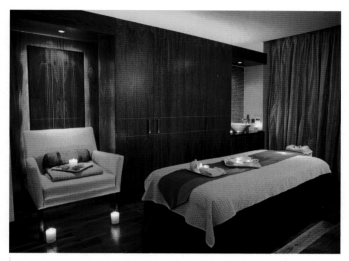

Suitable lighting will enhance the treatments clients receive

The core body temperature should be maintained at 37°C, which allows the body to function and the enzymes involved in metabolism to work efficiently. Should the temperature drop to 27°C, then the enzymes work half as fast, which is insufficient to keep the body alive. If the temperature rises to 41°C, the enzymes die in the heat and are unable to work, stopping bodily functions.

Think about it

Under the Workplace (Health, Safety and Welfare) Regulations 1992, the minimum temperature in the workplace should be 16°C one hour prior to work commencing (see 'You, your client and the law', page 68).

For a general body treatment involving electrical equipment, good lighting is essential so that you are able to see and be in control of the machine, but for massage, where the aim of the treatment is relaxation, softer lighting is appropriate. Many salons have dimmer switches on the wall lights enabling the lighting strength to be adjusted to suit the individual treatment.

There is a medical condition called SAD (Seasonal Affective Disorder) — a type of depression caused by a chemical imbalance in the brain due to a lack of sunlight. Although a therapist cannot offer an opinion on SAD as it is a diagnosis for a doctor, it is probable that clients will be prescribed a course of treatment on a sunbed to help the condition and may come into the salon with a doctor's referral.

Think about it

If you are unsure of the comfort of the lighting in your treatment area, try lying on the couch. Can you close your eyes comfortably? Do you have harsh lighting in your eyes? If necessary, make some adjustments where you can – a darker lampshade perhaps, or turn off the strip lighting for the duration of the treatment.

Heating

Correct levels of heating are essential in the salon, as temperature has a direct effect on the body, and the effectiveness of the treatment depends on the correct, comfortable temperature.

If your treatment room is too hot or too cold it will not be conducive to a pampering treatment, and the client will want to leave as soon as possible!

If the treatment room is too cold	If the treatment room is too hot
The blood capillaries constrict, less blood passes through, as the blood is sent to the internal organs to keep in warmth – therefore the client's skin goes pale through lack of bloodflow	The blood capillaries in the skin widen to allow blood to flow through them and the skin becomes very red
Sweat production in the skin stops and the skin begins to dry out, and feel cold to the touch	The sweat glands produce a lot of sweat, sitting on the skin surface to evaporate and cool – this makes the client feel moist and sticky
The muscle fibres contract and will start involuntary shivering to generate heat	Hair lies flat against the skin and mixes with the sweat
The metabolic rate in the body increases slightly to generate more heat	The metabolic rate is reduced, so less heat is produced, and the breathing rate increases, so more is lost through expired air
The client will be reluctant to disrobe and relax, ready for treatment	The client will want to get undressed, but will feel hot and flustered and may not want to be touched
The client's mental state or attitude is likely to be altered to one of agitation rather than relaxation!	The client's mental state or attitude will probably be one of lethargy, they may have a headache and want to go outside for fresh air and to cool down

Most modern buildings have gas-fired central heating, with a central boiler and radiators placed in every room, much like a domestic heating system, only on a larger scale. The boiler needs to be well maintained. The hot water supply will also come from the boiler, and the salon would cease to function without either heating or hot water.

Temperature control is governed by either:

- a wall-mounted control panel for all the radiators, with a temperature dial, or
- individual thermostatic controls on each radiator, which can be adjusted to suit the room and its needs, for example it can be turned up for clients coming in from the wet area, or having massage.

There are other methods of heating, including storage heaters, gas fires, electric under-floor heating and electric plug-in radiators, but gas central heating is likely to be most economical and the preferred method in a modern salon. It is also the safest method for fire prevention.

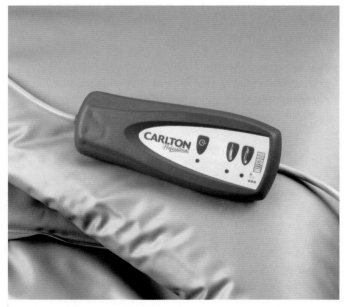

A heated over-blanket will keep the client comfortable and warm

Heat may be lost through:

- poor insulation
- walls and ceilings
- single-glazed windows
- open doors and windows.

As it is expensive to heat the salon, make sure that you do not waste money by leaving doors or windows open on a cold day — you may also create a draught on the client.

Keeping the client warm is essential, and you should have adequate bedding — blankets and large, warm bath towels — to wrap the client in. Muscle fibres relax in heat and constrict in cold, so you will be undoing all the benefits of heat treatment if the client is allowed to become cold. Once the client is on the couch, there are a number of electronically heated under- or over-blankets which offer safe, professional individual heating, designed to suit the client. These are similar to an electric blanket on a bed at home, and offer a cosy and gentle sedation prior to massage and body treatments. The client is literally cocooned in a warm envelope of blanket, heated to his or her own optimum level.

Ventilation

Air movement is essential to comfort, and ties in with the heating of the salon. Too little air movement in the salon or one room can create a stuffy atmosphere, while too much can make a room seem draughty. All humans exhale carbon dioxide and if this builds up in a busy salon, combined with heat and odours, clients and the therapists will feel very lethargic and may develop a headache.

Good ventilation also prevents a build-up of chemical fumes (if your salon has a nail extension bar) and stops unpleasant odours accumulating, especially if there is a staff room or relaxation area where clients are permitted to smoke. (Most salons would discourage smoking, on health grounds.)

Ventilation can be:

- natural
- mechanical or artificial.

Natural ventilation

This takes place when windows and doors are opened and also occurs with the movement of air through cracks or gaps in windows and doors. The obvious disadvantages to natural ventilation are possible cold draughts, noise and odours from external sources coming in and ruining the atmosphere, and draughts blowing papers about.

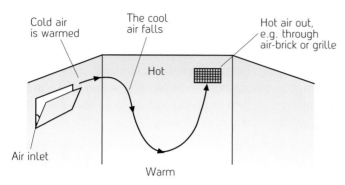

Natural ventilation by convection

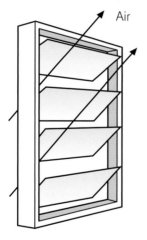

A louvre window can be used to direct airflow into the room

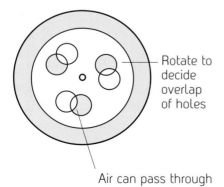

A coopers disk allows natural ventilation

Natural convection can be used for ventilation. This is where a small window, high up on a wall, is open, which allows cold air into the room. As it is high up, the cold air is warmed by the hot air it meets (heat rises) and the warmed air then drops into the room. As this air heats up, it rises and a ventilator grille, or airbrick, on an opposite wall draws it out. This keeps the air circulating without creating draughts.

Older windows sometimes have a double disc cut into them with two sets of holes (called a coopers disc). When the holes line up, the airflow is allowed to enter into the room. Louvre windows were a feature of many buildings of the 1970s. The slates of glass can be opened as widely as is required and are easy to clean. However, they are also easy to remove, making them a security risk.

Mechanical or artificial ventilation

Mechanical or artificial ventilation using electric extractor fans is more desirable as it is a controllable system, more efficient and cost-effective to run, with no draughts on the clients. Most modern extractor fans can take air in from outside, as well as extracting the stale air in a room. Ideally, they should be fixed to an outside window or wall, but not near open windows or doors, as they will simply extract the fresh air coming in.

Free-standing fans can be used to refresh a room or salon on a hot day, but these are not very safe as they are not stable and may be knocked over easily if in the main traffic flow of a room. Air conditioning, which passes air over filters and coolers, is a very effective method of ventilation but is the most expensive.

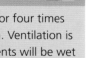

Think about it

In a busy salon the air change should be three or four times per hour, depending upon the size of the room. Ventilation is especially important in the wet area, where clients will be wet – they should not be allowed to get cold due to draughts and poor heating facilities.

General comfort

If the salon has appropriate heating, lighting and ventilation, the environment is well on the way to being suitable for a pampering, relaxing treatment. The general comfort of the client should also be considered, and often makes all the difference to a treatment.

You and your working environment

Towels, bedding and gowns can be warmed on a radiator, just before the client arrives, for that extra luxurious feeling of warmth.

- Ensure that the salon has a pleasant aroma, neither too chemical nor antiseptic based. Plug-in air fresheners are very acceptable, and you do not need to be qualified in aromatherapy as you would if you use an oil burner. Flower-based fresheners such as rose or lavender are associated with relaxing, so can be used throughout the salon.

- The salon décor should be soothing on the eye, with colour coordination and matching bedding, towels, and so on. Warm colours such as pink, peach and lavender are harmonious and create a calm and enticing look to the treatment rooms. Harsh, loud colours are not conducive to relaxation. If you are aiming to attract a male clientele, avoid an image that is too feminine in your colour scheme and accessories, as male clients may be put off by such a setting.

- Be ruthless with things past their best, such as chipped cups, old towels and threadbare gowns! Not only are they unhygienic, they create a poor impression. Throw away odd cups and invest in matching china. Keep cutlery and china in mint condition — no one wants to drink from a dirty cup and saucer. When offering the client water after the treatment, use a glass, rather than an old beaker, and regularly wash glasses so they shine like crystal!

- A selection of up-to-date magazines in reception will make a good first impression.

- Replace failed light bulbs as soon as they go, both for safety reasons and to maintain the professional image of the salon.

- To enhance the look of the salon, invest in some good quality houseplants, but remember to tend them well — poorly kept, or dying, house plants, look depressing. If you are not green-fingered, then invest in some nil-maintenance, artificial plants.

- Clients appreciate good quality toilet paper and soap dispensers.

Think about it

It is the attention to detail which makes the difference to clients. They need to feel cosseted and cosy, and valued.

Suitable music and sound

Music and listening to relaxing sounds, such as whale calls, can create a relaxing atmosphere, but always ask individual clients for their preferences. Musical choice is personal, and while one client may like the sound of a cascading waterfall to fall asleep to, another client may find it irritating.

Some large training salons have piped music put through to all salons via a central sound system, from a CD player, usually in reception. The disadvantage to this is that you have to listen to the receptionist's choice of music, rather than the client's choice. A small sound unit in the treatment room is better, allowing volume and choice to be personalised, and some clients just prefer to have complete quiet, so they can really drift away.

There are several things to remember when choosing music:

- Use of music in the treatment room, reception or in exercise groups is classed as a public performance. Phonographic Performance Ltd (PPL) collects licence payments on behalf of artistes and record companies from people wishing to play recorded music in public. Legally, all salons and exercise/aerobic instructors must purchase music that has a built-in licence (see 'You, your client and the law', page 81, for information on the Copyright, Designs and Patents Act 1988). While more expensive to purchase (a CD can cost about £30), it will prevent liability to a heavy fine. Most good specialist music shops have a section of licensed music — ask the shop assistant if in doubt.

- Compilation CDs can be very repetitive when played over and over, as the brain starts to anticipate the next track. This can be very irritating to the client. It is far better to vary the music and invest in several different CDs.

- Look at the length of time the music runs for. Nothing is more disruptive than the music ending just as the client is floating away and you are halfway through the treatment. You may have oily hands and should not break contact with the client, so you will have to end the treatment in silence. If you are doing a full body massage, check you have at least a one-hour CD playing before you start the treatment.

- Remember that your choice is not always the same as the client's. Always ask.

- Radio stations are not very suitable for easy listening as there is too much variation in the sound: the DJ may talk, adverts come on, weather, news and traffic are regular slots, and the client may be listening to roadwork information, instead of mentally relaxing.

You and your working environment

Atmosphere

A salon can have perfect facilities, be pretty and chic, with all essential ingredients in place, and yet if there is a poor atmosphere between staff, with tension and bad feeling, the client will pick up on it immediately. Often, the client will say, 'I don't know, it just didn't feel right' if the overall ambience of the working environment is poor.

The atmosphere in the salon needs to feel friendly. The staff should be approachable, work together as a team and make the client feel wanted and the most important person. No clients equals no business, so you will need to work hard to create a good working atmosphere which encourages clients to enter, stay and recommend you to others. (For more information on working together, solving difficulties and being mature in your working outlook, see 'You — the therapist', page 4.)

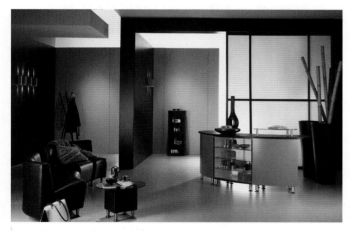

A soothing colour combination is vital in creating an appropriate atmosphere

Fire precautions and evacuation procedures

Using electrical equipment means there is a higher risk of a fire starting, so all Level 3 therapists should know the legislation involved and the actions to take should a fire occur.

Fire Precautions Act 1971

This Act is concerned with fire prevention and the provision of escape routes should an evacuation be required. The employer is responsible for fire safety in the workplace and he or she must ensure the workplace complies with the fire regulations.

The employer should have a fire certificate if:

- there will be more than 20 people working on the premises at any one time
- there will be more than 10 people working anywhere other than the ground floor.

Fire Precautions (Workplace) Regulations 1997 (amended 1999)

The regulations require all premises to undertake a fire risk assessment. If five or more people work together as employees, the risk assessment must be in writing. Employers must also take into account all other persons on the premises, not just employees.

There must also be a fire and evacuation procedure. In every period of one year there must be at least one fire drill which involves everyone. All staff must be fully informed, instructed and trained in what is expected from them and some people will have special duties to perform. Employees, trainees, temporary workers and others who work in any undertaking must, by law, agree to co-operate with the employer so far as is necessary to enable them to fulfil the duties placed upon them by law. This means co-operating fully in training courses and fire drills, even when everyone knows they are only a practice!

Most large training establishments will have their own policy on fire evacuation procedures and may carry out a fire drill once a term, that is three times per year. This is especially important with large groups of people or students, and any disabled persons who will need special consideration. Many fire-training exercises are organised with a fire safety officer from the local fire station. Often the fire engines will take part in the exercise to test their own attendance time from the station to the premises. Everyone should be made aware of his or her own particular rules for evacuation.

When joining any business/establishment the new employee should be briefed regarding all health and safety issues, and especially fire evacuation procedures. It is standard practice to include the information in a handbook containing all the establishment's policies.

Emergency procedures

Fire drill relevant to the working area

- Switch off all electrical equipment.
- Close windows.
- Clients should be led by the therapist to a safe area. If necessary, wrap clients up warmly using blankets and towels — this is especially important where a client has been having a body treatment.

You and your working environment

Building evacuation procedures in the event of fire or bomb alert

The following procedure has been agreed and must be followed. Any staff member who does not comply is committing an infringement of the college disciplinary code. Whenever a fire occurs, the main consideration is to get everybody out of the building safely. Protection of personal or college property is incidental.

Raising the alarm

Anyone discovering a fire must immediately raise the alarm by operating the nearest fire alarm and report to the controller the fire location.

On hearing the alarm the receptionist will immediately contact the emergency services and then evacuate the building.

In the event of a fire being discovered when the reception is unmanned – the premises officer on duty will contact the emergency services and assume control.

On hearing the alarm

All those in senior positions proceed to the control point, normally at a main entrance to the building – where one person must take control of the proceedings.

All other staff: close windows; switch off machinery and lights, and close doors on leaving the room.

Assist less able colleagues, leave the building by the nearest marked route and proceed quickly to the appropriate assembly point. Staff must supervise their class.

Staff evacuating the building must check their locality is clear.

Assembly points

Everyone must remain at assembly points well away from buildings and clear of access roads.

Report to control in person or via two-way radios where allocated.

Everyone must remain at assembly points until further instructions.

DO NOT re-enter the building until you are told it is safe to do so.

An evacuation procedure

- If possible, clients should take their valuable possessions with them, such as handbag and jewellery, but not if these are safely locked away, or if it puts the client or therapist in any danger. (Usually clients' belongings are kept under the trolley and therefore are within easy reach.)

- Be aware of the treatment being performed during the evacuation – if the client has chemicals on the skin, it may be easier to remove immediately. (This would need to be at the judgement of the lecturer in charge of the workshop – certainly a client having an eyelash tint will need to have it removed before being able to proceed to the assembly point.)

- Take appropriate remover and damp cotton wool or tissues to remove products on the skin such as facemasks. While not dangerous to the skin if left on, the client will probably be more comfortable, and the skin

less dry, if it can be removed. Be aware of the client's footwear, and if possible encourage the wearing of shoes to prevent an accident during the evacuation.

- If there were a real fire with a real risk of injury the fire service always recommend you get out as fast as you can – and let the experts, i.e. them, fight the fire. It is better to evacuate quickly and be safe.

Bomb alert

Act quickly if an abandoned parcel or bag arouses concern. Follow the procedures for a fire drill. Do not look inside a suspicious package.

Gas leak

- Open all windows.
- Evacuate the building following the fire drill procedure.

- Do not turn off or switch on any electrical equipment (including light switches) — this may cause a spark which could ignite the gas.

- Have in place sensible fire precautions

- Be informed — know what to do and where to go when the evacuation begins.

- Be sensible and do not panic — this will only make the client feel panicky, too.

- Make sure that you know the location of the fire bell, fire extinguishers and fire exit.

- Never ignore smoke or the smell of burning — it is far better to have a false alarm. Better safe than sorry!

- Do not misuse or mistreat electrical appliances that are a potential hazard — a healthy respect is needed.

- Do not ignore manufacturers' instructions for the storage and use of highly flammable products, which are very common within the salon.

- Do be sensible with naked flames and matches or disposal of cigarette ends — a smouldering tip can burst into flames that would destroy the salon in minutes.

- Check that all clients have been evacuated — the appointment book can be taken outside, as a check on which clients should be present. A college lecturer or trainer should do the same with the class register to check that the right number of students are present.

- Do not use a lift for the evacuation — it may be that the fire affects the electric mechanism and that then becomes another emergency.

If you are not at the correct location for the fire evacuation, report to your allocated assembly point. Otherwise you may not be accounted for. This may mean a fire fighter risking his or her life to go into a burning building to check — when all the time you were safe.

Fire-fighting equipment

Fire extinguishers

Only a person specially trained in the use of a fire extinguisher should attempt to use one. Never be at risk. Personal safety is more important than saving material items that can be replaced — a human life cannot be replaced. It is better to evacuate the building and call the fire service than it is to use the wrong extinguisher. Fire service safety leaflets recommend you never endanger life or stay in an area with a fire in an attempt to put it out — it is safer to leave it to the professionals.

In small premises having one or two portable hand-held extinguishers of the appropriate type readily available may be all that is necessary. In larger more complex premises larger equipment will be needed, training should be given and the location should be indicated. This is usually in a conspicuous position on an escape route near the exit doors.

Fires are classified by the type of material that has caught alight. The class of fire determines which fire extinguisher to use.

Class of fire	Fire extinguisher
Class A: Fires involving solid materials, e.g. wood, paper or textiles	Extinguishers with an 'A' rating, e.g. 13A Water extinguisher, foam extinguisher, dry powder extinguisher (size according to risk) **Water extinguishers** are the cheapest and most widely used, but are not suitable for Class B fires or fires involving electricity
Class B: Fires involving flammable liquids, e.g. petrol, diesel or oils	Extinguishers with a 'B' rating, e.g. 34B Foam extinguisher, CO_2 extinguisher, dry powder extinguisher (size according to risk) **Foam extinguishers** are more expensive than water, but can be used on both Class A and Class B fires
Class C: Fires involving flammable gases, e.g. propane, butane	Foam extinguisher (according to risk). Seek specialist advice **Dry powder extinguishers** are multi-purpose and can be used on Classes A, B and C fires. However, they can obscure vision
Class D: Fires involving metals	Special powder extinguishers (size and type according to risk), dry sand (quantity according to risk). Seek specialist advice
Class E: Fires involving electrical apparatus	CO_2 extinguisher
Class F: Fires in cooking appliances, e.g. oil	Extinguishers with an 'F' rating, e.g. 15F Wet chemical extinguisher

A quick guide to selecting an extinguisher:

Type of fire	Type of extinguisher	Colour	Uses		NOT to be used
Electrical fires	Dry powder	Blue marking	For burning liquid, electrical fires and flammable liquids		On flammable metal fires
	Carbon dioxide	Black marking	Safe on all voltages, used on burning liquid and electrical fires and flammable liquids		On flammable metal fires
Non-electrical fires	Water	Red marking	For wood, paper, textiles, fabric and similar materials		On burning liquid, electrical or flammable metal fires
	Foam	Cream/yellow markings	On burning liquid fires		On electrical or flammable metal fires

Different types of fire extinguisher

Fire blankets

Fire blankets are made of fire-resistant material. They are particularly useful for wrapping around a person whose clothing is on fire. A fire blanket must be used calmly and with a firm grip. If the blanket is flapped about, it may fan the fire and cause it to flare up, rather than put it out. The hands should be protected by the edge of the cloth and the blanket should be placed, rather than thrown, into the desired position.

Think about it

Never lean over the fire to find out how it started or why.

If you cannot control the fire, leave the room, close the door and phone the fire and rescue service.

Fire blankets conforming to British Standard BS6575 are suitable for use on small fires. These will be marked to show whether they should be thrown away after use or used again after cleaning in accordance with the manufacturer's instructions. Fire blankets are best kept in a central location for easy access.

Sand

A bucket of sand can be used to soak up liquids which are the source of a fire. If the fire is too large for you to contain, or you are in any doubt, never risk injury. Get out and phone the fire and rescue service.

Even small fires spread very quickly, producing smoke and fumes, which can kill in seconds. If there is any doubt, do not tackle the fire, no matter how small.

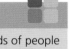

Think about it

Remember – hundreds of people die and thousands of people are injured in fires each year, caused by lack of concentration or carelessness. It is better to prevent a fire starting in the first place.

First aid

The Health and Safety (First Aid) Regulations 1981 set out the essential aspects of first aid that employers must address, because people at work can suffer injuries or fall ill. It does not matter whether the injury or illness is caused by the work they do. It is important that they receive immediate attention and that an ambulance is called in serious cases.

First aid can save lives and prevent minor injuries becoming major ones. First aid in the workplace is the initial management of any injury or illness suffered at work. It does not include giving tablets or medicines to treat illness.

This means that sufficient first aid personnel and facilities should be available to:

- give immediate assistance to casualties with both common injuries and illnesses and those likely to arise from specific hazards at work
- summon an ambulance or other professional help.

You and your working environment

This will depend upon the size of the workforce, the type of workplace hazards and risks, and the history of accidents in the workplace.

Two aspects of first aid need further consideration: trainees and the public.

- *Trainees* — students undertaking work experience on certain training schemes are given the same status as employees and therefore are the responsibility of the employer.

- *The public* — when dealing with the public these regulations do not oblige employers to provide first aid for anyone other than their own employees. This means the compulsory element of public liability insurance does not cover litigation resulting from first aid to non-employees. Employers should make extra provision for this themselves. Education establishments must also include the general public in their assessment of first aid requirements.

First aid kits

The minimum level of first aid equipment is a suitably stocked and properly identified first aid container.

First aid containers should be easily accessible and placed, where possible, near to handwashing facilities. The number of containers will depend upon the size of the establishment and the total number of employees in that area. The container should protect the items inside from dust and damp and must only be stocked with useful items. Tablets and medications should not be kept in there.

There is no compulsory list of what a first aid kit should contain but the following would be useful:

- a leaflet giving general guidance on first aid (such as the HSE leaflet 'Basic advice on first aid at work')
- 20 individually wrapped sterile adhesive dressings (assorted sizes) appropriate to the type of work
- two sterile eye pads
- four individually wrapped triangular bandages (preferably sterile)
- six safety pins
- six medium-sized individually wrapped wound dressings
- two large sterile individually wrapped unmedicated wound dressings
- one pair of disposable gloves
- antiseptic cream or liquid
- eye bath
- gauze

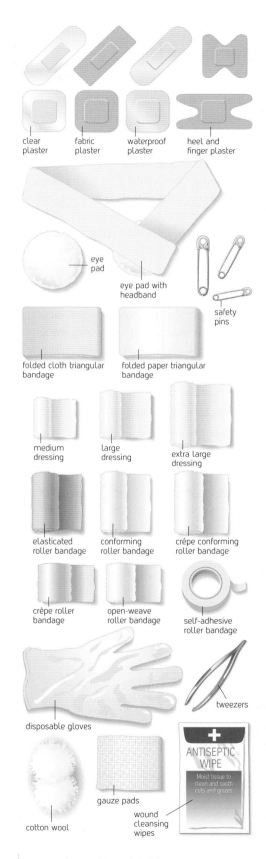

clear plaster · fabric plaster · waterproof plaster · heel and finger plaster

eye pad · eye pad with headband · safety pins

folded cloth triangular bandage · folded paper triangular bandage

medium dressing · large dressing · extra large dressing

elasticated roller bandage · conforming roller bandage · crêpe conforming roller bandage

crêpe roller bandage · open-weave roller bandage · self-adhesive roller bandage

disposable gloves · tweezers

cotton wool · gauze pads · wound cleansing wipes

ANTISEPTIC WIPE · Moist tissue to clean and sooth cuts and grazes

Items a first aid box should contain

You and your working environment

- medical wipes
- a pair of tweezers
- cotton wool.

Do not forget that if in doubt, do not treat — phone for an ambulance immediately.

First aid training

First aid certificates are only valid for a certain period of time, which is currently three years. Employers need to arrange refresher training with re-testing of competence before certificates expire. If a certificate expires, the individual will have to undertake a full course of training to be re-established as a first-aider. Specialist training can also be undertaken if necessary.

Records

It is good practice for employers to provide first aiders with a book in which to record incidents which require their attendance. If there are several first aiders in one establishment then a central book will be used.

The information should include:

- date, time and place of incident
- name and job of the injured or ill person
- details of the injury or illness and what first aid was given
- what action was taken immediately afterward (e.g. did the person go home, go to hospital, get sent in an ambulance?)
- name and signature of the first aider or person dealing with the incident.

Think about it

All activities should be continuously reviewed for accident potential.

If equipment is continually being broken because of lack of storage space or because a trolley is too close to a windowsill, then a review should take place. If the same accident repeatedly occurs, then it is important to ask why.

For your portfolio

Find out your establishment's set procedure to follow in the event of an accident. Include it in your portfolio – you need to know who your fire officer is and what the procedure is for helping a client safely out of the salon

Accident reporting procedures

Accidents happen, even to the most careful of people. The key is to react in the correct manner, stay calm and follow the establishment's accident procedures. You should be aware of every possible risk in all aspects of salon life, as shown in the diagram below.

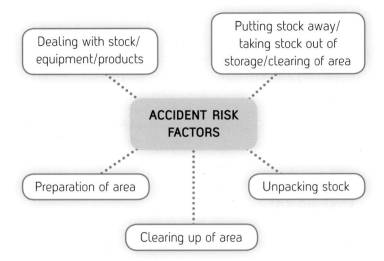

You, your client and the law

In this section you will learn about:

- legislation
- local by-laws
- insurance
- independent regulators
- industry codes of practice
- salon guidelines.

There are many regulations and lots of legislation covering you and your work in the salon. Any person dealing with members of the public and working with other people has to be aware of the law, and how to use it to be safe. You do not need to know all the regulations in detail, but you do need to know what your responsibilities are.

Legislation

All businesses are covered by laws as set down by the government in Acts of Parliament. These Acts of Parliament are continually being updated to fit into modern society, so you will find that Acts have dates after their title stating when they were updated.

These Acts are the law of the land. Breaking or ignoring them is therefore an offence, and can lead to punishment. You could be fined, your business could be closed or you could go to prison.

As well as UK law, there is European Union law to follow, too. The European Union (EU) is made up of 27 countries, including the UK, which joined the EU in 1993. EU laws are decided in Brussels, where the European courts are based, and all EU member states follow the same legislation.

Key terms

Legislation – laws passed by parliament.

Insurance – whereby the beauty therapist (or salon) pays an annual fee to an insurer (insurance company) to compensate them in case of loss incurred during the course of their work.

In order to be fully competent in employment it is essential that you have a sound knowledge of the basis of consumer protection and health and safety legislation. You need to understand how these laws protect you, your colleagues and your clients. The specific legislation that you need to know is given below.

Think about it

None of us can get away with claiming ignorance about the law. We should each take responsibility for our deeds and actions and must face the consequences if we act recklessly or endanger others. Insurance cover may be null and void if you are proven to be negligent or if legislation or establishment rules have been broken or ignored. An accident or injury to others could be the result, with serious implications to you personally and to your employers.

Health and Safety at Work etc. (HASAW) Act 1974

The employer's duty is to provide safe:

- premises – a safe place to work
- systems and equipment
- storage and transport of substances and material
- access to the workplace exits
- practices in the workplace.

The employer's duty to other persons not in employment includes not exposing them to health and safety risks – this includes contractors, employees, and self-employed people.

The employee has a responsibility to:

- take care during time at work to avoid personal injury
- assist the employer in meeting requirements under the Health and Safety at Work Act
- not misuse or change anything that has been provided for safety.

The employee has a duty to herself/himself, to other employees, and to the public.

The Act allows various regulations to be made, which control the workplace. It also covers self-employed persons who work alone, away from the employer's premises.

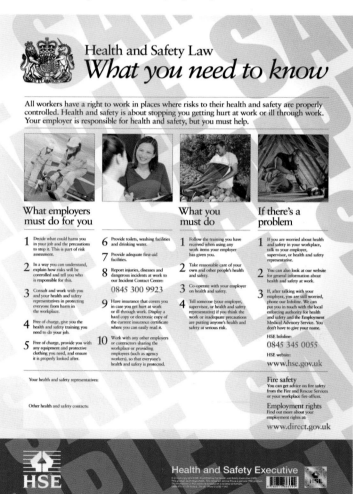

This requires all employers to provide systems of work that are, as far as is reasonably practicable, safe and without risk to health. (Source: Health and Safety Executive)

Employers' responsibilities	Shared responsibilities	Employees' responsibilities
Planning safety and security	Safety of all individuals in the workplace	Correct use of systems and procedures
Providing information about safety and security	Safety of the working environment	Reporting flaws or gaps in the system or establishment procedures
Updating systems and procedures with five or more employees	Never knowingly endangering anyone	Taking reasonable care of themselves and others
Regular training and information for all staff	Following all Health and Safety at Work Act directives	Co-operating with employers in the discharge of their obligations

Health and safety responsibilities

European Union directives

In 1992 EU directives updated legislation on health and safety management and widened the existing acts. These came into force in 1993. There are six main areas:

- Provision and Use of Work Equipment
- Manual Handling Operations
- Workplace Health, Safety and Welfare
- Personal Protective Equipment at Work
- Health and Safety (Display Screen Equipment)
- Management of Health and Safety at Work.

Some provisions of the EU directives are:

- the protection of non-smokers from tobacco smoke
- the provision of rest facilities for pregnant and nursing mothers
- safe cleaning of windows.

The Management of Health and Safety at Work Regulations 1999

These regulations place responsibility firmly on the employer to make significant risk assessments for the health and safety of employees and others working in the salon, record any significant findings, and instruct and train employees in the correct way to ensure all are protected. Codes of practice and systems need to be monitored, reviewed and adjusted to suit. All employees should be informed of these, and a statutory poster for health and safety displayed in the workplace.

The regulations cover a great deal of information for employers including:

- risk assessment
- principles of prevention to be applied
- health and safety arrangements
- health surveillance

- health and safety assistance
- procedures for serious and imminent danger and dangerous areas
- contact with external services
- information for employees
- co-operation and co-ordination
- persons working in host employers or self-employed person undertaking work
- capability and training
- employer's duties
- temporary workers
- risk assessments for new or expectant mothers
- protection of young persons
- exception certificates
- provisions of liability
- exclusion of civil liberties
- extension out of Great Britain
- amendments to The Health and Safety (First Aid) Regulations 1981.

Employment Rights Act 1996

This Act covers all aspects of an employee's terms and conditions after they have been employed for a month or more. After two months' employment, an employee should have a written contract with their conditions of work including:

- details of payment, along with commission and incentives
- hours of work and expected holiday entitlement
- the amount of notice an employee is expected to give
- the amount of notice the employer expects the employee to give

- the date the employment started
- a full job description
- the employee's workplace location.

If an employee does not receive a contract of employment in writing, they can apply to an industrial tribunal and the employer is obliged by law to provide one.

The Workplace (Health, Safety and Welfare) Regulations 1992

The employer should ensure the workplace complies with the requirements of these regulations by:

- maintaining the workplace and all equipment and systems used there
- ensuring adequate ventilation
- keeping the workplace at a reasonable temperature (minimum 16°C)
- making sure employees have sufficient light to work comfortably
- keeping the workplace clean and tidy
- ensuring employees have enough space to work comfortably
- keeping floor and 'traffic routes' in a reasonable condition (no holes, slopes or uneven surfaces)
- ensuring workstations and seating are suitable
- providing suitable washing and toilet facilities (with soap and a means of drying hands)
- making sure employees have accommodation for clothing (worn at work) and changing facilities
- providing employees with facilities for resting and eating (if meals are to be eaten on the premises)
- providing clean drinking water and cups
- regularly removing waste materials
- keeping employees safe from falling objects
- making sure all doors and gates are suitably constructed and fitted with any necessary safety devices
- making sure windows are protected against breakage, and signs (or similar) are incorporated where there is a danger of someone walking into them
- making sure escalators and moving walkways have safety devices fitted so they can be stopped in an emergency.

(For further information on the safe disposal of waste products, refer to page 76.)

> ### Think about it
>
> In most settings separate toilet facilities must be available for men and women. However, in small, mostly female salons, men and women can use the same facilities as long as the toilet is a separate cubicle and it can be locked. In larger health clubs and spas the toilet and locker facilities would be separate.

The Manual Handling Operations Regulations 1992

The Health and Safety Executive (HSE) has drawn attention to skeletal and muscular disorders caused by manual handling and lifting, repetitive strain disorders and unsuitable posture causing low back pain. The regulations require certain measures to be taken to avoid these types of injuries occurring.

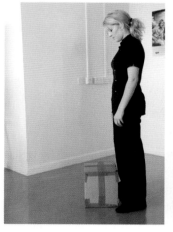
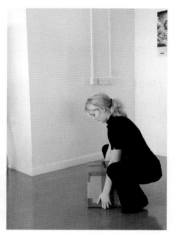
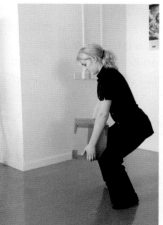
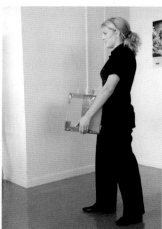

Safe lifting procedures must be followed

You, your client and the law

Think of all the situations that may apply in the salon:

- stock unpacking and storage — lifting heavy objects
- couch height adjustable for individual therapists
- chairs or stools used in the treatment rooms
- trolley height
- reception desk and chair
- rotation of job roles so that the therapist is not in the same position for every treatment
- height and size of nail art desk.

Think about it

It is worth considering all the factors listed above when purchasing equipment, as you then have to work with the consequences!

When purchasing a couch for home or mobile use, it is worth pretending to carry out a facial, complete with client lying on the couch, to find the right height. Working at a couch at the wrong height is very bad for the back in the long term, and may cause considerable discomfort.

Heat stress

The HSE draws attention to heat stress at work. The best working temperature in beauty therapy is between 15.5°C and 20°C.

Humidity (the amount of moisture in the air) should be within the range of 30 to 70 per cent, although this will vary if your salon has a sauna and steam area. These should be in a well-ventilated area away from the main workrooms, while still being accessible to clients. There should also be sufficient air exchange and air movement, which must be increased in special circumstances, such as chemical usage. Treatment rooms used for nail art, aromatherapy, bleaching or eyelash perming will need specialist ventilation methods.

- Mechanical ventilation — extractor fans, which can be adjusted at various speeds.
- Natural ventilation — open windows are fine, but be careful of a draught on the client.
- Air-conditioned ventilation — passing air over filters and coolers brings about the desired condition, but of course this is the most expensive method!

See page 60 for more information on ventilation.

A build-up of fumes, or of strong smells (for example from manicure preparations), will cause both physical and psychological problems, which affect not only clients but staff, too!

Physical effects	Psychological effects
Headaches	Irritability
Sweating	Aggressive behaviour
Palpitations	Fatigue — resulting in mistakes being made
Dizziness	Lethargy
Nausea, vomiting	Lack of concentration
Feeling faint	

The effects of heat stress

The Personal Protective Equipment at Work Regulations 1992

Every employer and self-employed person must ensure that suitable personal protective equipment is provided both for themselves and for their employees in situations where they may be exposed to a risk to their health or safety while at work. This is particularly relevant to micro current and epilation and the use of micro lance (for milia or in-growing hair removal), where there is a risk of contamination by body fluids (see also Environmental Protection Act 1990, The Controlled Waste Regulations 1992, amended 1993 and The Special Waste Regulations 1996 on page 76).

Protective clothing

This covers both equipment and protective clothing provisions to ensure safety for all those in the workplace. The regulations also provide that workplace personnel must have appropriate training in equipment use. Protective clothing, such as white overalls for work wear, ensures cleanliness, freshness, and professionalism. For certain treatments it may be advisable to wear extra disposable coverings. The client's clothing must also be protected.

Think about it

Research what your Awarding Body states about protective clothing. It may invalidate your insurance if you do not follow the rules — and it may ruin your own clothing if tint or wax were to be spilt on your uniform or trousers, for example.

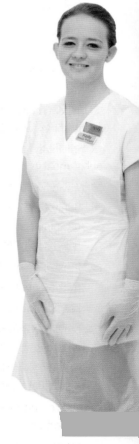

PPE regulations will protect the therapist too

Protection against infectious diseases

It is essential to protect against all diseases that are carried in the blood or tissue fluids. Protective gloves should be worn whenever there is a possibility of blood or tissue fluid being passed from one person to another, that is through an open cut or broken skin. Two specific infectious diseases to mention are:

- *AIDS (Acquired Immune Deficiency Syndrome)* – this disease is caused by HIV (Human Immunodeficiency Virus). The virus is transmitted through body tissue. Most people are aware of AIDS because of media coverage. The virus attacks the body's immune system, and therefore carries a strong risk of secondary infection, such as pneumonia, which could be life threatening. As there is no known cure, prevention through protection is vital.

- *Hepatitis (variants A, B and C)* – hepatitis is an inflammation of the liver. It is caused by a very strong virus transmitted through blood and tissue fluids. This can survive outside the body, and can make a person very ill indeed; it can even be fatal. The most serious form is hepatitis B and you can be immunised against this disease by a GP. For those who can prove they need this protection for their employment there is no cost involved. Most training establishments will recommend this.

Think about it

Always cover cuts with a plaster to prevent cross-infection.

The Control of Substances Hazardous to Health (COSHH) Regulations 2002

COSHH is the law that requires employers to control substances that are hazardous to health. One can prevent or reduce workers' exposure to hazardous substances by:

- finding out what the health hazards are
- deciding how to prevent harm to health by carrying out a risk assessment
- providing control measures to reduce harm to health
- making sure they are used
- keeping all control measures in good working order
- providing information, instruction and training for employees and others
- providing monitoring and health surveillance in appropriate cases
- controlling exposure to hazardous substances in the workplace
- planning for emergencies.

This law requires employers to control exposure to hazardous substances in the workplace.

Most products used in the salon are perfectly safe, but some products could become hazardous under certain conditions or if used inappropriately. All salons should be aware of how to use and store these products.

For your portfolio

A COSHH essentials information document is downloadable from www.coshh-essentials.org.uk

Employers are responsible for assessing the risks from hazardous substances and must decide upon an action to reduce those risks. Proper training should be given and employees should always follow safety guidelines and take the precautions identified by the employer.

The COSHH regulations require that the containers of hazardous substances are labelled with warning symbols. These symbols are shown below.

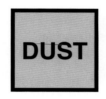
Dust

Toxic

Flammable

Irritant

Corrosive

Oxidising agent

Symbols showing types of hazardous substances

Here are some examples of potential hazards.

- Highly flammable substances, such as solvents, nail varnish remover or alcohol steriliser, are hazardous because their fumes will ignite if exposed to a naked flame.

- Explosive materials, such as hairspray, air freshener or other pressurised cans, are also highly flammable and will explode with force if placed in heat, such as an open fire, or even on top of a hot radiator.

■ Chemicals can cause severe reactions and skin damage – if chemicals are misused, vomiting, respiratory problems, and burning could be the result.

COSHH precautions

Employers must, by law, identify, list and assess in writing any substance in the workplace. This applies not only to products used for treatments in the salon but also to products that are used in cleaning such as bleach or polish. Potentially hazardous substances must be given a hazard rating or risk assessment, even if it is zero.

It is essential that you read all of the COSHH sheets used in the salon, and be safe: follow what they say, never abuse manufacturers' instructions and attend regular staff training for product use. You never know when you might need it!

Think about it

- Manufacturers have to supply a COSHH sheet containing product data for each product. The COSHH sheets should be kept together in a central folder in the salon so that everyone can refer to them.

- A reaction can happen if a client has recently used a chemical at home and it reacts with the products used in the salon, for example home hair colours.

- Clients on long-term medication are more likely to have a reaction. Triggers include hormone replacement therapy, the contraceptive pill, heart and blood pressure medication – this should be recorded on the client's record card.

For your portfolio

Obtain all the latest leaflets and information regarding COSHH from your local Health and Safety Executive Office.

Keep up to date – and keep safe!

Health Act 2006

This law has been introduced to protect employees and the public from the harmful effects of 'second-hand' smoke inhalation (passive smoking). Below is a summary of its key points.

■ From 1 July 2007 it has been against the law to smoke in virtually all enclosed and substantially enclosed public places and workplaces.

■ Public transport and work vehicles used by more than one person should be smoke-free.

■ Non-smoking signs should be displayed in all smoke-free premises and vehicles.

■ Staff smoking rooms and indoor smoking areas are no longer allowed, so anyone wanting to smoke will have to go outside.

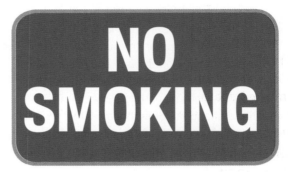

■ Managers of smoke-free premises and vehicles have legal responsibility to prevent people from smoking.

■ Anyone not complying with the smoke-free law is committing an offence and can be issued with a fixed penalty notice – up to a maximum of £200 if prosecuted and convicted by a court.

■ Failure to display non-smoking signs carries a fixed penalty of £200, or a maximum fine of £1000 if prosecuted and convicted by a court.

■ Failing to prevent smoking in a smoke-free place has a maximum fine of £2500.

The Gas Safety (Installation and Use) Regulations 1998

These relate to the use and maintenance of gas appliances. You may think that this does not apply to you as a therapist, but read on! The Gas Safety (Rights of Entry) Regulations 1996 give gas and HSE inspectors the right to enter premises and order the disconnection of any dangerous appliances. The inspectors themselves are not usually trained gas fitters, so they will instruct you to contact your local service engineer. Gas fumes are silent, with no smell, and deadly.

The Fire Precautions (Workplace) Regulations 1997 (as amended 1999)

The Fire Precautions (Workplace) Regulations brought together existing Health and Safety and Fire legislation. Its objective was to achieve a risk-appropriate standard of fire safety for persons in the workplace. These regulations were amended in 1999 to emphasise that the employer had unconditional responsibility for the safety of employees. As a result, most workplaces are now subject to the legal requirements of the above regulations.

New regulations now require small business owners to adequately assess the fire risks associated with their work activities and to decide what needs to be done to control these risks. The steps to be taken for a fire risk assessment are similar to those taken for general risk assessments, though you also have a general duty to the public (refer to Unit G22 monitor procedures to safely control work operations, page 88).

Staff need to be aware of the procedures involved in the event of a fire, preferably through the displaying of a notice. It is recommended that you have some form of fire-fighting equipment – even if it is just a fire blanket. Contact the fire authority in your area who will be happy to assist you.

The Provision and Use of Work Equipment Regulations 1998

The key points here are to ensure that all equipment at work is properly maintained, fit for purpose and in a good state of repair, as explained below.

Suitability of equipment

Employers must ensure that equipment is suitable for the purpose for which it is used or provided. When selecting equipment, they need to be aware of the working conditions and the risks to health and safety in the premises in which the work equipment is to be used and any additional risk posed by the use of the equipment.

Maintenance

Equipment must be maintained in efficient working order and good repair. Wherever possible, maintenance should take place when equipment is switched off to avoid risks to the person's health and safety; if maintenance can only take place when the equipment is switched on, precautions should be taken to protect the person carrying out the work. Where equipment has a maintenance log, this must be kept up to date.

Inspection

Where the safety of equipment depends on the installation conditions, it must be inspected after installation and before being put into service for the first time; or after assembly at a new site or in a new location, to ensure that it has been installed correctly and is safe to operate. This is also to ensure that health and safety conditions are maintained and that any wear and tear is detected and remedied in good time. Inspections that take place under this regulation should be recorded and kept until the next inspection takes place and is recorded.

Equipment should be used only for the purposes of the employer's business, and if equipment is obtained from another business, it should be accompanied by an inspection certificate.

Specific risks

Where the use of equipment is likely to involve a specific risk to health or safety, the equipment must only be used by staff trained to operate it. Where appropriate, employers need to provide training.

Any repairs, modifications, maintenance or servicing should only be carried out by a competent person.

Information and instructions

Staff operating equipment must be provided with adequate health and safety information and, where appropriate, written instructions on how to use it. This also applies to employees who supervise or manage the use of equipment.

Training

For health and safety reasons, staff should be given adequate training to operate equipment, including training in the methods which may be adopted when using the equipment, any risks involved and precautions to be taken. This also applies to employees who supervise or manage the use of equipment.

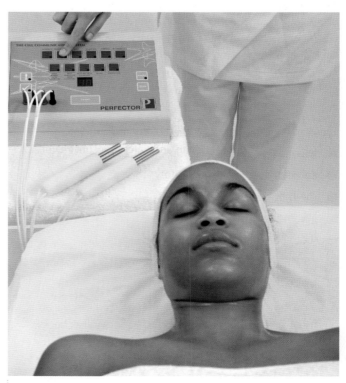

You must follow regulations in your Salon when using equipment

Protection against specified hazards

Employers are responsible for taking measures to ensure that staff using equipment should be protected from hazards that might endanger their health and safety. If it is not possible to prevent the risk, then it needs to be adequately controlled.

High or very low temperature

Where equipment, or any article or substance produced, used or stored in work equipment, is at a high or very low temperature, it needs to be protected so as to prevent injury to any person by burn, scald or sear.

Controls for starting equipment

Where appropriate, equipment should be provided with one or more controls for the purposes of starting it (including restarting after a stoppage for any reason).

Stability

Equipment should be stabilised by clamping, or another method, where necessary for health or safety purposes.

Lighting

The work area where equipment is to be used should have suitable and sufficient lighting.

The Electricity at Work Regulations 1989

These regulations affect the use of electrical equipment in every salon, clinic or health club. Regulation 4 states: 'All electrical equipment must be regularly checked for electrical safety.' In a busy salon this may be every six months. The check must be carried out by a 'competent person', preferably a qualified electrician. All checks must be recorded in a book kept for this purpose only.

Types of equipment to be checked would include:

- wax heaters
- autoclaves
- thermal booties
- infrared lamps
- foot spas that plug in
- paraffin wax heaters
- fast nail UV dryer boxes.

A 'competent person' need not be a qualified electrician, but must be capable of attending to basic safety checks. Manufacturers often supply their own technical staff to attend to safety checks.

PAT Testing (Portable Appliance Testing)

All companies and organisations should comply with The Electricity at Work Regulations.

Each electrical appliance should be comprehensively tested to meet the exacting requirements of the IET (Institution of Engineering and Technology) Code of Practice for In-Service Inspection and Testing of Electrical Equipment.

Ideally the electrician or competent person should be a member of both NICEIC (an independent voluntary body) and NAPIT (The National Association of Professional Inspectors and Testers). All engineers should undertake a NAPIT technical assessment and be subject to regular inspection and monitoring of their work and records.

All electrical equipment to be tested has to be disconnected from the mains supply. This may be inconvenient so ideally it should be carried out outside normal salon hours.

If electrical apparatus is found to be faulty, the equipment must be withdrawn from service and repaired. An electrical safety record book should be used to record dates, the nature of the repair and by whom it was done. It should also contain a list of tests carried out on the equipment under inspection, the results of those tests, and be signed by the competent person who carried them out.

This is essential for public liability insurance purposes and in case of legal action being taken for accidents due to negligence.

The Pressure Systems and Transportable Gas Containers Regulations 1989

Steam sterilising autoclaves fall under this act. You are required to have a written scheme of examination carried out or certified by a competent person.

The Controlled Waste Regulations 1992 (as amended 1993)

This requires that all clinical waste (for example, used needles, soiled dressings and used swabs) is collected by a licensed contractor and disposed of in an approved incinerator.

The Special Waste Regulations 1996 (as amended)

This legislation requires all clinical waste to be kept apart from general waste and to be disposed of at a licensed incinerator or landfill site, by a licensed company. This includes:

- waste which consists wholly or partly of animal or human tissue

- blood or other body fluids
- swabs or dressings
- syringes or needles.

The Reporting of Injuries, Diseases and Dangerous Occurrences Regulations (RIDDOR) 1995

These regulations cover the recording and reporting of any serious accidents and conditions to the local environmental health officer, whose remit covers beauty therapy and hairdressing salons. This officer will investigate the accident and make sure that the salon prevents the accident from happening again in the future. The officer can also assess the risk factors in each instance.

An accident or death at work must be reported within ten days. If the accident does not require a hospital visit, but the person is absent from work for more than three days, a report still needs to be made.

If an employee reports a work-related disease, a report must be sent: this could include occupational dermatitis or asthma. Any infection with hepatitis associated with skin piercing or special treatment must be reported to the local authority Environmental Health Officer immediately. There is a special form (F2508A) on which to confirm the details. Accidents as a result of violence or an attack by another person must be reported. A car accident when on company business is reportable in the same way as an accident at work.

A dangerous occurrence in which no one was actually injured must also be reported: for example, if the ceiling of the salon collapses overnight.

If you are a mobile therapist working in someone's home and you have an accident yourself or you injure the client you must report it.

The Health and Safety (Display Screen Equipment) Regulations 1992 (as amended 2002)

These regulations were written to implement an EU Directive and amended in 2002. They place a duty on employers to minimise risks associated with VDU (visual display unit) work. Employers must make sure that their workplaces are well designed and that consideration is given to how monitors are positioned and the relative height of the user's chair. You can also help to avoid problems by reporting any problems with your workplace design and taking frequent short breaks when using a computer for long periods. Prevention is better than cure.

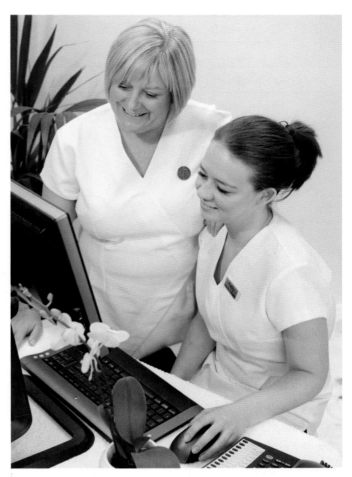

Position yourself correctly when using a VDU

Some people who use a VDU for long periods of time may experience discomfort in their hands, wrists, arms, neck, shoulders or back. This kind of pain is often referred to as repetitive strain injury (RSI) but this can be misleading as it means different things to different people. For that reason, it is often better to describe the group of conditions as 'upper limb disorders'. Usually these disorders are temporary but for a few people they can last for much longer and seriously disrupt their ability to carry out day-to-day tasks.

Although there is no evidence from the research carried out that VDUs can cause disease or damage to the eyes, long periods of time in front of a computer screen can make your eyes feel tired or sore temporarily.

Remember that all of the different terms you may hear — VDU, VDT, monitor, display screen equipment (DSE) — all mean the same thing: the part of the computer that shows what you are working on.

You, your client and the law

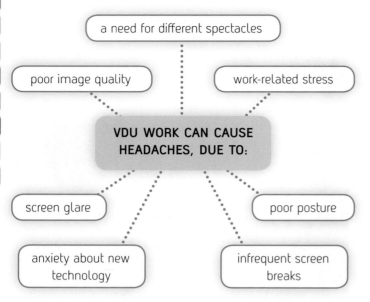

a need for different spectacles

poor image quality

work-related stress

VDU WORK CAN CAUSE HEADACHES, DUE TO:

screen glare

poor posture

anxiety about new technology

infrequent screen breaks

Once the employer recognises these issues, they are easily put right. People who suffer from photo-sensitive epilepsy are susceptible to flickering lights and striped patterns and they may be affected by the use of VDUs in some circumstances.

For more information on VDUs in the workplace, check out the Health and Safety Executive Leaflet 'Working with VDUs' available at www.hse.gov.uk/pubns.

Employers have to analyse workstations, and assess and reduce risks. They should look at:

- the whole workstation including equipment, furniture, and the work environment — workstations need to meet minimum requirements
- the job being done
- any special needs of individual staff
- planning work so there are breaks or changes of activity
- arranging eye tests, on request, and providing spectacles if special ones are needed
- providing health and safety training and information, so that employees can use their VDU and workstation safely, and know how to make best use of it to avoid health problems, for example by adjusting the chair.

Employers' Liability (Compulsory Insurance) Act 1969

Employers and self-employed persons must by law hold employer's liability insurance. This will reimburse them against any legal liability to pay compensation to employees for bodily injury, illness or disease caused during the course of their employment.

Employers must insure for at least £2 million per claim, but check with your own insurance company. Also follow the recommendations of your professional association.

It is worth remembering the following points.

- A legal claim made against your salon could result in very large financial losses and possibly the sale of the owner's business or even private home.
- Public prosecution results in a heavy fine for those not having this essential insurance cover.
- Damage to the salon could be so great that the business might never recover.
- Some cases can take up to ten years to come to court and with inflation the claim against you could be very much more than your original cover, if you only take the minimum requirements.

Consumer Protection Act 1987

This Act follows European laws to safeguard the consumer in three main areas: product liability, general safety requirements and misleading prices.

Before 1987 an injured person had to prove that a manufacturer was negligent before suing for damages. This Act removes the need to prove negligence.

An injured person can take action against:

- producers
- own brand manufacturers
- importers
- suppliers such as wholesalers or retailers.

In the salon this means that only reputable products should be used and sold. Care should be taken in handling, maintaining and storing products so that they remain in top condition.

It is important that all staff are aware of consumer protection laws when selling products and when using products in a treatment.

The Consumer Protection (Distance Selling) Regulations 2000

These regulations were introduced to increase consumer confidence. They will apply to you if the salon where you work sells goods or services via the Internet, by phone, by fax, or mail order. The key points of the regulations are as follows:

- The consumer must be given clear information about the goods or services on offer. This information includes the price, delivery, costs, arrangements for payment, and so on.

- The consumer must be sent confirmation after making a purchase.

- The consumer must have a seven-day cooling-off period (this is meant to equate to the time the consumer would spend in the salon deciding whether to purchase).

It is unlikely that these regulations will apply to your salon if you do not usually supply clients in this way, but agree to do so as a one-off request. However, if the business regularly handles such requests, it is likely the salon should comply with these regulations. If this is the case, the salon should also ensure it has registered with and is fulfilling the requirements of the Data Protection Act 1998 (see page 81).

The Cosmetic Products (Safety) Regulations 2003 amended 2008

Cosmetic products are governed by the rules as set out in The Cosmetic Products (Safety) Regulations 1996.

These regulations define a cosmetic product as any substance/preparation that is used on the skin, teeth, hair, nails, lips, with the intention to cleanse, perfume, change the appearance of, or to protect, keep in good condition or to correct body odours. So, everything found in a salon, basically!

Before a cosmetic product can be placed on the market it must be safe. All cosmetic products must be labelled with the following information.

- *A list of ingredients* – this should appear on the outer packaging of the item, or if there is no outer packaging, on the container itself. In relation to small items such as lipsticks and mascaras, this information can appear on a label attached to the product or in the near vicinity of it.

- *The name and address of the manufacturer/supplier* – these details must be of someone within the EEA (European Economic Area). If a full postcode is sufficient to identify the address then this is acceptable.

- *A minimum durability indication* – this should appear on both the outer packaging and the container itself. Storage instructions should also be given to enable the consumer to keep the product at its best until this date.

- *Warnings and precautionary statements* – these should appear on both the outer packaging and the container itself.

- *Batch number or lot code* – this unique number will help a manufacturer to recall a batch of products if need be.

- *The product function* – this may be given, where appropriate, unless the function is clear from the presentation of the product.

- *Weight marking* – this is required under the Weights and Measures Act 1985.

All of the above information must appear in a visible, legible and indelible form. This must also be given in English.

Medicines Act 1968

This Act deals with the supply and use of topical anaesthetics and is enforced by the police and the Medicines and Healthcare Product Regulatory Agency (MHRA). Product licence conditions are for medical application only and not for cosmetic use, therefore their use by a beauty therapist can be unlawful.

Trade Descriptions Act 1968

It is illegal to mislead the general public. This also applies to verbal descriptions given by a third party and repeated. So, if a manufacturer's false description of a product is repeated you are liable to prosecution. The law states that the retailer must not:

- supply information that is in any way misleading

- falsely describe or make false statements about either a product or a service on offer.

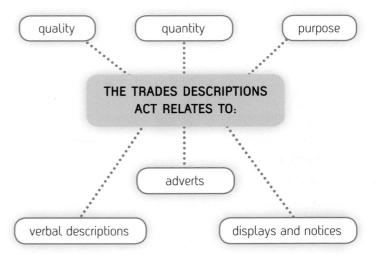

The Consumer Protection from Unfair Trading Regulations 2008

The European Union adopted the Unfair Commercial Practices Directive (UCPD) in May 2005 in order to strengthen laws for trades descriptions within Europe, as they varied from country to country, In the UK the directive was implemented as The Consumer Protection from Unfair Trading Regulations, which came into force on 26th May 2008.

The regulations maintain good practice and are specific about what retailers may or may not do.

The retailer may not:

- make false contrasts between present and previous prices
- claim to offer products at half price unless they have already been offered at the full price for at least 28 days prior to the sale.

Be mindful of using statements saying something is 'our price'. Comparison of prices can be misleading and can be illegal — be sure that the product is identical in every way. You should also check that products are labelled with their country of origin.

Related Acts: Sale of Goods Act 1979; Supply of Goods and Services Act 1982; Sale and Supply of Goods Act 1994; The Sale and Supply of Goods to Consumers Regulations 2002

- Wherever goods are bought they must 'conform to contract'. This means they must be as described, fit for purpose and of satisfactory quality (that is not inherently faulty at the time of sale).
- Goods are of satisfactory quality if they reach the standard that a reasonable person would regard as satisfactory, taking into account the price and any description.
- Aspects of quality include fitness for purpose, freedom from minor defects, appearance and finish, durability, and safety.

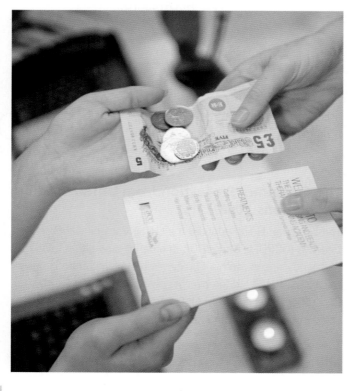

- It is the seller, not the manufacturer, who is responsible if goods do not conform to contract.
- If goods do not conform to contract at the time of sale, purchasers can request their money back 'within a reasonable time'. (This is not defined and will depend on circumstances.)
- For up to six years after purchase (five years from discovery in Scotland) purchasers can demand damages (which a court would equate to the cost of a repair or replacement).
- A purchaser who is a consumer (that is, they are not buying in the course of a business) can alternatively request a repair or replacement.
- If repair and replacement are not possible or too costly, then the consumer can seek a partial refund, if they have had some benefit from the good, or a full refund if the fault(s) have meant they have enjoyed no benefit.
- In general, the onus is on all purchasers to prove the goods did not conform to contract (for example that they were inherently faulty) and should have reasonably lasted until this point in time (that is, perishable goods do not last for six years).
- If a consumer chooses to request a repair or replacement, then for the first six months after purchase it will be for the retailer to prove the goods did conform to contract (for example that they were not inherently faulty).
- After six months and until the end of the six years, it is for the consumer to prove the lack of conformity.

Disability Discrimination Act 1995, as amended by the Disability Discrimination Act 2005 and the Equality Act 2010

This Act makes it unlawful to discriminate against disabled people in employment, the provision of goods, facilities and services, education, and the buying or renting property or land. In 2007, the promotion of civil rights for disabled people became the responsibility of the new Equality and Human Rights Commission.

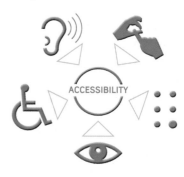

It is illegal for an employer (employing 20 or more staff) to discriminate against a disabled person or prospective employee on the grounds of their disabilities. If a person is suitable for the job, it is up the employer to make the necessary arrangements and adjustments in the workplace to ensure there is no disadvantage for the disabled person.

It is also unlawful to harass a person on the grounds of their disability. All employers must take positive steps to avoid harassment happening in the workplace.

Think about it

How user-friendly is your salon? Have a good look around; does it discriminate against disabled people in any way? Is there adequate wheelchair access? Does anyone employed in the salon know sign language? Do you have a price list in Braille?

How could your salon better accommodate the disabled client?

The Equality and Human Rights Commission is there to give advice on these important aspects of law and good customer service.

The Working Time Regulations 1998 (incorporating the European Working Time Directive and amended in 2003)

This controls how the employer organises the average working week, minimum daily and weekly rest breaks, and paid holiday entitlement – which before this Act was introduced, was left very much up to what the employer wanted to do. The law applies to full-time, part-time and casual workers. You should not work more than 48 hours in a week, with a rest period of 11 hours between each working day, with a minimum of one day off a week. If working for more than six hours, you are entitled to a 20-minute break.

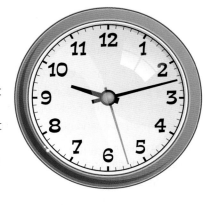

Performing Rights – within Copyright, Designs and Patents Act 1988

This Act is designed to protect the people who write music but then do not get the royalty payments they should when the music is played! Any use of music in the treatment room, reception or in exercise groups is classed as a public performance.

PPL is the body that is responsible for collecting licence payments from people wishing to use music on behalf of artists and record companies. Under the Copyright, Designs and Patents Act 1988, PPL can take legal action against anyone who does not pay a licence fee to use music – and it does! This can mean a considerable fine for those who try to avoid paying. So all salons and exercise/aerobic instructors need to purchase music that has a built-in licence. Although more expensive to purchase in the first place (a CD can cost up to about £30) it does save all the worry of a heavy fine, if caught!

Most good specialist music shops have a section of licensed music – just ask. (See the section in 'You and your working environment' for advice on choosing suitable music, page 62.)

Data Protection Act 1998

The Data Protection Act 1998 states that every organisation (data controller) that uses and processes personal information (personal data) must notify the Information Commissioners office, unless they are exempt. Failure to do so is a criminal offence. The main purpose of registration is to ensure that the eight principals of 'good information handling' are being followed.

Data should be:
1. Fairly and lawfully processed
2. Processed for limited purposes
3. Adequate, relevant and not excessive
4. Accurate
5. Not kept longer than necessary
6. Processed in accordance to the person's rights
7. Secure
8. Not transferred to countries outside the European Economic Area (EEA) without adequate and proper protection.

Any person can ask to see the information held by an organisation about him or her within 40 days for a fee that is now only £2. It is possible to gain compensation through a civil court action if you feel there has been any infringement of rights, in which information that was given for a specific purpose has been abused.

For your portfolio

You can visit the website of the Information Commissioner – www.ico.gov.uk

You, your client and the law

The Care Standards Act 2000

This Act is all about making provision for the protection of children and vulnerable adults and safeguarding them. It applies to any organisation that has contact with children, for example, schools and colleges, children's homes or care homes. It also links in with The Children's Act 2004, The Protection of Children Act 1999, and The Children (Leaving Care) Act 2000.

The key word is 'safeguarding' and the main guidelines for ensuring the wellbeing of young people under 19 are covered in the Government initiative Every Child Matters. The Government's aim is for every child, whatever their background or their circumstances, to have the support they need to:

- be healthy
- stay safe
- enjoy and achieve
- make a positive contribution
- achieve economic wellbeing.

Local Government (Miscellaneous Provisions) Act 1982

This relates to the local authorities in your particular area. Section 8 of this Act is concerned with the registration of any practitioners who pierce the skin. This applies to:

- acupuncture
- tattooing
- ear and body piercing
- epilation.

It applies to both salons and mobile therapists.

The concern of most local authorities is that through registration they will be able to keep some control of hygiene regulations and ensure that people have recognised qualifications. The enforcement of these regulations will depend upon the individual authority, as does the amount of inspection that takes place, and the scale of fees for registration.

This does not include people working in hospitals.

Local by-laws

Key terms

By-laws – laws decided by the local authority for your area.

Local government by-laws are laws decided by the local authority or borough council of an area, and they can differ from region to region. Therefore, Manchester has different local by-laws from Birmingham. However, both these authorities have a register of salons offering body massage as a treatment. This is to maintain a professional, qualified salon base and to eliminate the 'massage parlour' image.

You need to investigate the by-laws in your own area from your borough council – these by-laws relate to hygiene, and the registration of salons that perform ear piercing and/or epilation, as well as tattoo parlours.

London Local Authorities Act 1995 – amended 2004 & 2008

This Act requires all premises in London that carry out treatments to be licensed by their local authorities. This is for any skin piercing treatments, acupuncture, tattooing and ear piercing – and some local authorities also expect salons to register if they offer massage too.

Contact your local authority to check whether you need a licence when you start your new salon.

Insurance

Professional indemnity insurance

Every single professional beauty therapist should have this insurance protection, regardless of how few or how many treatments they carry out.

The best deal for these kinds of insurance policies can usually be found via your professional body – professional bodies are often able to offer the best rates because they negotiate on behalf of members and get a considerable discount.

As an employee you need to check with your employer whether you are covered on the company's business insurance, or if you need to organise your own cover. A salon owner or employer should include this in the public liability policy, so that all employees are protected against claims made by clients.

Public liability insurance

This insurance is not compulsory, but it is certainly advisable. It will protect the employer should a member of the public be injured on the premises. This could be something as unexpected as a roof tile hitting the client on her way into the salon. If this results in the client being unable to work for a long period of time, the client can sue the salon owner for compensation.

Insurance is important – so protect yourselves and your clients. Contact your professional association for guidance on all aspects of insurance.

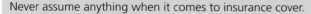

Never assume anything when it comes to insurance cover.

Always check whether you have cover as a therapist working in a salon. Would you be personally liable if things go wrong?

Check you are covered if you are a mobile therapist entering clients' homes. What if you were to spill wax on their new bedroom carpet? Are you covered?

If you are running a business from home, do not automatically think your household insurance will cover your work and clients coming to your home. What if a client were to fall in the driveway, and hurt herself? Would you be covered?

Accidents can and do happen – and many clients have heard of these 'no win, no fee' solicitor firms willing to take legal action against you. Better safe than sorry! Be covered and you have security and peace of mind. One of the advantages of joining a professional association is that they negotiate better and reasonably priced insurance cover.

Independent regulators

Advertising Standards Authority (ASA)

The ASA is an independent body set up to regulate the content of advertisements, sales promotions and direct marketing in the UK.

It is responsible for maintaining the quality of advertising standards through codes of practice for television, radio and other types of adverts, such as interactive adverts. The ASA can stop misleading, harmful or offensive advertising, ensure that sales promotions are run fairly, and help to reduce unwanted advertising sent through the post, by email or by text message. It also deals with mail order problems. Part of its role is to investigate complaints made about advertising, sales promotions or direct marketing.

The advertising standards codes especially apply to beauty products. Advertisements must be careful not to mislead or misdirect the consumer into believing that wrinkles will disappear, that skin will look ten years younger or that lines can be permanently removed. Adverts may refer to temporary prevention of the skin drying out, but any long-term or permanent correction of the lines or wrinkles is not possible and therefore not allowed in advertising.

ACAS (Advisory, Conciliation and Arbitration Service)

ACAS is an independent organisation that offers impartial advice to individuals and organisations to help resolve disputes or disagreements at work. It aims to encourage better and more direct workplace communication and to help businesses improve their employment practices. From April 2009, ACAS will concentrate less on how to manage disciplinary issues, grievances and dismissals and more on resolving problems in the workplace at an early stage, so saving businesses time and money.

BSI British Standards

BSI British Standards is the UK's national standards body, which brings together representatives from a range of organisations to develop formal standards for the benefit of UK business and consumers. Standards are there to help industry and society at large. So even if you are not involved in developing or manufacturing products, you are bound to come into contact with BSI Standards every day. The aim of the Standards is to:

- promote and share best practice, so designers can focus on developing better products
- set benchmarks for performance, quality and safety
- ensure similar products work together (for example making sure all CDs are the same dimensions)
- make technical requirements
- reduce risks
- reduce costs.

Industry codes of practice

Industry codes of practice or ethics are guides for correct procedures and etiquette as dictated by professional therapists' associations, of which there are several. Which professional body you join is a matter of personal choice, and may depend upon the one favoured by your training establishment.

The cost involved in joining depends on your level of entry – a student membership is normally available and with your joining pack you will be given a code of ethics or a code of practice.

Key terms

Industry code of practice – a guide for correct procedures and etiquette within a particular industry.

This code is a book of rules that the therapist agrees to abide by, as part of the contract of membership. If these rules are broken or ignored, membership can be withdrawn.

Being a member of a professional body brings benefits, which can include:

- a good insurance deal negotiated on the members' behalf
- support and advice upon leaving college
- a monthly magazine, with useful articles and adverts for jobs and equipment
- regular legal updates
- free legal helplines, for all aspects of your business
- discount cards for suppliers
- a business guide for setting up on your own.

The following is an extract from the FHT Code of Ethics and Professional Practice which is a typical set of rules and regulations for a professional therapist organisation.

Federation of Holistic Therapists Code of Ethics and Professional Practice

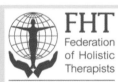

The UK and Ireland's largest professional association

The Federation of Holistic Therapists (FHT) is the UK and Ireland's largest and leading professional association for beauty, complementary and sports therapists. Professional therapist members of the FHT agree to abide by the FHT Code of Ethics and Professional Practice and any amendments or additions that may be made in the future.

Duties as a professional therapist

The definition of a professional therapist concerns the welfare of clients and the protection of the public from improper practice. This includes:

- making the care of your client your first concern
- providing a high standard of care at all times
- clients being treated with respect, as individuals
- professional knowledge being kept up to date
- acting lawfully in your professional and personal practice
- personal accountability for your professional activity

Failure to abide by this Code will result in disciplinary procedures being applied by the FHT Professional Conduct Panel ranging from a warning with sanctions according to conditions of practice, suspension until further training is completed, or termination of membership, depending on the nature of the breach. When an allegation is made against a professional therapist, the FHT will always take account of the standards set out in this Code when considering that allegation.

Guidelines to advertising your services

All advertising undertaken in relation to professional practice must be accurate and must not be misleading, false, unfair or exaggerated. Personal skills, equipment or facilities cannot be promoted as being better than anyone else's. Advertising any product or service requires promoting knowledge, skills, qualifications and experience in an accurate and professionally responsible way without making or supporting unjustifiable statements. Any potential financial rewards should be made explicit and play no part at all in the advice or recommendations of products and services that clients and users receive.

Limits of competence

A professional therapist must only carry out treatments and give advice within their area of training and competence. Clients' consent should be obtained before introducing new treatments into their existing treatment programme. A professional therapist has the right to refuse to treat a client if the treatment is outside of their competency level. In such circumstances they should refer to an appropriately qualified professional therapist or suggest that the client contact their GP.

Regulation

Beauty therapies are not currently regulated by statute that provides protection of title. Protection of title prevents anyone calling themselves a 'doctor', physiotherapist, chiropodist, chiropractor etc, without being registered with the relevant statutory regulator under the provisions of an Act of Parliament. Membership of a professional association for a therapy that is not regulated enables the therapist to demonstrate to clients that they are suitably qualified, insured and participating in Continuing Professional Development (CPD).

(Source: Federation of Holistic Therapists; www.fht.org.uk)

Salon guidelines

All the legislation mentioned in this Unit should be considered within the normal working life of the beauty therapist. Working safely and following the correct legal procedure is very important.

It is also very important to follow the salon guidelines for the particular establishment you are in – be it a training establishment, salon or health farm, ocean liner or a rented room in a health suite.

Key terms

Salon guidelines – policies and procedures followed within the salon.

It is vital that you are aware of the policies on health and safety, safety training and what exactly is expected within the job role. Normally salon rules are very similar, regardless of where the salon is located, but the safety procedures to follow if your salon happens to be floating in the Caribbean Sea will be very different.

It is very important that the salon expectations and the required behaviour for therapists are set out at the beginning. This could be at your induction training, or even at the initial interview.

Regular reviews of policies and regular training for updates are essential, as is your attendance. If a member of staff continually ignores safety requirements, whether through negligence or through ignorance (if they have not attended training), this could form the basis for dismissal. Worse still, should an accident happen through negligence, injury may occur, and the person responsible may be found liable.

Health and safety rules

These will encompass all aspects of the Health and Safety at Work Act, plus COSHH guidelines and the Electricity at Work Act.

As a professional therapist you should be in no doubt about:

- therapists' responsibilities
- salon procedures
- treatment safety
- equipment safety
- protection against cross-infection.

Client safety	Storage procedures	Stock regulations
Positioning of client	Electrical equipment	COSHH regulations followed
Minimum risk of hazard for bed height – getting on and off	Chemicals	First aid procedures in place
Correct use of equipment and products	Valuables	Stock rotation
Correct diagnosis for treatments	Stock	Spillage management
Correct evacuation procedures	Money	Correct storage and containers

Salon procedures for health and safety

Your employer or head of your training establishment should have all these standard procedures in place. If you are not instructed within your first few weeks of beginning your new post – then ask.

Check your knowledge

1 Who is responsible for ensuring that personal protective wear is worn, for example gloves during some microdermabrasion?
   a) The client
   b) The receptionist
   c) The manager
   d) The therapist

2 Who is responsible for adequate ventilation in the salon, to avoid build-up of fumes?
   a) The employer
   b) The receptionist
   c) The caretaker
   d) The employee

3 The Trade Descriptions Act protects the client against:
   a) unsafe practice in the salon
   b) unsafe products in the salon
   c) false claims on goods or services
   d) health and safety.

4 COSHH stands for:
   a) Control of Safety, Health and Hygiene
   b) Control of Students' Health and Hygiene
   c) Control of Substances Hazardous to Health
   d) Consideration of Services, Hazards and Harm.

5 What is sterilisation?
   a) The removal of dirt and being ultra clean
   b) The removal of bacteria
   c) The removal of viruses
   d) The removal of bacteria, spores and viruses

6 An example of a viral infection is:
   a) athlete's foot
   b) a cold sore
   c) scabies
   d) impetigo.

7 A bacterial infection causes:
   a) ringworm
   b) diarrhoea
   c) warts
   d) boils.

8 The Cosmetic Products (Safety) Regulations are concerned with:
   a) labelling and listing of products
   b) the price of products
   c) the size of products
   d) the colour of products.

9 A dry powder fire extinguisher is coloured with:
   a) black marking
   b) blue marking
   c) green marking
   d) red marking.

10 Chicken pox is a disease caused by:
   a) a virus
   b) a fungus
   c) a bacteria
   d) a cut.

Section

2

The workplace environment

Unit G22

Monitor procedures to safely control work operations

What you will learn

Check that health and safety instructions are followed

- Related legislation and keeping up to date
- Hazards and risks
- Monitoring your workplace through risk assessment
- Promoting a safe working environment
- Responsibilities – who does what?
- Communicating workplace instructions to others
- Communicating workplace policies and information
- Responding to breaches of health and safety
- Maintaining records
- Making recommendations for change
- Using electrical equipment

Make sure that risks are controlled safely and effectively

- Keeping accurate and legible records of workplace risks
- Reporting the existence of hazards and confirming precautions to control risks
- Informing others and minimising risk
- Reviewing operational controls to eliminate and control risks

Workplace policies

- The premises
- Stock and products
- Use of materials and hazardous substances
- Smoking, eating, drinking and drugs

Introduction

Monitoring the operation of **workplace** health and safety **procedures** is the legal responsibility of *all senior staff* in a salon not just that of the owner or manager — and good health and safety practice is everyone's collective responsibility.

This unit will help you to identify and examine the **hazards** in your workplace, check and evaluate the **risks** and look at ways to reduce those risks, through careful monitoring and sensible precautions.

This unit is for everyone at work, regardless of whether they are a paid worker, a volunteer, part-time or full-time employee, or a self-employed therapist in a mobile business. Everyone within the workplace has an obligation by **statutory law** to secure their own and others' health, safety and welfare, so this unit is about identifying the factors that contribute to you becoming a responsible employee, and a senior therapist. As a senior Level 3 student you need to be able to review and react to operational controls for workplace hazards, respond promptly and actively make recommendations for change.

As a Level 3 student, you will be dealing with others, with responsibility for more junior Level 1 and 2 students. You will also use the majority of the electrical equipment in the salon, which has a higher risk factor attached to it than manual treatments.

This unit is not a full guide to completing a full risk assessment — that should be done by a trained professional who specialises in that field. The purpose here is to give you an appreciation of the significant risks in the beauty salon, how to identify them and deal with them appropriately.

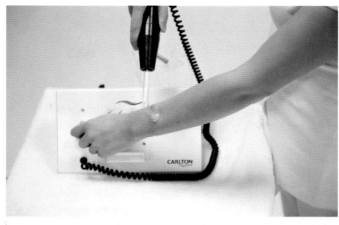

Testing equipment on yourself first helps reduce risk

G22 is a totally integrated unit and is wholly performance related. You can only make sure risks are controlled safely if you understand the risks themselves, and relate them to your competencies, capabilities and the scope of your job role.

This unit therefore contains some additional information that underpins the performance criteria, without being range specific. The ability to monitor procedures to safely control work operations is embedded within all practical units and therefore the information here is generic to all other units.

Each practical unit will have its own particular hazards which will be identified within the specific unit. General hazards in the salon and your actions and responsibilities are covered within this unit.

Think about it

On average 25,000 people leave the workforce every year, never to return, because of harm suffered at work.

Key terms

Workplace – this includes all areas of the salon, not just the 'front of house' which the clients see. It includes the staff room, the toilets, kitchens and storage rooms.

Procedure – a course of action or a step-by-step guide of how to complete a task/carry out a duty, as laid down by a policy.

Hazard – may be defined as anything that can cause harm, or which has the potential to cause harm. For example, a spillage or a faulty appliance.

Risk – the chance, however great or small, that the hazard has the potential to cause harm. For example, a spillage or a faulty appliance.

Statutory Law or instructions – laws and regulations which are created by Acts of Parliament, or the European Union. Governments may introduce a bill to update existing laws (which is why the dates of laws often say 'as amended…') or develop new ones to respond to changes in society.

Think about it

As a senior therapist what are your responsibilities to managing safety?

You have the following obligations:

- *Moral obligation* – it's just not acceptable for workers to suffer injury or ill health through their employment.
- *Legal obligation* – the law requires responsible people to have controls in place for health and safety and managers are liable to prosecution in court, and may even go to prison, if these are not in place, or negligence is proven.
- *Financial obligation* – as well as reducing fines and personal injury claims, insurance premiums are reduced and employees work better when health and safety is taken seriously – all good for the financial health of the business. By looking after the health of workers, productivity is increased and fewer sick days are taken.

Check that health and safety instructions are followed

In this section you will learn about:

- related legislation and keeping up to date
- hazards and risks
- monitoring your workplace through risk assessment
- promoting a safe working environment
- responsibilities – who does what?
- communicating workplace instructions to others
- communicating workplace policies and information
- responding to breaches of health and safety
- maintaining records
- making recommendations for change
- using electrical equipment.

Related legislation and keeping up to date

The **Health and Safety at Work etc. (HASAW) Act 1974** covers the legal requirements of an employer, and the Health and Safety Commission will give advice to those considering going into business and employing others. You should refer back to 'You, your client and the law' on page 68 for all the latest legislation for health and safety, so that you understand and can work within the employers and employees' main legal responsibilities for health and safety in the workplace.

Think about it

The law requires you to assess 'reasonable, foreseeable' risks. The three tests you can apply are:

- The employer has a **duty of care**
- Duty of care was breached
- The breach caused an accident.

For your portfolio

You need to check that your information is safe and from a reliable source. The Internet offers the opportunity to go onto the health and safety sites and look up the latest legislation. Downloads are available and the **Health and Safety Executive** (www.hse.gov.uk) have lots of leaflets and newsletters available which you can get copies of for your portfolio.

Civil law

Under **civil law**, victims of harm (claimants) can seek compensation if they feel that they have come to harm or suffered loss by the fault or negligence of another person (defendants). Usually, any legal action must be started within three years of an accident or when the injured person found that the injury was the fault of the other person.

Key terms

Health And Safety At Work etc. (HSAWA) Act 1974 – places duties on employers, directors, managers, manufacturers, and employees to ensure, so far as is reasonably practicable, good health and safety in relation to their activities.

Duty of care – the legal requirement which states that employers must do everything that is reasonably practicable to protect others from harm.

Health and Safety Executive (HSE) – the British Government body responsible for regulating risks to health and safety in the UK. It reports to the Health and Safety Commission.

Civil law – the section of the law which deals with disputes between individuals or organisations.

In civil law actions, a court is not making a decision based on a law being broken, but by listening to both sides of the argument. The amount of compensation or damages will depend upon the severity of injuries and the quality of life after the accident, and if the claimant is able to earn a living. The claimant has to show that negligence has taken place (this is called 'the **burden of proof**') and to satisfy a judge that on 'the balance of probabilities' the defendant was guilty of negligence.

For the claimant to be successful they have to show three things:

1 That the defendant owed the person a duty of care
2 That the duty of care was breached
3 That the injury was caused by a breach of the duty.

Criminal law

In **criminal law** the case against the defendant must be proven by the prosecution, in this case the state or its representatives, which uphold Her Majesty's Government's laws. The state brings cases against people, companies or organisations who have broken the health and safety laws as long as it is proved 'beyond reasonable doubt'. The courts also follow **precedent** when making their decisions. Penalties for criminal offences are high and can be fines and/ or imprisonment for the managers in charge. If a company is fined for an accident or death of an employee and it is not covered by insurance, it comes out of the profits, and can be thousands of pounds. Not worth the risk to bodily harm or the finances!

Key terms

Burden of proof – an obligation to prove what is alleged.

Criminal law – the section of law which punishes criminals for committing offences against the state.

Precedent – a previous case in law, the decision of which must be followed (also called 'case law'). Precedent is used to make sure the same principles for making decisions are used and consistent conclusions are reached.

Public Liability Insurance (see also 'You, your client and the law', page 82)

Within the beauty therapy industry we are able to protect ourselves with employers' liability insurance for any claims made against us, because of an injury received as a result of a treatment. Being covered by liability insurance is compulsory for many organisations except the health service and other public sectors. Most beauty therapy professional

bodies offer insurance cover – and it will protect you against claims of up to five million pounds – depending upon your experience and training.

To avoid a negligence claim under civil law a therapist should always:

! Do a full consultation with the client
! Fill out and update client record cards
! Work within the codes of practice
! Follow manufacturers' instructions
! Keep full guidance documents
! Be trained in first aid

For your portfolio

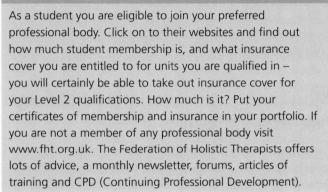

As a student you are eligible to join your preferred professional body. Click on to their websites and find out how much student membership is, and what insurance cover you are entitled to for units you are qualified in – you will certainly be able to take out insurance cover for your Level 2 qualifications. How much is it? Put your certificates of membership and insurance in your portfolio. If you are not a member of any professional body visit www.fht.org.uk. The Federation of Holistic Therapists offers lots of advice, a monthly newsletter, forums, articles of training and CPD (Continuing Professional Development).

Hazards and risks

It has been said that all actions have a consequence, and that is very true when looking at possible problems that may compromise health and safety.

The two key areas to consider are:
1 hazards in the salon
2 the risk that the hazard will cause harm.

A *hazard* may be defined as anything that can cause harm, or which has the potential to cause harm.

A *risk* is the chance, however great or small, that the hazard will actually cause harm to someone.

For example, a galvanic unit has the potential to be hazardous – there is a danger of electric shock, chemical, electrical or heat burns to the body, and allergic or sensitivity rashes from active products used. However, the risk of damage would be greatly minimised in the hands of a fully qualified therapist, who is following the manufacturer's instructions, using equipment which is regularly maintained, following all safety rules, and who has given a full consultation. For someone untrained, who has no qualification in beauty therapy, and has never used the machine before, the risk is much greater. This is the fundamental difference between a hazard and a risk.

The skill is not only to recognise the potential of the hazard to cause injury or harm, but to know how to act in the most sensible manner to neutralise or significantly reduce the risk.

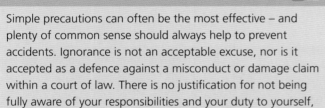

Think about it

Simple precautions can often be the most effective – and plenty of common sense should always help to prevent accidents. Ignorance is not an acceptable excuse, nor is it accepted as a defence against a misconduct or damage claim within a court of law. There is no justification for not being fully aware of your responsibilities and your duty to yourself, clients and colleagues.

Monitoring your workplace through risk assessment

Carrying out and acting upon risk assessment does not have to be complicated, but it does need to be thought through thoroughly. Be logical and do not look too hard – the obvious route is often the right one to take. Imagine making a cup of tea. What is the most hazardous part? Boiling the water and pouring it into the teapot is the most obvious answer, as boiling water has the potential to seriously burn the skin. Other risks include: a stomach upset if the milk has gone off, the handle on the teacup breaking, the teapot spout leaking – but these are secondary possibilities. Go for the main hazard, even if you think it is probably too obvious, and you cannot go far wrong.

Overview

A risk assessment is simply a careful examination of what, in your workplace, could cause harm to people, so that you can weigh up whether you have taken enough precautions or should do more to prevent harm. You are legally required to assess the risks in your workplace so that you put in place a plan to control those risks. The law does not expect you to eliminate all risk, but you are required to protect people as far as is 'reasonably practicable'.

Key terms

Management of Health and Safety at Work Regulations 1999 – legislation placing additional general requirements on employers to carry out risk assessments of reasonable foreseeable risks and to implement risk controls so far as is reasonably practicable.

Reporting of Injuries, Diseases and Dangerous Occurrences Regulations 1995 (RIDDOR) – legislation that requires the reporting of certain types of accidents and incidents.

The most important pieces of legislation concerning risk assessment for you to know about are the **Management of Health and Safety at Work Regulations 1999** and the **Reporting of Injuries, Diseases and Dangerous Occurrences Regulations 1995 (RIDDOR)**.

See 'You, your client and the law' on page 68 for detailed information.

The Health and Safety Executive is also an important source of information and support. See the five steps to risk assessment on their web site: www.hse.gov.uk.

Follow the five steps:

When carrying out a risk assessment you need to:
Step 1 Identify the hazards – make a list of the work tasks that are your responsibility
Step 2 Identify the risks – decide who might be harmed and how
Once you have recorded this information you can then:
Step 3 Evaluate the risks and decide on precautions
Finally you should:
Step 4 Record your findings and implement them
Step 5 Review your assessment and update if necessary

Steps 1 and 2 require a good look at everything you do in the salon, the equipment you use and working areas, who enters the building and so on. When that has been completed and you have identified the risks, you can then work out the likelihood of a problem occurring.

The likelihood or *probability rating* is:	**1** – *Highly unlikely* – there's a 1 in 1 million chance of the hazardous event happening **2** – *Unlikely but possible* – there's a 1 in 100,000 chance of the hazardous event happening **3** – *Probable/fairly likely* – there's a 1 in 10,000 chance of the hazardous event happening **4** – *Likely* – there's a 1 in 1000 chance of the hazardous event happening **5** – *Highly likely* – there's a 1 in 100 chance of the hazardous event happening
The consequence or *severity rating* is:	**1** – *Insignificant* – trivial injury (no first aid required) **2** – *Minor injury* – first aid required **3** – *Moderate injury* – up to three days off (or hospitalisation) **4** – *Major injury* – more than three days absence or to many persons **5** – *Catastrophic* – resulting in death (of one or more persons)
The *risk rating* is as follows:	*Low* = 1–7 *Medium* = 8–16 *High* = 17–25

The way of estimating and evaluating a risk is called a 'risk matrix' approach — it's a commonly used tool. In it you multiply the consequence of the risk by the likelihood of it occurring and you get the risk rating — see the table below.

Consequence					
5	10	15	20	25
4	8	12	16	20
3	6	9	12	15
2	4	6	8	10
1	2	3	4	5
		Likelihood		

17–25	**UNACCEPTABLE** Stop activity and make immediate improvements – someone will get hurt
10–16	**TOLERABLE** Look to improve within a specific timescale
5–9	**ADEQUATE** Look to improve at the next review
1–4	**ACCEPTABLE** No further action required, but ensure controls are maintained to a high level

Getting it right

	Where there are hazards with high likelihood and high consequences they should be managed and monitored proactively. If the machinery used is dangerous and in constant use – where there is a need for cleaning and maintenance, then it should be a high priority, e.g. a galvanic machine in a salon, or a sun bed .
	High consequence but low likelihood issues are suited to a good set of emergency plans and contingency rules. Say an electrical failure in a hospital, where it is essential that power is kept going. The same could be said for a salon – you do need a set of candles and torches for a power cut, but it is unlikely to happen.
	Low consequence issues with high likelihood are usually the ones we would come across in a salon – slips, trips and falls, things falling, and storage accidents – these can generally be solved by good housekeeping, and a little more thought.
	Low consequence and low likelihood issues are really the things we monitor for change, but can live with – there is a risk one light bulb will blow out, but it won't affect the whole salon.

So, using these ratings we can assess any of the work areas, jobs to be done and equipment. Risk assessment is really a judgement call and a risk matrix just helps reinforce what you think is a danger and what isn't. Do involve as many of the relevant people as possible, so you can view risks from all perspectives, especially if you do not actually work in the area.

The five key parts to any safety management system are:
1 Policy – have one in place to start with
2 Plan and organise – the possible people at risk and how to minimise that risk
3 Implement and operate – a safe system of working which everyone knows about
4 Measure performance – how good is it at prevention?
5 Review and control performance – has the control been sufficient to prevent an accident?

Page 94 shows a risk assessment combined with unit B20 for electrical equipment used within body massage.

Unit G22 Monitor procedures to safely control work operations

RISK ASSESSMENT

Name of equipment: infrared lamp

Step 1 what are the hazards?

- Faults with the electricity supply/faulty equipment
- Position of equipment/trailing wires/extension plugs being dangerous
- Incorrect set-up of equipment/wrong bulb being chosen or bulb not fixed in place
- Full consultation not carried out/contra-indications ignored/thermal sensitivity testing not carried out
- Treatment causing discomfort to client/skin damage caused by leaving lamp on for too long in same area/lamp too close to the skin/treatment not timed
- Risk of burning skin from the outer casing which becomes very hot

Step 2 who might be harmed?

- Client
- Therapist
- Others – in the case of fire being caused by electrical faults/burning from outer casing or touched when moving the equipment

Step 3 what is already in place?

- Equipment is PAT tested/Risk assessment book regularly updated
- Correct storage of equipment/bulb replaced regularly
- Manufacturer's instructions are always followed
- Supervision of use by a trained person
- Therapist to have correct training and follow it at all times
- Cover lamp after use with towel to warn people that it has been used
- Log time of lamp use to check the life of the bulb

Step 4 what further action could be taken?

- Risk assessment book regularly updated and easily accessible
- Regular training days/Regular PAT testing
- Allow a place where lamp can be stored safely after use, when still hot

Step 5 how will you put this assessment into action?

- Keep risk assessment book up to date
- Safe storage space for lamp to be allowed to cool down prior to moving it
- Update client details in case of adverse reaction or contra actions to treatment
- RIDDOR = Reporting of Injuries, Diseases and Dangerous Occurrences Regulations

The risk rating is:	The probability rating is:	The severity rating is:
medium	2 – possible	2 – 3 burning may occur from outer casing or from lamp bulb

A sample risk assessment form

For your portfolio

Using the risk assessment example on page 94, with the same ratings, look at one piece of equipment that you use on a regular basis. Complete the risk assessment and put it into your portfolio as an example of a risk assessment .

Promoting a safe working environment

We each have a right to work in a safe environment. A key question to ask when attending a job interview for any salon position is what staff training is available, not just for advancement of skill areas but also for health and safety training. Regular guidance for all levels of staff will help to identify and minimise the hazards.

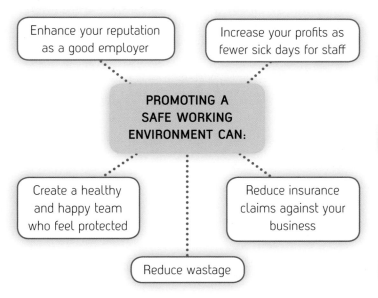

Think about it

As a Level 3 student you may be placed in a training situation and responsible for Level 1 or 2 students. If so, you will need to identify and meet their health and safety needs and ensure that they are competent in the activities they are about to carry out. It may be something as simple as using the hoover in a safe manner, or a more complex procedure such as dilution of eyelash tint or preparing an enzyme peel mask for a microdermabrasion treatment.

If you identify any additional training needs, they should be reported to the relevant person.

The salon workplace policy

A salon's workplace policy should include:

- workplace/environmental factors
- safe working methods and equipment use
- the safe use of all hazardous substances (not just for your particular job role)
- general policies for eating, smoking, drinking and drugs
- expected personal presentation
- what to do in the event of an accident, breakage or spillage
- all emergency procedures
- behaviour policies for all personnel
- corrective action where required.

If you are told at interview not to worry about any of the above, and that they really do not matter, then ask yourself, 'Do I really want to work in a place that has so little regard for the safety of its staff and clients, as well as breaking health and safety laws?'.

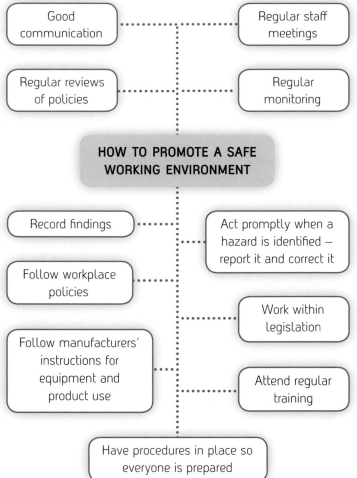

Think about it

Health and safety regulations apply to all businesses, and they should not be something merely brushed-up on where there has been an accident or near-accident at work – it should be a full-time concern.

Monitoring of the workplace

Processes and procedures need to be in place to ensure that your working environment is fit for work and does not endanger anyone coming into it. These need to be:

- carried out on a regular basis
- thorough and carefully checked
- relevant and appropriate for the hazard
- reviewed on a regular basis.

Your training establishment should also carry out a risk assessment for each class — you may not see it, as it is carried out by the lecturer, but it is regularly done.

A college monitoring sheet may look like this:

Course:		Course Code :		Day:	Time:
Hazard – likelihood	**Tick if applies**	**Tick if info leaflet given**	**Tick if specific advice given**	**Tick if formal assessment made (Head of Curriculum only)**	**Controls in place**
Slips, trips and falls					
Electrical equipment in use					
Blockage of fire escape					
Use of furniture as a hazard					
Hazardous substances					
Trailing wires					
Increased fire risk					
Fumes					
Physical exercise					
Manual handling					
Lone working					
Tools being used					
Sharp objects being used					
Ergonomics (IT)					
Food and drink (IT)					
Electrical equipment owned by tutor/student must have a valid Portable Appliance Test (PAT)					
At risk student(s) *(Give name and nature of risk - Please use separate sheet if more room is required)*					
Signature:			Date:		
Job role:					

Risk assessment for a class

Responsibilities — who does what?

The Health and Safety at Work etc.(HASAW) Act 1974 is largely about employers' responsibilities and duties, but if you are planning to run your own business one day, then you will need to know about the Act.

The general duties of employers to their employees are set down in Section 2(1) of the Act:

'It shall be the duty of every employer to ensure, so far as is reasonably practicable, the health, safety and welfare at work of all his employees.'

In addition to responsibilities to employees, an employer also has a duty to protect other persons, for example members of the public. These are stated in Section 3(1) of the Act:

'It shall be the duty of every employer to conduct his undertaking in such a way as to ensure, so far as is reasonably practicable, that persons not in his employment who may be affected thereby are not thereby exposed to risks to their health or safety.'

Self-employed people also have responsibilities under the Act which are dealt with in Section 3(2):

'It shall be the duty of every self-employed person to conduct his undertaking in such a way as to ensure, so far as is reasonably practicable, that he and other persons (not being his employees) who may be affected thereby are not thereby exposed to risks to their health or safety.'

Even if you are not planning to set up your own business, as an employee you will still have responsibilities under HASAW (see 'You, your client and the law', page 69, for your own and shared responsibilities).

Think about it

Responsibility leads to accountability — you may be able to delegate a job to someone else, but you cannot give away your accountability. You are ultimately responsible.

It is important for you to know who you should report any health and safety issues to in the salon. Salons will have different staff members covering various areas of responsibility, for example one or two staff will be trained in first aid, one person will assume responsibility for filling out the accident and report book and keeping health and safety records up to date, another will be responsible for building maintenance and replacement of light bulbs, and so on.

For your portfolio

Find out who covers which areas of responsibility in your salon. Compile a list or a flow chart of responsibility so that in the event of an incident you will know who to report any health and safety issues to.

Communicating workplace instructions to others

Not only should you be checking the workplace for risk assessments and safe practice — you should also be able to pass safe practices on. It may be as simple as a sign in the reception area, asking clients that if they have an illness or infection they should inform staff so as to prevent the spread of infection, or a sign asking clients to hang their coats up in the hall cupboard, so as not to cause obstruction, or a sign that states this is a fire door — keep clear.

Regular staff meetings will ensure that all workers understand the importance of safe working practice — and that should include all staff: caretakers, technicians, therapists, cleaners and if you are in a big health club, it should include the fitness trainers, maintenance staff and even the gardeners. In fact, the more staff and the larger the organisation, the more important good communication is.

Key terms

Workplace instructions – the salon's policies and procedures.

For your portfolio

Go to www.hse.gov.uk/betterbusiness/download.htm and customise your own HSE poster. There are seven to choose from and you can enter your own details and put in what you want it to say. You can then download it and print it off for your salon or training establishment (and put a copy in your portfolio too).

Communicating workplace policies and information

All professional salons should have a set of rules and procedures for everyone to follow. This should be common knowledge within the salon for the safety and protection of all.

By law, the salon has to display:

- health and safety rules and regulations on the wall in a prominent position
- fire evacuation procedures.

Professionally, the salon will also have:

- codes of practice to follow from its professional body with regard to set procedures
- a set of standards to maintain for insurance cover to be valid – usually linked to the codes of practice.

Legally, the employer is responsible for putting into place the rules covering the health and safety of all employees and clients and ensuring that safe practice is followed by all staff. The employee is obliged to carry out these practices by law. This will involve:

- regular training, with staff meetings to update on safety issues
- clear outlines given at the initial interview as to what is expected
- maintaining records of injuries or first aid treatment given
- monitoring and evaluating health and safety arrangements regularly
- obtaining a written health and safety booklet
- consulting the experts and being knowledgeable – ignorance is not an excuse.

Workplace policies relevant to your working practice

A salon has a legal requirement to have written risk assessments and documentation if it employs five or more people, but the sensible salon owner will have these in place regardless of how many staff are employed. Many insurance companies insist on written risk policies before they will agree to insure the business.

The other health and safety requirements for a small business are:

- to inform the Health and Safety Executive's area office or the **local authority**'s environmental health department of the business's name and address
- to inform the HSE's area office or the local authority's environmental health department of any new employees
- to display the health and safety law poster (available from the government's Stationery Office) or hand out leaflets containing the equivalent information

- to make an assessment of the risks in the workplace – which must be acted upon, and kept as a written record if there are five or more employees (this includes fire risks)
- to bring to the attention of employees a written statement of the business's health and safety policy, and keep it up to date
- to register with the local health authority, if appropriate – this will apply in particular to therapists who carry out skin piercing such as epilation.

When you inform the HSE that you are setting up a business, it may wish to check out your business premises. This will depend on the authority within your own area, and the HSE's requirements would affect you whether you work from home or in a salon.

Key terms

Local authority – local council. They employ Environmental Health Officers (EHOs) who try to protect people from environmental health hazards in their living and work surroundings. They enforce legislation such as the Health and Safety at Work Act 1974, the Food Safety Act 1990 and the Environmental Protection Act 1990. They also advise householders, shopkeepers, business owners, managers, and workers in industry.

Think about it

Although the Health and Safety Executive (HSE) is primarily concerned with the salon owner, remember that the salon owner is your employer, and therefore health and safety regulations will have a direct effect on your working environment. It is advisable to be aware of the owner's commitment to protecting you – it might influence whether you want to work in the salon, or not.

Workplace policies relevant to your job role

Take a closer look at your specific job role within the salon – could any part of your job harm yourself or others? This is not just about the treatments you carry out. For example, you could be in charge of changing light bulbs. When a bulb fails in a well-lit salon, it is not a problem, but if the only light bulb illuminating a dark stock room blows, then there is a greater risk of harm to everyone. Everyone has a responsibility to take their job role seriously – from the junior in charge of washing cups who may spread infection if her duties are not performed correctly, to the person in charge of maintaining the electrical equipment, with the potential to cause burns to a client.

Responding to breaches of health and safety

In order to respond promptly to any breaches of health and safety regulations or workplace instructions, you must first understand the types of workplace hazards you may come across. You will then be able to fully report the existence of hazards.

How many hazards are there in a beauty salon? Some of them are shown in the diagram below.

Although these are all identified as possible hazards, not all of them will occur, and certainly not all at the same time!

Some may be low risk, others may be high risk. For example, an experienced therapist may never have experienced a fire caused by faulty equipment overheating and bursting into flames. The important point is that the therapist will have recognised the possibility of faulty equipment becoming a hazard and will have her equipment checked regularly by a competent person, keep a safety log book with all equipment checks dated and signed (see Electricity at Work Regulations 1989 in 'You, your client and the law', page 76). The risk will have been minimised, and should a fire start, the logbook will show that responsibility has been taken, and the therapist/salon owner has not been neglecting their duty.

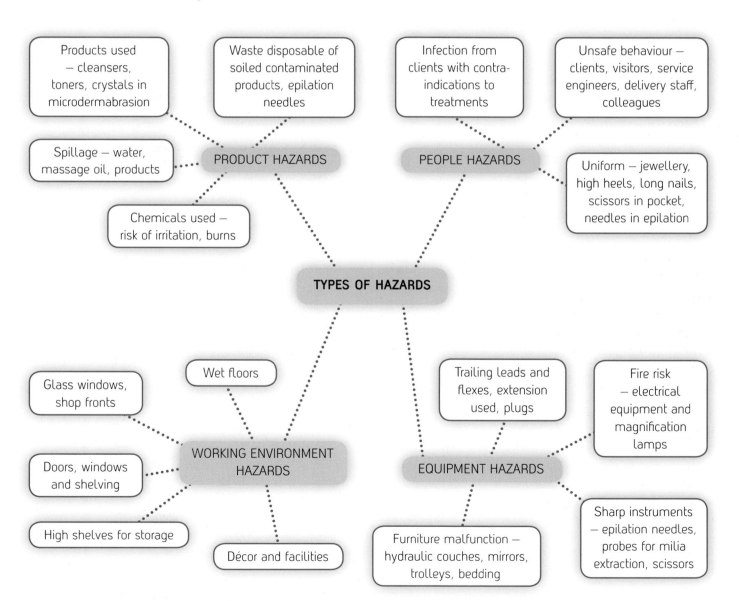

Identifying hazards in the salon

The following table gives some examples of general hazards.

Hazard and risk rating	Hazard and risk rating
The building – high risk	Floors – high risk
Checks – questions for assessment	**Checks – questions for assessment**
Is the building safe and stable? Is there any asbestos present in the roof or walls? Is the outside of the building in good repair, with no likelihood of anything falling on the client or passers-by? Is the sign for the salon secure? Are there stickers on the large salon window to avoid anyone walking into the glass? Has safety glass been used to minimise damage should an accident happen?	Are they clean and dry? Is there any spillage? Are they over-polished to become slippery? Are there any loose carpet edges or rugs to trip on? Are they hygienic and easy to clean?
Hazard and risk rating	**Hazard and risk rating**
Doorways and hallways – high risk	Windows and curtains – medium risk
Checks – questions for assessment	**Checks – questions for assessment**
Are they clear of obstructions? Is a fire exit being blocked? Are the doors too heavy to open safely?	Is any electrical equipment near a curtain which could catch fire? Are the windows safe and lockable, both for security and for sufficient ventilation and airflow?
Hazard and risk rating	**Hazard and risk rating**
General décor and facilities – low risk	Offices – medium risk
Checks – questions for assessment	**Checks – questions for assessment**
Is the paint on the walls lead-free? Are the light fittings secured? Has the wiring for lighting and plug sockets been recently checked for safety? Is the boiler regularly maintained and serviced? Are there modern gas mains and water pipes, and are they working properly?	Any trip possibilities from wires or cables? Is there any floor damage? Is the working temperature satisfactory? Any fire risk from piles of paper or over-flowing waste bins? Are fire exit routes clear? Is fire-fighting equipment in place and working? Are desks, filing cabinets and seating safe?

Identifying general hazards in the workplace

General hazards in the workplace are often out of the control of the therapist, and should be the responsibility of the salon owner, but if the sign to the salon was hanging off, ready to drop on to an unsuspecting passer-by or client, you would be neglectful if you did not report it and prevent an accident. Structural damage does happen to older buildings, and having a salon in an old building may mean that the amenities will not be modern. Older buildings can be very expensive to maintain and may present many more hazards.

The tables on the following pages give examples of hazards connected with equipment and products, and those connected with people.

Hazard and risk rating	Hazard and risk rating
Couch – high risk	Chairs – high risk
Checks – questions for assessment	**Checks – questions for assessment**
Are the brakes on? Is it at the right height for the therapist to work comfortably, and not too high for the client to get on? Is the bedding a danger by being too long and trailing on the floor ready to trip someone up? Is the bedding easily cleaned, protected during the treatment and hygienic?	Are they secured and at a suitable height? If hydraulic, are they regularly maintained? Are they stable? Are they on castors? Are they hygienic and easy to keep clean?
Hazard and risk rating	**Hazard and risk rating**
Trolleys – medium risk	Electrical appliances – very high risk (refer to individual pieces of equipment within the facial or body treatments units for specific dangers)
Checks – questions for assessment	**Checks – questions for assessment**
Are they glass-topped and liable to shatter? Are they secure on their castors? Are they regularly cared for? Are they hygienic and easy to keep clean? Are they up to the job given to them – is the equipment too heavy?	Are they regularly maintained by a competent person? Are they placed on a stable surface, rather than balanced on a window sill? Are they used by qualified personnel only? Are they stored safely? Are they used with the correct products only? Were they bought from a reputable manufacturer, to ensure safety? Are they used at the correct socket with the right plugs and fuses? Are any leads trailing?
Hazard and risk rating	**Hazard and risk rating**
Disposal of waste products – high risk	Products – very high risk
Checks – questions for assessment	**Checks – questions for assessment**
Are the correct bins available for different waste products? Is contaminated waste separated from the rest (e.g. body fluids, blood from milia extraction)? Who is responsible for disposing of the waste products and how regularly? Is infection control in place to minimise risk?	Are they clearly labelled? Are they stored safely and correctly (including toxic products)? Has a COSHH (Control of Substances Hazardous to Health) sheet been completed for each product? Do therapists know how to use them, and are they being used correctly? Are they stored in the proper containers, not in other bottles? Is the shelf life taken into account? Are lids secured properly? Is a designated first aider available in case of accidents? Do staff know what to do in case of personal injury caused by poor product use? Are correct patch tests being carried out to prevent allergic reactions? Is regular product training being offered?

Identifying equipment and product hazards

Hazard and risk rating	Hazard and risk rating
You – the therapist – high risk	Other people and visitors to the salon – very high risk
Checks – questions for assessment	**Checks – questions for assessment**
Do you lead others by showing good examples of safe working? Does your behaviour endanger others? Are you fully trained to use the equipment/products? Are you as hygienic as possible to avoid cross-infection? Do you follow the correct procedures for the workplace? Do you actively take part in regular training sessions for health and safety? Do you report possible hazards to the correct person? Is your uniform a health or safety hazard? Do you have safe shoes on? Are you wearing lots of jewellery? Do you walk around with sharp scissors in your pocket? Do you look out for the safety of others? Do you keep up-to-date client record cards? Do you use the correct lifting position when carrying heavy items?	Should they be there? Are they going to create a hazard? e.g. a service engineer carrying out a repair, with tools lying where clients are walking Do they know where they are going? Are they aware of steps, and the salon layout? Is their behaviour suitable for the salon, or are they using threatening behaviour? Is there a risk that they could steal something?

Identifying people hazards

Maintaining records

Once you understand the type of risk assessment questions you should be asking, you can then minimise the time it take you to record these findings and how you record them. All of the above questions would make a very lengthy checklist, so you need a concise safety chart with which to record your checks.

All the information above can be recorded upon a central sheet like this one:

AREA	VISUAL CHECKS	INITIALS WHEN CHECKED 8.30AM daily						ACTION REQUIRED/TYPE	URGENT YES/NO	DATE	ACTION TO:
		M	T	W	Th	F	S				
The building											
Floors											
Doorways											
Hallways											
Light bulbs											
Windows											
Curtains											
Décor											
Facilities											
Couches											
Chairs											
Trolleys											
Electrical											
Waste											
Products											
Therapists											
Other people											

WEEK BEGINNING:

Reporting hazards

Hazards can and do happen and everyone should be aware of the safety implications. As part of your personal responsibility, you will need to know which hazards you can deal with yourself immediately, or when help may be needed, and the hazard should be reported to a supervisor/lecturer/technician/manager. You need to know the level of your own authority and who else will need to be informed — doing nothing about a safety issue is not an option.

Type of hazard	Ways to avoid	When referral may be necessary
Breaches of security	Shut windows, lock cupboards and doors	When something is found open or something is believed to be missing. Full stock check required
Faulty/damaged products, tools, equipment, fixtures, fittings	Correct handling, correct storage, treat with care, follow manufacturers' instructions	When something is found to be broken
Spillage	Take care when mixing, pouring and filling, etc. – try to do it over a sink or draining board to catch any spillage	When spillage material is corrosive or irritant. When it is in the main traffic area where people may slip
Slippery floors	Make others aware by blocking the area with a chair or cone to prevent an accident, sweep up powder spills, mop up spills of liquid, refer to COSHH sheets for correct method	When acid, grease or polish is spilt
Obstruction to access and exit	Move large equipment away from doorways if able to do so, put bags and coats on a rack or shelving	When object is too heavy to be moved

Examples of hazards that should be reported

These hazards should be reported to a manager or the health and safety officer within your workplace, but there are hazards that will need to be reported to the local health officer or the HSE (see 'You, your client and the law', page 77).

Additional knowledge

Simulation

To simulate something is to recreate or mock up something. In this unit you are not permitted to simulate your evidence, so your evidence will be from actual performance and reports and carrying out risk assessments. However, simulation within the workplace is a very useful tool, and many large companies use it. For example, a company cannot set the building on fire every time they want to test their evacuation procedures, so they do a dummy run and often the local fire officers get involved, as it tests their engine response times to a fire, too. Simulation is also good when training in first aid or bomb evacuations, and the main emergency services simulate disaster scenarios so they are fully organised should a real emergency occur.

The key to these rehearsals is that you record and learn something from them — if you realise that a fire door is blocked or locked during the simulation, you learn from it and improve — after all it may saves lives in a real evacuation.

Making recommendations for change

Low-risk hazards

This is largely common sense. If the risk is low and you can deal with it straight away, then do so, and prevent an incident occurring. It could be something as simple as a client's handbag causing a minor obstruction where someone might trip over it. Pick it up off the floor, asking the client's permission where necessary, put it under the trolley out of the way and carry on with what you were doing. While this low-risk hazard does not need reporting, it still requires prompt action to prevent it becoming a more serious problem.

Always act within the policy of your workplace, so if there is a policy on where clients' handbags and coats may be stored to prevent congestion in the salon, then use the correct place.

High-risk hazards

You will need to be aware of the high-risk hazards associated with using electrical equipment, and how to deal with them. They are shown in the table below.

Identify the hazard	What is the risk?	What should I do to prevent the hazard from becoming a risk?
Frayed leads, cracked plugs, live wires showing	Electric shock/ electrocution	DO NOT USE Remove appliance from general use Label it as faulty Report it to the designated person
Trailing leads	Tripping over Electrocution Pulling the appliance over on top of the therapist or client Pulling the plug out of the socket	Use a socket nearer to you, to avoid overstretching the lead Use an extension lead and keep the flex around the perimeter of the working area
Equipment/ appliances left on after use, e.g. facial steamer or infrared lamp	Heater may burn dry Steam may scald Equipment may be an obstruction	Turn off the appliance and remove plug from socket Insulate the heated area by putting a towel over it, to show others it is hot Allow to cool and store safely

Electrical equipment hazards

For your portfolio

- What would you consider to be a low-risk hazard in your salon? Find out your salon procedure for dealing with this type of hazard.

- What do you consider to be a high-risk hazard? Write down how you would deal with this type of hazard and keep it as supplementary evidence in your portfolio.

- Where is your accident report book? What is the last entry? Fill out a sample page for a spillage incident.

Using electrical equipment

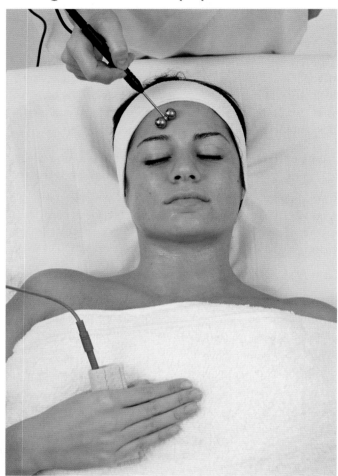

You must always consider the risks while using electrical equipment

As a Level 3 student, you will be using a large number of electrical appliances during your working day. These carry their own specific risks and records should be scrupulously maintained. Items may include:

- high frequency unit
- galvanic unit
- faradic unit
- microcurrent unit
- microdermabrasion unit
- gyrator massager
- vacuum suction unit
- infrared lamp
- audio-sonic unit
- sun beds.

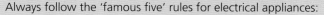

Think about it

Always follow the 'famous five' rules for electrical appliances:

1 Full consultation
2 Full contra-indication checklist
3 Always follow the manufacturer's guidelines
4 Always test equipment on yourself first
5 Never exceed client tolerance of current

This will always ensure that your treatments are risk free!

You will need to carry out sensible risk control at all times. Here are the general safety rules for all electrical appliances (for more specific ones for each individual piece of equipment, refer to the relevant unit — facial or body treatments).

General electrical safety rules

- Make sure your equipment is in a safe position in relation to your client.

- Only use equipment you have been trained and insured to use — do not 'have a go' with a piece of equipment, just because you have seen someone else do a treatment with it.

- Always follow manufacturers' instructions for treatment use, appropriate products used and storage and cleaning.

- If your salon policy for a piece of equipment varies from the manufacturers' instructions, then you must notify the designated person immediately, as there could be significant risk attached.

- Inspect equipment regularly in accordance with the Electricity at Work Regulations 1989, keep a safety check book and never use equipment you suspect may be faulty.

- Visually check the equipment prior to use — plugs and sockets should not be cracked or broken, no bare wires should be visible.

- Always carry out a full consultation and contra-indication checklist on the client prior to treatment.

- Always carry out a thermal and sensitivity test on the area to be treated.

- Always test on yourself before using the equipment on the client.

- When you have finished with equipment return all dials and settings back to '0' and leave it clean, sterile and ready for use.

- Do not overload plugs or extensions.

- Buy equipment from a reputable manufacturer who can offer after-sales and repair facilities, provide the accompanying correct products and regular updates for training.

- Store equipment safely to prolong its life and reduce fire risk. Never stack equipment on top of each other as this may break dials and knobs, reduce the effectiveness of the machine and ultimately endanger the client if the dials are not functioning correctly.

- Be careful to avoid trailing leads, which may trip people up, and moving equipment that is still plugged in.

- Always use the correct fuse in the plug — some galvanic machines, for example, require a 13-amp fuse, while some small equipment only needs a five-amp fuse.

- Never allow the client to interfere with your settings or dials — keep the controls out of reach.

- Remove all jewellery and metal objects from yourself and the client to prevent the current being attracted to the metal and causing a burn.

- Do not apply any electrical current over an open wound or broken skin, as the current will be attracted to the moisture content in the wound and cause a concentration of current to the area or a burn.

- Never exceed the client's tolerance to the intensity of the current — turn up the dials slowly and watch the client's reaction all the time. Ask for feedback on the comfort of the sensation.

- Always time the treatment and never exceed the recommended treatment time.

Make sure that risks are controlled safely and effectively

In this section you will learn about:

- keeping accurate and legible records of workplace risks
- reporting the existence of hazards and confirming precautions to control risks
- informing others and minimising risk
- reviewing operational controls to eliminate and control risks.

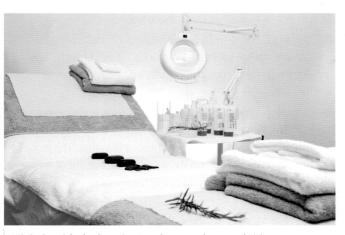

Minimise risks by keeping work areas clean and tidy

This section looks at ways of recording and controlling the risks for the hazards you identified earlier in the unit. You will need to know how to carry out risky tasks safely, following both manufacturers' instructions and your workplace requirements. You must also have a thorough understanding of the health and safety policies within your salon that affect your working day.

In the first part of this unit you looked at the various hazards and what to check for. Now you will look again at those hazards and see how to control or eliminate those risks and how to record your findings.

Keeping accurate and legible records of workplace risks

Why bother to keep records? Well, not only do you have a responsibility or moral duty to others to do so, it is also the law!

There are many ways to keep health and safety and risk assessment records:

- accident books
- control tables
- accident and illness forms for personnel
- personnel training records for first aid and risk assessment
- minutes of staff minutes
- health and safety logs for evacuation simulation
- checklists for observation risk assessments.

They don't have to be very complicated, but they do need to record the facts, dates, time of incident and they need to be legible — should a situation arise where you needed to prove that fire evacuation took place, for example.

For your portfolio

Go onto the health and safety executive website (www.hse.gov.uk/forms/) and investigate some of the ways of recording various health or safety issues. There are many forms for industry and some obviously won't relate to beauty therapy – but a lot do. There is one for communicative disease reporting, one for manual handling and the risk factors involved in lifting a heavy load, and many more. Research what is applicable to our industry and fill one out.

Reporting the existence of hazards and confirming precautions to control risks

These controls need regular reviewing to decide whether they are effective and if not, how they can be improved. There are no perfect answers, it is always a work in progress, and being refined and improved — but you cannot afford to have no controls in place and put workers and clients at risk.

For your portfolio

Using the table on page 107, work out what controls you need for the following:

lack of appropriate resources, poor performance at work, inadequate staffing levels, inadequate training, instruction or information, inadequate maintenance, inadequate policy/ procedure.

Think about it

Refer back to Professional basics, 'You, your client and the law', page 68, for a refresher on the relevant legislation relating to hazards and risks. But remember not to exceed your level of authority when identifying and reporting the existence of hazards. You will need to keep the appropriate person informed, i.e. the health and safety officer, who will confirm that appropriate precautions have been taken.

Work area _____   Date of assessment _____

Assessor's name _____   Position _____

Hazard Potential to cause harm	Does this apply ? (tick)	Precautions to control risks Some examples have been given here
1 Fall of client from the couch, bed or chair – risk of personal injury		Falls assessment, use of cot sides, use of adjustable height beds and electronic couches, never leaving the client unsupervised
2 Fall of object or material from a height – risk of personal injury		Good housekeeping arrangements, tidy storage of materials in cupboards, using a step to reach higher shelves to prevent over-stretching
3 Slip, trip or fall of person – risk of personal injury		Falls assessments, access routes kept clear, surfaces maintained in good repair, use of warning signs
4 Manual handling of large or heavy objects – risk of personal injury, non-compliance with health and safety legislation		Manual handling policy, handling risk assessments, training and use of appropriate handling aids
5 Use of electrical equipment – risk of personal injury, non-compliance with health and safety legislation		Regular electrical checks and safe use training
6 Fire – risk of personal injury, damage to property, non-compliance with health and safety legislation		Fire policy, fire risk assessments, fire prevention techniques, training and fire drills to assess effectiveness of evacuation procedures
7 Exposure to noise – risk of personal injury, non-compliance with health and safety legislation		Risk assessment of noise levels, allocation of noise zones, and provision and use of PPE
8 Exposure to/contact with biological agents e.g. clinical waste – risk of personal injury, ill health, non-compliance with health and safety legislation		Infection control policy, training, provision and use of PPE and appropriate storage and collection procedures
9 Inappropriate lighting levels – risk of personal injury, non-compliance with health and safety legislation		Risk assessment, monitoring of lighting fixtures, fittings and light bulbs, and PPM
10 Work in confined spaces – risk of personal injury, non-compliance with health and safety legislation		Safe working system, provision and use of safety equipment
11 Use of display screen equipment (DSE or VDU) risk of personal injury, non-compliance with H&S legislation		Display screen equipment (DSE) policy, risk assessment, safety training and provision and use of 'fit for purpose' equipment
12 Lone working – risk of personal injury, ill health,		Personal safety policy, risk assessment, training, use of appropriate equipment e.g. mobile phones, panic alarm button
13 Exposure to violence or aggression – risk of personal injury, ill health		Personal safety policy, risk assessment and training, environmental audit programme
14 Exposure to needles or other medical sharps – risk of personal injury, ill health		Infection control policy, needlestick procedure, immunisation programme, provision and use of suitable containers and disposal processes
15 Poor communication – organisational risk which could result in a lack of understanding with adverse consequences		Effective communication skills training, adequate record keeping and clear lines of responsibility
16 Lack of consultation/contra-indications for client – risk to the client leading to a possible adverse outcome, risk to organisation for adverse publicity and/or compensation claim		Competent staff and adequate skill mix, full training, use of appropriate diagnostic tests and equipment, correct paperwork generated, record cards up to date, legible, correct and thorough, effective lines of communication with staff
17 Lack of appropriate policy/procedures – risk to the client leading to a possible adverse outcome, risk to organisation for adverse publicity and/or compensation claim		Risk assessment, policy development, implementation and monitoring programme
18 Lack of training – organisational risk which could lead to a personal injury/ill health, non-compliance with health and safety legislation		Risk assessment, adequate resources, suitable training venues and attendance monitoring programmes
19 Breach of confidentiality – organisational risk which could result in legal action or adverse publicity		Data Protection legislation, training, suitable record keeping and storage arrangements
20 Client record cards unavailable for consultation – risk to client of inappropriate treatment/care, risk to organisation, adverse publicity and/or compensation claim		Timely appointment scheduling, effective lines of communication, receptionist training, suitable access arrangements for client record cards with central storage
21 Consent – organisational risk which could result in adverse publicity, and/or compensation claims		Consent policy, use of correct consent forms for minors, and training
22 Stress – risk of ill health to staff, non-compliance with health and safety legislation, compensation claims against the business		Risk assessment, monitoring of workloads, and working conditions, good communication with line managers, regular appraisals for training needs and support given Adequate financial resources and a recruitment programme

An example of a work area safety assessment form

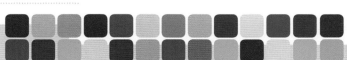

ACCIDENT / ILLNESS
REPORT FORM

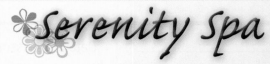

Serenity Spa

This form is to be completed by the injured party. If this is not possible, the form should be completed by the person making the report. If more than one person was injured, please complete a separate form for each person.

Completing and signing this form does not constitute an admission of liability of any kind, either by the person making the report or any other person.

This form should be completed immediately and forwarded to the Health and Safety Officer and Salon Manager.

If it is possible that an accident has been caused by a defect in machinery, equipment or a process, isolate / fence off the area and contact the Health and Safety Officer or Manager immediately.

SECTION 1 PERSONAL DETAILS

Surname: _Fabrizio_ (Mr/Mrs/Ms/Miss) Forename(s): _Julia_

Date of birth: _29/01/57_ Address: _27 Ash Grove, Birmingham_

STAFF ☐   CONTRACTOR ☐   VISITOR ☐   GENERAL PUBLIC ☑

SECTION 2 ACCIDENT / INCIDENT / ILLNESS DETAILS

Accident (Injury) ☑   Illness ☐   Date: _19/04/10_   Time: _13:07_ (24-hour clock)

Location: _Saloon room 4_

Nature of injury or condition and the part of the body affected:
Slipped on floor, hit elbow on trolley, possible dislocation

Account

Describe what happened and how. In the case of an accident state clearly what the injured person was doing. _Small patch of water on the floor - client got off couch_
and slipped on it

Name and address of adult witness(es): _Camilla Neal, Serenity Spa_

Details of action taken

Ambulance summoned ☑   Taken to hospital ☐   Sent to hospital ☐

First aid given ☐   Taken home ☐   Sent home ☐   Returned to work ☐

SECTION 3 PREVENTATIVE ACTION

Recommended: _to ensure that all spillages are mopped up straight away_

Implemented: (Yes)/ No   Date: _19/04/10_

Report raised by

Name: _Willena Simons_

Position: _Therapist_

Signature: _W Simons_   Date: _19/04/10_

FOR OFFICE USE ONLY
Copy sent to: Salon Manager ☐
Health and Safety Officer ☐

An accident report form

Informing others and minimising risk

There are many methods of informing other people of risks and you should take care to pass on information quickly and clearly. You must also know the actions you can take to minimise risks, without exceeding your level of authority.

The following tables contain ideas on controlling general risks in the workplace, risks from equipment and products, and from people.

Hazard	Control by taking the following actions
The working environment (the building)	Property owner's liability insurance, often known as buildings insurance, guards against claims relating to damage to the outside of the salon building, roof repairs, wall repairs, etc. Internal major fittings such as toilet facilities and kitchens are also often covered. Regularly maintain and check the outside of the property and repair minor damage before it becomes a major hazard.
Floors	Only use the correct products for floor cleaning and allow plenty of time to dry. Major stripping and recovering of the floor surface can be done outside normal salon times. Repair or avoid carpets and rugs with frayed edges and those not easily kept clean. Pay for professional cleaning companies to chemically clean carpets outside of normal salon hours.
Doorways and hallways	Have a regular inspection from your local fire safety officer who will advise the salon on the correct exit route in case of fire. Keep corridors tidy and clutter free.
Windows and curtains	Keep all electrical equipment away from the window area. Employ a tradesperson to ensure the windows open, are hinged properly and are safe and secure. Invest in double-glazing if possible, or carefully maintain older-style windows. Loose windows are the ideal entry for a potential thief.
General décor and facilities	Invest in safe decorating products bought from a reputable DIY store. Regularly check and maintain the utility services – many of them provide a regular service agreement for a yearly maintenance of gas and electricity parts (boilers and central heating, etc.).

Minimising risks in the workplace

Hazard	Minimise risk by taking the following actions
Couch	Buy from professional suppliers only, with guarantees and maintenance and repair agreements. Ensure the couch is the correct height to avoid back problems and buy an adjustable one where possible. Use protective coverings, which are washable, and minimise the risk of cross-infection by regularly disinfecting the couch and covering.
Chairs	As above. The recommended chair for use by professionals is the five-castor movable chair with adjustable height and backrest, often called the 'super secretarial chair'. Test out whether the height of the chair is suitable for you by sitting squarely with your bottom at the back of the chair, and your feet firmly flat on the floor. Regularly maintain the chair and lubricate the castors.
Trolleys	Ensure that all legs are secure and that castors are properly fixed. Never use a glass-topped trolley for equipment that becomes hot. Never overload a trolley. Evenly distribute the weight of equipment. Never push a trolley containing hot equipment – if you drag it, you will have more control. Always remember that a trolley can move – never use it as a work surface.
Electrical appliances	As above. Always buy from a reputable manufacturer who provides training, suitable products, an after-sales service, repairs and servicing. Have the equipment tested by a competent person, keep a log book of testing, dated and signed, with a system of labelling and for removing faulty equipment from use. Regular training updates for all staff as well as fire-fighting training, use of an extinguisher, and knowledge of who to report to in case of an electrical fire.

Continued

Hazard	Minimise risk by taking the following actions
Disposal of waste products	Clinical waste (waste which consists wholly or partly of animal or human tissue, blood or other bodily fluids, swabs, dressings, syringes or needles) to be kept apart from the general waste and be disposed of to a licensed incineration or landfill site by a licensed company. Subcontract the disposal of waste to a local firm, who will take away yellow bins with contaminated waste and replace them either daily or weekly. This can be expensive, but is a good service.
Products	Keep manufacturers' data sheets and ensure that their products are used in accordance with the manufacturers' recommendations. COSHH sheets have a space for the recommended first aid treatments if the product comes in contact with the skin, is ingested or spits into the eye. Learn these and be prepared for any eventuality. Ensure caustic ingredients are stored in clearly labelled and easily identifiable bottles or tubs. Keep thorough and up-to-date record cards for clients' treatments and products, especially if there has already been a reaction or allergy to a particular product, or if the client has a severe allergy to a specific substance such as nuts. Regularly attend commercial training courses to keep abreast of new products, and never guess a product use or equipment usage.

Minimising equipment and product risks

Hazard	Minimise risk by taking the following actions
Visitors	Be informed about visitors to the salon. Many salons employ a badge system to identify visitors, sales reps, tradespeople, delivery drivers, and so on. Do not be intimidated by a person shouting or abusive behaviour. Firmly ask them to leave, or consult with the manager/salon owner, and if necessary, call the police. Minimise the risk of client harm by asking tradespeople to carry out repairs in the quieter part of the day or when the salon is closed. Major repairs would necessitate the salon being closed, as the clients' safety must not be compromised.

Minimising risks from people visiting the salon

You should now begin to see that you can minimise the risk of harm, by following some basic steps, being responsible and thinking about your actions.

Refer back to Professional basics, 'You — the therapist', page 5, for information on ensuring your personal presentation does not present a risk.

Think about it

Occupational accidents kill over 300 people and injure over one million every year. Over two million people suffer illnesses caused, or made worse, by their work.

Young workers have 50 per cent more accidents than older workers (European Agency for Safety and Health at Work 2006).

Preventing accidents and ill health caused by work is a key priority for everyone at work. Competent employees are valuable.

Reviewing operational controls to eliminate and control risks

Remember to regularly review your operational controls. This will ensure that workplace hazards can be quickly eliminated or controlled to a manageable level whilst not endangering yourself, other staff or the public.

Hazard notices

- Vehicles and transport
- Lighting
- Computer workstations
- Bullying
- Doors
- Temperature
- Housekeeping
- Heights
- Slips and trips
- Electricity
- Aggression or violence
- Fire
- Noise and vibration
- Stress
- Manual lifting
- Chemicals, and harmful substances

Vehicles and transport

When people and transport are put together there is always potential for an accident. If your salon or training establishment has a car park, it should be well lit and well signposted, with traffic flow in one direction and speed restrictions, with well defined road markings and parking bays. All of this minimises the hazards.

Lighting

Poor quality lighting, whether it be too bright and blinding or too dim, can lead to any number of hazards, especially on stairs and in storage cupboards, or working with equipment. Outside the salon, pavements may be uneven and if unlit, a hazard.

Computer stations

Eye strain, back injuries and upper limb disorders can occur after extended periods of computer use. Keep an eye on reception staff and make sure their workstation is at the right height, user friendly and that they have enough breaks.

Bullying

Bullying can take many forms — constant criticism of a staff member who is actually competent, blocking promotions, racism, shouting at staff, persistently picking on one person, ignoring people, making jokes at another's expense. None of these occurrences should be tolerated in the workplace. Symptoms of bullying show as: anxiety, headaches, skin rashes, irritable bowel syndrome, tearfulness and a loss of self-confidence. If a staff member is off sick due to stress, they may be a victim of bullying.

Doors

Be aware of staff facing hazards when they open a door, especially if it is two-way traffic and someone is coming the other way, perhaps with a hot wax pot in their hand. Heavy doors and very light doors present a hazard.

Housekeeping

Keeping any work area clean and free from spillages can reduce all sorts of hazardous events occurring. Encourage team members in the salon to be clean, tidy and hygienic — right down to cups being washed promptly and rubbish being emptied on a regular basis.

Temperature

Make sure staff have a comfortable temperature to work within, and take care in very hot tasks and working areas, such as a sauna, swimming pool or wet area, or a room with no outside ventilation or light. (See 'You, your client and the law', page 72, for further information on heat stress and symptoms.)

Heights

Although it is fairly obvious, height is a real danger — both to work within or for storage of equipment. If you do need to go up a ladder, make sure you are properly trained and heavy items are not stored at such a height that is dangerous to retrieve them.

Slip and trips

You cannot afford to ignore trips and slips — we constantly remind students about trailing leads with electrical treatments and pulling equipment along when it is still plugged in at the wall — but that is exactly how a hazard causes broken bones and other injuries. Avoid uneven surfaces, follow designated routes, and mop up spillages at once. According to the HSE, slips and trips account for 33 per cent of all reported major injuries.

Electricity

Electricity is such a hazard and yet we all use it every day with quite a casual attitude! We tend to take it for granted, but it can cause shocks, burns and fires. Most beauty equipment relies on electricity as its source of power so hazard warnings should be used to alert users to the danger.

Aggression and violence

Verbal abuse, threats and even physical attacks are a hazard when people work with other people and the general public. You are more at risk of violence if you handle money, deal with complaints, work alone or work unsociable hours — so a receptionist should be aware of the hazards of going to the bank at the same time every day, and have a change of routine. Some form of protection, another person, or a better system — such as the bank providing a collection service and coming to the salon — could also be considered.

Fire

You can reduce the hazards of fire in two main ways — by preventing a fire starting in the first place, and by having procedures in place for safe evacuation with regular practices.

Chemical and harmful substances

Chemicals can be absorbed through the skin, breathed in and/or swallowed, causing ill health and injury. Know the dangers, use caution, and wear appropriate protective equipment.

The warning signs shown on page 112 are used to identify different types of harmful substances.

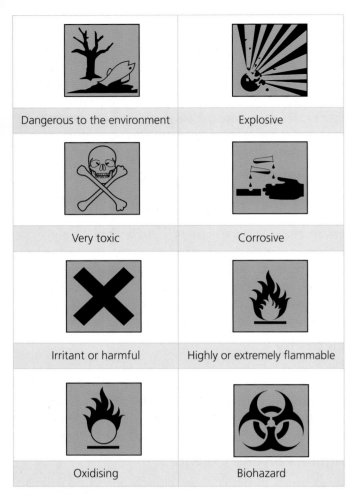

Dangerous to the environment	Explosive
Very toxic	Corrosive
Irritant or harmful	Highly or extremely flammable
Oxidising	Biohazard

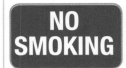

Red signs – these are prohibition signs. This means you are not allowed to do something (such as smoking, as shown here). Other common prohibition signs are no access for pedestrians or vehicle access. Red signs are also used for fire-fighting equipment.

Blue signs – these are mandatory signs. Something you must do (like washing your hands as illustrated). All PPE would come under these signs.

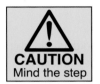

Yellow or amber signs – these are used as warning signs for hazards such as a step, a wet floor, electricity, radioactive materials and biological risks.

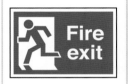

Green signs – these signs are for emergency escape routes in the event of a fire, and first aid provisions, such as first aid posts or emergency showers.

Stress

Excessive pressure and demanding workloads can cause both emotional and physiological problems, so try and keep stress under control – this is a valid hazard in the workplace and although it is invisible, it can be highly damaging to health.

Manual handling

Lifting, lowering, carrying, pushing, pulling or twisting are major causes of muscular and skeletal damage. Hazard signs will make people aware of this and training should be given – and proper steps put in place – for safety.

Safety signs

Safety signs play an important part in communicating health and safety information to everyone. Signs need to be provided whenever there is a hazard that hasn't been fully controlled in other ways. Make sure all of the team understands the meaning of the signs.

Think about it

If during the course of your commercial training you discover any conflict between manufacturers' instructions and your workplace/legal requirements, it must be reported immediately to people responsible for health and safety. If instructions conflict, confusion will result and possibly endanger yourself or others.

Workplace policies

In this section you will learn about:

- the premises
- stock and products
- use of materials and hazardous substances
- smoking, eating, drinking and drugs.

Most colleges and workplaces have policies on the following issues.

The premises

For insurance and mortgage applications, the salon owner must have adequate security measures in place. It is advisable to consult the local crime prevention officer who will come and survey the premises and give advice regarding the most vulnerable areas and the most common forms of entry by a burglar.

Externally

- Deadlocks on all doors and windows will make it more difficult for a burglar to enter the premises.
- Double-glazing is expensive but is more difficult to break into — the older the window and frame, the easier the entry.
- A burglar alarm, or even a dummy box on the wall, often deters a burglar.
- Closed circuit television (CCTV) may be available if the premises are in a shopping area with other stores.
- Premises with metal shop-front shutters offer the most effective deterrent to a burglar.

Internally

- Internal doors can be locked at night to prevent an intruder moving from room to room.
- Fire doors and emergency exits should be locked at night and re-opened by the first person in at the start of business every morning.
- A light left on in reception may also deter would-be burglars who might feel that well-lit premises will make them more visible.
- Stock and money should be locked away or put in the bank. Nothing should be visible to entice a burglar to break in in the first place!
- Expensive equipment should be locked away in treatment rooms or in the stock cupboard.

Very large businesses often employ security guards to patrol their premises at night, but along with alarmed infrared beams, these are not affordable for the average small salon owner. If, however, the salon is situated within a shopping centre or business park, night patrols may be included in the lease or purchase agreement or be offered for a set fee per year. Costs would need to be considered, but it may be an investment and save money in the long term.

Stock and products

This includes products on display and those used in the treatment rooms. Of all the temptations to the thief, these smaller items may prove irresistible — they are small enough for a pocket, and are very accessible. Unfortunately, this form of shoplifting costs many businesses a great deal of money, as stock can be expensive to replace and can be a big part of the capital outlay of a salon.

Another sad fact is that the average 'thief' may be rather closer to home than is comfortable. Staff may 'borrow' an item of stock for home use, and think that this behaviour is acceptable. Also, some clients may like the look of a lipstick and 'forget' to pay for it!

Whether items are shoplifted or pilfered, either way it means the salon has bought an item of stock from the wholesaler that it has not been paid for by its customer, so it has to absorb that financial loss. If left unchecked, this could eventually bankrupt the business.

Tight precautions are called for, including the following.

- Make one member of staff, usually a senior therapist or senior receptionist, responsible for stock control — she should be the only one with keys and access to stock.
- Carry out a regular stock check — daily for loss of stock and weekly for stock ordering and rotation.
- Use empty containers for displays, or ask the suppliers if they can provide dummy stock — this will also save the product deteriorating while on display.
- Encourage staff and customers to keep handbags away from the stock area, usually reception, to stop products 'dropping' into open bags.
- Have one member of staff responsible for topping up the treatment products from the wholesale-sized tubs.
- Hold regular staff training on security and let staff know what the losses are and how it may affect them — some companies offer bonus schemes for reaching targets of both sales and minimising pilfering. Heavy losses may affect potential salary increases.
- Carry out banking of money in the till at different times of the day and do not keep too much money in the till at any one time.

Reducing risks to staff safety

See 'You — the therapist', page 10, for information on personal security and safety.

Use of materials and hazardous substances

There are numerous substances within the salon which are considered to be hazardous to health, from caustic cleaning products and dishwasher tablets, to beauty products used in Level 3 treatments.

For your own and others' safety, follow these safety rules.

- Always follow manufacturers' instructions.
- Always read instructions and mixing labels carefully to get the correct and safe recipe.
- Report any differences between the manufacturers' instructions and your salon guidelines.
- Be informed and knowledgeable on COSHH regulations and read the COSHH sheets for your particular area of work.
- Use personal protective equipment (PPE) where possible — it should be provided for you.
- Never use products or chemicals on broken skin.

Provide eye pads for the client (cotton wool rounds) when using products on the face, especially exfoliants, brush cleansing or when carrying out treatments such as direct high frequency. Provide goggles for ultraviolet and infrared treatments. Be trained and be safe!

Think about it

If there is any doubt about the client's tolerance to a product, do a skin test 24 hours prior to the treatment. Some galvanic gels, for example, are quite strong, and may cause reactions on more sensitive skins. Check for any reaction, erythema, itchiness or stinging and burning sensations on the area of the patch test.

Store products correctly to stop them deteriorating and reacting. A cool dark place is essential, in containers with tight lids. Those products which react to temperature changes or to heat will need to be kept in a fridge.

Decant products with a spatula into a smaller bowl or dish, and never pour used products back into the main jar — the contamination will ruin the whole lot. Never use your fingers in products for the same reason.

Never use a product past its use-by date or one that has started to deteriorate or react, has an unpleasant odour or has lost its natural consistency. If a product starts to separate and become watery, then it is not useable and may cause a reaction.

Do not guess quantities or measurements, or substitute chemicals if what you require is unavailable.

Smoking, eating, drinking and drugs

Smoking

Cigarette smoking is recognised as a potential health risk, and there are safety risks attached to the use of chemicals and products. Not only has smoking been proven to be dangerous to the health of the smoker, it also has implications for the passive smoker, the person inhaling the smoke just by being in the area.

In a beauty salon it would be unusual to allow smoking, both for staff and for clients, not only for the health and safety risks but also for hygiene reasons and the lingering odour of cigarette smoke. A beauty salon is all about cleansing and nourishing the body, relaxing the mind and replenishing the soul — a smoky atmosphere would be in direct conflict with this ethos.

From the therapist's point of view, it is unprofessional to smoke at work — it leaves an unpleasant odour on clothing, on hair and on the breath. A client having a body massage or facial would certainly not appreciate the essence of smoke oozing from the therapist's every pore! A salon owner or manager might recommend to employees who smoke that the risks are too great at work, but they cannot dictate what the therapist does during her spare time.

The introduction of the Health Act 2006 also makes it illegal to smoke in enclosed work spaces — i.e. buildings. A beauty salon certainly comes under this classification. See 'You, your client and the law' for more details on the Act, page 74.

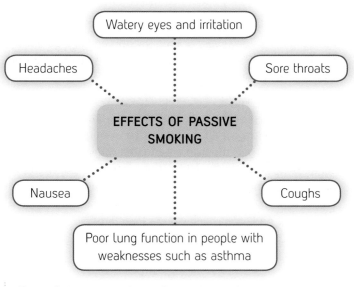

Effects of cigarette smoke on the passive smoker

For the client, smoking may undo all the good work carried out by the therapist and act against the treatment. Smoking robs the skin of vital oxygen; it causes dehydration, and can prematurely age the skin on the face. The therapist can only strongly recommend to the client that, like a healthy diet, moderate exercise and drinking lots of water, giving up smoking would greatly improve the client's health and sense of well-being.

Your employer has a duty under the Health and Safety at Work etc. Act 1974 to protect non-smoking employees from the hazards of tobacco smoke. Their duty of care also extends to clients and others who enter the salon (see 'You, your client and the law', page 68).

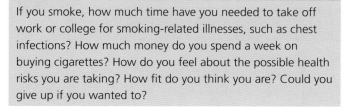

Think about it

If you smoke, how much time have you needed to take off work or college for smoking-related illnesses, such as chest infections? How much money do you spend a week on buying cigarettes? How do you feel about the possible health risks you are taking? How fit do you think you are? Could you give up if you wanted to?

Think about it

Discarded, still-lit cigarettes and accidentally dropped cigarettes on furniture or in a paper bin, are among the most common causes of fire, certainly domestic fires. A smoke detector which is in full working order can and does save lives.

Eating

Eating in the salon is very unprofessional, and is a potential health risk for germs, with the added risk of spillage, causing slippery floors.

Therapists should have an eating area and proper storage facilities for food, such as a fridge and cupboards, but it needs careful management to prevent stale food accumulating and causing a health risk. One staff member needs to be in charge of kitchen duties, cleaning out the fridge weekly and replenishing tea, coffee, milk, and so on. Some salons offer drinks and light refreshments to clients, and care must be taken to minimise the risk of infection, by thoroughly washing all glasses, cups and cutlery, ideally on a hot cycle in a dishwasher.

Drinking

Providing drinks in the salon for clients has a high risk factor for spillage and infection from dirty cups and glasses. A hot drink may be split onto a client, causing scalds, and drinks may easily be spilt on the floor, causing a hazard. There should be a staff member in charge of the drinks arrangements, as electric kettles and coffee percolators also have an electrical risk factor, and need to be regularly maintained and replenished when necessary.

Alcoholic drinks are consumed less frequently in business. Many companies are alcohol-free and expect staff not to consume alcohol during the working day. Alcohol lowers concentration levels, relaxes the body and lowers the reflexes, which is a considerable risk to the client, salon and therapist, especially when using electrical equipment. The traditional cheese and wine opening of a salon has largely been replaced with soft drinks and demonstrations, which also discourages the client from drinking and then driving home. Certainly, no machinery should be operated under even the smallest influence of alcohol.

Too much alcohol can have health effects which may act against salon treatments. Going over the recommended 14 units per week for a female or 21 units for a male (a unit being half a pint of lager, or a small glass of wine) can affect the absorption of vitamins, dull the hair and skin, dehydrate the skin, and stop the liver from functioning properly. Moderation should be the advice given to clients, so that their salon treatments give the body maximum advantage.

Think about it

A hangover from the previous night out can mean you are still over the drink-driving limit in the morning, and may seriously affect your capacity to work correctly.

Drugs

If you have to take medication prescribed by a doctor, ask about all the possible side-effects. For example, hay fever tablets can leave you feeling drowsy and tired, affecting concentration levels — this is a possible risk. If you combine those with a mild sleeping tablet, or an over-the-counter preparation to calm you down, the effects are doubled, as they are both sedatives, and you should not be driving, let alone operating electrical equipment on a client. If in doubt, do not mix medicines, and ask your local pharmacist about possible side-effects. You should always inform your

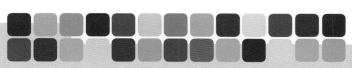

employer about any medication you are taking, and your workload may have to be adjusted for the duration of the treatment.

Using recreational drugs while working in the salon is just not safe. All recreational drugs are hazardous as they stay in the system for up to 48 hours, which can lead to accidents, errors in judgement and poor performance. There is a strong possibility of absenteeism, which affects every member of staff and inconveniences clients, through cancellations and late appointments, and it is not good for the reputation of any business. Drug-taking affects the personality, producing mood swings, hyperactivity, depression, and manic episodes — none of which create the right customer care environment to enhance and develop a business.

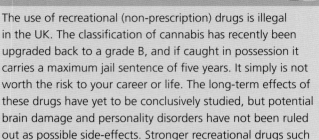

Think about it

The use of recreational (non-prescription) drugs is illegal in the UK. The classification of cannabis has recently been upgraded back to a grade B, and if caught in possession it carries a maximum jail sentence of five years. It simply is not worth the risk to your career or life. The long-term effects of these drugs have yet to be conclusively studied, but potential brain damage and personality disorders have not been ruled out as possible side-effects. Stronger recreational drugs such as ecstasy and cocaine have caused death.

Check your knowledge

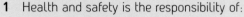

1   Health and safety is the responsibility of:
   a) the salon owner
   b) the therapist
   c) everyone
   d) the manager.

2   A hazard is defined as:
   a) something which has the potential to cause harm
   b) something which is a risk
   c) an action which reduces or controls or minimises
   d) an obligation to prove what is alleged.

3   Criminal law deals with:
   a) disputes between individuals or organisations
   b) punishing people for committing offences
   c) bullying in the workplace
   d) punishing people for poor performance.

4   How many people leave the workforce every year through harm suffered at work?
   a) 30,000
   b) 10,000
   c) 25,000
   d) 5000

5   The law concerned with carrying out risk assessments is:
   a) Management of Harm and Risk Regulations 1999
   b) Management of Work and Employers 1999
   c) Management of Hazards and Risk Regulations 1999
   d) Management of Health and Safety at Work Regulations 1999.

6   HSE stands for:
   a) Hazards and Safety Equality
   b) Health and Scary Equity
   c) Hazards and Safeguard Executive Council
   d) Health and Safety Executive.

7   Environmental Health Officers (EHOs) work for:
   a) the local authority
   b) the Health and Safety Council
   c) the local cleaning company
   d) the National Health Service.

8   RIDDOR stands for:
   a) Reporting of Incidences, Death and Dangerous Occupations Regulations 1995
   b) Reporting of Injuries, Diseases and Dangerous Occurrences Regulations 1995
   c) Reporting of Important Diseases and Dangerous Occasions Regulations 1995
   d) Reporting of Incidents, Death and Dangerous Occupancy Regulations 1995

9   Public Liability Insurance covers a therapist from:
   a) a possible action for harm caused in a treatment
   b) a road traffic accident
   c) the building catching fire
   d) a possible action against the shop sign falling on a client.

10 The number of steps in a risk assessment is:
   a) 4   c) 6
   b) 5   d) 7

Getting ready for assessment

As Unit G22 covers the importance of health and safety in the workplace and taking action to control workplace hazards, it is likely that this unit will link into all the other areas of your practical assessments. For example, if you are being assessed for the safe use of electrical equipment in Unit B14, link in a G22 assessment – especially if you need to maintain records of faulty equipment, spillage, faulty or damaged goods which may cause harm or if you identify any one at risk; for example, an elderly client with limited mobility who needs to go down some steps. There may be quite a few everyday occurrences in the salon which will qualify as evidence for Unit G22. You will be assessed on your competency and capability to deal with these types of health and safety responsibilities.

You will also be assessed via direct observation from your assessor and you may also contribute to your portfolio with witness testimony from your workplace, any courses you may have attended regarding health and safety and specialty training. Professional discussion, questions and answers, personal reports and risk assessment reports are also valid evidence.

Unit H32

Contribute to the planning and implementation of promotional activities

What you will learn:
- Making recommendations
- Identifying your SMART objectives
- Target groups/client profiles
- Agreeing requirements for the activity
- Producing a plan
- Meeting your planned timescale

Implementing promotional activities
- Implementing and adapting promotional activities
- Promotions and methods of communication
- Essential features and benefits of products and services
- Logical steps in promotion
- Clearing away to meet the venue requirements

Participating in the evaluation of promotional activities
- Methods of feedback
- Collating and recording information
- Participating in discussions

Introduction

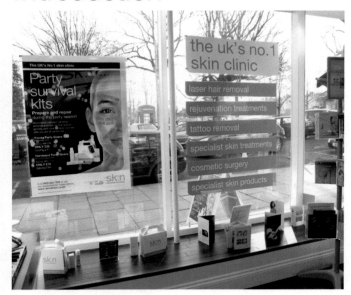

Level 3 treatments offer a vast range of additional products and services for the benefit of the client. It is essential for the growth of the business to keep the client knowledgeable and informed about all the possible treatments and products available within the salon. This should be done by having a **promotional strategy** for the year, for new products being launched and for the promotion of business when trade is slow. It is not only helpful for the client, allowing him or her to make informed choices, it is also essential if the business is to survive in a very competitive market place.

Promotions generate enthusiasm in the team and give therapists a chance to showcase their skills. This unit looks at the promotional side of the beauty therapy business. Think of promotion as information for your clients: it is for their benefit and to enhance their treatment choices, and to ensure they gain maximum benefit from the range of treatments on offer. It's not just about selling products to clients — although that is an essential part of the business; it is about promoting your services, enhancing your business image, informing clients who and where you are and expanding your business.

Contributing to the planning and preparation of promotional activities

In this section you will learn about:

- making recommendations
- identifying your SMART objectives
- target groups/client profiles
- agreeing requirements for the activity
- producing a plan
- meeting your planned timescale.

Making recommendations

Planning a suitable, workable promotion takes a lot of time and effort. Careful planning is essential for it all to go smoothly and the devil is certainly in the details! Once you have an idea or the beginning of one, you need to take it to the right person and book an informal appointment to discuss your ideas and how you intend to carry them out. That person may be a marketing manager in a large organisation, or your salon manager or owner, but all managers will be open to suggestions on increasing sales and making the public more aware of your business. However, your idea should be well thought through, and not just a vague scheme of advertising on the moon surface or something equally unachievable!

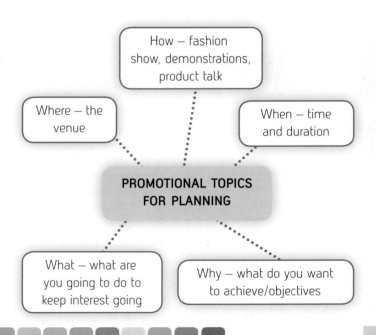

Unit H32

Contribute to the planning and implementation of promotional activities

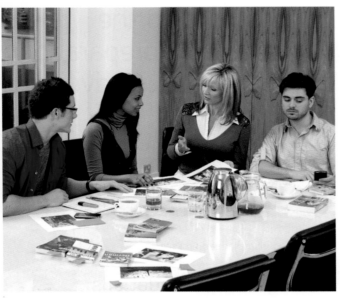

Planning together will produce more ideas

The legal aspect
— health and safety,
insurance

Potential hazards —
parking, transport, easy
access, packing and
unpacking stock

The cost
involved/budget

Stock to support
promotion

Materials — price
lists, flyers, discount
vouchers, gift
vouchers

**THE DETAILS OF
THE PROMOTION**

Team work — who
does what

Payment of staff —
cleaners, decorators,
caretakers

Tools, equipment
and materials

Linking your
promotion with
others, e.g. bridal
shops, florists,
chiropractors or
health clubs

Advertising — How
to promote the
promotion

Almost the first thing a manager is going to want to know is how much it will cost. Admittedly, some of the top cosmetic and perfume houses spend millions of pounds on television promotions and advertising, especially at Christmas time — but that is unrealistic for the average salon. After all, the end result is to make the business more profitable and increase brand awareness, not bankrupt it through spending too much.

Often a brainstorming session with lots of staff in a meeting will bring up good ideas, and as a team you can verbally plan things through before you commit to pen and paper. There are key things you need to think about and agree on or discount, before you move on to the nuts and bolts of planning.

Your notes may well look something like this:

Topic	Things to plan for and consider
The Where	Which venue? In the salon or hiring a hall or hotel suite to accommodate more people? The practical requirements: health and safety, fire evacuation, first aid cover, parking, disabled access, seating arrangements, lighting, heating, PA sound systems, music, microphones, **by-laws** and legislation, potential hazards such as steps and a stage. People to support the venue: cleaners, caretakers, catering staff, kitchens, locking up and cleaning up.
The When	What is the best time and duration? Daytime or evening? How long, to keep clients interested? Which events will do this? Changing of demonstrations to keep interest keen. Not too early so that people are still at work, not too late so that people won't want to come out. Weekday evening or weekends, term time or in the school holidays, drop-in sessions or specific timed events, e.g. 7pm demonstration of non-surgical face lifting.
The How	What is the best forum? Fashion shows, demonstrations, product talks, linked to a bridal event, spa day, trade show, sales of products and accessories; linked to a hair show, open day drop-in, cheese and wine tasting, champagne and canapés, hat show. Calendar-linked events: Mothers Day promotion, Christmas, Valentine's Day, birthdays, Yom Kippur, Diwali, New Year resolutions!

Topic	Things to plan for and consider
The Why	What to do you want to achieve? Increased sales of a product, increased treatment bookings, introduction of a new talented staff member, new product launch, showing off new premises, linked treatments – buy one get one free, courses of treatments, or specific health benefits. Cross-promotions, as in a spa for fitness linked in with facials, weight loss, toning treatments, hair treatments, or the wet area: sauna steam and Jacuzzi.
The What	What are you going to do to keep interest going? Change of pace through the evening with a programme of events at specific times. Demonstrations, talks, followed by free consultations, workshops with client involvement (therapist makes up half her face, the client does the other), step-by step facials with samples, sample goody bags at the end of the evening, talks, raffle with nice prizes at the end of the evening.

Identifying your SMART objectives

When you are ready to plan out your intended promotional activity you need to follow the SMART rules to provide you with clear objectives and to set out how you are going to realise them. SMART stands for:

- **S**pecific
- **M**easurable
- **A**chievable
- **R**ealistic
- **T**imed.

Specific objectives

Be clear on what you want to achieve. It is much better to focus on one or two key areas rather than make it all about everything in the salon, which is too much for a customer or client to take in. A specific goal would be the promotion of a new product line, a launch for a new machine (for example microdermabrasion), the introduction of a new staff member, or a new salon premises opening. Streamline the promotion to be clear, exact and a memorable event for clients.

Measurable

You need to be able to measure the success and judge the value of your promotion so that you can either improve and refine it, or not do it again, if it was not that successful. Obviously an increase in business will be a measure of the success, as will increased sales of the products or bookings for the treatments promoted. You may wish to give out limited-time discount vouchers, redeemable against treatments in the salon — these can be totted up to show how many people did take advantage of the promotion. The attendance of lots of people is a good sign of interest but it doesn't automatically follow that they will all spend lots of money with you.

Achievable

This is a lot to do with logistics. Can you organise the event to the high standard you require within the timescale? Is it realistic and practical, affordable, do-able and viable? Can you reach the targets you are setting?

If you aim too high, you are setting yourself up for failure and a poor result, so there has to be a happy medium between thinking big and being unrealistic. You may wish to use a local celebrity to open your salon: you have all the promotional materials printed and advertise the event in the paper — only to find that the celebrity has other plans on the day, because you didn't give them enough notice or book it with their manager.

During planning, never assume anything — unless it is that it will go wrong in some way — then, you will have a **contingency** or back-up plan for these eventualities and be covered!

Key terms

Contingency – unforeseen event or possible occurrence.

Realistic

Is your plan going to work? Are you being sensible and practical about it? Be rational and think it through. You may not have a film star to open your salon, or be holding a five-star party at the National Gallery for the launch of your new machine, but if you are down-to-earth about opening the salon with refreshments, giving treatment demonstrations and inviting a good selection of clients, with good advertising, there is nothing to say it won't be a great success. Don't plan too grand an event; be reasonable. Top party planners in the middle of celebrity land may be able to attract top names to your event, but that needs a large budget to support it! Would it pay off or would you have to accept that it is money that is not recoverable?

Timed

Be prepared to invest a lot of time to fully prepare for your event – some film premieres take a year to plan, even before the film is shot! The longer you have, the better – you will be more prepared. If you rush things then silly mistakes will catch up with you. If it is quite short notice for an event, keep it simple, then there is less to go wrong. You also need to think about your targets. You may have to recoup your first payment against your machine in three months' time, so you need an event to promote it within that time frame.

Taking account of all of these considerations should ensure that your event is a resounding success!

Target groups/client profiles

These are the groups of people you want to attract with your event: your audience. You need to have a clear idea of who they are, but keep it simple. You may have a general target in mind, for example, all clients, but are they all suitable for the treatment you want to promote?

You can break down your target audience with all sorts of subheadings to focus your market – age, suitability to treatment, links to specific events such as bridal or teenage prom make-up, men's grooming products or a new brand launch – but do try to have a target in mind. In recent years awareness of salon products and services has grown rapidly; it is no longer only the very rich clients who regularly visit the beauty salon – people of all ages have more disposable income. The general public are better informed about beauty treatments and their effects through articles in newspapers and magazines by beauty editors, and/or celebrity endorsements about treatments and results.

Some treatments will undoubtedly appeal to all ages and some will not, but be sure that your invited audience is the right one for the event, to avoid disappointment for everyone.

Agreeing requirements for the activity

When you have got the 'who and where' sorted out, you need to agree on the type of event and the requirements you will need to support it. After the budget, this should be the second thing your manager or salon owner agrees to: what is required. It is no good launching the new equipment if it is not ready, or has not arrived from the supplier, or if no one is trained to use it, or if the publicity materials are still at the printers. This will make your event look badly managed. You need a full list of requirements and it should be agreed in writing that they will be provided for you, by agreed dates, to make the event a success. These should include:

✓ Advertising for the event

✓ Publicity materials, leaflets, flyers

✓ Finances to pay for the venue, staff, insurance and so on

✓ Fees for a guest appearance, if booked

✓ Stock and equipment used

✓ Free gifts or sample bags to take away

✓ Refreshments provided and staff to serve and clear up

✓ Catering hire for cups, plates and glasses

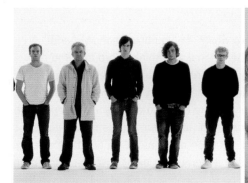
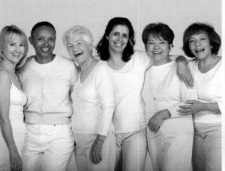
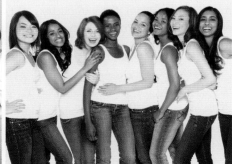

Your target group will have distinct features and attributes

✓ Caretakers for locking up

✓ Seating

✓ Parking

✓ Time to organise this

Producing a plan

Keep your objectives simple and achievable and focus on one or two areas rather than a huge event which could get out of hand. Planning is key.

Type and objectives

Once your objectives are agreed with the management and the event is going ahead, look at your objectives and find the best route to achieve them. Involve all the staff. A big company will have a marketing manager and it is their job to allot jobs to specific tradespeople, and co-ordinate all the support materials required.

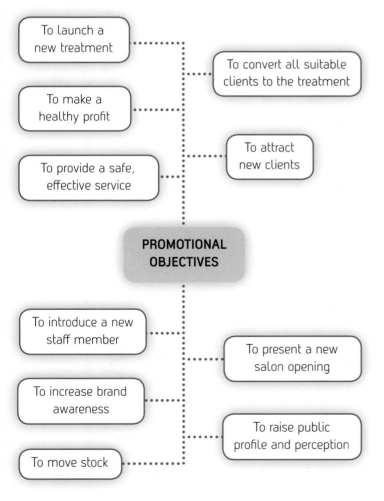

Roles and responsibilities

Even one promotional evening involves a lot of work and management should make it clear that all staff should actively participate. It is in everyone's interest to keep the business refreshed, current and profitable. No sales and clients = no jobs!

Working together on an outside project also helps people to bond as a team, and brings out individuals' talents. One team member may be good at organising but too shy to man the microphone and speak in public, or carry out a demonstration. The more extrovert member of the team, who is willing to go out in front and do a talk, may be no good at finer details, so would need to be helped with that aspect. Play to people's strengths and let them all get involved. Good delegation and division of labour depends on staff being reliable and informed of your expectations — so keep a list of roles and responsibilities.

This could tie in with timescales and your list should have a countdown of days until the big event. This means you can coordinate everything to time and you won't miss anything, for example paying the deposit for the hall two months before the event, but the catering deposit three weeks before the event.

Unit H32

Contribute to the planning and implementation of promotional activities

Promotional checklist

Team leader: Victoria; promotional manger   **Team:** Nadine, Anya and Petra

Timescale	Job needing action	By whom	Competed /proof
Six months before	Planning meeting Brainstorm activities, agenda and agree objectives. Submit plan for approval. Victoria to agree with management All to agree job allocation with SMART outcomes	Victoria All team	Contract drawn up Objectives outlined Budget confirmed
Three months before	Book Priory suite within hotel via general manager Speak to catering manager to supply staff and refreshments Ask to use PA system and music in situ through hotel system Establish running order for overview	Anya and Nadine	Agreement passed to Victoria Time and date confirmed Running order and programme
Two months before	Order publicity material from printer: flyers, tickets, vouchers and posters Check health and safety arrangements with hotel staff Organise **public liability and indemnity insurance** Choose and book models	Victoria and Petra	Risk assessment forms Insurance certificates Mock-ups from printer Signed contracts/written confirmation of booking
One month before	Advertise the event: contact the local paper for an advert or editorial piece, place posters in the window and point of sale material at reception Plan running order and how the event will flow	Anya and Nadine	PR materials and advertising in view
Two weeks before	Double check all of above and confirm Hold meeting for run-through Order additional stock	All the team	A tick list of what has been achieved to date and prioritise what still has to be finalised
Week before	Pick up the programme and publicity materials from printer Buy raffle tickets Pick suitable prizes for the raffle Check everything is in order for next week Report back to Victoria	Anya and Nadine	As above
Day before	Set up hall – including lighting, heating, music Full dress rehearsal – to time the talks so they marry up to the programme to create a sequence or running order Fill goody bags and add promotional materials Wrap raffle prizes Check models are suitable and in attendance	All the team	Completed checklist and ironing out of teething problems Have contingency plans for potential problems: extra models, a second music system, back-up mike
23rd Sept 2010	Day of event Transport promotional materials to venue Everyone to suite to display and set up couches for demonstrations	All the team	Video camera to record the event for future promotions and the evaluation
After event	Discuss and evaluate evening Give out and collect event questionnaires as clients visit the salon for treatments	All the team	Questionnaires for clients Responses from management File away all pertinent material to reuse and refer to in future planning

An example of a promotional checklist

Key terms

Public liability and indemnity insurance – insurance that covers you if someone is accidentally injured at your event or if property is damaged. It will include any legal fees and expenses which result from any claim by a third party.

Roles

It is always a good idea to have two or more people working together on the same topic, and then if one is ill the others can continue and the planning does not halt. Everyone should know their job roles and who they can go to in case of a problem. Always give your team the confidence to be able to speak up and identify possible problems so that they can be dealt with early on. This stops them becoming too large and ruining the event – and allows a contingency plan to be put in place.

Some staff may want sole responsibility, to take ownership of a task and often ask family and friends to help, too. That's good if they are reliable, but if a boyfriend (unknown to you) volunteers to organise the PA system, then you are totally dependent upon their help and commitment. It can also make managing the whole thing slightly awkward – you are not employing the helper and therefore may feel you cannot direct them as you would if you were. Of course, many hands make light work, so not all help should be disregarded, just be careful your helpers will not lose interest and not turn up on the day!

Resources required

Resource requirements need careful consideration for both the viability and the financial restraints of your plan. Having pink flamingos in the foyer of the hotel is both eye-catching and a good publicity stunt, but in reality is neither realistic, practical nor within the average budget range! A comprehensive list is required to support your objectives and when a running order of the event is drawn up, then your list of resources will begin to evolve and appear from it. Be logical – you need to think of absolutely everything, from the smallest detail of having enough tissues and cotton wool for demonstrations, to the larger issues of the correct lighting and sound system .

Legal requirements and planning

For a full explanation of legislation, please refer back to 'You, your client and the law' on page 68 of the Professional basics unit, where all the legal requirements are comprehensively covered.

All of the topics in the spider diagram below are covered in the Professional basics unit (see pages 2–86).

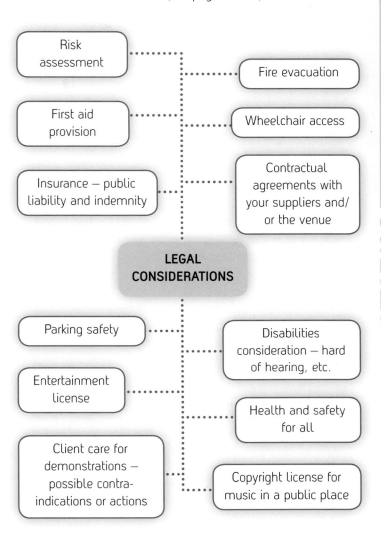

Unit H32 Contribute to the planning and implementation of promotional activities

Preparation and implementation of activities

Preparation of the event will ensure that its implementation will go smoothly. The amount of time planning the event will seem disproportionate to the event — say six months for one evening's work, but it will pay off with a well publicised, trouble-free and exciting evening. Poor planning means mistakes will be made and the event will not look as professional or as polished as you would wish. This will reflect badly on the salon and the business: the exact opposite of what a promotion is all about. Larger companies employ events and public relations managers who make a living out of planning parties and launches. They have lots of contacts and are very practised at putting events together in a short time, and this may be an option, if the budget will stretch to it. The advantage of being in the hands of a professional is that it takes the worry away from the salon owner — the disadvantage may be the cost of hiring them!

Budget

A fixed budget should be set right from the very beginning and then sub-divided into the areas required. You need to put everything into the budget planning, as small things can easily mount up and take the financial costs well above the original figure. It's not just the big costs that need to be thought about, such as room hire and advertising, but the smaller total costs such as flowers or goody bags which may sneak up in price. Other incidentals such as glass and crockery hire can be a hidden cost, so a comprehensive list is essential. It is always a good idea to have a bit of an emergency fund, too, as incidentals have a way of entering the budget. A cash float is ideal for this. You may need to buy something quickly to make the evening flow, for example at the dress rehearsal you discover you really need another extension lead — a minor problem that could be disastrous if there is no lead for a microphone or machine. Keep a record of everything spent, with receipts, both for accounting and auditing and so that you can learn from the event for next time. You will also need to be very accountable to the budget holder and prove that expenses have not got out of hand.

Try and negotiate discounts with your suppliers and build up a reputation as a good payer of bills — suppliers are more willing to help out a customer who pays on time. If you need flowers or an advert or a printing job done, use the same company as you would usually and ask for a special rate for block bookings or a bulk order. Paying for three or four adverts over a year with the local paper or radio station will often be much cheaper than a one-off.

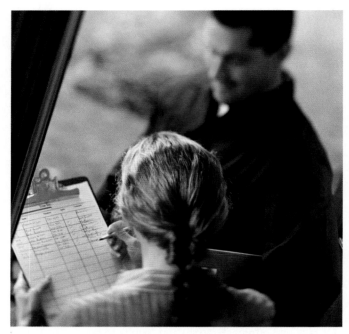

Developing a relationship with your suppliers is important

Planning your method of evaluation

How you evaluate your event will largely depend upon the type of event it is. Think about how you are going to **quantify** your event at the planning stage because you will need to prepare questionnaires, client feedback sheets or a record system for vouchers used. All of these methods will tell you how much the client enjoyed, learned and gained from the event. Obviously an increase in sales, treatment bookings and new clients walking in the door will also indicate the event was a success, but you need to record somewhere if it was as a direct response to the promotion or just a random coincidence. Asking the client on the record card during consultation would also be a valid method of evaluation: 'How did you hear about us?' or 'Did you come to our open evening?' will give an idea of how far-reaching your publicity is. It is wonderful to be able to clarify that business for the month of January increased by 50 per cent because of an event you planned!

Key terms

Quantify – measure.

Meeting your planned timescale

This is a vital part of your planning process — the use of resources should be merged into the timescale of your event. Having price lists and publicity materials delivered three days after the event is just a waste of money and if due to a lack of co-ordination is just not acceptable. To maximise the event you should have everything ready well in advance. This gives you 'wiggle room' if things are delayed, allowing you time to implement your back-up plan.

Implementing promotional activities

In this section you will learn about:

- implementing and adapting promotional activities
- promotions and methods of communication
- essential features and benefits of products and services
- logical steps in promotion
- clearing away to meet the venue requirements.

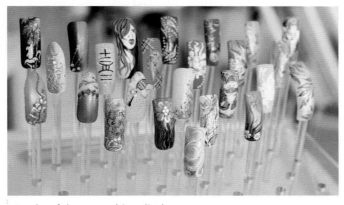
A colourful, eye-catching display

Think about it

Review the resources you are planning to use in your promotion. Are you using everything as effectively as you could? Remember a resource can be: people, stock, tools and equipment or time.

Promotional activities enable you to:

- allow clients to try treatments or products they have not experienced before
- retain customer loyalty
- convey an impression of activity and change within the salon
- attract new clients
- reinvent the ethos and feel of the salon
- show the salon is under new management

- improve customer satisfaction
- improve your public relations.

Implementing and adapting promotional activities

So, your planning stage is over and you now need to implement your strategy for your practical event. This is where all your hard work comes to fruition, so that you can create a seamless and professional event. If your planning has been done correctly, then it should be an effortless event that looks well managed and, above all, is fun for clients. Keep high levels of good communication going throughout the implementation so everyone knows what is expected of them, to avoid misunderstandings or misdirection. There may be minor last-minute changes to make, so you need to be a little flexible to adapt to changing circumstances. If your contingency plans are in place, you will have an alternative to replace the problem – and this gives a certain amount of confidence and calmness to the proceedings. If you are leading the event and are unruffled and calm, then everyone else will be too! This is why a full dress rehearsal is so important – the teething problems are ironed out then, not on the day. Have enough resources to go around and use them wisely and effectively.

Resources required	Possible problems	How to adapt and rectify
People	Staff not turning up/ illness Models not showing up Catering staff late	Do not be dependent upon one member of staff – use and train a few to be ready as back-up. Agree to pick people up on the way to the event – nice and early – to ensure that transport is not the problem. Have back-up models, just in case. Prepare junior staff to help with catering, clearing away and helping the caretaker.
Suppliers and stock	Suppliers not delivering stock/ products Promotional materials not arrived	Insist on an early delivery date, but if they let you down on the day use an alternative local supplier and have additional stock in the boot of the car to call upon if necessary. Ideally check with the supplier 24 hours before the event so you can print off fliers from your own computer as a last resort and have a box to give out.

Continued

Unit H32

Contribute to the planning and implementation of promotional activities

Resources required	Possible problems	How to adapt and rectify
Tools and equipment	Failure of equipment to work Electricity supply faulty Tools missing	Have a designated member of staff for loading tools and transporting to the event. Have a complete spare kit in the car and more than one machine for demonstration use. If employing a trainer from a commercial company to demonstrate a technique or equipment (e.g. microdermabrasion) then ask them to bring their own equipment, too.

Promotions and methods of communication

Once you've decided on the type of promotional activity you want to undertake, such as a introducing a new treatment or therapist, you have to choose the most effective and suitable way to communicate your information.

Demonstration evenings

Rather than inviting your clients to *hear* about a new salon treatment where you talk them through it, you could do a demonstration and *show* how effective the treatments can be. If you have one therapist actually doing the treatment, another therapist can be describing the treatment, step-by-step, as the stages are shown.

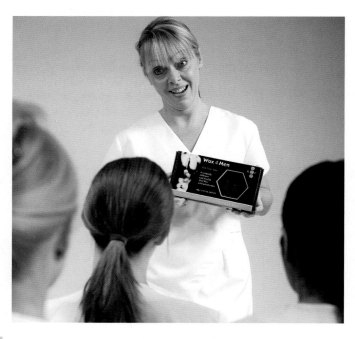

You need a public speaker:

- with self assurance
- who understands the techniques being shown
- who is confident to answer questions from the audience
- who can generate a good atmosphere and engage with the audience.

This can be in a small section in the salon or treatment rooms, or on a stage in a large auditorium, using a microphone and slides. Regardless of the size, do make sure everyone can see the demonstration and organise the chairs to facilitate that. You can combine the demonstrations with refreshments and a raffle, and get staff to mingle with clients to build rapport and talk through the price list and answer any questions they may have. A published programme will keep people informed about the format of the evening. Some larger events may be a combination of promotions, a trade show where the clients can buy items and a fashion show, with hairstyles and other retailers, such as bridal outfitters. Obviously the more tradespeople involved, the more organisation it will require, and the larger the premises needed.

Websites

The internet is widely available to everyone and with phone technology being ever more developed you can access the web anywhere, on the move. Planning and designing a web page or a complete site needs to be done by an expert in the field so that it looks professional, is easy to follow, flows with links to the right topic, is creative and represents your salon and products. When a website is designed properly, it can be wonderful and easy — when it is badly or inexpertly designed, it is the most frustrating thing! As a generalisation, the younger generation are more used to working on the internet — so a website alone may not attract the older or the technophobic client!

Newspaper advertising

Here are some local advertising tips.

- Use suppliers' or manufacturers' additional marketing support information and packages whenever possible.
- Make sure you have a chance to see your completed advert before it is printed and keep a copy of the proof.
- Request a good position in the paper. If you advertise regularly, the paper will probably do this for no extra charge.
- If you have a choice of publications, find out which one best covers your area, and suits your needs.
- If you pre-book a number of issues, ask for a discount — just as clients do when they book a course with you.

One other method is to advertise in the local Yellow Pages or in other local directories. This is a measurable way of reaching potential clients in your area. It can be expensive but it is a universal method of finding tradespeople.

Journalists

Invite a local reporter to visit your salon for a treatment. This may result in a feature article written about the salon and the treatment given. The following tips may help when dealing directly with the media.

- Avoid answering questions with a simple 'yes' or 'no'. Provide as much relevant information as possible, which will allow the journalist to write an interesting article full of useful information.
- Try to anticipate what the journalist will ask. You will then be able to prepare answers to likely questions.
- Remember to be positive. Tell the journalist what you do offer, not what you don't.
- Keep your communication suitable for the consumer — avoid technical terms. Use language that everyone will be able to understand.

Press releases

Use simple statements with a strong headline. Always cover the key facts, avoid using jargon and include a quote.

- If you are successful, your information may be included in the editorial content of a local publication.
- Editorial is more effective than advertising.
- Two to three days after sending your press release to the beauty editor, phone and check that it has been received. Invite the editor for a complimentary service at the same time and start to build a relationship.
- If you are prepared to offer a competition prize, let the editor know. Newspapers love to offer prizes to their readers.
- If a journalist comes to see you, make sure your salon looks at its best and that you make his or her time as enjoyable as possible.
- If you are holding an event at your salon, let the local paper know in advance.

Radio advertising

There are numerous local radio stations operating from town or city centres and hospitals. The radio station may wish to cover a beauty therapy topic and this would be a good opportunity for you to participate and lend your expertise. This will often attract clients and is good experience for you.

Mailings

There are many different types of mailings, including:

- distributing leaflets through letterboxes
- negotiating an 'insert' of your leaflet within the local newspaper
- approaching local businesses who may consider supplying leaflets to their employees.

Leaflet drops could be questionnaires which, when completed, the prospective client could drop into the salon in return for a gift. This will give you invaluable information for future marketing strategies and possibly gain a new client.

If you concentrate distribution of leaflets in small controlled areas, you will be able to assess the feedback quite easily, and this will allow you to work out a systematic method for future mailings.

Newsletters

In the run-up to Christmas, a newsletter detailing special offers and Christmas gift vouchers should help to increase sales. It does not have to be professionally produced — you could produce your own leaflet on a computer — but it does need to look professional and be spell-checked!

How often should you send newsletters? The answer is as often as is profitable. Analyse the results, and if sales go up, you have it right, so keep doing what you are doing!

Local clubs and groups or charities

Local clubs and societies often struggle to find interesting speakers. You could offer to give a talk for the local women's groups and other groups, or give demonstrations of various treatments your salon offers, to tempt members into the salon. Supporting a local charity also promotes goodwill in the community and helps raise the profile of the charity.

Promoting the business locally

Local shop owners and workers will be more willing to help you with promotion (and more enthusiastic about your services) if you offer them a complimentary service or two. Include their services with your own — work with hairdressers, florists, bridal outfitters and so on.

Existing clients

Clients love to know everything that is going on in 'their' salon. Suggestions for news might be:

- a new treatment at the salon
- a new therapist joining the salon
- a therapist with advanced training techniques

- special offers or promotions
- advanced information regarding an open evening
- a review of a previous open evening
- a reminder to book early for Christmas, the summer holiday season, etc.

Give leaflets to all salon clients. Offer them a discount or a complimentary treatment when they introduce a friend. Open evenings are an excellent way to attract new clients to the salon. To make sure the evening goes well, you should:

- advertise the evening well in advance
- have enough staff on hand to talk to the clients
- run a competition to win free treatments, or give special offers on products or services, to encourage prospective clients
- offer good quality, complimentary refreshments
- capitalise upon an occasion (for example, summer holidays) — try to have a theme and encourage sales by selling gifts and offering free gift-wrapping
- dare to be different — organise a male-only night
- offer loyalty schemes and bonus-point incentives.

Vouchers

You could also try marketing ideas such as vouchers. For example, when clients make a purchase they will be given three or four vouchers with offers relating to their next visit

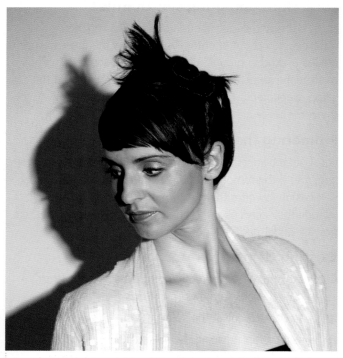

A makeover is a special treat to celebrate a milestone birthday

or possibly money-off vouchers to try a new treatment. Alternatively, a customer loyalty scheme, where clients are rewarded under a bonus-point system, could increase their loyalty and number of purchases. This way you encourage the clients to try things they may not have considered before. These schemes have been tremendously successful and encourage both brand and salon loyalty.

Capitalising on celebrations

Father's Day, Mother's Day, Easter, Valentine's Day, birthdays, Christmas, Yom Kippur, Diwali, New Year and New Year's resolutions — the list of special occasions when clients may be encouraged to bring you extra business is endless!

Testimonials

Written recommendations, known as testimonials, are the best advertising you could ever achieve as long as plenty of people get to read them. Ask your happy, satisfied clients to write a comment on the treatment and how pleased they are with the salon and its services. Have a comments board in reception for the best letters, which others will read!

Email

Record email addresses whenever available. Email is now a common form of communication and the great thing about using it in marketing is the low cost. It costs very little to send an email, so you can send details of special offers or promotions to all your clients for no more than a fraction of your monthly internet package. Alternatively, if you use an external marketing company, it is now possible to send full-colour email bulletins or 'e-bulletins', including full-colour photographs, for less than the price of a first-class stamp.

Think about it

Sending too many emails, and emails that take too long to download with huge pictures, are annoying, and can cost the client extra money. You will put the client off by sending SPAM emails.

Dynamic displays

Displays must be eye-catching and attractive, regularly updated, topical and spotlessly clean. Think about what you want to say about your salon and yourself — does your window display do you justice?

Essential features and benefits of products and services

To promote them effectively, you have to know and understand the features and benefits of the products and services that the salon offers. Everything you offer has a feature and a benefit. A product's attributes or characteristics are its features. The advantages to the client of the product are its benefits.

The features and benefits of a facial cleanser are shown in the table below, as an example.

Features	Benefits
Unbreakable packaging	Cleanses the skin
Pump action convenience and control	Prevents facial blemishes
Variety of sizes	Removes make-up
Economical when purchased in larger sizes	Helps exfoliate
Exclusive products unavailable on high street	Helps regulate the acid mantle

Features and benefits of a facial cleanser

Logical steps in promotion

Whichever method of promotion you decide upon, make sure you follow the planning and objective-setting steps outlined in the beginning of this unit. This will help it all go smoothly. Be logical in your delivery, especially if it is a demonstration: have a beginning or introduction, a middle – when you talk about features and benefits, and a conclusion. Ensure that you know everything there is to know about your product or treatment to anticipate questions and give full answers. Specify at the beginning of the demonstration whether you will answer questions throughout, or whether they should be held until the end of the demonstration.

Do remember that you cannot lecture your clients and that everyone has a limit to their attention span: three hours of demonstrations will mean an audience gets fidgety and loses interest. It is much better to have twenty-minute or half-hour demonstrations and allow people to move around and ask questions. Keep the information relevant to the topic, quite straightforward and as simple as possible. The more confused the clients become, the less likely they are to purchase or to book treatments. Try and go for a 'wow' factor of before-and-after treatments and show how wonderfully beneficial the treatments are.

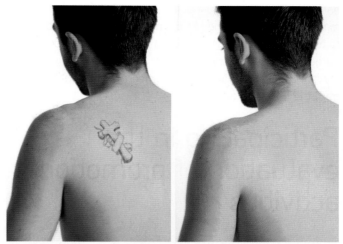

Showing before-and-after photographs of clients is an effective way of promoting treatments

You want clients to feel they can approach you and are comfortable enough with your skills to book treatments. Be enthusiastic, animated and passionate about your topic, because enthusiasm is infectious and your clients will catch it! Encourage questions about services and products and respond to queries in a friendly and open manner. This will give a positive and friendly feel to the promotion and enhance goodwill in your relationship with your potential clients. If you are asked something you can't answer, ask a colleague or offer to get back to the client with an answer (remember to take their details if you do not know the client personally).

Clearing away to meet the venue requirements

After your event, be sure to leave everything as you found it and be careful not to over extend the hire agreement – you may find you get charged an additional twenty-four hours of hire if you run over your allotted time. All equipment should be cleaned and put away, following both health and safety and manufacturer's instructions. If you have used the kitchen and catering facilities, they must be cleaned and returned to the hire company in the same good condition you picked them up in. You may be charged for breakage of glasses or crockery and you should always check to see if they pick up the hired equipment or you deliver it back to them.

This is part of your professionalism and your reputation may be harmed if you leave a mess – as well as possibly being refused permission to use the venue again. Thorough clearing up includes taking rubbish with you for disposal and locking up the premises. If the event is in the salon, the rooms should be returned to the normal state ready for the following day's trading — make sure all staff are responsible for helping. Don't allow some staff to go home early and leave it to a few — this is not fair when everyone will benefit from the boost in trade.

Participating in the evaluation of promotional activities

In this section you will learn about:

- methods of feedback
- collating and recording information
- participating in discussions.

So, the event is over, all went according to your extensive planning, and it is the morning after. How do you know if your event was a success?

Methods of feedback

You need to use an agreed method to gain feedback, collate and record it and then draw accurate and clear conclusions from all you have learned. The more events you take part in, the better you become at judging the success, but it does also need a tangible outcome to justify all the expense and effort you went to. Your event may have been well attended, but it doesn't automatically follow that the people are going to spend money with you.

There are several methods of evaluating a promotion's effectiveness:

- increase in clients' general attendance because of raised profile
- increased treatment bookings
- increased sales of products promoted
- verbal questions with clients
- business reply with evaluation sheet
- telephone survey.

If the event is a small one, the salon owner or manager can go around speaking to clients as the event draws to a close, asking if they enjoyed the evening and what they especially liked about it.

Questionnaires can be left on the chairs for clients to fill in — but keep the questions short and with a tick for yes/no, as people don't have a lot of time to write a full critique of the evening. A box with an enquiry for future events will help with planning — and try to capture clients' contact details to put them on your mailing list. Always make sure they understand your intention and that you gain their permission to have their details. (See data protection legislation in 'You, your client and the law' on page 81.)

A telephone survey is a good idea if you have the staff to devote the time to it, but if it is carried out within salon hours you are unlikely to catch people at home. This may have to be a designated evening job for several staff — depending, of course, on having the attendees' telephone numbers.

Speak to your clients when they are in reception if they attended the promotion and then ask if they can spare a moment to run through a questionnaire.

A discount voucher given out on the night and then redeemed against a treatment or product is always a good way to capture attendance, as you can keep it when presented against the cost of a treatment. Over a period of a month you should be able to calculate the increase in sales or treatment bookings and then put it into a report. Go back to the five basic steps of who, what, when, why and how and evaluate them all. Did they all work well? Would you choose somewhere else next time — was the venue big enough? Too big and not very cosy? How was the ambience? Too cold? Too hot? Too cramped?

Another important task is to compare the projected budget against the actual expenditure — this is a good indication of your planning skills. Were there lots of incidental costs not originally planned for? Were you over budget from under-estimating the cost of the required resources?

It's not just the clients' perception of the event that needs to be included within the feedback — staff involved should also be able to comment on how it went, whether it was well organised, if they felt their contribution went well and how to improve it for the future.

All the feedback should be collated into a document freely available to all — and you may be asked to present it to the senior management team, so it needs to be constructive, non-personal and objective in its analysis.

Collating and recording information

How you present the feedback report will depend upon your IT skills — there is nothing wrong with a handwritten report, but if a spreadsheet or database is used then it can be presented in a variety of ways, and bar charts, pie charts or graphs give a quick visual indication of the results. You should include all findings (positive and negative) and cover the following topics:

- The reaction of clients — did they enjoy, engage and learn?
- Are clients encouraged to come into the salon for treatments/sales?
- The response from staff — were they fully used and actively involved?
- The suitability of the format — what to change for the future
- Suitability of the venue
- The budget and whether it was appropriate and used wisely
- Outgoing costs measured against **return**
- Whether the objectives were met
- What problems, if any, occurred and what contingency used
- Was the planning, timescale and activity appropriate and adequate
- Increase in client attendance, bookings or sales for the specific event.
- How to improve it for the next event.

Key terms

Return – profit or loss, but also any benefits gained which may not be purely financial, for example the generation of team spirit through an event.

Participating in discussions

A review of the event should involve everyone who took part and could be either a formal presentation or a staff meeting in a discussion with management in attendance. Be non-judgemental in your evaluation, i.e. do not applaud/blame any one person for the success or failure but try to be impartial and detached, to gain as much as you can from other people's perceptions. You may consider it a huge success but others may see things from a different angle. Encourage staff to comment and then all staff can learn from it. Use your report as an agenda for the discussions and this will keep the meeting focused and well-structured.

This meeting and the conclusions you draw will also form the basis for your future recommendations, what you need to change, and what you have learned through the whole process. You should add a summary of the discussions to your report and keep it for the salon's future reference.

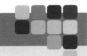

Check your knowledge

1 The function of a promotional evening is to:
   a) raise the profile of a business
   b) keep on top of health and safety requirements
   c) make sure staff are working hard
   d) make sure price lists are up to date.

2 The mnemonic for objectives when planning promotions should be:
   a) SMILEY
   b) SMART
   c) START
   d) CLEVER.

3 Types of insurance required for promotions are:
   a) fire, theft and damage
   b) third party
   c) public liability and indemnity
   d) copyright and licensing insurance.

4 Which of these is not necessary when planning the event?
   a) Risk assessment
   b) Health and safety
   c) Fire procedures
   d) Medicines Act

5 A benefit of a product is:
   a) what it does for sales
   b) what it does for the client
   c) whether it is unbreakable
   d) whether it comes in large sizes.

6 A feature of a product is:
   a) what it does for sales
   b) what it does for the client
   c) whether it is unbreakable
   d) whether it is a free gift.

7 A target group is:
   a) the point of the promotion
   b) the average age of the audience
   c) the quality of the audience
   d) those who the promotion is aimed at.

8 Who is in charge of health and safety for an outside event?
   a) The salon owner
   b) The hall owner
   c) The caretaker
   d) The event's organiser.

9 www stands for:
   a) World Wide Web
   b) World Wide Women
   c) World Wide Windows
   d) World Wide Waves.

10 Evaluation allows you to:
   a) check the effectiveness of the promotion
   b) change the promotion once it's finished
   c) withdraw vouchers once they have been given to the customer
   d) fire staff if it wasn't effective.

Getting ready for assessment

Evidence for planning and implementation of promotional activities should occur naturally as you are carrying out demonstrations of products, managing displays within the reception or salon area, and working with your product companies to devise and implement advertising campaigns, or any additional activities you run to promote your workshops to clients.

You must be assessed at least once and you must cover both the objectives of enhancing the business image and increasing the business growth; this could be through your job within an external salon (you will need an employer statement to show how you undertook actions to increase salon trade) or it could be within your training centre. You need to keep a copy of any adverts, aftercare leaflets or treatment plans you make which increase revenue for your salon and event plans, posters or price lists you draw up which you can demonstrate have had a positive effect on sales of products or treatment bookings. You will also be directly observed.

Unit G11

Contribute to the financial effectiveness of the business

What you will learn

How to contribute to the effective use and monitoring of resources

- Types of resources
- Following salon and legal procedures
- Stock
- The principles of stock control and ordering
- Checking deliveries and order documentation
- Managing people
- Indentifying and resolving resource problems

How to meet productivity and development targets

- Setting and agreeing productivity and development targets
- Reviewing and recording your progress
- Promotions and opportunities to achieve targets

Introduction

The key to a successful business is making and maintaining a **profit**. A profit is the amount of money left after all the outgoings of a business have been paid, including stock and wages. To be able to make a profit, a business must monitor its outgoings very closely, and a small business is only as good as its resources management. A sad truth is that regardless of how good your skills are — you may be a very competent therapist — the business may fail if you do not look after your resources correctly .

A beauty therapy salon is a great user of resources — people, stock, tools, equipment and time. All have to be managed and coordinated so that the business grows and flourishes, and a healthy balance is maintained through vigilant supervision, with all members of staff appreciating their responsibilities for resources.

Key terms

Profit – income or earnings, or turnover or revenue after all the outgoings have been paid.

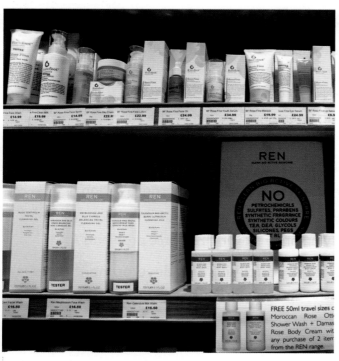

Selling complete skill care regimes benefits the client and is profitable for the salon

How to contribute to the effective use and monitoring of resources

In this section you will learn about:

- types of resources
- following salon and legal procedures
- stock
- the principles of stock control and ordering
- checking deliveries and order documentation
- managing people
- indentifying and resolving resource problems.

Types of resources

A beauty salon is only as good as its resources. It may surprise you to realise exactly what is classified as a resource — have you ever thought of yourself as a core resource? Resources in a busy salon include stock, tools and equipment, people and time.

Staff — therapists, cleaners, caterers, maintenance, accountants

Energy — electricity, lighting, heating, washing machine, dryers

Stock — salon sizes, retail sizes, display

TYPES OF RESOURCES

Equipment

Time

Hygiene resources — laundry, equipment, cleaning materials, decoration

Hidden resources — tissues, couch roll, cotton wool, sponges

All these resources have to be paid for and managed

Think about it

Maximum profit goes hand in glove with minimum waste.

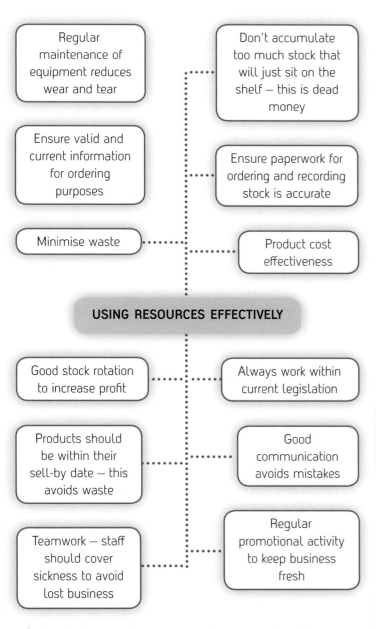

The effective use of resources contributes to profitability

Resource responsibility does not just stop at using stock carefully. Turning appliances off will reduce your energy outgoings — and your carbon footprint. Being effective with your time and working within commercially acceptable treatment times will also help your business.

Following salon and legal procedures

There are numerous general legal requirements relating to safe working practices concerning resources:

- The Health and Safety at Work Act 1974
- The Manual Handling Operations Regulations l992
- The Reporting of Injuries, Diseases and Dangerous Occurrences Regulations (RIDDOR) 1995
- The Electricity at Work Regulations 1989
- The Cosmetic Products (Safety) Regulations 2003, amended 2008
- The Control of Substances Hazardous to Health (COSHH) Regulations 2002.

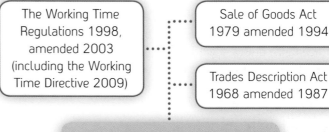

The principles of good business

The principle of keeping track of what comes in and what goes out is the same, regardless of whether your eventual aim is to become a salon owner or you are happy to stay an employee, or even if you intend to become a mobile therapist. Your role in monitoring resources may vary, as a salon manager has more resource responsibility than a junior therapist, but all staff should avoid wasting materials and try to be cost-effective, even if their job role does not include stock taking or ordering the required goods. Every staff member should contribute to the effective use and monitoring of resources.

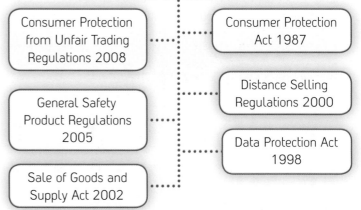

Key legislation relating to consumer protection and working conditions

(See 'You, your client and the law', page 68, for information on the above legislation.)

Salon procedures

Salon procedures for managing resources will vary according to the size of the salon, the type of business and services it offers, the level of staffing and the efficiency of its management. There are no hard and fast rules for organisation of resources but all large national corporations and beauty groups will have policies in place so that all their salons use universal paperwork regardless of who is in charge of the individual salon. The self-employed therapist will need a smaller-scale method of resource management, but the principle of the system is the same.

Stock

Stock is both:

- the second largest investment of money – the first is people
- the lifeblood of the business, as no stock to perform treatments equals no clients.

Controlling stock is often seen as tedious and boring, and the relevance is rarely appreciated by the younger therapist, who is often given the job of checking all stock held, the arrival of deliveries and for damaged or broken goods. However, the importance of this should not be underestimated. Running out of best-selling stock through poor stock control is lost revenue, which may be reflected in lower commission for sales for individual therapists.

Stock levels

The first thing a salon has to decide is the level of stock to be held. This will, of course, depend upon the treatment ranges that are to be offered, the number of therapists using the products and the product suppliers. It is common practice

to open an account with your choice of supplier and, initially, many of the larger suppliers have a minimum ordering level of either monetary value or stock level – a £2000–£5000 investment in stock is not unreasonable. They will supply in bulk for larger salons, but once you are a proven reliable customer, smaller orders will be accepted, albeit with a higher delivery charge. The advantage of going to a larger company is once you have made the investment; they will advise you on best-selling lines and give you a guide to the most popular retail products. They will organise the promotional materials, point of sale leaflets and price lists, and often take part in promotional events with your salon to boost sales. However, there is no guarantee that they will not discontinue your favourite lines.

For the smaller business of a single therapist, it is often a matter of trial and error and experience with the client base that will reveal the fast-moving product lines and those that gather dust.

Stock is not just the retail products kept in reception for sales; it also includes the bulk purchase of products used at the workstations, which are often purchased in litres and then decanted into convenient sizes. Many suppliers will provide both trade and retail size products and new therapists soon learn it is far more cost-effective to order trade sizes for treatments while keeping a smaller level of retail stock for sale.

The principles of stock control and ordering

Small salons will perform a manual stock-take; larger salons with computerised tills will electronically count stock, rather like a supermarket, and automatically adjust stock levels according to the bar code of the product when scanned through the till. Whichever method is used, the principle is the same.

1. You must regularly count existing stock, including displays, retail, samples and salon sizes in the treatment rooms.
2. Compare that to the minimum stock level set and if it is below, reorder as required to keep up levels.
3. Coordinate this information with the salon ordering system so that minimum levels do not drop so low that an item goes out of stock.
4. Speak to colleagues to ensure you have all relevant information relating to stock levels so stock control is accurate.

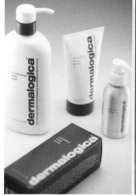
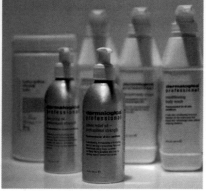

Trade and retail sizes of products

Date:	13 May 2010							
Code	Description	Size	Minimum stock level	In stock	Sold	On order	Date ordered
	Retail skin care						
1000	Cleanser	200 ml	14	2	12	12	15/05/10
1010	Toner	200 ml	14	5	9	9	
1020	Moisturiser	200 ml	14	6	8	8	
	Salon skin care						
1001	Cleanser	400 ml	14	4	10	10	
1011	Toner	400 ml	14	3	11	11	
1021	Moisturiser	400 ml	14	3	11	11	
	Aftercare pack						
2050	BioSkinJetting 1 and 2	Pack	20	8	12	12	
	Retail camouflage						
3100	Cover Crème Coffee	10 g	6	4	2	2	
3101	Cover Crème Apricot	10 g	6	7	0		
3102	Cover Crème Brown	10 g	6	2	4	4	
3103	Cover Crème Tan	10 g	6	4	2	2	
3104	Cover Crème Barley	10 g	6	4	2	2	
3105	Cover Crème Natural Tan	10 g	6	1	5	5	

Stock control sheet

Points 1–4 should be carried out sequentially on a regular basis — small salons may do this at the end of the working day, others weekly and larger salons as a monthly or bi-monthly operation.

Ordering

Stock can be ordered in a variety of ways:

- By post — the top copy of the duplicated stock sheet can be sent off to the supplier.

- By telephone — this is the quickest method but can prove unreliable if you are misheard, and if making a big order it can prove expensive.

- By fax (if available) — the drawback of using this method is that the copy is not always clear, so write in black pen as pencil or light pen does not copy well.

- By email.

- Computer — a program linked up to the till which automatically generates an order.

- In person — give your order to a visiting representative of the supplier.

Checking deliveries and order documentation

The method of delivery will vary depending on the size of the order. Small items will come through the post in a padded envelope; large orders will arrive in boxes via specialist companies dealing in deliveries; local suppliers will have a delivery van that brings the stock to your door. If your supplier is local, it is possible to pop in personally and pick up stock on the way to work. You may also drop into your local wholesale supplier if you run out of stock — but remember to account for additional purchases in your overall financial accounting.

Checking stock on arrival

It is important that all deliveries are checked accurately and completed against the order documentation, with any inaccuracies or damage immediately reported to the relevant person. The supplier must be notified immediately and will usually despatch a replacement the same day. Depending on the company's **policy** and how much the supplier values your custom, this may be free of charge. If the goods are hand delivered, damaged goods will be taken back to the supplier by the delivery person; otherwise you will need to post them.

Key terms

Policy – a set course of action, a plan, or principle or procedure within the salon for decisions and actions that everyone must follow for the good of the business. This could be for health and safety, selling, customer complaints and so on.

Quantity	Description	Sterex initial	Customer initial
1	Salon BioSkinJetting Lotion Size 1	EFS	JH
1	Salon BioSkinJetting Lotion Size 2	EFS	JH
1	Salon BioSkinJetting Cleanser (400 ml)	EFS	JH
1	Salon BioSkinJetting Toner (400 ml)	EFS	JH
1	Salon BioSkinJetting Moisturiser (400 ml)	EFS	JH
3	Retail BioSkinJetting Cleanser (200 ml)	EFS	JH
3	Retail BioSkinJetting Toner (200 ml)	EFS	JH
3	Retail BioSkinJetting Moisturiser (200 ml)	EFS	JH
18	Assorted BioSkinJetting Retail Cover Crème 10 g	EFS	JH
5	BioSkinJetting Finishing Dust 35 g	EFS	JH
1	Surgical Hand Piece	EFS	JH
25	Microprobes (15 x 3s and 10 x 4s)	EFS	JH
1	BioSkinJetting Cover Crème Palette x 18 shades	EFS	JH
5	Client Aftercare Kits	EFS	JH
10	Client Information Leaflets	EFS	JH
1	Sharps Box	EFS	JH
1	BioSkinJetting Badge	EFS	JH
1 pack (25)	Consultation Cards	EFS	JH
1 pack (50)	Aftercare Leaflets	EFS	JH
1	Smoothing Ice Ball	EFS	JH

Date: 9.6.2010   **Checked by:** E F Stoddart

BioSkinJetting package checklist

Think about it

Most large suppliers pass responsibility for goods while in transit to the delivery service. It is only when the salon signs for the delivery that it becomes the responsibility of the salon. It is worth checking your own insurance for liability for in-transit stock should it go astray. Do not automatically assume that the wholesaler accepts responsibility for lost goods.

Managing people

Managing people is probably one of the most difficult tasks, but good staff are essential for a growing business. The key to success is to employ the right people in the first place — those who are enthusiastic, show commitment and a willingness to work as part of a team. Once the right team is in place, it will need nurturing. Staff need:

- a professional environment in which to work (see Unit G22 Monitor procedures to safely control work operations, page 88, and 'You, your client and the law', page 68)
- a sense of self-esteem through a defined job role, incentives and good staff training

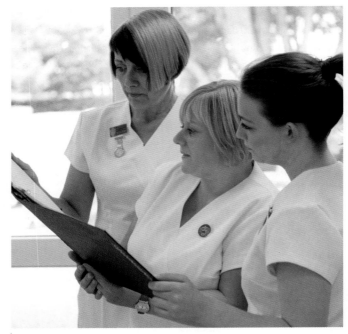

Good teams lead to more efficient salons

- respect from peers and management as a professional
- financial recognition — a fair wage for a skilled professional
- appreciation from clients, colleagues and management.

(See 'You — the therapist', page 17, for further information on managing resources, tools and equipment, dealing with others, how to cope with conflict and personal time management.)

Think about it

Records for which you are responsible should be accurate, legible and up to date.

Identifying and resolving resource problems

Most common problems can be resolved with a calm approach, a little thought and contingency planning. There should be plans in place for a number of unforeseeable difficulties such as staff sickness. Regular staff meetings will allow all staff to be informed of the procedure if a member of staff phones in sick. This may include rearranging appointments by phoning the clients, or drawing upon a bank of part-time staff, who may be available on the day, with minimum disruption to the client. Good quality, professional and efficient staff training will ensure that accurate records are kept, deliveries are correct, equipment repairs are carried out in good time and time is well managed. For unforeseen circumstances, ensure you know health and safety procedures.

The working therapist may spot a potential resource problem that the stock controller is unaware of, for example the therapist may notice a seasonal increase in a treatment or publicity in a magazine that may generate interest in a particular product. At the weekly staff meeting, there should be an opportunity for the therapist to recommend increasing stock levels of the particular item. This should not be viewed as challenging the authority of the stock controller, but rather as a positive contribution to the financial effectiveness of the business. The therapist will need to clearly show the benefits to the business and if agreed, implementation may well be immediate. It may be as simple as increasing the basic stockholding, or reinforcing the promotion with displays and demonstrations.

For further guidance on consulting the relevant person to resolve problems, see 'You and your working environment', page 54.

Think about it

Who in your salon is responsible for stock control?

How often is stock ordered?

How is it delivered?

What happens if something goes missing?

Think about it

You must always remember the limits of your authority when dealing with any stock problems. For example, it may not be your job to complain to the supplier. You might lose goodwill and upset a good working relationship if you interfere when it is not your place to do so.

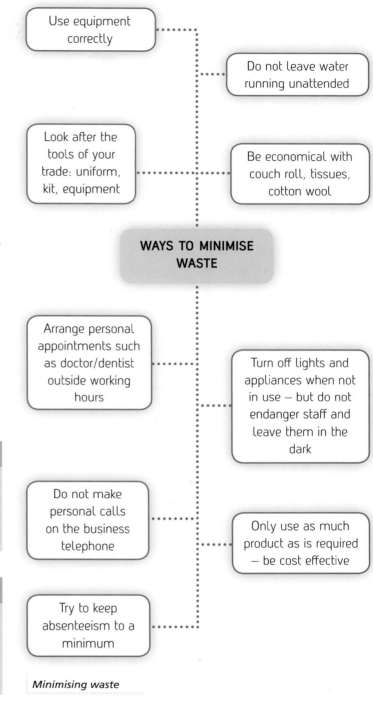

Use equipment correctly

Do not leave water running unattended

Look after the tools of your trade: uniform, kit, equipment

Be economical with couch roll, tissues, cotton wool

WAYS TO MINIMISE WASTE

Arrange personal appointments such as doctor/dentist outside working hours

Turn off lights and appliances when not in use — but do not endanger staff and leave them in the dark

Do not make personal calls on the business telephone

Only use as much product as is required — be cost effective

Try to keep absenteeism to a minimum

Minimising waste

Resolving common resource issues

Resource	Common problem	How to resolve it
Staffing	Staff going off sick Holiday cover Maternity leave	Accept that illness is inevitable, but keep a sickness record as continuous absenteeism is not acceptable, especially for minor illness. Have enough staff to cover or arrange a rota so everyone covers a little of the day to avoid letting clients down. Give clients sufficient notice of cancelled appointments, where possible. Keep a bank of staff who are flexible and able to provide sickness cover.
	Staff not all trained to the same level so gaps in treatments offered	Ensure that there are enough staff who are equally trained, to avoid specialist staff having a monopoly on certain treatments, but who can't be covered when sick.
	Workers and shirkers!	Rotate the training and jobs so that the responsibilities of work and duties are shared equally – this avoids some staff doing nothing whilst others work really hard and contribute to the growth or the business. It is important that all staff know all of the running of the business, and understand the processes.
Stock control	Running out of stock	This is down to lack of forward thinking. A system needs to be in place and should be stuck to, with the correct paperwork of stock rotation adhered to. Counting stock on a regular basis is key to knowing what you are running out of, and then ordering in advance so that you do not let a client down. You may have to do an emergency trip to your local wholesaler to pick up missing stock.
	Having too much stock	Stock which is not moving or bringing money back into the salon is dead stock. Organise a promotion, get all staff on board to push the sales and make a prominent display of it, so that clients want to purchase it. Ensure that it is not past its sell-by date. If it is, your company may have to write it off, or reduce it considerably, with a sign to give the reason it is reduced in price. Also, talk to the supplier or sales rep – if the products are still good, they may swap them for the same monetary value of goods that you do use on a regular basis.
	Having stock/equipment which no one is trained in using	Organise a training day or half-day and invite the sales trainer for the products to come in and offer the staff a **development** training day. Then have a sales promotion, with staff incentives and get the equipment in use and the products on sale.

Key terms

Development – growth, expansion or improvement of the business, or personal development through training for advancement.

Resource	Common problem	How to resolve it
Records	Inaccurate records or deliveries	Inaccurate records usually indicate that someone is not doing their job properly – this may be down to lack of training or lack of time. Training should be organised once the source of the problem has been identified. Time management needs to be realistic – if the therapist is given a big job, expect them to need the time to do it properly.
		Work on building rapport with your suppliers and ask them for help with inaccurate deliveries – it may be a mistake at their end so allow them time to put it right. Keep sending products back, and if they do not co-operate with you, you may need to think about changing suppliers
Tools and equipment	Broken equipment/tools which are old	Have a sufficient bank of equipment/tools so that having one out of action does not bring the business to a halt.
		Have a good relationship with your equipment supplier, so that a replacement machine can be used, whilst repairs are carried out. Sufficient insurance cover will make damage and breakages manageable and cover the cost of maintenance charges. Getting machines regularly checked will prevent damage and minor damage turning into major faults.
		Think about leasing equipment so that repairs and replacements are part of the deal.
		Replace and renew old tools before they break.
Time	Poor time management Overrunning with appointments Keeping clients waiting Not finishing jobs	Invest in some training for all staff, so they understand how to manage their time. Train receptionists so that they know the correct timings for treatments and can manage an appointment page for several staff and allot the correct spaces for treatments.
		Be reasonable in your expectations for treatment timings, sales targets and client turnover – if you put staff under too much pressure, nothing gets done. It is better to tackle one job well and finish it, than it is to start ten and not complete one of them.
		Share out the job roles evenly, and keep up teamwork so that no single person feels responsible for the running of everything – that leads to stress and sickness.

Think about it

The best service companies have a very simple philosophy: they do whatever is necessary to ensure that their customers have an excellent experience and are served beyond their expectations .This includes 'lateral service' – hidden support for fellow employees, stock control, resources and the treatment – altogether giving a professional ambience and ethos to the salon, which is very attractive to clients.

Think about it

The records you are responsible for should also be accurate, legible and up to date. For further detail and advice refer to Communication in Professional Basics, page 29.

How to meet productivity and development targets

In this section you will learn about:

- setting and agreeing **productivity** and development **targets**
- reviewing and recording your progress
- promotions and opportunities to achieve targets.

Key terms

Productivity – the amount of work achieved or expected over a period of time and the measure of worker efficiency.

Target – a set figure or projected sum of sales, treatments or products used over a period of time; a goal to work towards.

In most salons, productivity and development targets are set for retail sales, technical services and the staff's personal learning. These three key areas are all essential for the growth and development of the business.

Setting and agreeing productivity and development targets

We all react well to praise. By having goals to work towards, you will feel you have achieved something, knowing that your efforts will be recognised.

A keen therapist will want to increase her client base and/or product turnover if she knows that not only is her work to be rewarded with praise but there is an extra incentive to do so. Targets should be realistic and achievable. They should be mutually agreed between you and your manager, with a set target over a defined period of time. It could be monthly, every other month or every three months, depending on your terms of employment. Short-term goals are often a good idea too – they feel more achievable and reinforce the work ethic when reached.

Think about it

Rather than view targets as a negative aspect of work, most therapists look forward to the challenge – knowing that they can only benefit by trying their hardest to achieve. A large salon incentive can be anything from free products or treatments, to a weekend break, shopping vouchers or even a trip abroad. If you read the trade magazines, you will find some fabulous prizes given by commercial companies, rewarding a therapist who has become therapist of the year, or salesperson of the year.

Target setting will be both personal, for your own growth and development, and commercial for the salon, including sales targets, treatments per day, and so on.

It is important that you try to achieve your targets – doing so will not only keep you employed, it will also make you very commercial and give you invaluable experience should you decide to run your own salon or develop a mobile business.

The setting of targets is part of your action plan to improve your performance at work, which is incorporated within the **appraisal** system of monitoring your performance. You will find it easier to set achievable targets if you make sure they are SMART:

S = Specific. Have particular targets, or aims, in mind rather than too grand an idea. Set a goal specific to you, for example I want to complete two assessments each week.

M = Measurable. Make sure you are able to measure your aims with a start and a finish. Assessments can be measured against the NVQ performance criteria and ranges. Targets could be related to sales. You must know what you sell at present, and how much you want to improve, for example product sales might be on average £50 per day now, and a 10 per cent increase would raise them to £55 per day.

A = Achievable. Do not set a target that cannot be realised. A short-term target may be to complete an NVQ Level 3 unit by a set date.

R = Realistic. Doing ten treatments an hour is not realistic – be sensible with your aims. How long realistically will it take you to cover all the performance criteria and ranges in one unit?

T = Timed. For the target to be achieved, there should be a timescale for you to aim towards, e.g. by next month I will improve my timekeeping by 50 per cent or I am going to have my body massage assessment unit finished and ready to be signed off by Easter.

Key terms

Appraisal – an evaluation of a how effectively an individual is working within their job role. This may be related to bonuses from achieving sales targets and is a general performance review, carried out annually. The employee's strengths and weaknesses are identified, often with peer appraisals. This is then written up and agreed between the line manager and employee, signed by both parties, with mutually agreed objectives for training and target dates for any improvements required for an increase in good working practice or to gain promotion.

Retail sales

Retail sales are an important part of generating income for the salon as sales are not labour intensive and are very cost-effective. Being successful in selling requires sufficient stock, knowledge of the products and confidence to be able to sell. Retail sales are a major part of your profit and an integral part of your overall treatment and aftercare.

Successful retail selling:

- brings profits without taking up treatment time
- complements treatments, leading to increased client satisfaction
- helps clients keep up the good work between appointments
- encourages repeat buying when clients like a product
- adds to your exclusivity with professional-only products.

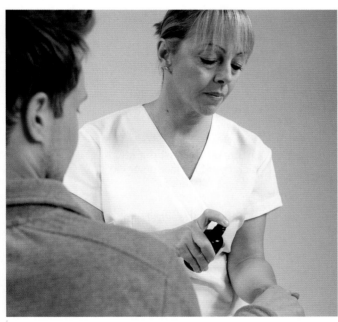

You can demonstrate suitable products during your consultation

Technical services

These refer to your skill areas and how much income you generate for the salon by giving the clients treatments. The appointments page is a good indicator of success in this area. The manager will be looking at the number of clients returning to the same therapist, new clients drawn to her and her treatment portfolio. There is a danger of the therapist favouring certain clients and offloading others, perhaps because they are not as generous. Some therapists like to stay in their comfort zone and ignore those treatments that require greater skills or more time to perform. The appointments pages will reflect this pattern should it emerge. Therefore, in your productivity goals agreed with your line manager, your treatment repertoire will be analysed and targets set for development and increasing your skills base.

Personal learning

Personal learning is your individual development within the existing salon structure and includes:

- selling
- treatments
- identifying gaps in the market
- new training
- working with others
- identifying your strengths and weakness and working to improve them (**self appraisal**)
- responsibility for training others
- taking on more responsibility
- time management
- planning and rescheduling your own work.

Key terms

Self appraisal – a judgement of your own performance at work, using a set form with headings such as communication skills, time keeping, performance, relationships with others and meeting targets.

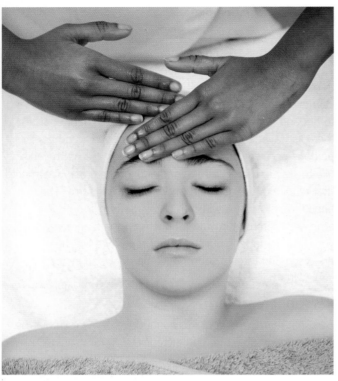

Some therapists enjoy performing hands-on treatments ...

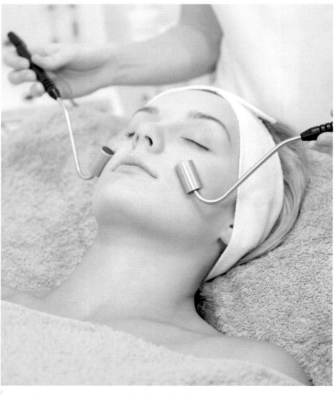

... while others may prefer electrical treatments

Agreeing targets

Agreeing targets for productivity and development with your line manager requires good communication, preparation and a willingness to accept the process and the feedback as constructive. (For detailed communication skills, see 'You and your client', page 29.)

A good manager will set realistic targets in discussion with you, and you should feel able to negotiate an achievable goal. If targets set are unachievable, staff become demotivated, relations become strained, the business is affected and a no-win situation results. It is important to regularly review targets to consolidate and to keep them SMART.

When achievable targets are not met, there will also be consequences for the business.

Targets not met

Unhappy and demoralised therapist

Pressure from superiors and peers

Stress/illness/time off sick resulting in worsening figures

Ineffectual/seen as not being team player

Costs to the business financially

Loss of job

Loss of business

The downward spiral: failure to achieve targets will affect the business

Improving your performance

Your performance will develop alongside your experiences in the salon, but you will also need to set a target for improvement.

Self-analysis is essential for growth and maturity of the therapist within a salon environment. This is often referred to as professional development, and some companies provide a continuing professional development folder (CPD) — rather like a record of achievement at school! All your training certificates and qualifications may be put in there, and it helps you spot where there are gaps in your training. Keep reading trade magazines to keep abreast of the trends within the business and ask if you can go on additional commercial training, to keep your skills current and create extra revenue for your salon.

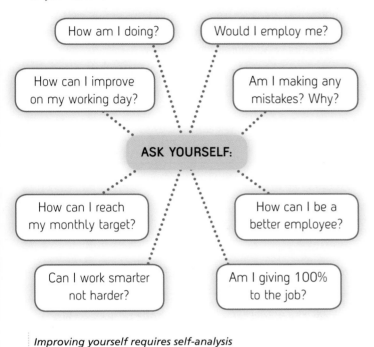

Improving yourself requires self-analysis

Inside diagram:

- How am I doing?
- Would I employ me?
- How can I improve on my working day?
- Am I making any mistakes? Why?
- **ASK YOURSELF:**
- How can I reach my monthly target?
- How can I be a better employee?
- Can I work smarter not harder?
- Am I giving 100% to the job?

Identifying training needs

If a therapist keeps making the same mistakes over and over, and clients complain or stop coming to the salon altogether, this indicates that something is wrong! Often, with age, it is easier to be reflective and spot our own mistakes and then make changes to put things right. Sometimes it is not so easy to be inward-looking, and this is where a good manager will help by giving regular work-related reviews. This is called an appraisal.

Many large companies provide both self-assessment sheets for the employee to fill in, throughout a set period, and then a joint review sheet with the manager, to help improve performance.

A self-assessment appraisal is not just about achievement within the job role and how many sales have been completed — that is really only a part of being a therapist. (However, it is an important aspect of remaining profitable.) It is also about short-term plans and development of

Think about it

Appraisal will give you the opportunity to learn, to progress in personal growth and to maintain good working relationships. It is important to react positively to any feedback or review. Nobody likes criticism, but it is important to listen carefully to what is said and take on board the suggestions and advice being offered to you. Appraisal should be viewed very much as a two-way discussion, not a reprimand. It is essential for your development as a therapist that you evolve and expand yourself to meet the demands of industry. An appraisal will help you do this.

the individual and it opens up many areas for discussion between a manager and an employee. It should highlight how well the individual is coping within his or her job role, whether the salon is asking too much of an employee, and provides an opportunity for the therapist to offer opinions on improvement.

Communication skills

In the Professional basics unit, there is a lot of advice about good communication skills with your clients and how to build rapport with them. This is an important aspect of any business, but it is also important to enjoy good and clear communication with other members of staff, too. To communicate effectively with team members and managers allows you to be seen and see others in a positive manner and to set developmental and productivity targets without personalities getting in the way. To be too emotional at work is not professional and being resentful about targets and job roles will not help you develop as a team player. If you can, try to be clear and accurate in your instructions to others, be receptive and open when instructions are given to you and be positive with those who are assisting you and encouraging good practice. Often, you need to lead by example and show that you can learn and grow from negative feedback — providing it is given in a constructive way. To be bullied over your work performance is not acceptable nor is it acceptable to harass others — so do make sure that you remain unemotional and professional in all your communications.

Think about it

When negotiating targets with your line manager it is beneficial if there is mutual respect. Avoid confrontation and taking things personally and try to appreciate the greater experience and wealth of knowledge your manager has. Consider the bigger picture — look, listen and learn. Your manager may be pressurising you because he or she is confident in your abilities to deliver, and they have greater responsibilities to ensure steady growth within the business.

An appraisal or team review should happen on a regular basis, perhaps once a month, or every three months.

- It should be at a mutually agreeable time.
- It should be constructive and open, not conducted in fear of job loss.
- It should be objective and as non-personal as possible.
- It should be a review for both parties, not just a performance judgement.
- It should be constructive and positive.
- It should leave the employee feeling enthusiastic, not depressed!

Reviewing and recording your progress

Spend some time preparing for your appraisal. Think back over your performance since your last review. How far have you progressed? Use the SMART criteria to evaluate your success and identify areas where you could have done better. A self-assessment form will help you identify your strengths and areas for improvement. Consider as well what you want to achieve in the future, for example new training requirements or additional responsibility.

Below is an example of a common format to get you thinking about the topics likely to come up in your appraisal.

Self-assessment form	
Salon: Blissed Out	**Date:** 5 July 2010
Position held: Beauty Therapist	**Therapist:** Amira Farhed
Please add comments on how you feel you are progressing in each area listed. Thank you.	
Appearance	Good. I do try to look professional every day.
Absences	Room for improvement as I have had 5 working days ill with flu this month. However, no other absences this year.
Time keeping	Could be better. I have been late twice this month as I have been relying on public transport. I have now organised a car share system with a colleague to ensure this will not be a problem in the future.
Job performance	Good. My regular clients always ask for me, and I have worked hard this month to attract new ones.
Sales targets	Good, as above. My sales are from my regulars but with the help of our recent sales meetings I am developing additional sales with other clients. My sales figure this month is in excess of target to date. My annual figures are well on target.
Treatment targets	In light of our recent training, I am not content to stay in my comfort zone and am actively encouraging my existing clients to try new treatments. This month I have had 3 clients book in for the new non-surgical face lifting treatment we have launched.
Strengths	I am confident with my treatments and I especially like facial electrical treatments. I am really enjoying them, and so are my clients.
Weaknesses	Time management. Treatment can over-run because of time spent on sales at reception, therefore I need one of the juniors to prepare my working area ready for the next client. I am happy to train whichever junior is designated to this task and will communicate my requirements daily.
Any areas of change	I have organised for Joanna to assist at the manicure station – we have lots of drop-in clients – this month, as Suki seems to have the flu bug that I had and is still off sick.
Staff development request	I would like to go on a BioSkinJetting training day if possible, as we have been asked for the treatment by several regular clients.
Action plan for next review	To improve on time management and complete my course.

An example of a self-assessment form

Feedback

It is important to get feedback on your performance, both good and bad, to help you grow into a commercial therapist and enable you to develop your skills and maturity. It also helps you become more employable, opening up new exciting avenues of opportunity in your career.

Think about it

Sarah and Caroline have both been working at Escape for the same amount of time, and are each due to have a review of their job role and performance by their manager.

Sarah is a hard worker, reliable, punctual and enthusiastic, and thinks of her review as an opportunity for further development. Caroline is not as reliable as Sarah, particularly her time keeping and punctuality, and she is not always motivated. Caroline is not looking forward to her appraisal – she feels threatened and feels sure she is going to get a reprimand.

1 Who needs the appraisal the most? Why do you think that?
2 How can both employees get the most from their appraisal?
3 If you were the manager, how would you handle each review?

Promotions and opportunities to achieve targets

As well as carrying out treatments to the very best of your ability, you must keep abreast of trends and innovations within the beauty industry. Beauty editors are sent hundreds of samples and given treatments to promote the latest innovative developments, as a favourable report generates free publicity in newspapers and magazines. Advertisements in both men's and women's magazines keep clients aware of the latest treatments, so expect your clients to ask for them.

You should find out how your salon keeps up with the latest trends, for example, visiting major trade shows is an excellent way of seeing demonstrations of new equipment and products. Entering national competitions is also a good way to meet like-minded professionals and share good practice. This can help to raise the standard of skill levels in the industry, and motivate and enthuse all who take part.

Work and time management

Time equals money in the salon and it is up to each therapist to recognise this, and if needs be, to supervise and direct others to help maximise time. If your treatments are booked in with a gap of fifteen minutes every time, that accumulates into at least two hours of gaps within a day! If you can instruct the receptionist to book your column with a much smaller gap, you not only cut down on wasted time, but your productivity goes up! Under the Supply Of Goods And Services Act 1982 you must complete your treatments within a commercially acceptable time (and you must do so for assessments too) because you have entered into a contract with the client to carry out that service with reasonable care and skill and, unless otherwise agreed, within a reasonable time and to make no more than a reasonable charge.

The diagram below shows the benefits of keeping within

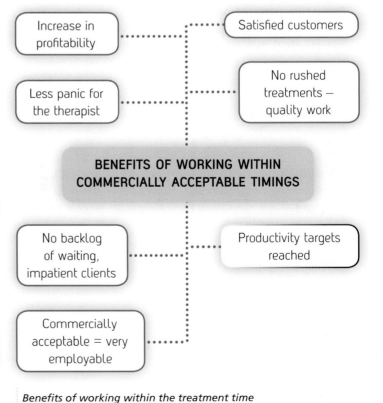

Benefits of working within the treatment time

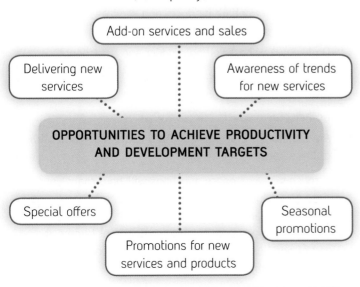

treatment times, as an example of good performance.

Opportunities to achieve productivity and development targets

Promotion

The first step is to allocate a percentage of the business's income to promotion and to use some of the profits generated by sales to help generate future sales and drive the business forward. Promotions are about perception – how your existing and potential clients see you and your business. It is about steady and maintained business growth and increased profitability.

Objectives

Your salon has to set objectives and keep up with trends and phases in the beauty industry. Marketing needs careful planning, for example a salon might set an annual **budget** and then plan advertising and promotions on a monthly basis. It can be as little as £50 per month or it could be set as a percentage of turnover, but it is essential to think ahead to maximise the return on the business's investment. The first thing to consider is the business's unique selling points (USPs). (Refer also to unit H32 Contribute to the planning and implementation of promotional activities, pages 128–130, for various types of advertising.)

Proactive promotion

A perfect way to boost sales, increase bookings and attract new clients is through sales promotion. It is important to put together a calendar of promotional activity at the beginning of the year so that you endeavour to promote your business throughout the year. Highlight quiet periods or the times when you are introducing something new. Ensure that there is always something happening within the salon.

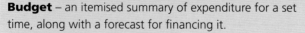

Key terms

Budget – an itemised summary of expenditure for a set time, along with a forecast for financing it.

Client profiles – the information which describes the groups you are marketing to – the demographic information such as age, gender, employment type, family situation etc, which will dictate how you approach them.

Using and converting existing clients

A large number of customers will be existing salon clients. It is therefore important to find out which treatments and products your clients would be willing to purchase. Identify your target market by asking yourself the following questions:

- What are my **client profiles**?
- Who are my ideal clients?
- What methods am I using to target clients, and are these achievable?
- What percentage of my business consists of existing clients?
- Do I keep my old clients?
- Do I know whether my clients are satisfied?
- Do I have an updated database, and if so, how frequently do I use it?
- Am I making the best possible use of the resources available (including media resources, the local community and financial services)?
- Are my opening hours suitable for the people I am trying to attract?
- Am I aware of current plans for the local area that might affect my business?
- Am I making the best use of the local community?
- Am I involved and aware of local activities that could be of benefit to the salon?
- What is the public view of the salon in the local community?
- Where are my main competitors located? Realistically, how much of a threat are they to my business?
- How do I differentiate products and services from competitor salons?
- Do I know my best-selling product and treatment?
- Do I have an adequate stock system in place?
- Am I cross-selling products?
- Do I display products effectively?
- Are there any niche markets that I could reach and attract to the salon?

All of these self-awareness questions will help make your business grow, and as an employee your contribution needs to keep evolving and developing so that the business can flourish. Meeting productivity and development targets is a big part of any business and it will contribute to the financial effectiveness of the business .

Check your knowledge

1   The main resources in any business are:
    a) time, stock, people and tools
    b) time, stock, tools and furniture
    c) time, tools, sales and stock
    d) time, tools, targets and furniture.

2   Good stock levels means having:
    a) lots of everything in stock
    b) lots of the most expensive items in stock
    c) lots of smaller items in stock
    d) the best-selling lines in stock.

3   Stock records for which you are responsible need to be:
    a) in a record handbook
    b) accurate, legible and up to date
    c) locked away in the safe
    d) held by the bank manager.

4   The profits in a business are:
    a) the money made through sales
    b) the money made in addition to treatments
    c) the money left after all the outgoings are covered
    d) the money left after the year has finished.

5   Good communication is essential for:
    a) all staff
    b) customer-facing staff only
    c) managers and salon owners
    d) customers only.

6   Time management is all about:
    a) working really hard to fill up the day
    b) looking as though you are working really hard
    c) watching the clock
    d) using your time efficiently.

7   You should regularly review your target setting to ensure:
    a) they are achievable and realistic
    b) you can make more commission
    c) you earn days off
    d) you can beat the other therapists.

8   Regular stock rotation is important to ensure that:
    a) new treatments can then be promoted
    b) the shelf for stock becomes clear
    c) the stock is within its shelf life
    d) the manager sees you are busy.

9   The purpose of a self-appraisal is to:
    a) monitor others' performances at work
    b) monitor your performance at work
    c) report others' behaviour to the manager
    d) report the manager to the salon owner.

10 The effect of good resources is to:
    a) keep stock levels very high
    b) manage staff and wages
    c) increase the profitability of the business
    d) stop products being stolen.

Getting ready for assessment

Unit G11 also links into other areas of your Level 3 assessments and treatments. This unit will not be completed until nearly the end of your course, as the ranges covered are quite detailed. You need to show you have successfully managed the following resources:

• People   • Stock   • Tools and equipment   • Time

You will need to act as a salon manager within your workshop time, supporting colleges in the salon and working with tutors and technicians to monitor the stock and resources required. This could involve taking part in a stock check or setting targets for yourself (for example, sales of treatments or training courses to enhance your repertoire of treatments) to help enhance the business. You can also use your external employment experiences to contribute towards your evidence but remember that you will need an employer statement or letter to show how you undertake actions to increase the financial effectiveness of the business. This evidence may link in with promotional activities you have undertaken for Unit H32. You will need at least one direct observation from your assessor and lots of supporting evidence. This could involve documentation from training, promotional events or problems you may have encountered with resourcing as well as how you overcame them.

Section
3
Anatomy, physiology and the skin

Related anatomy and physiology

What you will learn

Structure and functions
- Cells and tissues
- Skin
- Skeleton
- Joints
- Muscles
- Circulatory system (blood)
- Lymphatic system (lymph)

Basic principles
- Nervous system
- Endocrine system
- Respiratory and olfactory systems
- Digestive and excretory systems
- Reproductive system

Introduction

As a beauty therapist studying Level 3, you will perform a wide range of treatments, and each of these treatments will have specific benefits and effects on the client. For you to fully understand the effects of treatments on the body, you need to understand its underlying structures.

There are specific anatomical words you need to use and understand, so that you can describe either a position or a movement, when answering your examination questions.

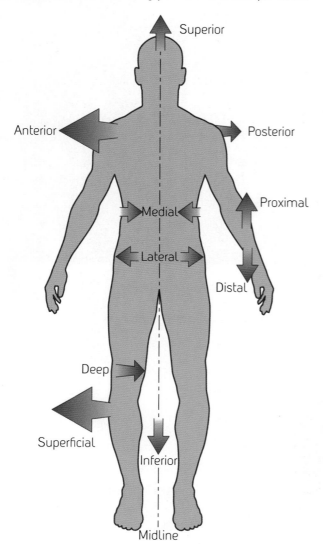

Anatomical positions and movement

Key terms

Anatomy – the study of the structure of the body.

Physiology – the study of the function of the body.

The structure and function of cells and tissues

The basic elements

The human body is an incredibly complex creation, but we can break it down into simple terms for study. The following are the main structures of which it is composed: **cells** which make up **tissues,** which help form **organs,** which make up **systems**.

For your exam

You will be expected to sit written papers for anatomy and physiology to prove competence and understanding. Most Awarding Bodies have external papers with set dates for you to sit your exams. There is no substitute for revision and you will have to put work in to remember key facts. You will be expected to label diagrams, draw simple structures and answer questions about all the topics listed.

Revision is the key to success.

Key terms

Cell – the basic structure and function unit of a living organism; a microscopic unit that combines with others to form tissues.

Tissue – a group of cells that act together for a specific purpose.

Organ – a structure that contains at least two different types of tissue that act together for a specific purpose.

System – two or more different organs that work together to provide a specific function.

Diffusion – when chemicals become concentrated outside the cell, this is the flow of small molecules that takes place through the cell's membrane until a balance exists. Cells lining the small intestines use diffusion to take in digestive products and pass them into the bloodstream for use throughout the body.

Osmosis – the movement of water through the cell membrane from areas of low chemical concentration to areas of high chemical concentration. The cell membrane is semi-permeable (meaning it will let some sized molecules through – a bit like a sieve) and osmosis allows the movement of water across the membrane until the concentration of solution equalises.

Anatomical positions		Anatomical movement		
Superior	Above	**Flexion**	Reducing the angle between two bones at joint	
Inferior	Below	**Extension**	Increasing the angle between two bones at joint	
Anterior	Front or in front	**Abduction**	Moving away from the midline	
Posterior	Back or back of	**Adduction**	Moving towards the midline	
Medial	Midline towards centre	**Rotation**	Moving a body part on its axis	
Lateral	Side or away from the midline	**Circumduction**	Moving a body part round in a circle	
Proximal	Nearest to a point of origin	**Supination**	Outward rotation away from the body	
Distal	Furthest from a point of origin	**Pronation**	Inward rotation towards the body	
Superficial	Nearest the body surface	**Inversion**	Turing a body part inwards towards the body	
Deep	Away from the surface	**Eversion**	Turning a body outwards away from the body	
Ventral	Front	**Elevation**	Lifting a body part	
Dorsal	Back	**Depression**	Lowering a body part	

These are then supported and joined by connective tissue — **membranes** and **cartilage** — to make the systems work smoothly and comfortably together.

Cells

The cell is the basic building block of all life forms. There are many types of cell in the human body, varying in size, structure and function, and as such there is no such thing as a 'typical cell'. However, cells do have certain structural characteristics in common.

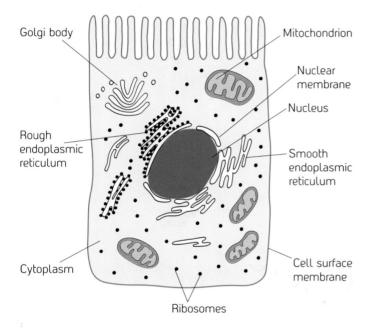

Golgi body

Rough endoplasmic reticulum

Cytoplasm

Ribosomes

Mitochondrion

Nuclear membrane

Nucleus

Smooth endoplasmic reticulum

Cell surface membrane

The structure of a cell

Key terms

Membranes – layers of material which act as selective barriers, letting some substances through but not others.

Cartilage – a stiff but flexible type of connective tissue.

Lipids – a category of organic compounds that includes fats.

Protein – a category of organic compounds that includes structural materials, enzymes and some hormones.

DNA – the genetic compound of the cell: it makes up the genes. DNA stands for deoxyribonucleic acid.

Gene – a hereditary unit composed of DNA which, combined with other genes, forms the chromosomes.

Chromosome – a thread-like body in the nucleus of the cell that contains genetic information.

Structure	Function
Cell membrane/ plasma	This encloses the cell and contains its contents, and allows substances to pass in and out of it. The outer or cell membrane is a layer of **lipids** sandwiched between two layers of larger **protein** molecules, which allows selective permeability, passive transport of fat-soluble substances, and active transport of charged particles.
Cytoplasm	A gel-like liquid consisting of 80 per cent water which fills the cell – it keeps the contents in place and contains the organelles (see below).
Nucleus	Master of the cell. It contains the cell's **DNA** (deoxyribonucleic acid) and controls growth and repair. A nucleus has a double membrane called a nuclear envelope. It is the largest cell structure, containing a double-layered membrane continuous with the ER (see page 157). It contains a tangled mass of chromatins made up of DNA and protein and controls all cellular activities, **genetic** material and nucleic acids (DNA and **RNA**).
Organelles	Mini organs in the cytoplasm. There are lots of organelles for different jobs, rather like mini factories. Two main types are mitochondria and ribosomes. Mitochondria are responsible for energy and cellular respiration. Often referred to as the power-houses of the cell, these rod-shaped structures consist of a double membrane. The inner membrane is folded into ridges which contain **enzymes** that break down **glucose** to form a compound rich in energy called adenosine triphosphate (ATP). Ribosomes manufacture proteins. Some are attached to rough ER (see page 157); some remain free in cytoplasm. They contain ribonucleic acid (RNA) and they manufacture enzymes and proteins both for export and for use within the cell.

Structure	Function
Golgi apparatus	These process, sort, then deliver proteins and fats to the membrane. Similar to smooth ER (see below) with vesicles that contain proteins and enzymes, lipids, collagen and **mucus**. They produce collagen and mucus, keep all secretions away from cytoplasm, and are best developed in secretory cells such as those in the pancreas and salivary glands.
Lysosomes	Powerful enzymes produced as vesicles from the Golgi apparatus. They break down bacteria and destroy damaged cell structures and extracellular matter, e.g. osteoclasts in bone formation.
Endoplasmic Reticulum (ER)	Endoplasmic Reticulum is a series of inter-connecting membranes – like canals – in the cytoplasm. A network of branches with similar structure to and continuous with plasma membrane. There are two types – rough and smooth: • Smooth ER synthesises fats and steroid hormones, detoxes some drugs and produces phospholipids and steroids. • Rough ER is studded with ribosomes – it produces proteins and enzymes. Its job is to synthesise proteins, enzymes and hormones which may go into other cells. The ribosomes contribute to cell support, and channel transport materials within the cell.

The structure and function of cells

The structure of cells

A cell is the smallest living unit in the human body. Cells adapt to the job role they have, but they all have the same vital processes of life; remember – MRS GREN:

Movement	Must be capable of some movement – it may not be far, but it will happen.
Respiration	This is the process of producing energy in order to carry out all the metabolic processes required.
Sensitivity/irritability	The ability to detect changes in the environment.
Growth and repair	The ability to increase in size and repair damage to cells as well as producing new, similar cells (by **meiosis division**).
Reproduction	The process by which new individual cells are produced (by meiosis division).
Excretion	The process by which the cell eliminates the waste products of **metabolism**.
Nutrition	The process by which food is obtained for use as energy for growth and repair to the body.

Key terms

Irritability – the response to stimulus on the muscle through nerve impulses.

Mitosis – cell division. A cell doesn't keep growing; it divides into two 'daughter cells', which further divide and so on (this happens billions of times). There are five phases of mitosis and then division is complete.

Meiosis division – cell division of the last stages of the sex cells in the womb, when the cell bodies divide twice, but the chromosomes separate from each other only once – so halving the number of mature cells. There are 23 chromosomes in an ovum (egg), and 23 chromosomes in sperm, so when an ovum and sperm join together to form a human being (fertilisation), there are 46 chromosomes. (This forms a zygote, which matures into a baby.)

Metabolism – the physical and chemical reactions that occur within an organism.

Cell respiration – the controlled exchange of nutrients, oxygen and glucose, as well as the elimination of waste such as carbon dioxide, to activate energy needed by the cell to function well.

Key terms

RNA – an organic compound involved in the manufacture of proteins within cells. RNA stands for ribonucleic acid.

Enzymes – organic substances which speed up metabolic reactions.

Glucose – a simple sugar that circulates in the blood – it is the main energy source for metabolism for all cells.

Mucus – a thick fluid secreted by cells in membranes and glands, which lubricates and protects tissue and keeps thing moving smoothly with no friction.

Related anatomy and physiology

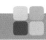

For your exam

You may be asked in a written paper to draw a simple cell, with all its components. Try to recreate the entire diagram and label all the structures in the table. Start from the inside and then work out – draw a simple nucleus, then enclose it in a square and then add the detail. Then remember MRS GREN to list the essential properties of any living organism.

Tissues

A group of cells that all perform the same function is called a tissue. Some cells have more than one function and can therefore be classified as more than one type of tissue, for example some cells of the immune system are also blood cells. Tissues can be classified into four main groups.

Type of tissue	Job role in the body
Epithelial	Covering for outside and lining inside of the body – known as endothelium when lining internal organs.
Connective	Supporting tissue includes fibrous and elastic fibres. **Ligaments**, cartilage, and bone-blood.
Muscular	There are three types: • Skeletal – called voluntary muscle as it is under a person's conscious control • Smooth – called involuntary muscle as it is found in organs over which we have no control (digestion, breathing, etc.) • Cardiac – specialist muscle forming the heart which never stops working, until death.
Nervous	A highly specialised tissue containing **neurons** which form: • the **central nervous system** • the **autonomic nervous system** • the **peripheral nervous system** as well as specialist sensory organs such as the retina of the eye.
	We should include blood here: it has a specialist role in the body but it is classed as connective tissue. However, it does not have a physically supporting role in the body, or any connective role, in the sense that it does not support or join muscles, bones or organs – but it is vital to life and is the transport system of the whole body.
Blood	A suspension of red and white blood cells (erythrocytes and leucocytes) in **plasma**. It contains 45% cells and 55% plasma. The blood's function is to: • transport food and oxygen to all the cells of the body • remove the waste from all the cells of the body • fight infection • clot by thrombocytes forming at the site of a wound.

The job roles of different tissue types

Key terms

Ligaments – strong dense flexible bands of connective tissues which link bones together at a joint. They strengthen the joints and allow a full range of movement.

Neuron – a cell which transmits electrical nerve impulses and carries information from one part of the body to another.

Central nervous system – consists of the brain and spinal cord.

Autonomic nervous system – made up of the sympathetic and parasympathetic nervous systems supplying the internal organs.

Peripheral nervous system – made up of the autonomic and somatic nervous systems.

Plasma – the protein serum content of blood, a thin yellow liquid containing fibrinogens for blood clotting, globulins to support oxygen transport of amino acids, albumin, carbon dioxide and hormones around the body.

Epithelial tissue

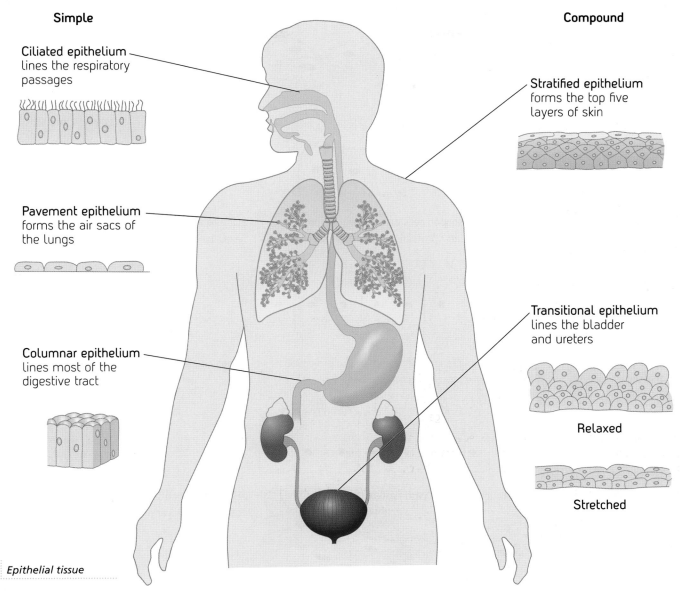

Simple

Ciliated epithelium
lines the respiratory
passages

Pavement epithelium
forms the air sacs of
the lungs

Columnar epithelium
lines most of the
digestive tract

Compound

Stratified epithelium
forms the top five
layers of skin

Transitional epithelium
lines the bladder
and ureters

Relaxed

Stretched

Epithelial tissue

Epithelial tissue (epithelium) provides the covering for outside and the lining for inside surfaces of the body, protecting it
from wear and tear and it is continually renewing itself as required. Epithelial tissue is also the tissue from which glands are
developed. Lining epithelia can be subdivided according to its structure. The various types are shown in the table on page 160.

Type of lining epithelia	Structure	Location/job
Simple squamous or simple pavement epithelium	Simple flat cells form a smooth lining	Lines blood vessels
Simple cuboidal epithelium	Simple cube-shaped cells	Produces secretions – for example, mucus – and covers the ovaries
Columnar	Tall, column-shaped cells on a basement membrane providing greater protection against wear and tear	Lines glands and digestive system; for example, the stomach and intestines
Ciliated columnar epithelium	Tall, column-shaped cells with hair-like projections which move mucus and other substances	Lines air passages and fallopian tubes
Stratified squamous epithelium	Many layers of cells with flattened surface	Horny stratified layer – no nucleus, creates the germinative layer of the skin
Transitional epithelium	Similar to stratified epithelium but with rounded surface cells which adapt to expansion	Waterproof organs, found in the bladder, capable of withstanding urine

Types of epithelial lining tissue

Glands

Glands develop from epithelial tissue and can be classified as exocrine or endocrine. Endocrine glands secrete hormones directly into the bloodstream (see page 207). Exocrine glands pass their secretions through a single duct (simple glands) or through several secretory ducts (compound glands). Many of these secretions contain enzymes which produce chemical changes in specific substances but remain unchanged by the reaction. The types of exocrine glands are shown in the table below.

Type of exocrine glands	Location in the body	Secretions	What they look like
Simple tubular glands	Walls of small intestine, stomach	Substances which aid digestion	
Simple coiled glands	Sweat glands in skin	Sweat to control body temperature	
Simple saccular glands	Sebaceous glands in skin	Sebum which lubricates skin and hair	
Compound tubular glands	Duodenum (first section of small intestine)	Substances which aid digestion	
Compound saccular glands	Salivary glands in mouth	Substances which aid digestion	

Types of exocrine glands

Connective tissue

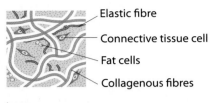

Connective tissue

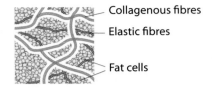

Adipose tissue

There are five types of connective tissue, as shown in the table below.

Type of connective tissue	Illustration	Structure	Job role
Loose connective tissue – areolar (e.g. **subcutaneous** tissue)	Elastic fibre / Connective tissue cell / Fat cells / Collagenous fibres	Loose network of collagen and elastic fibres, few blood cells and nerves, some fat cells	Packing tissue combination of white fibres, yellow elastic and cells. Forms tough transparent lining between and within organs
Adipose or fatty tissue	Collagenous fibres / Elastic fibres / Fat cells	Similar to areolar tissue but with network of fat cells which provides food reserves for the body and insulates against heat loss	Similar to areolar, but containing many fat cells. Protects delicate organs such as the kidneys
White fibrous – dense connective tissue or fibrons tissue (e.g. ligaments, collagen fibres, reticular and elastic fibres)	Fibroblast nuclei / Collagen bundles	Bundles of strong collagenous fibres and fibroblasts arranged regularly or irregularly	Collagen fibres Regular bundles in tendons, ligaments; irregular arrangement in fascia surrounding muscles
Cartilage – hyaline, elastic fibrocartilage	Pure cartilage / Cartilage cell	Cells called chondrocytes separated by fibres, no blood vessels, tough and elastic	White fibrous and yellow elastic Intervertebral discs
Bone tissue Compact and cancellous	Channel (for nerves and blood vessels) / Bone cells	Specialised type of cartilage which has undergone ossification, collagenous fibres provide strength and mineral salts provide rigidity; has a rich blood supply	Bones of the human skeleton

Types of connective tissue

As the name suggests, connective tissue connects and supports all other types of tissue. It consists of living cells as well as non-living matrix and fibres. There are two types of fibres, **collagen** and **elastin**. Collagen fibres develop from cells called fibroblasts which secrete collagen, the main supporting cells of the body. These form coarse fibres which are grouped into bundles. Elastin fibres allow for the stretchy or elastic properties required in some areas of the body such as **tendons** and internal organs.

Key terms

Collagen – main protein of connective tissue, providing strength. It is the main component of cartilage, ligaments, tendons, bone and teeth; it also strengthens blood vessels and skin.

Elastin – a protein similar to collagen, it is the main component of elastic fibres in the skin and other areas of the body which need to be able to stretch.

Tendons – tough white fibrous cords of connective tissue which attach muscles to bone (the fibrous covering of the bone is the periosteum). Tendons allow the bones to move when the skeletal muscles contract.

Subcutaneous – deepest layer of the skin, the fatty layer which consists of adipose tissue.

Adipose – located under the dermis, this is the body's energy store, made up of loose connective tissue in which fat cells (adipocytes) are suspended. Adipocytes are essential to health around the eyes, and give the internal organs warmth, energy and protection – but too much adipose tissue is not good for health and obesity may occur.

Fascia – fibrous connective tissue that envelopes a muscle and provides the pathway for nerves, blood vessels and lymph flow.

Cartilage

There are three different types of cartilage, as mentioned in the table on page 162.

Type of cartilage	Description	Location
Hyaline	This is the most common in the body. It is firm and elastic, so gives support and flexibility thus reducing friction; it acts as a shock absorber within the joints	Joints; also the ear, larynx and between the ribs and sternum (forms the C-shaped rings that keep the windpipe open, preventing it from collapsing in on itself)
Elastic cartilage	Also called yellow elastic because it is constructed of yellow elastic fibre	Tip of the nose, and upper ear
Fibrocartilage	Also called white fibrocartilage because it is made up of fibres with cartilage cells in between	In the discs of the spine where great strength is required

Types of cartilage

Membranes

There are also three types of membrane in the body, which make body parts run smoothly, reduce friction and prevent passages drying out.

Type of membrane	What it does	Location
Mucous membrane	Produces a slimy sticky fluid (mucus) to lubricate surfaces and prevent them from drying out – makes passages run smoothly	Lines all the surfaces which open onto the outside of the body: the airways and the digestive, urinary and reproductive tracts
Synovial membrane	Produces synovial fluid which is thick and viscous to cushion and ensure joints work smoothly	Lines the spaces around the joints, e.g. knee and hip
Serous membrane	Produces a more watery fluid, for the organs to slide against each other, to prevent friction internally	Surrounds the lungs, heart and all the organs in the abdomen

Types of membrane

Muscle tissue

Muscle cells (often called fibres) are long and thin. Muscle contraction produces skeletal movement. Muscle tissue can contract without first being stretched, unlike elastic connective tissue fibres.

There are three types of muscle tissue, which are shown in the table below.

Type of muscle tissue	Structure	Function	Illustration
Skeletal muscle, often called voluntary muscle or striped muscle	Long muscle cells/fibres containing striped myofibrils of actin and myosin bound together by connective tissue, with rich blood supply provided by capillaries running between muscle cells	Contracts strongly when stimulated to provide voluntary movement	Skeletal muscle fibre — Striations, Nuclei
Smooth muscle, often called unstriped muscle	Spindle-shaped cells bound together by connective tissue, supplied by automatic nerves	Contracts automatically without conscious thought (contractions) over long periods of time	Smooth muscle cells, Nucleus, Connective tissue
Cardiac muscle	Short, cylindrical branched fibres bound together by connective tissue which allows nerve impulses to spread from one to another and along the muscle. Involuntary and irregularly striped	Contractions are controlled by nerves and occur automatically throughout life in the heart wall only	Cardiac muscle cell, Striation, Nucleus, Connective tissue

Types of muscle tissue

Nervous tissue

Nervous tissue consists of nerve cells called neurons. Neurons have a large cell body containing a nucleus as well as several short projections called dendrites and one long projection called an axon. The function of nervous tissue is to transmit messages or nervous impulses from inside or outside the body to other tissues, in a process of communication. The dendrites import nervous impulses from other cells and tissues while the axon exports nervous impulses away from the cell body to other structures. You could think of dendrites as taking incoming calls and axons as making outgoing calls from a single neuron!

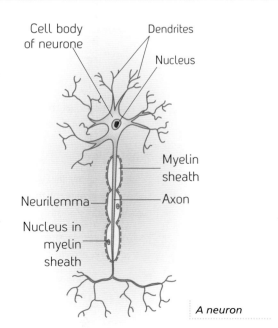

A neuron

Organs and organ systems

A group of tissues functioning together is called an organ. The skin is an example of an organ which consists of epithelial tissue, connective tissue and muscular tissue. Organs can be classified as tubular or compact and while each type shares some common structures, none are identical. All organs contain a blood supply.

Type of organ	Structure	Example
Tubular	Three common layers – outer epithelium, middle muscular layer, inner endothelium – plus unique layers associated with its individual function and a space called a **lumen**	Heart, small intestine
Compact	Superficial layers called the cortex; deeper layers called the medulla; no lumen	Liver, kidney

Types of organ

Key terms

Lumen – the inner open space or cavity of a tubular organ such as a blood vessel or an intestine.

One or more organs functioning together is called an organ system. The structure and function of each organ system is shown in the table below.

Type of organ system	Structure	Function
Circulatory	Blood, heart and blood vessels – arteries, veins, arterioles, venules and capillaries	Transports oxygen and nutrients to the tissues in blood and carries waste away
Respiratory	Mouth, nasal cavities, trachea, bronchii, bronchioles, lungs	Facilitates gaseous exchange (oxygen and carbon dioxide) between body and environment
Lymphatic	Lymph, lymphatic vessels, lymph nodes, spleen	Filters and eliminates harmful bacteria and waste, produces lymphocytes, which fight infection
Digestive	Mouth, oesophagus, pancreas, liver, gall bladder, stomach, small and large intestines	Breaks down food and facilitates the absorption of nutrients and elimination of waste
Urinary	Kidneys, bladder, ureter, urethra	Main excretory system, storage and elimination of urine
Nervous	Central nervous system – brain and spinal cord, peripheral nervous system and sense organs	System of communication within body and between the body and the environment
Endocrine	Endocrine glands – hypothalamus, pituitary, thyroid, adrenals, gonads and pancreas	Produces hormones which control many functions and facilitate **homeostatic** regulation
Skeletal	Axial and appendicular skeleton, joints, cartilage and tendons	Supporting framework which provides protection and facilitates movement
Muscular	Skeletal muscles	Facilitates movement in conjunction with skeletal system
Reproductive	Male – penis, testis, epididymis, scrotum, sperm duct; female – ovaries, uterus, vagina, mammary glands	Hormonal regulation, menstrual cycle, fertilisation, pregnancy, birth, lactation, continuation of the species

Types of organ system

You will learn more about each of these systems now.

Key terms

Integumentary system – term often used to refer to hair, skin and nails. It protects the body like a suit of armour, preventing harmful invaders from getting in.

Homeostatic – being in a steady state, a condition of internal stability and constancy. All cells want to be in homeostasis as it is the peak condition. Any disruption and the cells will adjust: take on more water, energy and so on. With long-term disruption, ill health can occur. The main organs for homeostasis in a human are the lungs, skin, liver and kidneys. Bodily activities need to be controlled to maintain good health – water levels, salt and sugar levels, temperature and so on.

Related anatomy and physiology

The skin

You will learn about:
- the functions of the skin
- the structure of the skin.

The function of the skin

Skin has six main functions:

- sensation
- heat regulation
- absorption
- protection
- excretion
- secretion.

Think about it

Remember SHAPES from your Level 2 book? To remind you of the skin's functions, think SHAPES: **S**ensation, **H**eat regulation, **A**bsorption, **P**rotection, **E**xcretion and **S**ecretion.

Sensation

The sense of touch is often thought of as the most important function of the skin. We touch ourselves a countless number of times each day when we wash, dress, apply products, rub an aching limb or scratch away an itch. Touch is also an important way in which we communicate our feelings with others and, of course, it is the basic technique of most, if not all, beauty and complementary therapy treatments. It is the underlying principle of manual or 'hands on' treatments.

In the same way that people transmit and receive messages through touch, the skin is involved in a communication process with the brain via sensory nerves, which carry messages around the body. There are thousands of sensory nerve endings in the skin which send and receive messages to and from the brain. They recognise sensations of pain, pressure, touch, heat and cold on the skin and carry messages about these sensations to the brain, which sets off a reaction. For example, if the finger is pricked with a pin, the sensory nerve endings in that area will recognise the skin damage and send a message to the brain. The brain will send a message back to the finger which is recognised as pain and instructs the finger to move. Of course, this all happens very quickly! Some messages do not travel as far as the brain, but instead produce automatic and immediate reflex actions in response to the stimulation of the nerve endings. So, the skin's function of sensation is a two-way process of receiving and transmitting information between the external world and the internal systems.

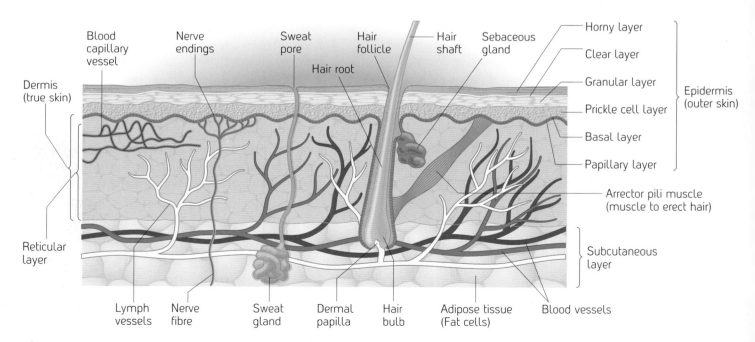

The skin

Heat regulation

The skin plays an important role in helping to maintain the optimum body temperature for normal functioning of its systems. Normal body temperature, which is measured by a thermometer either under the tongue or in the **axilla**, is 36.8°C. Body temperature is slightly higher at night than in the morning and higher in younger than older people as they tend to be more active, but it fluctuates slightly as a response to internal or external factors. Extreme changes in body temperature can be dangerous, even fatal. Like sensation, temperature regulation is controlled as the brain stimulates specific nerve endings in the skin.

Body temperature is regulated internally in two ways, by sweating and **vasodilation**.

Sweating

Sweat comprises water and waste products, and the amount excreted varies according to changes in temperature. The body is producing small amounts of sweat all the time, which we are usually unaware of, and this serves to maintain the temperature of the body. When body temperature increases, more sweat is produced in an attempt to lower the body's internal temperature through the process of evaporation. Body temperature can increase as a response to external or internal factors such as a hot climate, vigorous activity, stress or illness.

Vasodilation

The skin, like the entire body, contains a network of vessels which transport blood. The smallest and most superficial of these vessels are capillaries. To lower body temperature the capillary walls expand (vasodilation), resulting in a larger surface area. This brings more blood close to the surface of the skin, causing it to cool down more quickly, cooling the body at the same time. When the body feels cold the opposite happens. The capillary walls get narrower (**vasoconstriction**) which results in a smaller surface area and less blood volume close to the skin's surface, so less heat is lost. Another change that occurs on the surface of the skin when the body feels cold is the appearance of 'goose bumps' which make the little hairs on the skin stand up on end. These hairs trap warm air close to the skin's surface, providing insulation to help to maintain the body's normal temperature.

Absorption

One of the skin's most important properties is its ability to repel moisture and bacteria and, on the whole, act as a waterproof seal. To this end, the skin has the ability to absorb only a small amount of oily substances. The outermost layer of the **epidermis**, the stratum corneum or horny layer (see page 166), acts as a barrier against water, though a tiny amount can be absorbed, and oily substances can be absorbed via the hair follicles. Many molecules are simply too big to penetrate the skin at all. Manual massage and electrical current (which is applied in some salon treatments such as **galvanism** or **high frequency**) aids absorption by dissolving larger molecules and thus assisting their passage through the layers of the skin.

The varying thickness of the stratum corneum affects the absorption of substances. Where it is thickest, on the soles of the feet, there is limited absorption. Where it is thinner, on the face and neck, absorption is greatest. Absorption is further assisted by manual or mechanical exfoliation, which helps to remove the outer keratinised layers of the stratum corneum.

Key terms

Epidermis – the thin, top layer of the three sections which form the skin (epidermis, dermis and subcutaneous layer). It has no blood supply and sits on top of the dermis.

It is made up of five layers: stratum corneum, or horny layer; stratum lucidum, or clear layer; stratum granulosum, or granular layer; stratum spinosum, or prickle cells layer; stratum germinativum, or basal layer. These layers form the outer protection of the body and are constantly renewing and shedding, forming new skin that repairs itself when necessary.

Galvanism – the use of a piece of electrical equipment for treatment that provides a constant direct current on the negative or positive polarity. It can be used in three ways: on the face to deep cleanse an oily or blemished skin (desincrustation) and to introduce products deep into the skin for a specific purpose such as hydrating, soothing or healing (iontophoresis). On the body it helps in the treatment of cellulite.

High frequency – an alternating electrical current that oscillates (changes direction) at very high speed. It may be applied directly or indirectly to the body and face.

Key terms

Axilla – or armpit, the area of the body between the upper humerus and thorax. It provides a passageway for the large, important arteries, nerves, veins and lymphatics which ensure that the upper limb functions properly.

Vasodilation – widening of blood vessels.

Vasoconstriction – narrowing of blood vessels.

Related anatomy and physiology

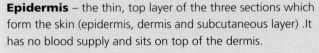

Protection

The skin serves to protect the body and its internal structures in a number of ways. Physical sensation alerts the sensory receptors to environmental factors which may cause damage through the perception of heat, cold and pain. Skin is also a water-tight container. If it were not, the body would absorb the water it came into contact with whenever a person went swimming or took a shower, and also the water inside the body would escape. The stratum corneum, together with a layer of fatty adipose tissue, provide this water-tight seal. The adipose tissue has a further protective quality. It cushions the body against knocks and blows, protecting the bones and internal organs from injury.

Ultraviolet (UV) light is a well-documented enemy of the skin and exposure to it can cause severe, irreversible damage such as burning or skin cancer. When the skin is exposed to the sun, melanocytes are stimulated to produce increased levels of the colour pigment melanin. This darkens the outer layers of the epidermis and slows down penetration by ultraviolet rays to the deeper layers of the **dermis**. Melanin production protects the skin by blocking out some of the harmful effects of UV.

The skin and sunlight also work together to benefit the body. Exposure to ultraviolet rays stimulates the production of vitamin D by the skin, which is necessary to promote healthy bone tissue. The skin requires protection from harmful bacteria and other disease-forming micro-organisms. The stratum corneum blocks the invasion of foreign bodies, while sebum has a mild antiseptic quality and so can destroy some bacteria. Sweat and sebum combine to form the **acid mantle** which helps to prevent invasion by bacteria and fungi.

Key terms

Dermis – the second of the three layers of the skin, found between the basal layer of the epidermis and the adipose or subcutaneous tissue. It contains all the blood and nerve supply to the skin, as well as the hair shaft, sebaceous and sweat glands.

Acid mantle – often termed the hydro lipid film (hydro = water, lipid = fat), so it is the thin coating of the skin, made up of sebum and sweat. Its job is to help prevent bacterial growth. It has a pH value of 4.5–5.5.

pH – potential hydrogen. This is the degree of alkalinity and acidity measured on the pH scale of 1–14, where 1 is a strong acid, 7 is neutral and 14 is a strong alkali. The pH of the skin is 4.5–5.5.

The acid mantle

The skin has the ability to balance acid and alkaline factors and maintain a pH of 4.5–5.5. This makes it slightly acidic and the light oil that coats the skin is what is known as the acid mantle.

The acid mantle plays a part in the function of protection as it prevents the invasion of harmful micro-organisms which could cause infection. Because of the alkaline content of cleansing products, excessive or incorrect use will have the effect of stripping the skin of its natural oils. As sebum has an antibacterial effect, the disturbance of the pH balance combined with the drying effect can leave skin prone to infection and irritation.

Nourishing products	
pH	Similar acidic pH to skin (4.5–5.5)
Examples	Moisturisers, cuticle conditioners, massage mediums, nourishing masks, hair conditioners
Precautions	Use correct product for skin/hair type to avoid over-nourishment
Cleansing products	
pH	Alkaline pH
Examples	Cleansers, exfoliators, cleansing masks, soap, shampoo
Precautions	Overuse can have a drying effect

The pH of nourishing and cleansing products

Excretion

The skin eliminates waste products by excretion. The sweat glands excrete sweat which contains salt, urea and other impurities which would be hazardous to the body if not expelled. Excretion of sweat is minimal under normal circumstances.

Secretion

The skin secretes substances from specialised cells and glands which are beneficial to the health of the skin. For example, the sebaceous gland secretes sebum which is an oily substance made up of fatty acids and waxes. Sebum serves the purpose of nourishing the skin and hair and also plays a part in protecting against infection.

Additional knowledge

The process of keratinisation

It takes about 28 days for the cells to travel up from the basal layer to the top of the epidermis to be shed. This process of keratinisation is faster in exposed parts of the body, such as the hands and face.

Think about it

The skin is in fact, the largest organ of the body. People in quiz shows always say the liver – but the skin is the largest organ.

Think about it

We shed skin cells all the time – they are in our clothes, on bedding, and on any surface we brush up against. An amazing 60 per cent of the collection in a vacuum cleaner is made up of dead skin cells! The only time you really see skin shedding is when a suntan begins to peel off, or when there is a malfunction of the exfoliation process, as in psoriasis.

The structure of the skin

Some of the skin's structures such as sweat and sebaceous glands and blood vessels and nerves have been discussed on pages 166–168.

The skin can be divided into three distinct layers.

1 The outer layer is the epidermis.
2 Beneath it is the dermis. The epidermis and dermis are 'glued' together by the basement membrane.
3 Deepest of all is the subcutaneous or fatty layer which consists of adipose tissue.

Structure of the epidermis

The epidermis consists of five layers:

1 stratum corneum – the surface or horny layer
2 stratum lucidum – the clear layer
3 stratum granulosum – the granular cell layer
4 stratum spinosum – the prickle cell layer
5 stratum germinativum – the deepest or basal cell layer.

Stratum means layer and the second part of the name refers to its structure or function.

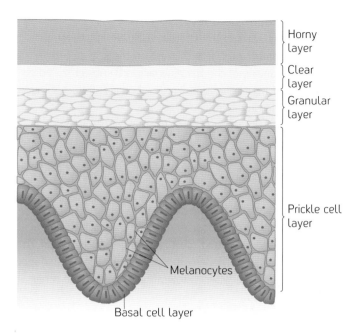

The structure of the epidermis

Think about it

Your Awarding Body may (or may not) insist you learn the Latin names for the epidermis, and they all begin with the term Stratum – which just means layer. A good way to remember the rest of their names is the mnemonic of **C**urvy **L**adies **G**et **S**ome **G**lances.

A mnemonic is just a short rhyme or phrase to help the memory – only good if you can remember what they mean! Some students like them, it's your choice, but they can be useful!

Stratum corneum/horny layer

The stratum corneum is a layer of cornified (thickened) cells which forms the surface of the epidermis. It is the visible part of skin and the area where skin is shed. Here the cells are flattened, consist mainly of keratin and overlap to protect the skin from damage. The stratum corneum is sometimes called the horny layer because of the thickness and roughness of the dead skin cells. Darker skins have a thicker stratum corneum than paler ones and therefore have greater protection from the damaging effects of UV light. The stratum corneum is thickest on the soles of the feet and thinner on the face, which affects the absorption of applied substances.

Stratum lucidum/clear layer

Lucid means clear and the stratum lucidum is a layer of dead, transparent cells. It is thickest on the soles of the feet and the palms of the hands which are subject to more wear and tear than other areas of the body. The thicker layer provides added protection.

Stratum granulosum/granular layer

This granular layer contains living cells which are beginning to wear down. The cells are much flatter than those in the deeper layers and contain less fluid.

Stratum spinosum/prickle cell layer

The stratum spinosum consists of living cells which are plump and filled with fluid. This is also known as the prickle cell layer because of the way the cells look. They are shaped like spines or spikes, which allows them to attach to other cells.

Stratum germinativum/basal cell layer

The deepest layer of the epidermis is the stratum germinativum, also known as the basal cell layer because of its position at the base of the epidermis. This layer consists of living 'parent' cells which reproduce by continually dividing to make new cells called keratinocytes. Keratinocytes produce the protein keratin, the main building block of skin, hair and nails.

Keratinisation

Skin is continually making new cells in the stratum germinativum and shedding them from the stratum corneum in a process called keratinisation. The three lower layers of the epidermis contain living cells which are fed by the dermis, while in the two uppermost layers the cells start to die. A new cell is formed when a parent cell divides. It moves up through the layers and changes in shape and structure to become flatter and more horny. By the time the cell reaches the stratum corneum, it is no more than a flat, empty shell which is shed away. This natural shedding process is called **desquamation**.

The process of keratinisation, which carries a new cell on its journey from the stratum germinativum to the stratum corneum, takes approximately 28 days. As a person ages, the process of keratinisation slows down. This explains why older people seem to keep a suntan for longer – they retain their dying skin cells so that there is a build-up of old skin cells in the stratum corneum as they wait for new ones to push through.

Beauty therapists use techniques to manually slough off dead skin cells, such as facial and body scrubs, electrotherapy such as galvanism, and **microdermabrasion** which makes the skin look brighter and fresher.

Structure and function of the dermis

The dermis contains many fewer cells than the epidermis and more connective tissue. The dermis is divided into two layers as well as a number of appendages such as sweat and sebaceous glands, hair follicles and nails.

The uppermost layer of the dermis is rich in nerves and blood supply, which exist to feed the lower, living layers of the epidermis. Blood carries nutrients and oxygen to the cells and carries away waste products. The deepest layer of the dermis is made up of two types of protein fibres – collagen and elastin. These fibres are tangled together and form the connective tissue of the dermis. Each has a separate structure and function.

- Collagen fibres are thick strands of protein which provide skin with structure and strength. Collagen fibres exist in bundles which run in different directions in different parts of the body.

- Elastin fibres are present in the dermis in tight bundles. Along with collagen fibres, they provide skin with its characteristic elasticity – the ability to stretch and return to its natural state.

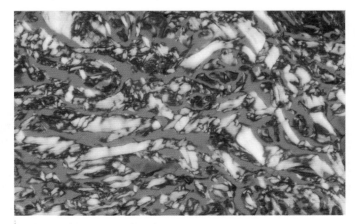

Collagen fibres viewed under a microscope

Key terms

Desquamation – exfoliation; the process of shedding flakes of skin.

Microdermabrasion – the removal of the stratum corneum by light abrasion to improve the condition of the skin.

A decline in the regeneration of collagen and elastin fibres of the dermis is the cause of lines, wrinkles and the less pronounced facial contours characteristic of mature skins.

Sweat glands

There are two types of sweat gland: eccrine and apocrine.

- Eccrine glands – these are found all over the body, but there are more of them in the palms of the hands and the soles of the feet. They are constantly excreting small amounts of sweat in order to maintain optimum body temperature.

- Apocrine glands – attached to hair follicles under the arms, in the groin and around the nipples. They are the larger of the two glands and are activated when we are excited, stressed or anxious. Apocrine sweat also contains pheromones, which are hormones that are thought to play a role in sexual attraction.

When sweat comes into contact with bacteria it causes an unpleasant smell which we recognise as body odour. Deodorants contain an antiseptic which decreases the activity of bacteria while anti-perspirants contain an astringent which reduces the pore size, as with a toner, and so less sweat reaches the surface of the skin. Both products commonly contain a perfume which masks body odour.

Sebaceous glands

Sebaceous glands secrete sebum, a natural oily substance, which moisturises the skin and helps protect against infection due to its antibacterial quality. There are no sebaceous glands on the palms of the hands, the soles of the feet or the surface of the lips. Areas containing the most sebaceous glands are the scalp, the back and the chest. There are more sebaceous glands in a man's body than in a woman's and more in black/dark Asian skins than in white/Caucasian, so males and people with black/dark Asian skin tend to have more oily skin.

Factors which increase sweat production	Factors which decrease sweat production
Warm external climate or warm clothing	Temperatures lower than 36.8°C, which result in vasoconstriction
Vigorous activity which increases muscle temperature	Limited activity, which results in a lowering of body temperature
Hot, spicy foods and alcohol which can cause vasodilation of the capillaries	Removing certain foods from the diet that cause vasodilation
Skin colour – black skin contains more sweat glands	Skin colour – white/Caucasian skin contains fewer sweat glands
Certain illnesses or medical conditions are accompanied by a fever which results in a high temperature	Certain illnesses result in a decrease in sweat production, such as low blood pressure and diabetes
Hot flushes and sweating are characteristic of the **menopause**	As the body ages, circulation becomes sluggish and the body has a tendency to feel cold
Certain forms of medication have side-effects which increase body temperature	With age the sweat glands eventually become redundant due to inactivity
Hormonal activity caused by an emotional response to fear or excitement, which causes vasolidation in all areas of the body	

Factors which affect sweat production

Key terms

Menopause – the end of the reproductive cycle in a female, when periods no longer occur due to a lack of oestrogen and progesterone, hormones from the ovaries that stimulate the menstrual cycle. Menopause can occur naturally with age (approx. 50–53 years) or through surgery, if the ovaries and/or uterus are removed during a hysterectomy, or through illness and the use of certain medication. Premature (early) menopause can occur in women who have hormonal or medical problems.

Structure and functions of the subcutaneous layer

The subcutaneous layer separates the dermis from muscles. The subcutaneous layer is therefore underneath the main layers of skin (the dermis and the epidermis). The subcutaneous layer functions as a storage area for fat. This layer of fat serves to protect the body against knocks and bangs by cushioning the blow. It protects the internal organs, the bones, the blood vessels and nerves. There is an abundance of nerves and blood vessels throughout the dermis and they are protected by fat cells.

The subcutaneous layer has another important function. As fat is a poor conductor of heat, it insulates the body by preventing heat loss — the same way that draught insulation works in the home when it is fitted around doors and windows. It keeps the cold on one side and the heat on the other. Female skin tends to retain more fluid than male skin and the subcutaneous layer is thicker, giving it a 'softer' appearance.

Skin colouring

The skin owes its colouring to the red haemoglobin found within the blood vessels, yellow carotenoids within subcutaneous fat and the dark brown pigment melanin. Various degrees of pigmentation are present in different ethnic groups. The differences are in the amount of melanin produced and are not dependent upon the number of **melanocytes** present (see below).

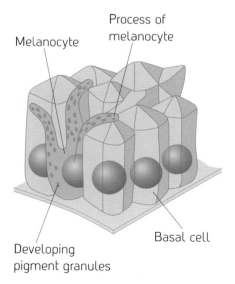

Melanocyte

Process of melanocyte

Developing pigment granules

Basal cell

Melanocytes in the basal cells

Key terms

Melanocytes – cells which make melanin.

Certain areas of skin are very rich in pigment, such as the genital area and the nipples, while practically no pigment is present in the palms of the hands and the soles of the feet (often referred to as 'glabrous' skin; it lacks hair follicles and sebaceous glands, and has a thicker epidermis).

The pigment is stored as fine granules within the cells of the germinative layer, although some granules may also be deposited between the cells. In white/Caucasian skin the granules occur only in the deepest cell layers and mainly in the cylinder-shaped cells of the basal row. In all other skin types pigment is found throughout the entire layer and even in the granular layer (stratum granulosum).

Melanin

All melanin is made in special cells called melanocytes and then distributed to the epithelial cells. The melanocytes are scattered in the basal layers of the epidermis and mature as the embryo is developing in the womb. They are influenced by the units of inheritance gene code which determines race and colouring.

Skin characteristics and skin types

Skin characteristics and skin types of different client groups come into six basic categories:

- White/Caucasian
- Black
- Asian
- Oriental
- Mixed race
- Mediterranean/Latino.

These are generalised only for purposes of identification. Always remember that there are many variations within these categories.

Additional knowledge

Albinism

Some people are born without the ability to produce melanin within their skins and with no hair pigment — a congenital condition called albinism. People with this condition have pure white hair, white skin and pink eyes.

A congenital condition describes a condition that is recognised at birth or that is believed to have been present since birth. Congenital malformations include all disorders present at birth, whether they are inherited or caused by an environmental factor.

White/Caucasian skin

How to recognise it	Features	Possible problems
White/Caucasian skin is the most delicate of all the skin types. It is light in colour with blue or green eye colouring. It has blue and pink tones from the blood capillaries, which can be seen through the pale epidermis, and its melanin content is not as high as other skin types. Most likely origin: Britain Northern and western Europe North America Canada New Zealand Australia. 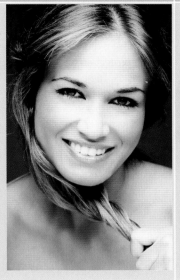	The skin of blond or red-haired people tends to have a fine hair growth, and as the hair colour is light or fair, it is not noticeable. It tends to be finer in texture and thinner than non-white skin.	Light skins do not tan easily and are at risk of skin damage, especially if there are large amounts of freckles present. Fair skins burn quickly and are less tolerant of ultraviolet light so care should be taken in hotter climates. It is prone to early signs of ageing and wrinkles, and may bruise easily. It can be more prone to broken capillaries, especially if the skin is very pale.

Origins and features of white/Caucasian skin

Think about it

People native to Canada, New Zealand and Australia have naturally darker skin. However, due to migration into these countries from Northern Europe, the population has a high proportion of white/Caucasian skin types. The indigenous people of Canada are Inuit and are related to the Eskimos in the Arctic; the indigenous people of New Zealand are the Maori and descended from Polynesians; and the indigenous people of Australia are the Aboriginals. Their darker skin offers greater protection from the sunlight.

Additional knowledge

Variations in white/Caucasian skin

Of course, not all white/Caucasian skin is very pale and delicate. Some skin tones are darker if the parents have brown or black hair, in which case the skin may tan more easily and be less prone to easy damage. Some white/Caucasian skins, noticeably the Irish and Scottish, have striking dark hair colouring with paler skin tone.

Think about it

All these basic skin categories provide a general overview and are not to be used to replace a thorough consultation with the client – and remember: there are always exceptions to the rule! Treat each client as an individual, not just a category of skin colour, as different factors come into play with each client: different lifestyles, dietary intake and use of products will determine how the skin behaves and reacts.

Black skin

How to recognise It		Features	Possible problems
Black skin has more evenly distributed melanocytes, which are larger and more active than in white/Caucasian skin. Black skin is also more robust: it has greater elasticity and strength of collagen fibres, giving support to the skin, so there is less possibility of dropped contours of the face. Black skin tends to be darker across the forehead and perimeter of the face but lighter in the middle on the cheeks. Most likely origin: Africa West Indies/Caribbean African American.	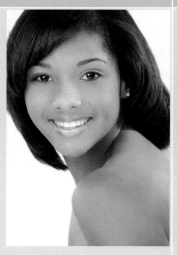	Black skins are the result of living nearest to the equator: the denser pigmentation is an added protection against the harshest of the ultraviolet rays. Sebaceous glands are larger and denser, giving good lubrication and moisture, making it less prone to premature wrinkles. This also means the ageing process is slower in a black skin, with less cell deterioration. Because black skin flakes and is shed more quickly than white/Caucasian skins, cell renewal is also faster.	Some black skins are quite sensitive to products and care should be taken to avoid harsh, abrasive products, or strong alcohol-based toners. These types of product are often used to treat an 'oily' skin, but black skin is not usually oily at all – the reflection of light against the black skin often gives the skin a glow or sheen. As the epidermis is thicker, black skins easily form scars, which can turn into keloid tissue (an over-thickening of the skin, in a pink or beige colour, which is more noticeable against a darker background).

Origins and features of black skin

Additional knowledge

Protected skin

Skin cancer is not as common in people with black skins, as they are protected from the harmful UV rays of the sun. Also, the epidermis is considerably thicker than in lighter skins, and it is therefore less reactive and not prone to allergies or infection: warts are rarely found on a black skin.

Asian skin

Asian skin can be broken into two types: light and dark. The features listed here are more relevant to the darker Asian skin type, while the features of lighter Asian skin are discussed with the Oriental skin type further on.

How to recognise it		Features	Possible problems
The sallow (yellow/olive) undertone of Asian skin is more pronounced with a darker tone in dark Asian skin. There is a higher proportion of melanin present. Most likely origin: Pakistan India Sri Lanka and Malaysia.	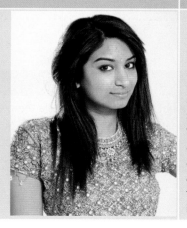	This skin has more sweat glands, which are also larger, to keep the body temperature at a manageable level in the heat. Do not confuse this sheen of sweat with oil – this skin generally has little problem with oil-related conditions such as acne. The skin is smooth and line-free, strong and adaptable, with the underlying fibres being supportive well into middle age.	There is minimal wrinkling, but this skin is prone to loss of pigmentation if care is not taken. It can have a tendency towards uneven colouring and pigmentation can cause dark circles under the eyes.

Origins and features of Asian skin

Oriental skin

The features of Oriental skin can also apply to lighter Asian skin.

How to recognise it	Features	Possible problems
Light Asian and Oriental skins have a yellow undertone, and can develop an olive tone, if they are Oriental. The base colour is cream and this skin is usually clear and fine. Most likely origin: Japan China Hong Kong Thailand Middle East.	The skin is smooth and fine, with minimal blemishes and this skin type rarely shows degeneration due to ageing. There is little or no face and body hair. The skin has good tolerance of ultraviolet and does not wrinkle early.	This skin scars easily and there may be irregularities in the skin's surface, seen as pitting or unevenness. Hyperpigmentation can also occur, and clients may be concerned about these age spots developing. As the skin is fairly oily, especially around the T-zone, this skin group may develop a problem with open pores and comedones along the nose.

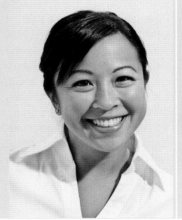

Origins and features of Oriental skin

Mixed-race skin

How to recognise it	Features	Possible problems
A client with mixed-race skin will need a very thorough consultation to ensure that the skin analysis is correct, as those in this category are not typical of any particular type. For example, a client with a black father and white/ Caucasian mother may have a combination of the skin colour, producing a darker tone to the skin, without necessarily having the sheen or tendency to develop keloid tissue which black skin has. Most likely origin: mixed parentage from any ethnic background.	These will vary entirely with the combination of the gene pool.	The skin will be more of a product of the mixture of parents and the environment. The correct product use will also dictate how clear the skin is, and whether the acid mantle is intact and doing its job correctly. This skin type is the easiest one to misdiagnose.

Origins and features of mixed-race skin

There is one other skin type you may come across which, although it is not a range for your NVQ, is still a recognisable skin type: Mediterranean/Latino skin.

Mediterranean/Latino skin

How to recognise it	Features	Possible problems
This skin has a golden colour with olive undertones. These darker, more olive tones are found in the warmer climes which produce dark, swarthy skins, which tan easily. Most likely origin: Spain Italy Southern France Portugal Greece Southern and central America.	This skin type tends to be oilier, due to the sebaceous glands producing more sebum to keep the skin lubricated in the heat. It therefore does not dry out too much, and is slow to form wrinkles. As the hair colour is also darker, facial and body hair is more noticeable and often grows thicker and is coarse in texture. This skin is robust and less prone to damage; it can withstand ultraviolet without burning.	There is a tendency for excessive facial and body hair, and skin can be fairly tough and thicken as it ages.

Origins and features of Mediterranean skin

Lesions

Lesions are growths or abnormal patches of skin. Many cause no ill effects, others are more serious and require treatment. The following table explains the different terms used to describe them.

Type of lesion	Description	Illustration
Bulla	A raised fluid-filled lesion larger than a vesicle	
Fissure	Crack or break in the skin	
Macule	A flat coloured spot	
Nodule	Solid, raised lesion larger than a papule, often a symptom of a systemic disease	
Papule	Small circular raised lesion at the surface of the skin	

Type of lesion	Description	Illustration
Plaque	A patch	
Pustule	A raised lesion containing pus – often in a hair follicle or a sweat gland	
Ulcer	A lesion resulting from the destruction of the skin and often as deep as the subcutaneous tissue	
Vesicle	Small, fluid-filled raised lesion, a blister	
Wheal	Smooth, rounded, slightly raised area, often itching and can be seen as hives (urticaria) when a person suffers an allergic reaction	

Types of lesions

Both the client's and the therapist's skin are directly affected during treatments.

Effects for the client	Effects for the therapist
The skin is deep cleansed and stimulated by massage and electrical treatments; therefore it is exfoliated, encouraged into fresh cell production and removal of waste. It then looks brighter, clearer and can function fully – offering protection to the body.	The use of products on the therapist's hands when applying products will help cell production, keep the skin on the hands soft and supple, which is essential for the 'tools' of treatment, and promote good health.

The skeleton

You will learn about:
- the functions of the skeleton
- bones and bone tissue
- the structure of the skeleton
- movement at joints.

Related anatomy and physiology

The functions of the skeleton

The human skeleton is a mobile, bony framework consisting of approximately 206 bones which establish its characteristic shape. As well as providing shape, the skeleton has other important functions linked to its structure, which are shown in the table below.

Function	Description
Support	Without a skeleton we would be a wobbly, floppy mass of cells and tissue, unable to stand, move or support ourselves. The bones in the pelvis, legs and feet support the weight of the upper body.
Attachment for skeletal muscles and leverage	Muscles attach to the bones of the skeleton and pull them into different positions so that the bones act like levers. This allows many types of movement at joints.
Development and production	1. Source of blood cells – Many bones are hollow and consist of spongy bone tissue which is filled with red marrow. Red marrow is the site for the production of blood cells in adults. 2. The facial bones have air sacs (sinuses) which are lined with epithelial tissue which produces mucus to keep bacteria at bay (see 'The skull' on page 181).
Protection	The various parts of the skeleton protect the underlying structures. The cranium protects the brain, the thoracic cage protects the heart and lungs, the pelvic girdle protects the reproductive and digestive organs, the spinal column protects the spinal cord and nerve pathways.
Allows movement	Through a series of muscles pulling on the bones and joints for movement.
Mineral stores	Store of calcium – calcium makes bone hard and is used to maintain the compact tissue of bones. Its release into the bloodstream, initiated by parathyroid hormone, is required to maintain heart rate, respiration and muscle contraction.

Functions of the skeleton

Think about it

Whenever there is a model of a skeleton, it is plastic, so you get the impression a skeleton is a dry, plastic, static structure inside the body. It isn't! It is a living structure, making blood cells and growing, replacing cells and working really hard to help the muscles with movement.

Think about it

Another mnemonic – for the functions of the skeleton remember SAD PAM: **S**hape, **A**ttachment, **D**evelopment of blood cells, **P**rotection, **A**llows moment, **M**ineral stores.

Think about it

If you can remember that there is a cell in can**cell**ous bone, it will remind you that red blood cells are made in the marrow of cancellous bone.

Bones and bone tissue

The skeleton of a human embryo consists of a flexible tissue called cartilage, which is made of strong collagen and stretchy elastin fibres. Nearly all cartilage is gradually replaced by hard bone tissue in a process called **ossification**, although some remains on the joint surfaces of most bones in the form of articular cartilage. Development of the skeleton continues until about the age of 25, by which time the final size and shape of the skeleton has been established. However, growth, destruction and repair of bone tissue continue throughout life to maintain the strength and health of the skeletal system.

Key terms

Ossification – to turn into bone.

Bone formation and growth

Bone tissue is rigid and non-elastic and consists of about 67 per cent calcium and 33 per cent organic matter, mainly collagen. The process of ossification depends on a delicate balance between the construction and destruction of bone tissue. This is maintained by specialist cells, as described on the next page.

Ossification and growth of bone

Osteoblasts make new bone tissue. They secrete collagen, which forms a strong yet flexible framework. Mineral salts, especially calcium, are then deposited within this framework to provide hardness in a process called calcification. Osteoblasts become trapped in the framework of bone tissue and develop into osteocytes, which release further calcium ions that become part of the bone tissue.

Osteoclasts contain lysosomes, which are enzymes that digest protein and also break down minerals in bone because of their acidic quality.

In this way the skeleton is maintained, as oscteoclasts destroy old bone tissue while osteoblasts construct new bone. The process also allows bone tissue to act as a storage medium for calcium.

Key terms

Osteoblasts – a cell that makes bone.

Osteoclasts – a cell that breaks down bone.

Structure of bone

There are two types of bone tissue: compact and cancellous.

Type of bone tissue	Characteristics
Compact	Hard, strong and relatively heavy. Forms the tough outer shell of most bones in the human skeleton.
Cancellous	Spongy texture (also known as spongy bone tissue). Spaces in the tissue contain red bone marrow where blood cells are formed. Lightweight.

Characteristics of compact and cancellous bone tissues

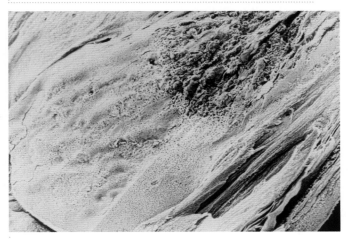

Cancellous bone

Classifications of bones

There are five types of bone:

- long
- short
- flat
- sesamoid
- irregular.

They have structures suited to their function and position in the human body.

Type of bone	Structure	Examples
Long	Consists of a shaft of compact bone tissue and two spongy extremities called epiphyses made of cancellous bone tissue	Femur (thigh) Humerus (upper arm)
Short	Short, irregular bones consisting of cancellous bone tissue surrounded by a thin layer of compact bone tissue; lightweight	Carpals (8 wrist bones) Tarsals (7 ankle bones)
Flat	Plate-like layers of compact and cancellous bone tissue make these bones strong yet lightweight	Frontal (forehead)
Sesamoid	Oval-shaped bone located in tendons	Patella (kneecap)
Irregular	Mass of cancellous bone tissue surrounded by a thin layer of compact bone tissue	Vertebrae (spine)

Classifications of bones

Effects of ageing on bone tissue

One of the greatest influences on skeletal development in infancy is nutrition. Vitamin A influences osteoblast and osteoclast activity, which is needed to maintain a homeostatic balance, and vitamin D is required to aid the absorption of calcium from the intestine. Vitamins C and B12 are also essential to bone growth.

Osteoporosis

Age-associated changes in the digestive system can radically affect the condition of the skeleton. Less calcium is absorbed from the diet, which appears to affect post-menopausal women more than men of the same age, adding to the tendency towards osteoporosis. However, more men are inheriting the condition and if they have a poor diet then they increase the probability of osteoporosis. Changes in the digestive system also affect the absorption of vitamin D and changes in the skin slow down the production of vitamin D activated by natural sunlight. As the function of vitamin D is to transport calcium from the digestive system to the bones, a deficiency means that new bone tissue is produced at a slower rate than existing tissue is destroyed. During middle age and into old age, bones start to shrink and the skin can become saggy as it fits less snugly on the internal framework. Bones in the face diminish in the same way as bones in the body and this bone shrinkage is partly to blame for the lack of tautness which is noticeable in mature skins.

How to help the skeleton

◼ Hormone replacement therapy (HRT) is commonly prescribed to women to treat the effects of the menopause. Treatment with the hormone oestrogen has been found to have a positive effect on calcium metabolism, which in turn reduces loss of bone density and lowers the risk of osteoporosis.

◼ Maintain regular gentle exercise, such as walking, which prevents bone mass loss and encourages the production of vitamin D in the skin via natural sunlight.

◼ Diet should contain adequate amounts of calcium, which the body needs to produce new bone tissue. The recommended daily intake is about 700 mg or one pint of skimmed milk.

The structure of the skeleton

The skeleton is divided into two parts:

◼ the axial skeleton

◼ the appendicular skeleton.

The axis of the body (axial skeleton) is made up of 80 bones of the skull, thoracic cage (rib cage) and vertebral (spinal) column. The appendicular skeleton consists of 126 bones found in the upper and lower limbs, the pelvic girdle (pelvic bones) and the shoulder girdle (clavicle, humerus, scapula).

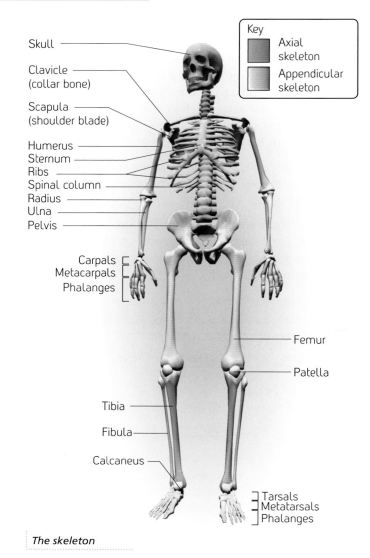

The skeleton

Axial skeleton		
1 frontal	4 nasal	7 cervical vertebrae
2 parietal	1 vomer	12 thoracic vertebrae
2 temporal	1 maxilla	5 lumbar vertebrae
1 occipital	1 mandible	5 fused bones of sacrum
1 ethmoid	2 zygomatic	4 fused bones of coccyx
1 sphenoid	2 palatine	24 (12 pairs) ribs
2 lacrimal	1 hyoid	1 sternum
Total: 80 bones		

Bones of the axial skeleton

Appendicular skeleton	
2 scapula	2 pelvic bones
2 clavicle	2 femur
2 humerus	2 patella
2 radius	2 fibula
2 ulna	2 tibia
16 carpals	14 tarsals
10 metacarpals	10 metatarsals
28 phalanges	28 phalanges
Total: 126 bones	

Bones of the appendicular skeleton

The skull

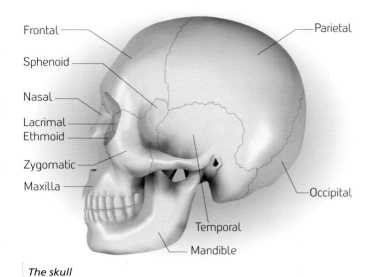

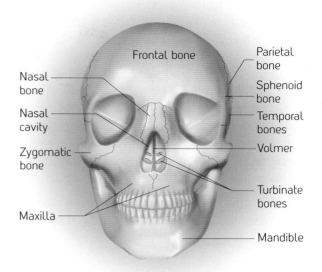

The skull

The skull, also known as the cranium, is a very hard structure that protects the brain. Although it looks like one bone it is actually made up of 22 separate bones that are fused together at ridged joints called **sutures**. Ten bones make up the skull and 12 form the face.

The skull has two parts: the cranium, which forms the roof and back of the skull and contains the brain; and the face, at the front of the skull, which contains the eyes and teeth. The cranium forms a deep cavity to protect the brain and is constructed of flat bones which are strong yet lightweight. The facial bones are irregular and formed into peaks and furrows to protect the eyes, nasal cavities, teeth and tongue.

There are many openings in the skull to allow blood vessels and nerves to enter and leave. The largest of these is at the base of the skull and this is called the foramen magum. This opening allows the spinal cord and blood vessels to pass to and from the brain. A baby's skull has soft spots called the fontanelles. Over a period of about 18 months the bones gradually join together. During this time, care should be taken to protect the baby's head.

Key terms

Sutures – ridged, fibrous joints of the skull.

Think about it

Skulls vary in size and shape. Your genes can dictate many features of your face shape, such a prominent cheek bones, square forehead or prominent jaw line. A forensic anthropologist looking at an old skeleton is often able to identify the country of origin of the person by the shape of the skull.

Bone	Position
1 Occipital bone (×1)	At the back of the skull
2 Parietal (×2)	Positioned at the back of the head and forms the roof of the skull
3 Frontal (×1)	Forms the front of the skull, forehead and upper eye sockets
4 Temporal (×2)	At the side, around the ears
5 Sphenoid (×1)	At the base of the skull, wing-shaped, forms the temple
6 Ethmoid (×1)	Positioned between the frontal and sphenoid bones and forms roof of the nasal cavities
7 Lacrimal (×2)	One in each eye orbit. These bones are fused together to form the shape of the skull, and their joins are known as sutures.

Bones of the skull

Related anatomy and physiology

The sinuses

The sinuses are the hollow spaces within the bones of the skull and face which open into the nasal cavity. There are four pairs of air sac spaces (frontal sinuses, sphenoid sinuses, ethmoid and maxillary) and their function is to make the skull lighter, to provide mucus and act as a resonance space in the head for speech. They are lined with mucous membranes and fill with air during respiration. The fine nasal hairs helps trap debris and prevents substances go into the lungs. Because they open out from the body they are prone to infections such as sinusitis and/ or they can become irritated with allergic reactions to pollen, chemicals and so on. The lining of the sinuses may become swollen and infected causing excessive mucus production. During a cold the sinuses can also be inflamed and the nose and cheek areas feel tender and sore. If the sinuses become blocked during a cold, it makes breathing harder, and it has to take place through the mouth, which alters speech patterns.

The skull is attached to the body via the vertebral column. The vertebral column enables the head to turn and tilt. The weight of the head is supported by the neck, the shoulder girdle bones and muscles.

The shoulder girdle

The shoulder girdle is formed by four bones — the two scapula and the two clavicles. The scapula is the large, flat bone at the upper back which sits flush against the rib cage, and the clavicle is the long thin bone, slightly S-shaped, from the sternum to the shoulder joint. The main function of the shoulder girdle is to allow a full range of movement in the upper body and arms.

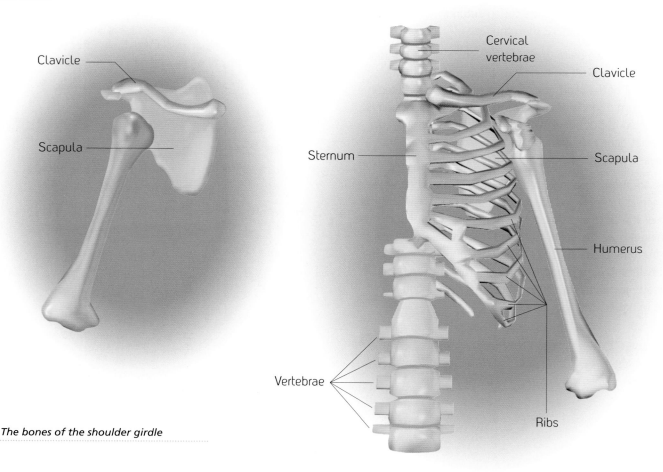

The bones of the shoulder girdle

The pelvic girdle

The pelvic girdle consists of two large innominate hip bones, joined at the back by the sacrum, and the pubis symphysis at the front. The three bones on each side are the ileum, ischium and the pubis — they are fused together to form a very solid structure for weight bearing and muscular attachment. The pelvic girdle in a female is wider and shallower to allow for pregnancy and childbirth.

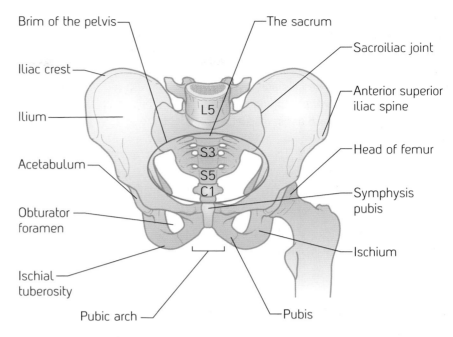

Brim of the pelvis
The sacrum
Iliac crest
Sacroiliac joint
Ilium
Anterior superior iliac spine
L5
S3
Acetabulum
S5
C1
Head of femur
Obturator foramen
Symphysis pubis
Ischial tuberosity
Ischium
Pubic arch
Pubis

The bones of the pelvic girdle

The spine

The vertebral column consists of 33 individual bones, though some are fused together. Between each vertebra is a pad of fibrous tissue called an intervertebral disc which acts as a shock absorber against gravity and injury. Each vertebra contains a hole in the centre and through this runs the spinal cord which forms part of the central nervous system (CNS).

Cervical
(7 bones)

Thoracic
(12 bones)

The first three types of vertebrae are known as true vertebrae because they move. They are separated by intervertebral discs. These are pads of fibrocartilage, which have shock-absorbing functions.

Intervertebral discs

Lumbar
(5 bones)

The **Sacral** (5 bones) and **Coccygeal** (4 bones) vertebrae are known as false or fixed vertebrae because they cannot move independently and there is no movement between them. Note that the coccyx does move in relation to the sacrum.

The vertebral column

> #### Think about it
>
> The spine and skeleton are key to body shape and height, as well as abnormalities – see the General pathway, page 335, for a description of the spinal problems of kyphosis, scoliosis and lordosis, and when to treat and when to seek medical approval.

Related anatomy and physiology

The thoracic cage

The thoracic cage consists of 12 thoracic vertebrae and 12 pairs of ribs, as well as one sternum. This cage protects the heart, lungs and major blood vessels and is a point of attachment for the diaphragm and intercostal muscles which assist respiration.

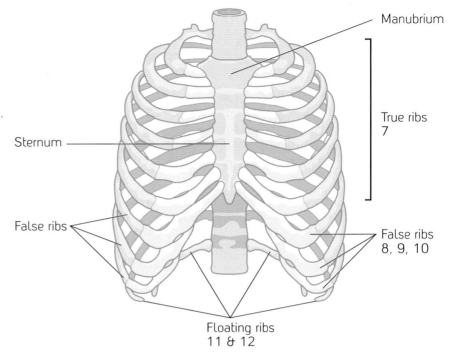

The thoracic or rib cage

Relation of bone structure and function

The axial skeleton has a central position in the structure of the body.

Axial skeleton	Function
Skull	• Cranium protects the brain • Base of the frontal bone and zygomatic bones form the eye sockets • Mandible forms the lower jaw and aids mastication (chewing) • Temporal bone protects the ear canal
Vertebral column	• Protects spinal cord • Provides attachment for ribs • Provides attachment for muscles
Thoracic cage	• Protects lungs • Protects heart and major blood vessels • Provides attachment for diaphragm • Provides attachment for intercostal muscles

Functions of the axial skeleton

The appendicular skeleton consists of the limbs, clavicles and scapulae. Together with muscles, the appendicular skeleton is responsible for voluntary movements. These can range from complex coordination involving the whole body such as walking and jumping to small, specific movements such as writing or wriggling the toes

Movement at joints

A joint is formed where two bones meet. Without them, the skeleton would be static and movement would be limited. Some joints are very strong, whilst others need to be more mobile — it is not possible to be both strong and mobile. Joints can be classified according to their mobility.

Category of joint	Name	Example
Immobile joint	Fibrous Often called synarthroses	The skull joints
Slightly mobile joint	Cartilaginous	Between the vertebrae and sternum
Mobile joint	Synovial Often called diarthroses	Knee joint. Most other joints of the body are synovial — there are seven types (see page 185)

Category of joint

Immobile joints

In infancy, many of the skull bones are not fully joined together, which allows the skull of the baby to pass through the birth canal and in two places, the anterior and posterior fontanelles, there are gaps between them. As the infant grows, these open joints join to form the rigid skull. The irregular, serrated edges of bone are bound together by tough, fibrous tissue at the suture lines.

Slightly mobile joints

Some joints require a small amount of movement but still have to be strong. This can be seen between the vertebrae of the spine and the pubis symphysis (the pelvis). The hormones during pregnancy soften the pubis symphysis, to allow a slight give during childbirth. In these joints there is a thick pad of fibro-cartilage between the bones held in place by a strong fibrous ligament. This pad acts as a shock absorber.

Mobile joints

Synovial joints are freely moving joints, though movements are limited by the shape of the articulating surfaces and the ligaments which hold the bones together. Because they have to be able to withstand the friction of movement these joints are complex. The surfaces of the bone are covered with **smooth cartilage**. The joint edge has a strong **fibrous capsule** surrounding a sac of **synovial membrane** between the bone ends. This membrane secretes lubricant fluid that allows frictionless movement and the **articular cartilage** keeps the bones apart. The joint has stabilising ligaments which bind and strengthen it.

Three types of movement are possible at synovial joints:

- angular movements including flexion and extension, abduction and adduction
- rotary movements including rotation and circumduction
- gliding movements where one part slides on another.

For more information on types of movement, see the table on page 186.

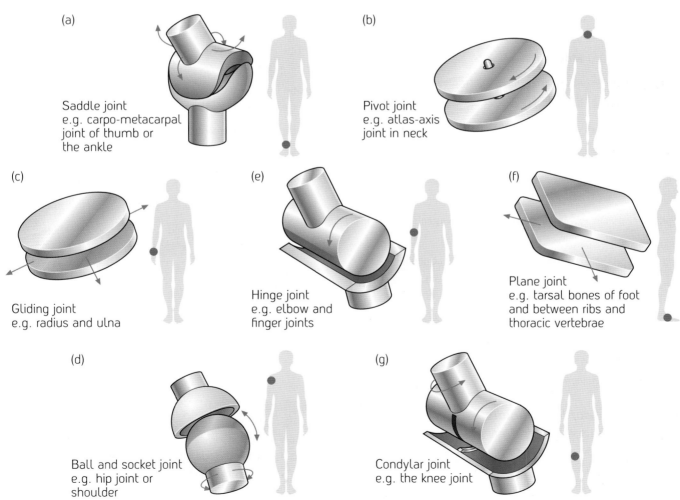

(a) Saddle joint
e.g. carpo-metacarpal joint of thumb or the ankle

(b) Pivot joint
e.g. atlas-axis joint in neck

(c) Gliding joint
e.g. radius and ulna

(e) Hinge joint
e.g. elbow and finger joints

(f) Plane joint
e.g. tarsal bones of foot and between ribs and thoracic vertebrae

(d) Ball and socket joint
e.g. hip joint or shoulder

(g) Condylar joint
e.g. the knee joint

Joint movements

Key terms

Smooth cartilage – a coating on bones that helps joints move freely.

Fibrous capsule – layer of connective tissue.

Synovial membrane – soft tissue that lines synovial joints.

Articular cartilage – smooth, strong white tissue which covers joints.

For your exam

During an exam you may be asked to describe a synovial joint, or give the different types of joints found in the body. It can be confusing. Remember that there are *three categories* of joint in the body: immobile, slightly mobile and mobile joints.

Then, there are *six types* of mobile joint. So, look closely at what the question has asked – do remember that synovial joints are only one of the three types.

Joint type	Movement
Ball and socket	Allows movement in any direction, e.g. the shoulder and the hips (although slightly limited as the socket is bigger)
Condyliod	Movement is slightly more limited, e.g. ankle and wrist
Hinge	Only suitable for flexion and extension, e.g. elbow and knee
Pivot	Where one bone pivots around another, e.g. radius and ulna
Plane/gliding	Has two surfaces which allows gliding movements in any direction, e.g. carpals and tarsal joints
Saddle	Has two concave surfaces of bone that work together for movement, e.g. metacarpal joint of wrist/hand

Joint types and movement

Homeostatic disorders of joints

Joints undergo a lot of wear and tear in a lifetime and it is common for older clients to complain of stiff, swollen or aching joints. However, it is difficult to separate age-associated changes from mechanical strain or injury. Repetitive actions of joints due to occupation, sporting

activities or strain caused by poor posture can certainly influence the stability of joints as we age. Cold weather and inactivity during sleep cause the body's circulatory system to slow down, which can lead to a build-up of fluid at the joints resulting in swelling or discomfort.

A further age-associated problem is the loss of water from cartilage. Think again about the intervertebral discs. These 'cushions' contain water which is squeezed out by the pressure of gravity over time which makes them less flexible and can cause problems with lifting and bearing heavy weight. As the discs lose water, they become flatter, which also explains why our height decreases with age.

Disorder	Description	Example
Arthritis	Inflammation of joints	Swollen, aching joints
Spondylosis	Degenerative disorder of intervertebral discs	Pain in cervical and lumbar region
Rheumatoid arthritis	Chronic, progressive disorder	Typically affects fingers, wrists, feet, ankles
Bursitis	Inflammation of **bursae**	Housemaid's knee
Torn cartilage	Damaged **menisci**	Footballing injuries to knee joint
Tendinitis	Inflammation of tendons	Caused by overuse, e.g. tennis elbow or repetitive strain
Sprain	Overstretched tendon, cartilage or muscle	Sporting injuries
Dislocation	Bones in joint become disconnected	Sudden or unnatural movements

Disorders of the joint

Key terms

Bursae – small fluid-filled sacs lined by a synovial membrane. They provide a cushion between bones and tendons and/or muscles around a joint.

Menisci – cartilage disks that acts as a cushion between the ends of bones that meet in a joint.

The muscular system

You will learn about:

- the functions of skeletal muscle
- the structure of skeletal muscle
- muscle tone
- attachment of muscles to the skeleton
- points of origin and insertion
- actions of chief muscles of the face and body.

Muscle categories

The naming of muscles is complicated. They can be named according to:

1 function — for example flexor or extensor, adductor or abductor — the movement they cause
2 **attachments** — where they are in the body, for example the sternocleidomastoid, which originates from the top of the sternum and clavicle and inserts into the mastoid process of the skull, behind the ears
3 shape — the trapezius is a kite-shaped muscle at the upper back
4 formation or how they are made — biceps (two heads) triceps (three heads)
5 position — intercostals are muscles are between the ribs.

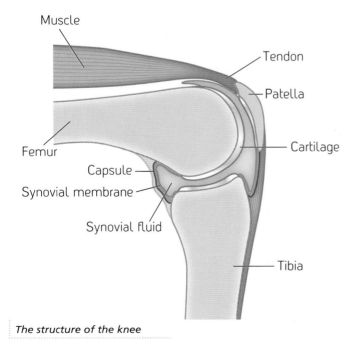

The structure of the knee

All types of muscle tissue have some characteristics in common:

- Excitable — responds to a stimulus
- Able to contract (shorten)
- Able to stretch (lengthen)
- Elastic — returns to original shape after contraction or stretching.

There are three types of muscle tissue:

1 Cardiac muscle — forms the heart
2 Smooth muscle (involuntary) — forms the internal organs
3 Skeletal muscle (voluntary) — attached to bones.

Cardiac muscle – the heart

- Only found in the heart
- Both involuntary and irregularly striped
- Short round fibres
- Contracts automatically throughout life
- Controlled by nerves
- Strongest type of muscular tissue within the human body

Smooth muscle – involuntary

- Not under the control of conscious thought
- Found in the walls of internal organs
- Unstriped and with no sheath
- Designed for slower contractions and does not tire easily
- Stomach, bowel and uterus are types of involuntary muscle

Skeletal muscle – voluntary

- Forms the flesh of the limbs and trunk, and moves the skeleton
- Most superficial
- Striped in dark and light bands often called striated muscle
- Bundles of muscle fibres form sheath of muscle

Key terms

Attachment – points of origin and insertion of the muscle. Muscles may be attached to bones via the tendons to produce movements of the joints, or they may be attached from other connective tissue such as cartilage or the fascia of other muscles.

Related anatomy and physiology

- Under the control of the conscious control
- Contracts quickly but tires easily too

The functions of skeletal muscle

Skeletal muscle has four main functions:

- It facilitates movement.
- It raises body temperature.
- It maintains posture.
- It assists venous return.

Movement

The most obvious function of skeletal muscle is to facilitate movement at joints and thereby increase or decrease the angle between two bones. Muscle is attached to bones via tendons at the points of **origin** and **insertion**. When a muscle contracts, the origin remains fixed while the insertion moves towards it, so reducing the angle of the joint. For example, sitting up from a lying down position shortens the angle between the trunk and the thighs as the abdominal muscles contract or shorten.

Body temperature

When muscles are working hard, they produce heat, and muscle fibres work best when warmed up — muscle contractions happen faster and blood circulation is increased. This is a continuous heat-generating cycle: the more work the muscles do, the more heat generated, the better the

muscles perform. The opposite is true when the muscle fibres are cold — so care must be taken when exercising to warm the muscles up gently prior to strenuous exercise, to avoid damaging them.

Posture

As well as enabling movement, skeletal muscle is responsible for maintaining posture, which is achieved by the same concept of contraction. Under normal, resting circumstances the muscles are in a state of partial contraction known as **muscle tone**. If our muscles were completely relaxed all the time, our bodies would not be able to hold themselves upright, as the weight of our bones and organs, particularly the skull and brain, would pull us over. Not surprisingly, the muscles with the greatest tonicity in humans are found in the neck and back. Postural muscles do not require conscious effort to carry out their function, although they can be affected by bad habits and improved through training.

Venous return

Veins take the deoxygenated blood back to the heart, but unlike arteries, which operate under high pressure, the veins are not self-propelling. The veins in our body rely on the pressure of the movement of the muscles to stimulate the flow of blood within them, using valves at regular intervals

Key terms

Origin – the end of the muscle which remains relatively fixed during contraction of the muscle. Often fixed to bone, but can be fixed to other muscles and fascia.

Insertion – the opposite end of the muscle origin, which moves towards the origin, moving the bone it is attached to. When the muscle fibres contract the insertion comes up towards the origin; this takes place over a joint to cause movement.

Agonists – the prime movers or main activated muscle.

Antagonists – opposite muscles which work together to allow movement; if one contracts the other has to relax its fibres to allow movement to take place.

Synergists – muscles on the same sides of a joint to perform the same movements and work together in the same direction.

Muscle tone – the muscle fibres are in a partial state of contraction, and operate a shift system, to avoid muscle fatigue.

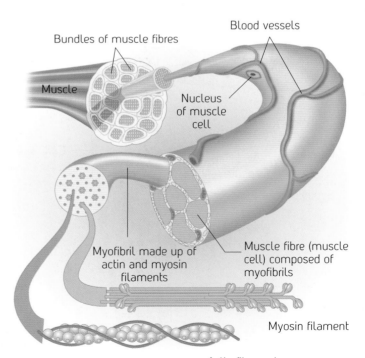

Bundles of muscle fibres

Blood vessels

Muscle

Nucleus of muscle cell

Myofibril made up of actin and myosin filaments

Muscle fibre (muscle cell) composed of myofibrils

Myosin filament

Actin filament

Muscle structure

to prevent the flow of blood back downwards. When these valves become congested with blood, varicose veins may occur. Disabled people and people with limited mobility need regular physiotherapy, passive exercise of the limbs, or massage to help circulation of blood back to the heart.

The structure of skeletal muscle

Muscle tissue consists of large striped cells which are elongated and highly specialised. They are bound together in bundles by connective tissue which contains collagen and elastin fibres that give muscle its strength and elastic properties. Running the length of muscle cells are filaments of the proteins actin and myosin. It is these fibres of protein that give muscle its characteristic striped appearance. Within the bundles of muscle fibres there is also a rich supply of blood vessels and nerve attachments.

Think about it

Muscle comprises:
- 75 per cent water
- 20 per cent actin and myosin
- 5 per cent mineral salts, glycogen and fat.

Muscle tone

Skeletal muscle is responsible for different types of contraction during dynamic or static activity.

Concentric muscle work	If the origin and insertion move closer together, the muscle is shortened or contracted and is said to be working concentrically.
Eccentric muscle work	If the muscle tries to halt a movement during exertion, it is said to be working eccentrically. The muscle attempts to contract but is extended by external forces which force the origin and insertion apart.
Static muscle work	If the muscle has to contract to prevent movement, it is said to be working statically.

Muscle contraction type

Concentric and eccentric contractions are also known as **isotonic** contractions. Static muscle work is known as **isometric**. The term isometric means equal measures, as in a muscle working in equal measures with an external force to prevent movement. Isometric exercises are used to increase muscle strength by increasing tension without causing contraction, usually by pushing against a solid,

immovable force. Isometric and isotonic contractions can be illustrated by considering the different types of muscle work involved in doing pull-ups on a high bar.

Think about it

The term 'muscle tone' leads you to think of a body builder, with well-defined muscles that you can clearly indentify. In physiological terms muscle tone really means the ability of the muscle to respond to stimulus and how quickly and efficiently it works –and how quickly it tires. Muscle fibres work in shifts, so that as one set of fibres gets tired and has a depleted supply of oxygen and nutrients then another set of fresh fibres takes over. This shift system keeps us walking and functioning all day long. So muscle tone is really about durability and effectiveness. It is the state of partial contraction of muscles under normal, resting circumstances.

Attachment of muscles to the skeleton

Skeletal muscles may be attached to bone, cartilage, ligaments or skin via tendons and aponeuroses. Tendons have the appearance of cords and consist of fibrous collagen tissues, while aponeuroses are a thin sheet of fibres which attach flat muscles, as in the abdomen. The most well-known tendon is the Achilles, which connects the calf muscles to the heel. Fibrous tissue also forms a protective and supportive sheath of connective tissue around muscles known as fascia, which contains a rich supply of blood and nerve fibres. Where muscles attach to each other the fibres of one interlace with the fibres of the other. In the muscles of the abdominal wall the fibres of the aponeuroses interlace, forming the linea alba, the shallow groove which leads from the umbilicus to the sternum.

Key terms

Isotonic contraction – here, the muscles contraction and force is constant but the muscle length changes, to overcome the opposing force – as in pushing something over.

Isometric contraction – this is when the muscle contracts but no movement takes place – as in maintained posture. The muscle length stays the same but the force may increase – as in pushing on an immovable object such as a wall.

Muscle fatigue – the failure of the muscle to contract fully once the food stores of glucose and oxygen have been used up, with the result of an accumulation of lactic acid.

Belly – thickest part or main body of the muscle, usually in the middle, half-way between insertion and origin.

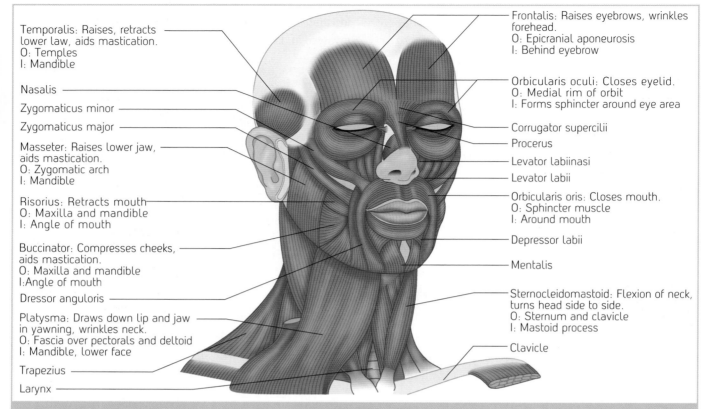

Temporalis: Raises, retracts lower law, aids mastication.
O: Temples
I: Mandible

Nasalis

Zygomaticus minor

Zygomaticus major

Masseter: Raises lower jaw, aids mastication.
O: Zygomatic arch
I: Mandible

Risorius: Retracts mouth
O: Maxilla and mandible
I: Angle of mouth

Buccinator: Compresses cheeks, aids mastication.
O: Maxilla and mandible
I:Angle of mouth

Dressor anguloris

Platysma: Draws down lip and jaw in yawning, wrinkles neck.
O: Fascia over pectorals and deltoid
I: Mandible, lower face

Trapezius

Larynx

Frontalis: Raises eyebrows, wrinkles forehead.
O: Epicranial aponeurosis
I: Behind eyebrow

Orbicularis oculi: Closes eyelid.
O: Medial rim of orbit
I: Forms sphincter around eye area

Corrugator supercilii

Procerus

Levator labiinasi

Levator labii

Orbicularis oris: Closes mouth.
O: Sphincter muscle
I: Around mouth

Depressor labii

Mentalis

Sternocleidomastoid: Flexion of neck, turns head side to side.
O: Sternum and clavicle
I: Mastoid process

Clavicle

Facial and neck muscles

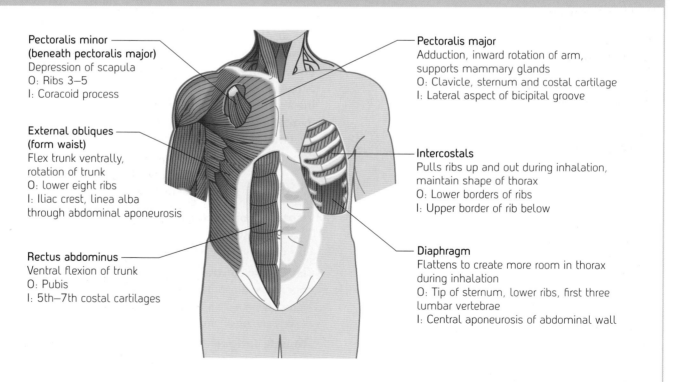

Pectoralis minor
(beneath pectoralis major)
Depression of scapula
O: Ribs 3–5
I: Coracoid process

External obliques
(form waist)
Flex trunk ventrally, rotation of trunk
O: lower eight ribs
I: Iliac crest, linea alba through abdominal aponeurosis

Rectus abdominus
Ventral flexion of trunk
O: Pubis
I: 5th–7th costal cartilages

Pectoralis major
Adduction, inward rotation of arm, supports mammary glands
O: Clavicle, sternum and costal cartilage
I: Lateral aspect of bicipital groove

Intercostals
Pulls ribs up and out during inhalation, maintain shape of thorax
O: Lower borders of ribs
I: Upper border of rib below

Diaphragm
Flattens to create more room in thorax during inhalation
O: Tip of sternum, lower ribs, first three lumbar vertebrae
I: Central aponeurosis of abdominal wall

Anterior muscles of the chest, neck and abdomen

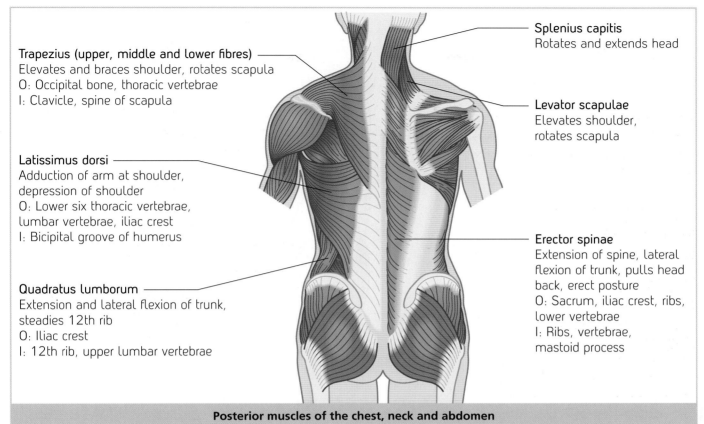

Splenius capitis
Rotates and extends head

Trapezius (upper, middle and lower fibres)
Elevates and braces shoulder, rotates scapula
O: Occipital bone, thoracic vertebrae
I: Clavicle, spine of scapula

Levator scapulae
Elevates shoulder,
rotates scapula

Latissimus dorsi
Adduction of arm at shoulder,
depression of shoulder
O: Lower six thoracic vertebrae,
lumbar vertebrae, iliac crest
I: Bicipital groove of humerus

Erector spinae
Extension of spine, lateral
flexion of trunk, pulls head
back, erect posture
O: Sacrum, iliac crest, ribs,
lower vertebrae
I: Ribs, vertebrae,
mastoid process

Quadratus lumborum
Extension and lateral flexion of trunk,
steadies 12th rib
O: Iliac crest
I: 12th rib, upper lumbar vertebrae

Posterior muscles of the chest, neck and abdomen

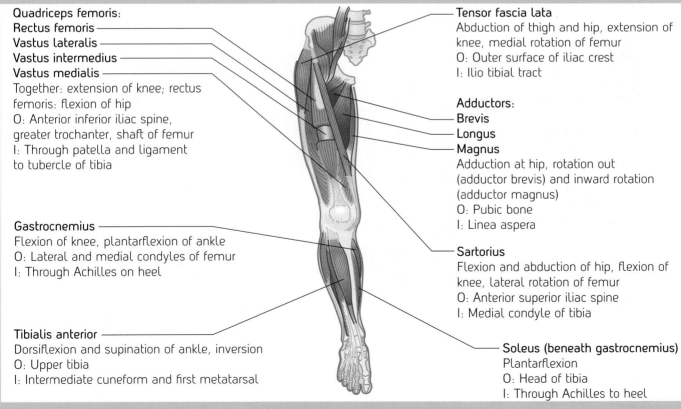

Quadriceps femoris:
Rectus femoris
Vastus lateralis
Vastus intermedius
Vastus medialis
Together: extension of knee; rectus
femoris: flexion of hip
O: Anterior inferior iliac spine,
greater trochanter, shaft of femur
I: Through patella and ligament
to tubercle of tibia

Tensor fascia lata
Abduction of thigh and hip, extension of
knee, medial rotation of femur
O: Outer surface of iliac crest
I: Ilio tibial tract

Adductors:
Brevis
Longus
Magnus
Adduction at hip, rotation out
(adductor brevis) and inward rotation
(adductor magnus)
O: Pubic bone
I: Linea aspera

Gastrocnemius
Flexion of knee, plantarflexion of ankle
O: Lateral and medial condyles of femur
I: Through Achilles on heel

Sartorius
Flexion and abduction of hip, flexion of
knee, lateral rotation of femur
O: Anterior superior iliac spine
I: Medial condyle of tibia

Tibialis anterior
Dorsiflexion and supination of ankle, inversion
O: Upper tibia
I: Intermediate cuneiform and first metatarsal

Soleus (beneath gastrocnemius)
Plantarflexion
O: Head of tibia
I: Through Achilles to heel

Anterior muscles of the leg and hip

Related anatomy and physiology

191

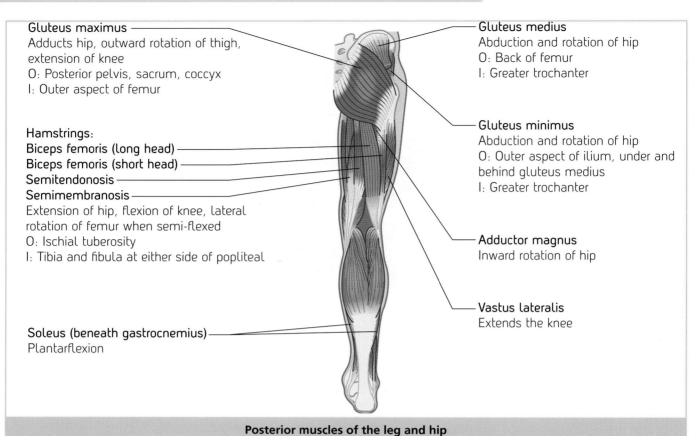

Gluteus maximus
Adducts hip, outward rotation of thigh,
extension of knee
O: Posterior pelvis, sacrum, coccyx
I: Outer aspect of femur

Hamstrings:
Biceps femoris (long head)
Biceps femoris (short head)
Semitendonosis
Semimembranosis
Extension of hip, flexion of knee, lateral
rotation of femur when semi-flexed
O: Ischial tuberosity
I: Tibia and fibula at either side of popliteal

Soleus (beneath gastrocnemius)
Plantarflexion

Gluteus medius
Abduction and rotation of hip
O: Back of femur
I: Greater trochanter

Gluteus minimus
Abduction and rotation of hip
O: Outer aspect of ilium, under and
behind gluteus medius
I: Greater trochanter

Adductor magnus
Inward rotation of hip

Vastus lateralis
Extends the knee

Posterior muscles of the leg and hip

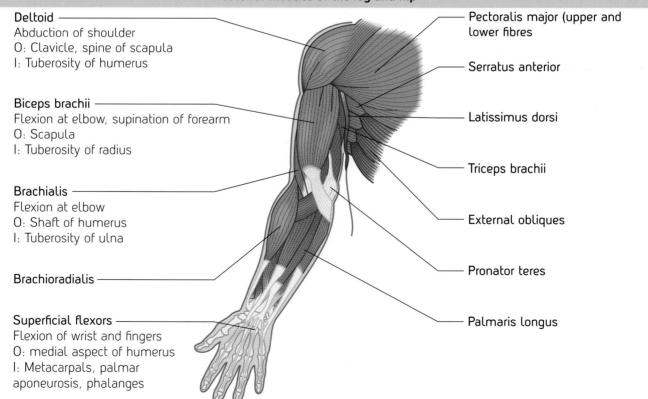

Deltoid
Abduction of shoulder
O: Clavicle, spine of scapula
I: Tuberosity of humerus

Biceps brachii
Flexion at elbow, supination of forearm
O: Scapula
I: Tuberosity of radius

Brachialis
Flexion at elbow
O: Shaft of humerus
I: Tuberosity of ulna

Brachioradialis

Superficial flexors
Flexion of wrist and fingers
O: medial aspect of humerus
I: Metacarpals, palmar
aponeurosis, phalanges

**Pectoralis major (upper and
lower fibres**

Serratus anterior

Latissimus dorsi

Triceps brachii

External obliques

Pronator teres

Palmaris longus

Anterior muscles of the arm and shoulder

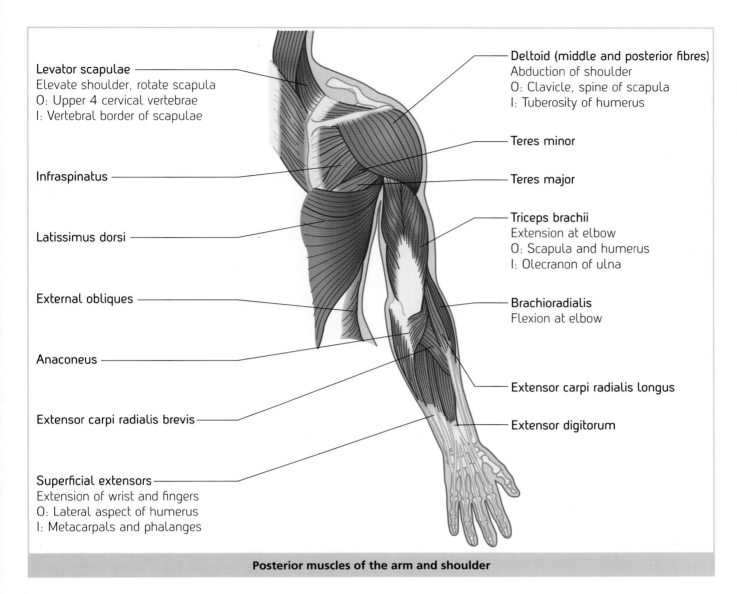

Levator scapulae
Elevate shoulder, rotate scapula
O: Upper 4 cervical vertebrae
I: Vertebral border of scapulae

Infraspinatus

Latissimus dorsi

External obliques

Anaconeus

Extensor carpi radialis brevis

Superficial extensors
Extension of wrist and fingers
O: Lateral aspect of humerus
I: Metacarpals and phalanges

Deltoid (middle and posterior fibres)
Abduction of shoulder
O: Clavicle, spine of scapula
I: Tuberosity of humerus

Teres minor

Teres major

Triceps brachii
Extension at elbow
O: Scapula and humerus
I: Olecranon of ulna

Brachioradialis
Flexion at elbow

Extensor carpi radialis longus

Extensor digitorum

Posterior muscles of the arm and shoulder

Origins, insertions and actions of the chief muscles of the face and body

Related anatomy and physiology

The superficial and deep muscles respond very well to manual massage and electrical treatments which have beneficial effects on both the client and the therapist:

Effects for the client	Effects for the therapist
Massage reduces the build-up of **lactic acid** within the muscles and can induce deep relaxation by bringing oxygen, blood and nutrients to the fibres. This also brings about mental relaxation – the client may even fall asleep during treatments. Smooth muscle will also be relaxed by massage, and on the abdomen can aid digestion and release tension. Muscles which have been over-used will relax and cellular regeneration can take place.	Skeletal muscle responds well to use and to stimulation – developing fitness and tone and treatments will help build strength and endurance in the muscles. By using muscles correctly, with correct posture and building up a routine of use, muscles will be taught to work effectively so that you will have stamina for a full day's treatments. Incorrect use of muscles will result in repetitive strain injury and pain in the muscles.

The cardiovascular system

You will learn about:
- blood
- the structure of the heart
- the structure of the blood vessels
- the functions of the cardiovascular system.

The **cardiovascular** system consists of:
- a fluid – blood
- a pump – the heart
- a network of blood vessels, arteries, veins and capillaries.

Key terms

Lactic acid – formed when the energy supplies of glycogen and oxygen in the muscle are used up. Adenosine triphosphate (ATP) is formed when glycogen and oxygen mix. ATP is a rich source of energy for the muscle. Oxidation occurs and pyruvic acid is created to feed the muscle. However, if there is no more oxygen, pyruvic acid is converted into lactic acid and can cause muscle fatigue and pain. Massage should remove the lactic acid and take it to the lymph nodes for conversion and disposal.

Cardiovascular – when the muscles cause movement and the blood flow and oxygen rate is increased.

Blood

Blood is a thick, alkaline fluid which appears bright red in the arteries and dark red in the veins, depending on the presence of more or less oxygen respectively. It makes up about 8 per cent of our body weight so that the average volume of blood in an adult is between 5 and 6 litres. Blood contains about 55 per cent fluid in the form of plasma and about 45 per cent solid in the form of blood cells.

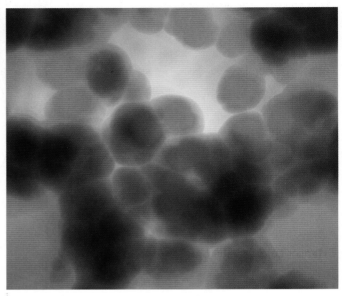

Blood cells under a microscope

Think about it

The mnemonic for blood contents and function is **O**ld **C**harlie **F**oster **H**ates **W**ild **W**omen **H**aving **D**ouble **C**hins = Oxygen, Carbon dioxide, Food, Hormones, Waste, Water, Heat regulation, Disease, Drugs and Clotting.

Blood transports:
- oxygen from the lungs to all the cells of the body
- carbon dioxide from the cells back to the lungs via the veins
- nutrients from the digestive tract to all of the body's cells
- waste products from the cells to be excreted
- hormones sent from the endocrine glands to regulate the cells
- medication into the cells.

It regulates:
- water content of cells
- body heat.

It protects:
- against infection and disease
- against blood loss by clotting.

Components of plasma	Function
Water = 90% of total volume	Renews cellular fluid
Minerals: chlorides, phosphates, carbonates	Maintain pH of blood at 7.4; maintain electrolyte balance for correct functioning of body tissues
Proteins: albumin, globulin, fibrinogen, heparin	Make blood viscous (sticky) which controls its flow and maintains blood pressure
Nutrients: glucose, amino acids, fatty acids, glycerol, vitamins	Required for energy, heat and raw materials
Gases: oxygen, carbon dioxide, nitrogen	Required for/produced by cellular respiration
Waste products: urea, uric acid, creatinine	By-products of metabolism
Antibodies and antitoxins	Protect against infection and neutralise some toxins which may enter the body
Hormones	See 'The endocrine system', page 207
Enzymes	Produce chemical reactions in other substances

Composition of plasma

Type of cell	Structure	Function
Erythrocytes (red blood cells)	Produced in red bone marrow of spongy bone, minute biconcave discs, about 5 million per cubic millimetre of blood. Contain the protein haemoglobin which attracts oxygen to form oxyhaemoglobin, which is bright red in colour	Carry oxygen to the tissues from the lungs and carry carbon dioxide away
Leucocytes (white blood cells)	Larger than red blood cells and less numerous. Three types: 75% granulocytes which can pass from bloodstream to site of infection; 20% lymphocytes made in the lymph nodes; 5% monocytes	Concerned with immunity. Granulocytes/ phagocytes: ingest bacteria and cell debris (phagocytosis); lymphocytes: produce antibodies; monocytes: phagocytosis
Thrombocytes (platelets)	Made in the bone marrow and are even smaller than red blood cells	Concerned with clotting the blood (haemostasis) which has three stages – narrowing of lumen in blood vessels, formation of platelet plugs, clotting and retraction of fibrin

Blood cells

The structure of the heart

The heart is a hollow, muscular, cone-shaped organ located behind the sternum, slightly to the left side of the body. It consists of four chambers: two upper chambers, called the left and right atriums, and the two lower chambers, called left and right ventricles. The heart also contains four main valves which are mechanisms to prevent blood from flowing in the wrong direction. The heart wall consists of three layers: the **endocardium**, the **myocardium** and the **pericardium**.

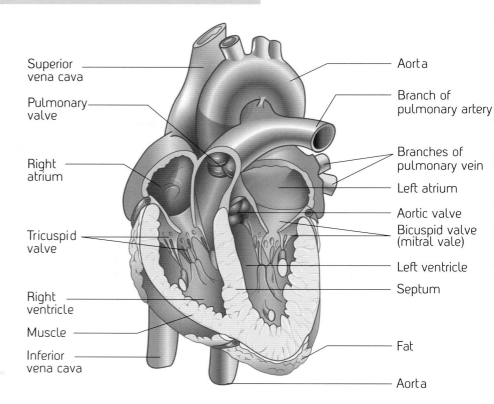

The heart

Structure and function of the heart

Structure	Location	Function
Left atrium/right atrium	Upper chambers	Receive blood flowing towards the heart from veins
Left ventricle/right ventricle	Lower chambers	Direct blood away from the heart through arteries
Right atrio-ventricular valve (tricuspid)	Between right atrium and right ventricle	Prevents backflow of blood into the right atrium during contraction of the right ventricle
Left atrio-ventricular valve (bicuspid) (mitral valve)	Between left atrium and left ventricle	Prevents backflow of blood into the left atrium during contraction of the left ventricle
Aortic valve	Between the aorta and the left ventricle	Prevents backflow of blood into the left ventricle
Pulmonary valve	Between the pulmonary vein and the right ventricle	Prevents backflow of blood into the right ventricle

Key terms

Endocardium – the inner layer of the heart wall.

Myocardium – the middle layer of the heart which contains cardiac muscle that contract to pump the blood.

Pericardium – the outer layer of the heart.

Pulmonary circulation – circulation between the heart and the lungs, as the blood is sent to pick up oxygen.

General (systemic) circulation – the pathway of blood from the left side of the heart to the rest of the body's tissues via the aorta.

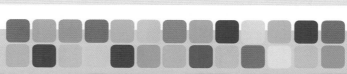

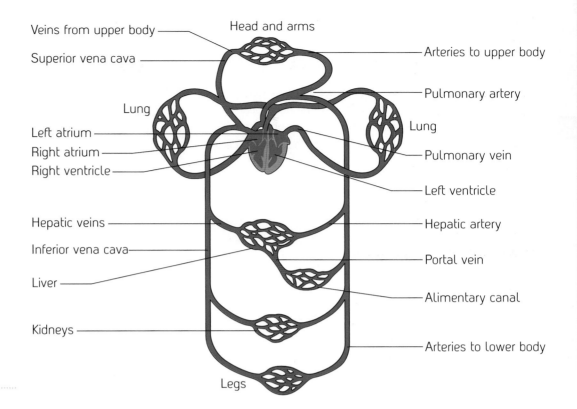

Veins from upper body

Head and arms

Superior vena cava

Arteries to upper body

Pulmonary artery

Lung

Left atrium

Lung

Right atrium

Pulmonary vein

Right ventricle

Left ventricle

Hepatic veins

Hepatic artery

Inferior vena cava

Portal vein

Liver

Alimentary canal

Kidneys

Arteries to lower body

Pulmonary circulation and systemic circulation

Legs

Pulmonary circulation

- Deoxygenated blood travels through the veins called inferior vena cava and superior vena cava into the right atrium.
- It flows from the right atrium through a valve into the right ventricle.
- From the right ventricle the blood passes through another valve and goes into the pulmonary arteries.
- From the pulmonary arteries the blood is carried to the lungs to pick up oxygen and get rid of carbon dioxide.
- This new oxygenated blood is then returned to the left atrium of the heart by the pulmonary veins.

Pulmonary artery

Superior vena cava

Aorta

Pulmonary valve

Pulmonary veins

Right atrium

Inferior vena cava

Left atrium

Bicuspid valve

Tricuspid valve

Tendons

Septum

Left ventricle

Right ventricle

Cardiac muscle

Deoxygenated blood

Oxygenated blood

General circulation

- The oxygenated blood passes from the left atrium through the valve into the left ventricle.
- It then gets pumped into the aorta, the main artery through the abdominal cavity.
- Under great pressure the blood is pumped all around the body, to give oxygen and nutrients to all of the cells.
- Once the exchange in the cells has been completed, the blood is deoxygenated and full of waste, so its journey begins again with a return to the right atrium of the heart by the inferior and superior vena cava.

Related anatomy and physiology

197

Factors which affect the heart

Adrenaline

In times of stress, excitement or anger the adrenal glands release adrenaline. This is the 'fight or flight' hormone which causes the heart rate to speed up so that you can face up to or run away from danger. The effect of the heart beating faster means you have a greater blood flow around the body, to feed the muscles ready for action, either to fight the foe or run away to safety.

Nerves

The cardiac muscle is special, it needs no stimulation from the brain to keep beating. If it did it would stop during sleep and unconsciousness. However, nerves can cause it to speed up or slow down — the sympathetic nerves will speed up the heart, if the body is under stress, and the parasympathetic nerves will slow the heart rate back down.

The structure of the blood vessels

Blood vessels are the tubes (our internal pipework!) which form a network around the body for the transportation of blood.

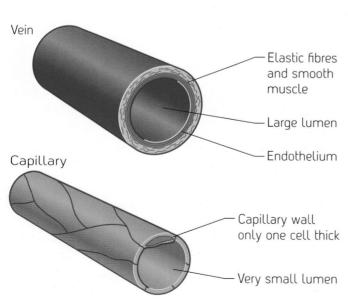

Artery

- Elastic fibres and smooth muscle
- Lumen
- Endothelium

Vein

- Elastic fibres and smooth muscle
- Large lumen
- Endothelium

Capillary

- Capillary wall only one cell thick
- Very small lumen

The structural differences of arteries, capillaries and veins

Arteries, capillaries and veins carry the blood to where it needs to go and respond to our supply and demand, depending upon our level of activity: if we are exercising or at rest.

Arteries

- Carry blood away from the heart
- Carry oxygenated blood (except the pulmonary artery)
- Have thicker muscular walls
- Have no valves
- Blood flow is rapid
- Blood pressure is higher
- Tend to lie deeper in the body
- Very small arteries are called arterioles

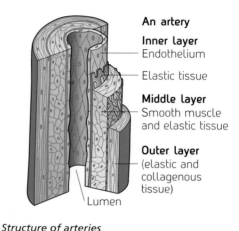

An artery
Inner layer
Endothelium
— Elastic tissue
Middle layer
Smooth muscle and elastic tissue
Outer layer
(elastic and collagenous tissue)
Lumen

Structure of arteries

Capillaries

- Arterioles are connected to capillaries
- Capillaries are the smallest of the vessels, and give nutrients to the smallest cells
- Capillaries are thin enough to allow substances to pass through them — called capillary exchange
- Oxygen and nutrients are delivered to cells
- Carbon dioxide and waste are removed from the cell
- Capillaries connect to venules (very small veins)
- Deoxygenated blood is picked up from venules to go into veins to go back to the heart

Veins

- Venules become veins
- Carry blood towards the heart
- Carry deoxygenated blood (except pulmonary vein)

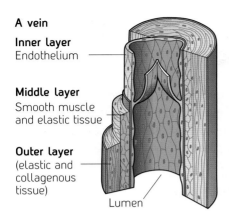

A vein

Inner layer
Endothelium

Middle layer
Smooth muscle
and elastic tissue

Outer layer
(elastic and
collagenous
tissue)

Lumen

Structure of veins

- Have thinner muscular walls
- Have valves
- Blood flow is slower
- Blood pressure is lower
- Tend to be more superficial in the body

> **Additional knowledge**
>
> **Coronary heart disease**
> There is a space at the centre of the arteries, veins and capillaries called a lumen. This is where the blood flows through. If the lumen in an artery gets blocked by cholesterol (a fatty substance) which clings to the lumen wall, the width of the space becomes smaller and smaller, until it becomes blocked up altogether. This is called coronary heart disease, and if blood flow to the heart is disrupted it can lead to heart attacks or angina. Exercise, a low cholesterol diet and regular medical checks will help keep cholesterol levels within the blood stream to a healthy level.

The pathway of blood

Capillaries form the link between arterioles and other tiny vessels called venules, which collect the blood from the capillaries. Venules then unite to form veins which carry blood on its journey back towards the heart. Arteries are thicker than veins and have a larger lumen (space at the centre). With one exception, they carry oxygenated blood away from the heart. Veins carry deoxygenated blood towards the heart, with one exception. (The exceptions are the pulmonary artery and vein, which take the blood to and from the lungs to pick up oxygen, and then return to the heart to be pumped around the body.)

Unlike arteries, veins contain valves which prevent the backflow of blood. The largest artery in the body is the aorta, which carries oxygenated blood from the left ventricle to all parts of the body (except the lungs). The largest veins in the body are the superior and inferior vena cavae. The superior vena cava carries deoxygenated blood from the upper parts of the body and the inferior vena cava carries deoxygenated blood from the lower parts of the body to the right atrium.

The pulse

The pulse can be felt in the wrist and in the neck, as these two arteries — the radial in the wrist and the carotid in the neck — are the most superficial to the skin. The number of beats per minute represents the heart rate, pushing blood through the artery.

The pulse is the rhythmic pumping of the blood around the body by the heart.

As blood is pumped from the left ventricle into the aorta, the aorta is already full of blood and so it becomes distended in order to accept more. The left ventricle contracts which causes vibrations along the arteries due to the expansion of the aorta. The expansion and contraction of the aorta causes a wave of similar movements throughout the arterial network which is known as the pulse.

The average resting pulse rate is approx 72–75 pulses per minute. It can vary between 60–80 and is also affected by:

- exercise — the pulse rate can double during strenuous exercise, but in a fit person, it will not increase as much as the heart is already used to exercise and does not have to work as hard
- age — children and babies have a higher pulse than adults
- gender — lower in females, higher in males

> **Additional knowledge**
>
> **Pulse rates**
> A fast resting pulse rate is called tachycardia, and this can indicate heart disease or be a reaction to drugs. Stimulants such as coffee, tea, alcohol and recreational drugs may also cause tachycardia, as will some phobias — fear of flying or spiders may cause the pulse to quicken. Bradycardia is the opposite and means a slow pulse rate of less than 60 beats per minute. Very fit athletes can train their body to slow down the pulse to avoid over-exertion during sports events, for example long-distance running.

- medication — certain drugs can affect the pulse
- emotional state — anger, fear, excitement can also affect the pulse rate.

Blood pressure

Blood pressure is the amount of pressure created by the blood on the walls of the arteries as it flows through them.

It is greatest in the large arteries leaving the heart, falls slightly in the arterioles and is hardly apparent at all in the capillaries. Blood pressure is even lower in the veins and in those veins entering the heart there is negative pressure, or suction, caused by the relaxation of the heart's chambers. Blood pressure fluctuates with each pumping action of the heart. It is highest when the ventricle contracts, forcing blood from the heart, and lowest when the ventricle relaxes. The maximum value is called systolic pressure and the lowest value is called diastolic pressure.

A doctor uses a sphygmomanometer to measure the blood pressure.

Blood pressure is measured by the weight of a column of mercury (Hg) it can support, calculated in millimetres. This used to be in a literal sense, and you could see the mercury being pushed up a scale, but it is now almost always done by digital machines.

The two phases of blood pressure are measured.

- *Systolic* pressure is the force exerted by blood on the walls in arteries during the contraction of the ventricles, which shows the highest pressure the heart can produce.
- This is the first reading and the first sound heard as the large heart valve closes.
- *Diastolic* pressure is the pressure on the walls of the arteries during relaxation of the ventricles. It is the second number in the blood pressure reading and it a quieter sound. The two together is a blood pressure reading — for example $110/70$.
- Normal arteriole pressure is 110–120mm Hg systolic pressure and 65–75mm Hg diastolic pressure.

Blood pressure problems

High blood pressure, known as hypertension, occurs when blood is forced through the arteries at abnormally high pressure which can damage the artery walls. This can lead to a stroke, where the blood flow to the brain is blocked, or a heart attack.

Low blood pressure, known as hypotension, can occur after shock, haemorrhage or heart failure and can be dangerous because there is an insufficient blood supply to the vital organs.

Blood pressure is used as an indicator of the health of both the blood vessels and the heart — that is why it is taken at regular intervals if a patient is in hospital. A weak heart will show as hypotension, and damaged blood vessels will show as hypertension.

Blood shunting

The body contains thousands of miles of blood vessels and there is not enough blood to fill all of them, all the time. So, there are certain points where small arteries have direct contact with small veins — a kind of short cut, missing out the capillaries. When needed, the blood can travel along these shunt vessels and go directly to the vein or artery, and this is often the case during exercise or after eating a heavy meal. The body is asking blood to be in the digestive tract, but then as the body leaves the dinner table, and decides a walk would be nice, more blood is needed for the muscles. So as a short cut, the blood uses the shunt vessel to get from A to B. This is a safety device for the body, to ensure adequate supplies of blood get where they need to be.

For this reason, it is not a good idea to carry out treatments on a client after a meal or strenuous exercise — especially if they are lying down. The demands of the blood flow may be so great that the blood flow to the brain is depleted and the client may faint.

Nearly all beauty therapy treatments affect the circulation in a positive way:

Effects for the client	Effects for the therapist
Most products and treatments within Level 3 have a stimulating effect on blood flow. This means cellular activity is quickened, as oxygen and nutrients are speeded to cells, and waste and CO_2 are taken away. The whole body benefits from this — as it would with exercise. The area being worked upon obviously benefits the most.	When performing treatments, especially any form of massage, the blood flow in the arms and hands is increased — and the effects of stimulation in this area means the skin and nails will get lots of oxygen and nutrients, so remain healthy with encouraged growth. It is somewhat ironic that therapists' nails grow quickly, as they need to keep them short to work safely!

Additional knowledge

Blood groups

All human blood has been classified as belonging to one of four groups: A, B, AB and O. The basis of classification is based upon the presence or absence of specific, genetically determined antigens on the surface of red blood cells. Not all blood mixes easily with another's blood, so a transfusion of blood from person to person needs care and attention. If the blood groups are not compatible then the red blood cells clump together (called agglutination) and this endangers life – any blockage of vessels can be fatal. Of the four blood types O is the most common. A person with O is classed as a universal donor because their blood can be given to all blood types and a person with AB is a universal recipient because they can receive blood from all groups.

There is also a category called the rhesus (Rh) factor. Blood is subdivided into rhesus groups of negative or positive. If a person with Rh negative blood is given Rh positive blood in transfusion, antibodies develop and will cause agglutination if another transfusion is given. This could also be fatal. It is especially important during childbirth; if a negative mother gives birth to a positive baby, it could be fatal to the child if their blood were to mix.

Do you know your own blood type?

Blood type	May give to	May receive from
O	Any blood group	O
A	A and AB	O and A
B	B and AB	O and B
AB	AB	Any blood group

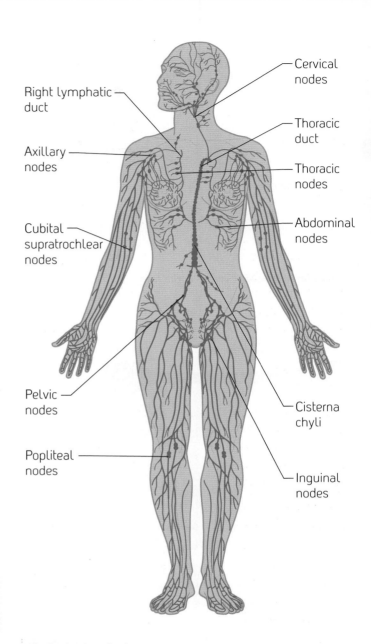

The body's lymphatic system

Labels: Right lymphatic duct · Cervical nodes · Axillary nodes · Thoracic duct · Thoracic nodes · Cubital supratrochlear nodes · Abdominal nodes · Pelvic nodes · Popliteal nodes · Cisterna chyli · Inguinal nodes

The lymphatic system

You will learn about:
- lymphatic circulation
- lymph nodes
- lymph vessels
- lymph ducts.

The lymphatic system consists of lymphatic capillaries, vessels, nodes and ducts. The capillaries and vessels form a network around the body which act as tunnels for the transportation of lymph fluid, in the same way that blood vessels provide a network for the transport of blood.

Lymphatic circulation

Blood does not flow into the tissues but remains inside the blood vessels. However, plasma from the blood is able to seep through the capillary walls and enter the spaces between the tissues. This fluid provides the cells with nutrients and oxygen, and has now become interstitial fluid. Interstitial fluid circulates through the tissues giving nutrients and oxygen to the cells and carrying waste back into the blood. Excess fluid which does not return to the blood is called lymph and it is collected and returned to the blood by the lymphatic system. Lymph travels from the lymphatic capillaries to the larger lymphatic vessels. Along its journey

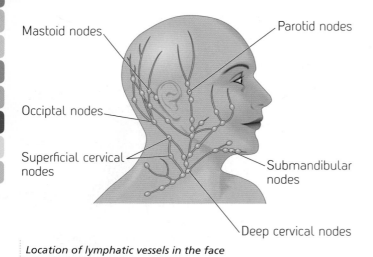

Location of lymphatic vessels in the face

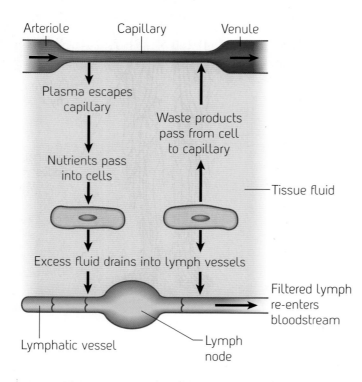

The relationship between blood and lymph

it passes through lymphatic nodes which are situated in areas of the body where there is a greater risk of infection. At these points, the lymph is filtered and cleaned and also lymphocytes are produced — these are antibodies that help prevent infection. Having passed through at least one lymph node, lymph fluid travels into lymphatic ducts. The ducts pass lymph back into the blood circulation where it becomes part of blood so that the cycle can begin once again.

The functions of the lymphatic system are to:

- help fight infection — it is part of the immune system and it produces specialised white blood cells called lymphocytes, which recognise harmful substances and destroy them

- distribute fluid in the body — lymphatic vessels can drain as much as 3 litres of excess fluid daily from tissue spaces

- transport fats. Carbohydrates and protein are passed from the small intestine directly into the bloodstream. However, fats are passed from the small intestine into lymphatic vessels called lacteals before eventually passing into the bloodstream.

There are approximately 600 small bean-shaped lymph nodes scattered throughout the body — in groups or clusters around the groin, breast, armpits, and knees and around the major blood vessels of the abdomen and chest. These are the glands which swell up and become tender if the body is fighting infection. The doctor will feel the glands in the neck to see if they are enlarged and tender — a good indication that infection is present. When the lymph glands are overwhelmed with infection the doctor will prescribe antibiotics to help the body fight infection.

The lymph nodes or glands contain specialist white blood cells called monocytes and lymphocytes.

- Monocytes destroy harmful substances by ingesting or eating them.

- Lymphocytes produce antibodies that stop the growth of bacteria and prevent their harmful actions. Lymph nodes enlarge to manage the infection and this causes the glands to swell up.

Structure of the nodes

Lymph nodes have a fibrous outer capsule containing lymphoid tissue. Lymph enters through the **afferent** lymphatic vessels and leaves the nodes through the **efferent** lymphatic vessels. There may be as many as five afferent vessels entering a node but only one or two efferent vessels carrying the filtered fluid away from the node.

Key terms

Afferent – carrying towards.

Efferent – carrying away.

Think about it

Lymph operates in a one-way system around the body, always towards the heart. This is why massage should also follow the same direction.

Feature	Structure	Function
Lymph	Straw-coloured fluid	Carries more waste than nutrients
Lymphatic capillaries	One cell thick, hair-like structures which combine to form lymphatic vessels	Transport lymph from the tissues
Lymphatic vessels	Larger and thicker than capillaries, contain valves which prevent backflow of lymph	Transport lymph through one or more lymphatic nodes
Lymphatic nodes	Vary in size from a pin head to an almond	Filter lymph to remove bacteria, so can become swollen and tender if infection is present. Produce some antibodies
Lymphatic ducts	Larger thoracic duct is about 45 cm long, has valves and is located at the back of the abdomen; smaller right lymphatic duct is about 1 cm long and formed by the joining of the vessels from the head, thorax and right limb	Collect lymph and return it to the bloodstream. Thoracic duct receives lymph from vessels in the abdomen and lower limbs and empties into the left subclavian vein; right lymphatic duct empties into the right subclavian vein

Structures and functions of the lymphatic system

The spleen

The spleen consists of lymph tissue and is part of the lymphatic system. It is found in the left-hand side of the abdomen, under the diaphragm and behind the stomach.

Functions of the spleen

- A reservoir for blood — if blood is required urgently anywhere in the body, due to injury, it can call upon the reservoir to help.

- Lymphocytes are produced here — the body can cope without a spleen, but if it has to be removed then the body has a much lower resistance to disease and infection.

- Filtering — old worn-out blood cells are filtered from the blood and destroyed in the spleen after roughly a 120-day cycle.

Conditions associated with the lymphatic system

- **Hodgkin's disease** — this is cancer of the lymph nodes.

- **Oedema** — fluid retention, often seen around the ankles, but can be anywhere in the body and is common in people who are stationary, or bed-bound. Massage is good to increase the movement of lymph, but as it is often a sign of systemic illness, such as kidney malfunction, GP approval should always be sought prior to treatment.

Key terms

Hodgkin's disease — cancer of the lymph nodes.

Oedema — swelling caused by fluid retention.

Lymphatic circulation and beauty therapy

The circulation of both blood and lymph is increased by manual and electrical beauty therapy techniques. Effleurage movements gently stimulate lymphatic flow and have a draining effect, which helps rid the body of toxins and waste products, as well as reducing puffiness. Electrical vacuum suction is particularly stimulating to the lymphatic system, which is why it is important to always work in the direction of lymphatic flow, towards the nearest lymphatic duct.

The digestive system

You will learn about:
- the structure of the digestive system
- the process of digestion
- excretion
- regulation of blood glucose.

The digestive system is designed to change the food we eat into small simple molecules that can be absorbed into the bloodstream and used by all the cells to produce energy and building blocks for growth and repair.

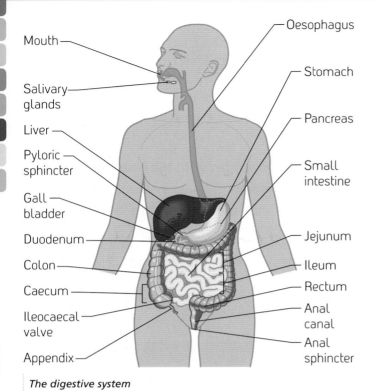

Mouth
Salivary glands
Liver
Pyloric sphincter
Gall bladder
Duodenum
Colon
Caecum
Ileocaecal valve
Appendix

Oesophagus
Stomach
Pancreas
Small intestine
Jejunum
Ileum
Rectum
Anal canal
Anal sphincter

The digestive system

To do this, the digestive system is made up of a number of organs and glands which facilitate the chewing, swallowing, digestion, absorption and elimination of food. It runs from the mouth, where food is ingested (taken in), to the rectum, where waste is expelled. Food is passed from one structure to another in a process which breaks it down into its component parts, ensuring that essential nutrients are absorbed into the bloodstream.

The structure of the digestive system

Name	Structure and location
Mouth	The taking in of food and liquid is called ingestion. The mouth is a cavity bound by lips and cheeks. It contains the tongue and teeth, which assist in **mastication**, and the salivary glands, which produce saliva, the functions of which include softening food, digestion of carbohydrates and cleansing of the mouth and teeth. Saliva lubricates the food and contains the enzyme salivary amylase, which begins to break down the starch in cooked foods such as bread, potatoes, grains and cereals. The tongue contains nerve receptors and is divided into four main areas which detect sour, salty, bitter and sweet flavours.

Name	Structure and location
Pharynx	The muscles of the pharynx, in the throat, push the food down into the oesophagus or food pipe. A flap of cartilage called the epiglottis prevents the food being swallowed from going into the lungs by mistake.
Oesophagus	This is the food pipe. A muscular canal which extends from the pharynx to the stomach, located behind the trachea and in front of the vertebral column. The food is propelled downwards towards the stomach by the process of peristalsis. Peristalsis is a wave of contractions occurring in the muscles which squeeze and relax to push food along the digestive tract.
Stomach	A J-shaped structure located below and to the left of the diaphragm. The upper opening from the oesophagus consists of a weak **sphincter** muscle, while the lower opening into the small intestine consists of a strong pyloric sphincter which prevents the regurgitation of food. The stomach churns the food and releases gastric juices to help break it down. • Hydrochloric acid – kills harmful bacteria and helps to dissolve the food. • Pepsin – begins the digestion of proteins. Some substances are absorbed directly through the stomach wall into the bloodstream, including water, alcohol and glucose. Food stays in the stomach for about four/five hours and leaves in a liquid form called chyme.
Small intestine	Consists of the duodenum, jejunum and ileum and is a long tube (6 metres) extending from the pyloric sphincter to the large intestine, located in the central and lower abdominal cavity within the curves of the large intestine. The inside of the small intestine is covered with millions of finger-like extensions called villi. Villi have a rich blood supply and food is absorbed across their whole surface area. The nutrients are passed into the bloodstream, with the exception of fat. Fat is absorbed directly into lymphatic capillaries called lacteals (which gives it a white milky colour) and is transported around the body and blood circulation.

Name	Structure and location
Pancreas	A gland approx. 12–15 cm long which lies across the posterior abdominal wall behind the stomach. As well as releasing hormones it also produces the following enzymes: • typsin – digests proteins and breaks them down into amino acids • amylase – which continues the digestion of starch molecules into the sugar maltose • lipase – breaks fats into fatty acids and glycerol. The pancreas also keeps a check on the amount of glucose in the blood.
Liver	The largest gland in the body, located in the upper-right section of the abdominal cavity, beneath the diaphragm. Most of the blood enters the liver through the hepatic portal vein, which carries blood from the stomach, intestine, spleen, pancreas and gall bladder. The blood in the portal vein carries nutrients: glucose, amino acids (which are protein chains), vitamins and minerals. Functions of the liver: • Stores and filters blood • Destroys bacteria and worn out red blood cells • Breaks down excess proteins into urea – excreted as urine • Secretes bile for the digestion of fat • Detoxes alcohol, drugs and other chemicals • Stores vitamins A, D, E, K and iron • Stores glycogen – which is then broken into glucose and used for energy • Converts nutrients – proteins (amino acids) into lipids (fats) or glucose (sugar) – when required by the body
Gall bladder	A pear-shaped organ located near the right lobe of the liver. The cystic duct of the gall bladder joins the hepatic duct of the liver to form the bile duct. This is a reservoir for the bile, from the liver, required for fat digestion. It can be removed if inflamed or infected or full of gallstones, which are accumulations of cholesterol crystals.

Name	Structure and location
Large intestine	A tube approximately 1.5 metres in length which extends from the ileum to the anus and consists of seven sections: caecum, ascending colon, transverse colon, descending colon, sigmoid colon, rectum and anal canal. Any remaining undigested food and roughage (fibre) become waste matter and can be expelled from the body. Any remaining nutrients and water are removed from this waste mater and reabsorbed back into the body. The large intestine contains million of bacteria, which produce vitamins K and B. These bacteria also ferment some forms of carbohydrates, such as onions, beans, pulses and lentils, a by-product of which is gas in the digestive tract.

Structure and location of the digestive system

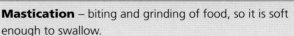

Key terms

Mastication – biting and grinding of food, so it is soft enough to swallow.

Sphincter – any circular muscle which contracts to constrict or close a natural passage or opening, for example the anus, the oesophagus opening into the stomach, or bile and pancreatic ducts opening into the digestive tract.

The process of digestion

The journey of food begins in the mouth with the process of ingestion. Food is broken down and softened by chewing and becomes mixed with saliva. Mechanical digestion is the term given to the physical breakdown of food in the form of biting and chewing. The churning of food in the stomach is also an illustration of mechanical digestion — it works a bit like a food processor, mashing up food and mixing it with digestive juices.

Chemical digestion involves the production of digestive juices which act on food and break it down into smaller molecules. During the process of digestion, nutrients are broken down into small, soluble molecules which can be easily absorbed into the bloodstream and later used as raw materials for cells and tissues or as energy for respiration.

- Starch digestion starts in the mouth — salivary amylase breaks down starch molecules to become the sugar maltose.

- In the duodenum the enzyme maltase breaks down each maltose molecule into two molecules of glucose. Sucrose is broken down by the enzyme sucrase into glucose and fructose (fruit sugar), and lactose (milk sugar) is broken down by the enzyme lactase into glucose and galactose.

- Proteins are made up of smaller molecule chains called amino acids. Protein digestion begins in the stomach with the enzyme pepsin, which breaks down most proteins into small units called polypeptides.

- In the duodenum the enzyme typsin, found in pancreatic juices, breaks down proteins and polypeptides into smaller substances called peptides. Peptides are broken down by enzymes to become amino acids.

Pepsin		Typsin	
Protein ➔	Polypeptides ➔	Peptides ➔	Amino acids

Excretion

The final part of food's journey is elimination, which takes place when 'food' passes from the colon to the rectum. In fact, the material which enters the large intestine contains very little food at all, as it has mostly been absorbed before it arrives. The material entering the large intestine contains water, salt, indigestible cellulose and bacteria. Most of the water and salts are absorbed by the colon, which causes the bacteria to die, leaving only cellulose and dead bacteria which form a paste. This paste forms the faeces, which consist of a little water and a solid part which is about 50 per cent dead bacteria and 50 per cent cellulose. The brown colour of faeces comes from the breakdown of old red blood cells.

Excretions of urine

The urinary system consists of the following:

- two kidneys which excrete urine
- two ureter which transport urine from the kidneys to the bladder
- the bladder where urine is collected and stored
- the urethra through which urine is discharged from the bladder.

The kidneys are bean-shaped organs lying on the posterior wall of the abdomen, either side of the spine. Because of the position of the liver, the right kidney is slightly higher than the left.

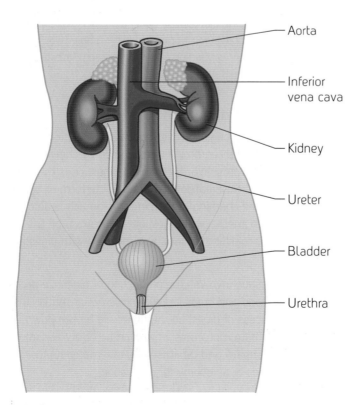

The female urinary system

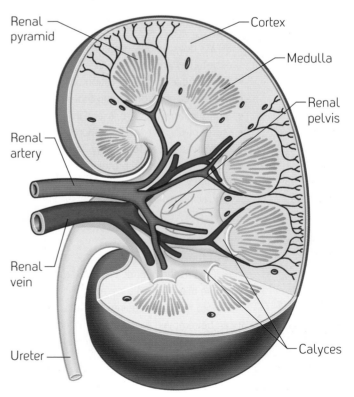

Cross-section of a kidney

A kidney has two main parts:

1 outer cortex — this is reddish brown and is the part where fluid is filtered
2 inner medulla — the paler colour made up of cone-shaped sections called renal pyramids. This is the area where some materiel is selectively reabsorbed into the bloodstream.

The renal pelvis is in the centre of the kidney, which is a funnel-shaped cavity which collects urine from the renal pyramids in the medulla and drains into the ureter.

The cortex and medulla contain tiny blood filtration units called nephrons. Nephrons are the functional units of the kidney and a single kidney has more than a million nephrons.

Functions of the kidneys

- Filtration of impurities and metabolic waste
- Regulation of water and salt balance
- Formation of urine
- Regulation of blood pressure and blood volume

Urine is produced by three processes:

- filtration — takes place in the Bowman's capsule, the collection point for the waste products carried in the blood
- selective re-absorption — the loop of Henle helps re-absorb urine (only 1% of liquid actually filtered is actually excreted as urine, the rest is re-absorbed)
- collection — a collecting tube in the medulla.

Composition of urine

Urine is a pale watery fluid but its colour varies depending upon what fluid is drunk and is a good indication of health — the right concentration of salts etc. is when it is pale yellow; dark urine means the body needs more water. Urine is slightly acidic, between 4.5—7.5 pH, depending upon the pH of the blood. The control of salt levels within the body is essential to life and the kidneys' role is vital. Urine concentration is also an indication of health problems and the presence of glucose is an indication of diabetes. Hormones indicating pregnancy and menopause can also be detected through urine.

Regulation of blood glucose

The typical blood glucose level is about 80—90 mg per 100 ml of blood. Glucose is present in higher levels after meals, particularly if they are rich in carbohydrates. This is known as the absorptive state, when blood glucose levels rise to a maximum of 140 mg per 100 ml of blood.

If glucose were transported immediately from the digestive system to other parts of the body, there would be a shortage of glucose between meals and blood sugar levels would fall dramatically. So some glucose is used immediately and some is stored for later. Glucose that is not immediately required for energy is converted into glycogen and triacylglycerols (fat) and stored in the liver, skeletal muscle and adipose tissue. Blood glucose levels typically return to normal within two and a half hours after eating, even though digestion continues for longer.

When the body needs energy but the stomach is empty, supplies built up in the liver, adipose tissue and skeletal muscle during the absorptive state are used. The breakdown of proteins also provides glucose.

The pancreas also plays an important role in the regulation of blood glucose (see 'The endocrine system', below). When blood sugar levels fall it produces a hormone to make the glycogen stores to convert to glucose. When blood sugar levels rise it produces insulin to make the excess glucose convert to glycogen for storage.

A deficiency in insulin results in high levels of blood glucose, and this is characteristic of the condition Diabetes mellitus. The diet for a diabetic should be the same as the recommended balanced diet for all adults — regular meals based on starchy foods which contain less sugar and fat. People suffering from diabetes might require more snacks in their diet to help maintain blood glucose levels, and they should make sure that these are of nutritional value.

The endocrine system

You will learn about:
- the functions of the endocrine system
- the pituitary gland
- the thyroid gland
- the pancreas
- the adrenal glands
- gonads.

Key terms

Hypothalamus – the part of the brain that links the nervous system to the endocrine system via the pituitary gland.

Pituitary gland – a gland in the brain which controls and regulates a number of endocrine functions. It maintains the body's homeostasis (internal stability and constancy).

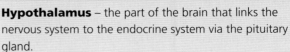

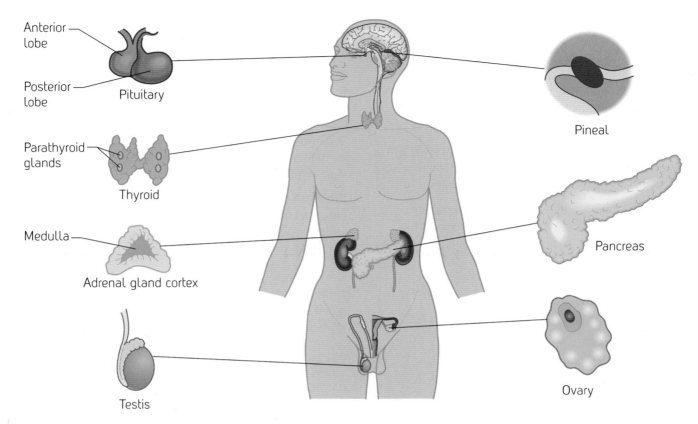

Anterior lobe
Posterior lobe
Pituitary
Parathyroid glands
Thyroid
Medulla
Adrenal gland cortex
Testis
Pineal
Pancreas
Ovary

The endocrine glands and their position in the body

The endocrine system is the series of glands in the body which make and control hormones, which in turn control all the metabolic processes within the body — from bone growth to body temperature.

The endocrine system is often described as functioning like an orchestra, with the **hypothalamus** acting as band leader and the **pituitary gland** acting as the conductor. The pituitary is sometimes referred to as the 'master gland' because of its regulating function although, as in an orchestra, all the components must work together. If one gland is not working efficiently, the others must become more active to compensate and maintain harmony.

The functions of the endocrine system

Endocrine glands could accurately be described as organs. They produce chemical compounds called hormones which are secreted directly into the bloodstream and carried to specific organs, glands or tissues in other parts of the body where they have a specific effect. Hormones are slow-acting chemical messengers which control many of the body's functions including growth, metabolism, sexual development and co-ordination. Endocrine glands continually secrete hormones, although the level of secretion is altered to

meet the body's needs. If glands over- or under-secrete hormones, the body reacts by displaying abnormal physical or physiological symptoms.

Disorders of the endocrine system are of concern to the beauty therapist as they can contra-indicate certain treatments, or a client's concerns, such as superfluous hair growth, may point to the presence of an endocrinological disorder.

The hypothalamus controls the endocrine and autonomic nervous systems and it therefore has an effect on many of the body's functions, including:

- emotion
- sexual activity
- secretion of pituitary hormones
- appetite
- autonomic nervous system
- body temperature
- metabolism
- water balance.

The pituitary gland

The pituitary gland is divided into two sections the **anterior** and **posterior** lobes, which have different functions and secretions, as shown below.

Hormone	Target	Function
Thyroid Stimulating Hormone (TSH)	Thyroid gland	Regulation of metabolism, breakdown of fat, control of water content
Somatrophic hormone (growth)	Long bones and muscles of the body	Increases rate of growth and maintains size in adulthood. Over-secretion in children can cause gigantism, under-secretion can cause dwarfism
Adrenocorticotrophic hormone (ACTH)	Adrenal cortex	This stimulates and controls the growth and hormonal output of the adrenal cortex
Follicle stimulating hormone (FSH)	Sexual organs	Controls maturation of ovarian follicles in females and sperm production in males
Gonadotrophic hormones	Sexual organs	These control the development and growth of the ovaries and testes
Luteinising hormone (LH)	Sexual organs	In women this helps prepare the uterus for the fertilised ovum, and prepares breasts for lactation in pregnancy. In men it acts on the testes to produce testosterone
Prolactin	The breasts	This stimulates the production of the milk from the breasts following birth
Melanocyte-stimulating hormone (MSH)	The skin	This stimulates the production of melanin in the basal cell layer of the skin

Secretions of the anterior pituitary gland

Key terms

Anterior – at the front of.

Posterior – behind or lower.

Hormone	Target	Function
Oxytocin	Pregnant uterus, breasts	Contraction of smooth muscle, stimulates the uterus during childbirth and stimulates the breasts to produce milk
Antidiuretic hormone (ADH) or vasopressin	Kidneys	Increase in absorption of water so less urine is excreted. Under-secretion can cause Diabetes insipidus, which is characterised by excess excretion of dilute urine

Secretions of the posterior pituitary gland

Endocrine glands have a feedback mechanism as a fail-safe for health which is coordinated by the pituitary gland. This gland is influenced by the hypothalamus and will increase output if either gland fails to produce hormones, or decrease production if either gland over-produces and floods the bloodstream with hormones.

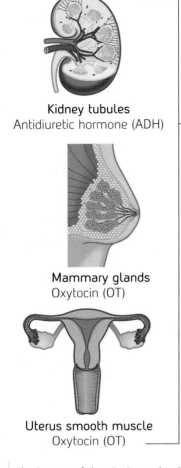

Kidney tubules
Antidiuretic hormone (ADH)

Mammary glands
Oxytocin (OT)

Uterus smooth muscle
Oxytocin (OT)

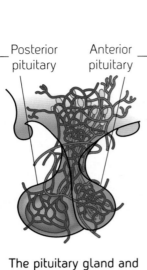

Posterior pituitary

Anterior pituitary

The pituitary gland and its master control

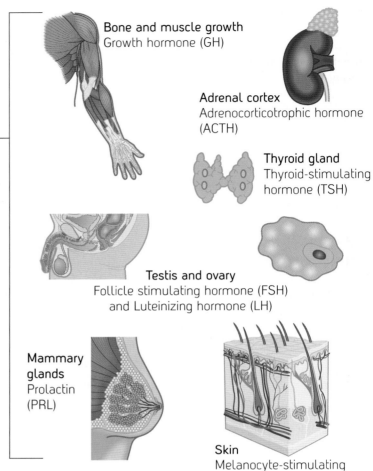

Bone and muscle growth
Growth hormone (GH)

Adrenal cortex
Adrenocorticotrophic hormone (ACTH)

Thyroid gland
Thyroid-stimulating hormone (TSH)

Testis and ovary
Follicle stimulating hormone (FSH) and Luteinizing hormone (LH)

Mammary glands
Prolactin (PRL)

Skin
Melanocyte-stimulating

The impact of the pituitary gland

The thyroid gland

The thyroid gland is situated just behind your collarbone in the centre of your lower neck. Its main job is to control the speed of the body's processes — the metabolic rate.

Hormone	Target	Function
Thyroxine and triodothyronine	Cells and tissues throughout the body	• Regulates metabolism in tissues • Influences growth and cell division • Influences mental development • Stores the mineral iodine, which it needs to manufacture thyroxin • Stimulates the involuntary nervous system and controls irritability • Increases urine production • Breaks down protein and increases uptake of glucose by cells
Parathormone		Distribution and metabolism of calcium and phosphorus

Secretions of the thyroid gland

The thyroid gland also has a feedback mechanism. It will increase production to meet demands for more thyroid hormones at various times, such as during the menstruation cycle, pregnancy and puberty.

Malfunctions of the thyroid gland

Under-secretion
Hypothyroidism – dry, coarse skin and hair, low metabolism, weight gain, low body temperature, feeling cold all the time, dry and brittle hair, muscle spasm (tetanus)
Over-secretion
Hyperthyroidism – anxiety, high pulse rate, increased metabolism, weight loss, heat intolerance, brittle and porous bones, kidney stones

Disorders of the thyroid gland

The pancreas

The pancreas produces pancreatic enzymes which play a part in digestion and are described as an exocrine function of the pancreas. The pancreas also has an endocrine function. An area called the **islets of Langerhans** produces two hormones from alpha and beta cells. The alpha cells produce glucagon and the beta cells produce insulin.

Hormone	Target	Function
Insulin	Blood sugar	Controls metabolism of carbohydrates, lowers blood sugar levels. The release of insulin prompts the liver and muscles to store glucose, in the form of glycogen. This helps bring down the sugar levels.
Glucagon	Blood sugar	Raises blood sugar levels. The release of glucagon prompts the liver and muscles to release glycogen stored within them into the blood stream, which helps restore levels.

Secretions of the pancreas

Key terms

Islets of Langerhans – groups of specialised cells in the pancreas that make insulin and glucagon.

The adrenal glands

The adrenal glands produce certain hormones. They consist of two separate endocrine glands:

- The adrenal cortex secretes mineralocorticoids, glucocorticoids and sex hormones.
- The adrenal medulla secretes adrenaline and noradrenalin.

Hormone	Target	Function
Mineralocorticoids, e.g. aldosterone	Water content of tissues	Regulate mineral content of body fluids, regulate salt and water balance
Glucocorticoids, e.g. cortisone, cortisol, hydrocortisone	Blood sugar, liver	Regulate metabolism of carbohydrates and proteins, conversion of protein to glycogen for storage in the liver, increase blood sugar level by decreasing use of glucose
Sex hormones (androgens and oestrogens) and steroids	Reproductive organs	Development and function of sex organs, physical characteristics in both sexes, psychological characteristics in both sexes
Adrenaline	In conjunction with and stimulated by the sympathetic nervous system	Fight or flight mechanism increases heart rate and supply of glucose, blood and oxygen to muscles, digestion slows down
Noradrenaline	Circulation	Contracts blood vessels, raises blood pressure

Secretions of the adrenal glands

Malfunctions of the adrenal glands

Over-secretion
Increased likelihood of ulcers, increased blood pressure
Cushing's syndrome – excess fatty tissue on trunk, oedema, male pattern hair growth, raised pH of blood (alkalosis)
An adrenal tumour in females produces male characteristics – male pattern hair growth, deepening of the voice

Under-secretion
Excess water loss from the body, lowered pH of blood (acidosis)
Addison's disease – anaemia, low blood pressure, muscle wastage, hyperpigmentation

Disorders of the adrenal glands

Additional knowledge

Fight or flight

Adrenaline is the hormone responsible for the 'fight or flight' reaction in the body — but it also kicks into action when the body is under stress, such as a pounding heart, increased ventilation rate and dry mouth with butterflies in the tummy. The effects can be frightening and some people would describe these as classic symptoms of a panic attack. The stress hormones are broken down slowly so the effects on the sympathetic nervous system are long lasting — the best way to counteract this is exercise — actually doing the physical act of working the muscles as they were designed to do — either facing up to or running away from danger!

The gonads

Gonads are the organ which makes gametes (reproductive cells). In women gonads are called ovaries and produce ova (eggs) and in men gonads are called testes and produce sperm. They are controlled by follicle-stimulating hormone (FSH) and luteinising hormone (LH). They produce the hormones oestrogen, progesterone and androgens.

Hormone	Target	Function
Oestrogen	Secondary sexual characteristics in females	Development of female reproductive system, development of external genitalia, uterus and breasts, regulation of menstrual cycle
Progesterone	Structures involved in pregnancy	Maintenance of pregnancy, development of placenta, prepares breasts for lactation
Androgens	Secondary sexual characteristics in males	Development of male reproductive system, male hair growth pattern, voice deepening, muscle bulk

Secretions of the gonads

Disorders of the ovaries

If the ovaries fail to respond to stimulation by the pituitary gland, the production of oestrogen and progesterone can be reduced or the secretion of androgens can increase. Such an imbalance is usually characterised by a masculine pattern of hair growth in females, which is known as **hirsutism.**

Primary hirsutism is caused by an increased sensitivity to normal levels of androgens in the blood, which usually begins during puberty and settles down during the thirties. Secondary, or 'true', hirsutism is caused by increased androgen production in the ovaries or adrenal glands and can begin just prior to or just after puberty.

Key terms

Hirsutism – a masculine pattern of hair growth in females caused by a hormonal imbalance of oestrogen and progesterone.

The nervous system

You will learn about:
* the central nervous system
* the autonomic nervous system
* sense organs.

The central nervous system

The nervous system provides a network of communication between different areas of the body and also acts as a

Related anatomy and physiology

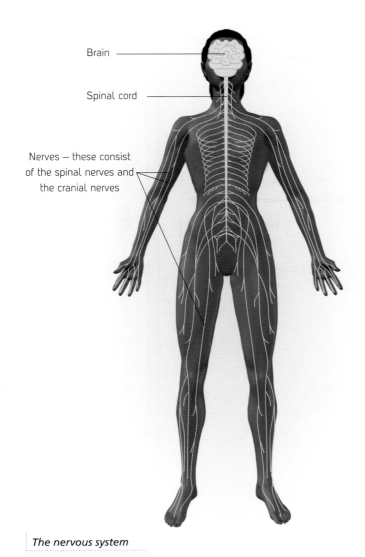

Brain

Spinal cord

Nerves — these consist
of the spinal nerves and
the cranial nerves

The nervous system

receptor for information from the internal and external environment, for homeostasis to be maintained. The central nervous system (CNS) consists of the brain and spinal cord. An example of the simplest circuit in the CNS involves communication between a single sensory nerve and a motor neuron in the brain or spinal cord. This then transmits an impulse to a muscle or gland causing a reaction. Some reflex actions involve several nerves, such as the knee-jerk reflex which is used to indicate the condition of the nervous system.

The autonomic nervous system

The autonomic nervous system (ANS) supplies the internal organs and is so called because these organs function without conscious effort — that is, their functions are automatic. There are two parts to the ANS:

- Sympathetic nervous system — this has nerves that supply the internal organs and run back to the spinal nerves, as well as nerves which supply the blood vessels, sweat and sebaceous glands and the **arrector pili** muscle in the dermis.
- Parasympathetic nervous system — it has branches which run to all of the internal organs.

Therefore each organ has a double nerve supply which provides opposing actions. This is a back-up supply system to maintain homeostasis and prevent illness.

Key terms

Arrector pili – tiny muscle fibres attached to hair follicles which contract to make the hairs stand on end, causing goose bumps.

How impulses are transmitted

The structure and functional unit of the nervous system is made up of fibres (called dendrites) that send impulses to the nerve cell, the nerve cell itself, and the fibres (called axons) that convey the impulses from the cell. These are classified according to their function:

- afferent — carry impulses from all parts of the body to the central nervous system
- efferent — carry impulses from the central nervous system to muscles and glands in the body
- interneurons — connect neurons within the nervous system.

These neurons send the messages or nerve impulses to neighbouring neurons for organs, muscles or glands, depending upon what is required. The neurons do not touch one another — there is a tiny gap over which the signal must jump, called a synapse. The nerve impulse is electronically fired to the next neuron by the release of chemicals, which diffuse across the synapse. The reaction continues along the network of neurons in this way until it reaches its destination, which could mean several thousand synapses firing away for just one small series of movements within the body (there are 500 metres or more if supplying the lower limbs). The neuron's function is dependent upon both enough water within the body for transmission, and enough salts and electrolytes within the bloodstream to function properly. Impulses from the synapses travel in one direction only. Any inflammation of the synapses is called neuralgia, and can be extremely painful.

Related anatomy and physiology

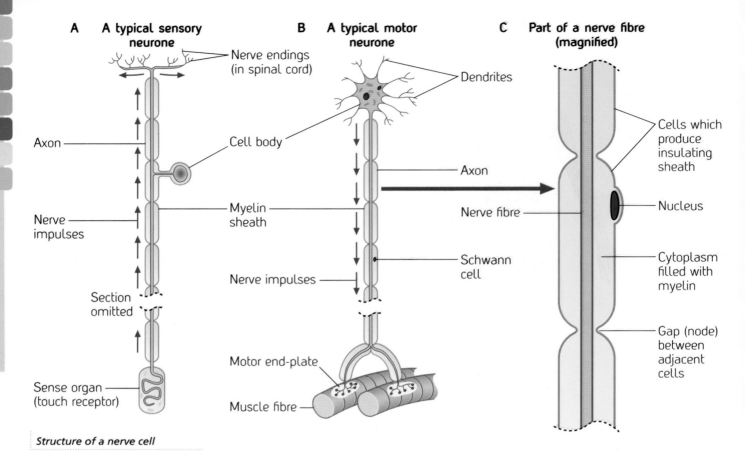

A A typical sensory neurone

Nerve endings (in spinal cord)

Axon

Cell body

Nerve impulses

Myelin sheath

Section omitted

Sense organ (touch receptor)

Structure of a nerve cell

B A typical motor neurone

Dendrites

Axon

Myelin sheath

Nerve impulses

Schwann cell

Motor end-plate

Muscle fibre

C Part of a nerve fibre (magnified)

Cells which produce insulating sheath

Nucleus

Nerve fibre

Cytoplasm filled with myelin

Gap (node) between adjacent cells

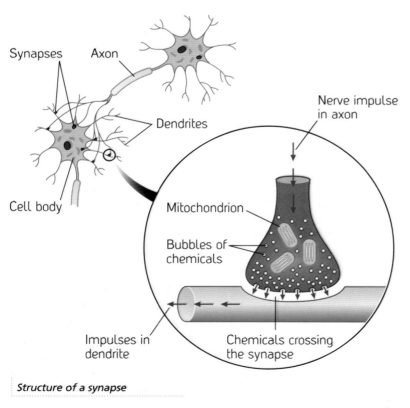

Synapses

Axon

Dendrites

Cell body

Mitochondrion

Bubbles of chemicals

Impulses in dendrite

Nerve impulse in axon

Chemicals crossing the synapse

Structure of a synapse

Nerves

The axons from a large number of neurons are arranged in bundles and form nerves — imagine lots of independent electrical wires surrounded by a cable, holding it all together.

A ganglion is a semi-independent band or mass of highly organised nerve cells working outside the brain and spinal cord, which forms a subsidiary nerve centre which receives and sends out nerve fibres, such as in the sympathetic system.

Unlike other cells, neurons cannot divide and reproduce themselves. If neurons are destroyed they cannot be replaced, although they are good at repair when damaged.

Neuropathy is the term used for any disease of the nerves, and would certainly be a contra-indication to treatment. Total damage to the nerve supply, if it has been crushed or severed, results in paralysis to the area. Diabetics often suffer with neuropathy, especially in the lower limbs, and GP approval prior to treatment should be sought for this reason.

Sense organs

The sense organs are the eyes, ears, nose, mouth and skin, and their function is to pass on the many impulses which are continually stimulating them. They receive sensory impulses from the external environment and transmit information to the CNS via nerves which stimulate a physical or a psychological reaction. Obvious illustrations of sensory impulses are those of sight, sound, smell, taste and touch – see the table below.

Sensory impulse	Path from sense organ to CNS	Point of interpretation
Sight	Optic nerve (2nd cranial nerve)	Interpreted in the visual areas of the occipital lobes
Hearing	Vestibulococlear nerve (8th cranial nerve)	Interpreted in auditory areas of temporal lobes
Smell	Olfactory nerve (1st cranial nerve)	Interpreted in the temporal lobe
Taste	Facial nerve (7th cranial) and glossopharyngeal nerve (9th cranial)	Interpreted in the temporal lobe with the corresponding smell. Few tastes can be interpreted without corresponding sense of smell
Pain, heat and cold	Nerve endings that transmit pain and temperature changes	Sensory nerve fibres run in the spinal nerves to the posterior nerve roots in the spinal cord
Light touch	Nerve endings that transmit light touch	Sensory nerve fibres run in the spinal nerves to the posterior nerve roots in the spinal cord
Firm pressure	Nerve endings that transmit firm pressure	Sensory nerve fibres run in the spinal nerves to the posterior nerve roots in the spinal cord

Sensory impulses

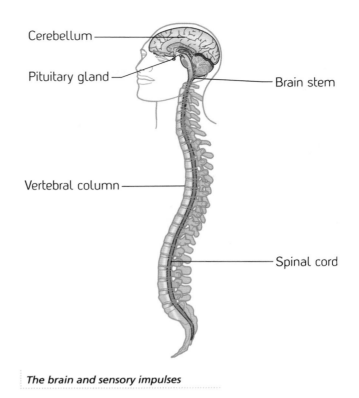

The brain and sensory impulses

Labels: Cerebellum, Pituitary gland, Brain stem, Vertebral column, Spinal cord

The respiratory system

You will learn about:
* the basic principles and structure of the respiratory system.

The lungs

The lungs are large organs situated at either side of the thoracic cavity separated by the heart. They are each enclosed in a membrane called the pleural membrane. This consists of two layers: the visceral pleura and the parietal pleura. Between these layers is a space called the pleural cavity, containing fluid. The fluid allows the membranes to slide over each other during breathing.

How the respiratory system works

The respiratory system consists of the structures leading to the lungs and the structures within the lungs. Every living cell in the body needs oxygen, which is obtained from the air that we breathe. Air is breathed in through the nose and/or mouth and travels along the respiratory tract to the lungs. As we breathe in, the chest expands, the diaphragm flattens and the intercostal muscles lift the ribs upwards and outwards. The lungs expand to fill the increased area and become filled with air. As we breathe out, the intercostal muscles relax

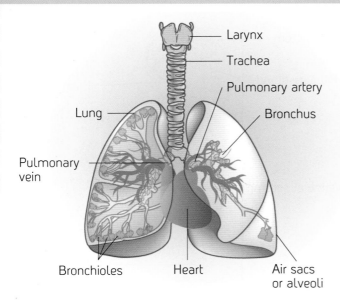

Cross-section of the lungs

and the diaphragm is dome-shaped. If the airways become blocked, accessory muscles assist the main muscles of respiration. The sternocleidomastiod raises the sternum while serratus anterior and pectoralis major pull the ribs outwards (see the chest muscles diagram on page 190). During forced exhalation, latissimus dorsi and the anterior abdominals help to compress the thoracic cavity.

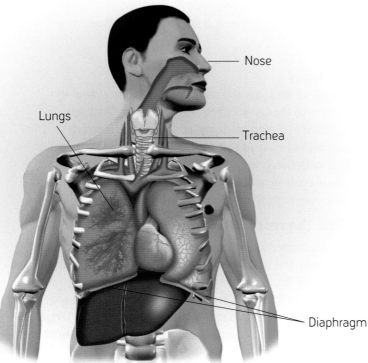

The respiratory system

Respiratory system	Structure	Function
Nose	Lined with mucous membranes which prevent the entry of foreign particles. Nostrils lead into the nose and posterior nares lead out to the pharynx	Vascular mucous membranes warm air as it passes through the nose, mucus moistens air and traps dust particles
Pharynx	Leads from nasal cavity and is continuous with the oesophagus	Auditory tubes carry air to the middle ear. The pharynx is part of the respiratory and digestive systems but cannot be used simultaneously so breathing ceases momentarily during swallowing
Larynx	Continuous with the pharynx above and trachea below, consists of several cartilages including the epiglottis	During swallowing the larynx shifts upwards and forwards so that the epiglottis blocks its opening
Trachea	Below the larynx extending down the front of the neck and into the thoracic region between the lungs. Consists of muscle, fibrous tissue and rings of cartilage	Epithelium lining the trachea secretes mucous, which combines with dust particles and is swept upwards by the cilia away from the lungs
Bronchii	Two structures, one on either side, leading from the trachea to the lungs. Left bronchii are narrower to allow room for the heart. Similar structure to trachea	Carry air from the trachea into the bronchioles

Respiratory system	Structure	Function
Bronchioles	Bronchi divide progressively into smaller bronchi, the finest of which are the bronchioles, which consist of muscular fibrous tissue. They then join onto the alveoli	Carry air from the bronchii towards the lungs
Alveoli	Bronchioles branch to form minute tubes called alveoli	Inhaled air reaches the alveoli via the respiratory tract
Capillary networks	Network of blood vessels surrounding the alveoli	Location of gaseous exchange between the air in the alveoli and the blood in the vessels

Structure of the respiratory system

Additional knowledge

Essential oils
Essential oils used in aromatherapy are also able to pass into the bloodstream through the respiratory system.

Additional knowledge

The neurological role in respiration
Although you can hold your breath and control the speed of breathing (a key part of relaxation during beauty therapy treatments), you can't actually interrupt the basic process of respiration: the body is hard-wired to keep breathing.

Breathing is controlled by the **medulla oblongata** in the brain and is part of the autonomic nervous system. Messages are sent from the brain, through phrenic nerves, to the diaphragm and by the intercostal nerves to the external intercostal muscles, and cause the muscles to contract. This causes inspiration (breathing in). When the message stops the relaxation of the muscles occurs, allowing expiration (breathing out) to take place. This is an automatic process, which keeps the body breathing when asleep or unconscious.

Key terms

Medulla oblongata – the lower half of the brain stem.

The olfactory system

The olfactory system provides the body with a sense of smell known as **olfaction.**

Key terms

Olfaction – the sense of smell.

The brain is able to distinguish about 20 000 different scents with the help of the nervous system, although a professional perfumer (called a nose!) can learn to distinguish 100 000 different smells. Smell is the most evocative of all the senses and can stir up memories, emotions and even the reflex action of vomiting, designed to protect us from harm. It is linked deep into our subconscious minds to help the body remember a possible danger.

Millions of olfactory receptors in the nose transmit messages in the form of nerve impulses to the brain. It is interesting to note that in most of the nerves in the body, the passing on of messages (or impulses) about the environment is done through the spinal cord, and from there to the brain. But, in the case of olfactory cells, the nerve fibres pass through the bony cribriform plate at the top of the nose, and connect directly with the area of the brain known as the olfactory bulb, situated in the cerebral cortex, so messages are passed to the brain directly.

The olfactory system is made up of:

Mucous membrane	This lines the nose, moistens the air passing over it and helps to dissolve the odorous gas passing through the cavity. The rich blood supply also helps to warm the air temperature as it comes in.
Cilia	The tiny hairs inside the nose covered in mucous. These are highly sensitive and are extensions of nerve fibres connecting with the olfactory cells.
Olfactory cells	These are embedded in the mucous in the upper nasal cavity. These are special sensory cells adapted to sensing smell. Each olfactory cell has a long nerve fibre called an axon, leading out of the main body of the cell, which picks up information received and passes it onto the brain for recognition.
Olfactory bulb	This is the area of the brain situated in the cerebral cortex, which perceives smell.

Parts of the olfactory system

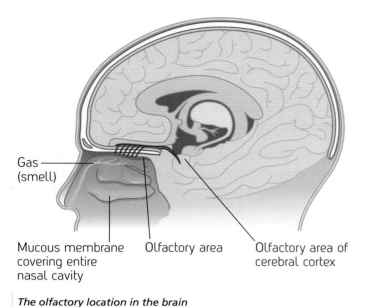

Gas
(smell)

Mucous membrane
covering entire
nasal cavity

Olfactory area

Olfactory area of
cerebral cortex

The olfactory location in the brain

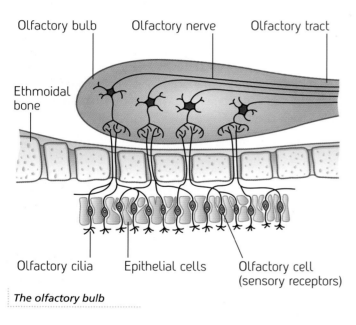

Olfactory bulb   Olfactory nerve   Olfactory tract

Ethmoidal
bone

Olfactory cilia   Epithelial cells   Olfactory cell
(sensory receptors)

The olfactory bulb

How we perceive smell

Substances such as essential oils or perfume give off smelly
gas particles. These are drawn up the nose during inhalation
and are dissolved in the upper part of the moist membrane
of the nasal cavity.

This mucus surrounds the cilia that stick out from the bottom
of the olfactory cells. The absorbed gas particles reach the
cilia and stimulate nerve impulses to travel along the axon
of the nerve cell (see 'Nervous tissue', page 214), through
bones in the skull and then to one of two olfactory bulbs.

Nerves from the olfactory bulb then carry nerve impulses
to the brain, many of which travel to the limbic system
in the rhinencephalon (the area of the brain that controls
complex emotional behaviour, such as pain, anger, pleasure
or affection, and also certain automatic functions). This
is why smells are so closely associated with memories
and emotional responses, for example cabbage smells
can remind you of school and evoke a positive or negative
emotional feeling.

Lesions in this part of the brain can result in a wide range of
abnormal behaviours.

Additional knowledge

Familiarity with smells

We can become immune to smells. If we spray
perfume, we soon stop noticing it because the olfactory
receptors will stop being stimulated, until a new smell
comes along. Strong smells will also cause a reactive
involuntary action, for example, a strong smell may cause
gagging or vomiting.

The reproductive system

You will learn about:
- the female reproductive system
- the male reproductive system
- menstruation and fertilisation.

The function of the reproductive system is to ensure the
continuation of the species.

The female reproductive system

The female reproductive system consists of the ovaries,
uterus, vagina, external genitalia and mammary glands.

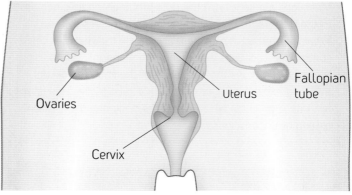

Ovaries

Uterus

Fallopian
tube

Cervix

The female reproductive system

Female reproductive system	Structure	Function
Ovaries	Two small glands the size and shape of almonds located on either side of the uterus	Release an ovum (egg) at monthly intervals and secrete the female hormones responsible for sexual development
Uterus	Hollow, thick-walled organ located between the rectum and the bladder at 90° to the vagina. Lined by the endometrium	Receives fertilised ovum, which grows to fill the uterus, then uterus grows with the foetus until birth
Vagina	Extends from uterus to labia, behind the bladder and urethra and in front of the rectum	Vaginal glands secrete lubricating fluid to moisten the vulva and assist penetration during sexual intercourse
External genitalia	Labia – two fleshy folds covered with skin and hair Mons pubis – pad of fat covered with skin and hair over the pubis symphysis Clitoris – small, sensitive organ of erectile tissue	Mons pubis and labia protect the internal structures such as the clitoris
Mammary glands	Consists of 15–20 lobes of glandular tissue which, in turn, consists of several smaller lobes called lobules	Act as reservoirs and secrete milk during lactation

Structures and functions of the female reproductive system

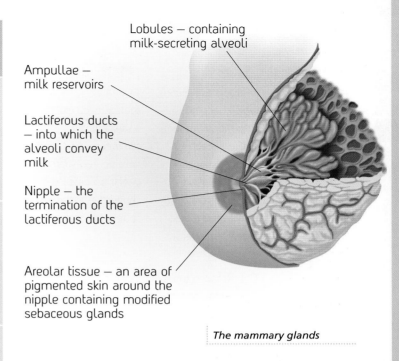

Lobules — containing milk-secreting alveoli

Ampullae — milk reservoirs

Lactiferous ducts — into which the alveoli convey milk

Nipple — the termination of the lactiferous ducts

Areolar tissue — an area of pigmented skin around the nipple containing modified sebaceous glands

The mammary glands

The male reproductive system

The male reproductive system consists of the testes, epididymis, scrotum, sperm duct and penis.

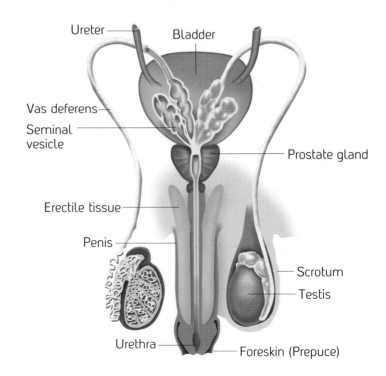

Ureter

Bladder

Vas deferens

Seminal vesicle

Prostate gland

Erectile tissue

Penis

Scrotum

Testis

Urethra

Foreskin (Prepuce)

The male reproductive system

Related anatomy and physiology

Related anatomy and physiology

Male reproductive system	Structure	Function
Testes	Reproductive glands which become suspended in the scrotum. Each testis contains 200–300 lobules which contain convoluted tubes called seminiferous tubules	To create spermatozoa (sperm) – the lining of seminiferous tubules develop into sperm; interstitial cells in connective tissue secrete testosterone
Epididymis	Tightly coiled tubes attached to the back of the testes	Seminiferous tubules open into epididymis which leads to the deferent duct of the seminal vesicle
Scrotum	Sac-like structure which hangs outside of the body	Contains the testes
Sperm duct	Formed by the deferent ducts and seminal vesicles, leading from the base of the prostrate to the urethra	Passage for seminal fluid and sperm
Penis	Tubular organ with plentiful supply of venous sinuses and a tip called the glans penis covered with foreskin	Becomes engorged with blood to cause an erection which facilitates sexual intercourse

Structures and functions of the male reproductive system

Menstruation and fertilisation

The female ovum is one of the largest cells in the body, measuring about one tenth of a millimetre in diameter. You might think that the production of a single ovum takes one month, the period of the menstrual cycle. In fact, it is a continual process which begins even before birth and continues until the menopause. Following puberty, a few ova are reactivated every day so that there is a steady supply to ensure the release of a single ovum each month. At the time of **ovulation**, the ovum is at the surface of the follicle. Increased fluid pressure within causes it to pop and the ovum is ejected into the fallopian tubes. If sperm are present, fertilisation can occur in this location.

Key terms

Ovulation – part of the menstrual cycle, the release of the ovum, which occurs 14 days into the menstrual cycle.

The menstrual cycle

This describes the (approximately) 28-day reproductive cycle that occurs in most females. Day 1 refers to the first day of menstruation and day 14 is the day ovulation usually occurs. The menstrual cycle is controlled by the relative levels of the hormones oestrogen and progesterone which determine whether an ovum is released. If the ovum is not fertilised, progesterone levels drop, the endometrium is shed as menstrual blood and the cycle begins once again. Menstruation usually begins between the ages of 12 and 15 and continues until the menopause.

Fertilisation

This describes the process of bringing together the male and female gametes (sexual reproduction cells) in the fallopian tubes. Natural fertilisation occurs following sexual intercourse when the male penis deposits seminal fluid in the vagina. The sperm in the fluid are helped by a number of physiological factors. The cervix, which is usually blocked by mucus, becomes more permeable during ovulation. Secondly, cilia lining the entrance to the cervix, waft the sperm through. Finally, sperm have a tendency to swim towards the tube containing the ovum rather than the empty tube, due to their response to chemical signals. At this stage, the membrane of one sperm fuses with that of the ovum. Immediately, the sperm stops swimming and the composition of the ovum membrane adjusts to prevent any other sperm from entering. Normal pregnancy in humans lasts 40 weeks and involves a series of changes in the mother as well as in the developing foetus.

Check your knowledge

1 The study of the body's *structure* is called:
- **a)** Physiology
- **c)** Psychology
- **b)** Anatomy
- **d)** Physiotherapy.

2 The smallest structure in the human body is:
- **a)** a cell
- **c)** an organ
- **b)** a tissue
- **d)** an organelle.

3 How many chromosomes are there in a normal, healthy body cell?
- **a)** 23
- **c)** 64
- **b)** 46
- **d)** 92

4 A collection of cells with a similar structure and function is called:
- **a)** an organ
- **c)** a tissue
- **b)** a colony
- **d)** a system.

5 Neurons are the cells found in the:
- **a)** kidney
- **c)** liver
- **b)** brain
- **d)** bone.

6 Which of the following is made up of epithelial tissue?
- **a)** Leg muscle
- **c)** Shoulder blade bone
- **b)** Lining of the lung
- **d)** Blood cells and fluid

7 Which of the following is connective tissue?
- **a)** Striated muscle
- **c)** Nerve fibres
- **b)** Bone
- **d)** Skin

8 Which of the following has a mucus membrane lining?
- **a)** Heart
- **c)** Intestine
- **b)** Abdomen
- **d)** Thorax

9 Which of the following cells are unable to multiply or repair themselves?
- **a)** Skeletal muscle
- **c)** Bone
- **b)** Epithelial
- **d)** Nerve

10 Which of these bones is part of the axial skeleton?
- **a)** Patella
- **c)** Ulna
- **b)** Sacrum
- **d)** Scapula

11 Which of these bones is part of the appendicular skeleton?
- **a)** Mandible
- **c)** Sternum
- **b)** Tibia
- **d)** Vertebra

12 Which of the following is a long bone?
- **a)** Scapula
- **c)** Carpal
- **b)** Radius
- **d)** Tarsal

13 Which of the following is a deficiency disease causing softening of bones?
- **a)** Scurvy
- **c)** Rickets
- **b)** Arthritis
- **d)** Rheumatism

14 Which of the following has a ball and socket joint?
- **a)** Wrist
- **c)** Hip
- **b)** Ankle
- **d)** Elbow

15 Muscles are connected to bones by means of:
- **a)** ligaments
- **c)** fascia
- **b)** tendons
- **d)** cartilage.

16 Which of the following chemicals collect in a muscle during strenuous exercise?
- **a)** Glucose
- **c)** ATP
- **b)** Lactic acid
- **d)** Glycogen

17 A sphincter muscle is found in the:
- **a)** arm
- **c)** abdomen
- **b)** leg
- **d)** mouth.

18 Which of the following muscles lies under the breast?
- **a)** Trapezius
- **c)** Pectorals
- **b)** Deltoid
- **d)** Latissimus dorsi

19 When the fingers bend towards the palm of the hand, the movement is called:
- **a)** abduction
- **c)** extension
- **b)** adduction
- **d)** flexion.

20 The point of communication between neighbouring nerve cells, across which the impulse is passed, is called the:
- **a)** nucleus
- **c)** synapse
- **b)** axon
- **d)** dendron.

You and the skin

What you will learn

- Individual skin characteristics
- How the environment affects skin
- Skin colouring
- The pH of skin
- Desquamation
- Allergic reactions and sensitivity testing
- Skin conditions and pigmentation disorders
- Contra-indications to treatments
- Recognising skin types
- Ageing of the skin
- Products and the skin

Introduction

An in-depth knowledge of the skin is essential if you are going to offer clients the full range of mechanical and electrical treatments and manual massage techniques. You will already have an understanding of how the skin behaves, how it grows and what its problems or reactions may be. For Level 3, this knowledge needs to be built upon, to enable you to be confident in your treatment planning, using more advanced techniques and electrical equipment.

You will also find parts of the following units useful in your study of the skin: for the structure of the skin, refer to Related anatomy and physiology, page 169, and Facial treatments, page 276; for facial consultation techniques and body treatments, see the General pathway, pages 256 and 324.

> ### Think about it
>
> Your individual characteristics are the result of four major influences:
>
> - the genes you inherit from your parents (called intrinsic factors, i.e. in-built)
> - the environment in which you live
> - how you look after your skin
> - your general health.

Individual skin characteristics

Skin colour, and to a large degree, how it behaves and ages, is determined both genetically and environmentally.

Genetics

From each parent, we inherit a set of genes — an arrangement of codes, known as our DNA. The instructions within the genes will produce our own unique set of features — often called units of inheritance. These will determine our hair colour, eye colour, skin colouring, and so on.

A simple way to visualise this is to think of a gene as carrying a set of instructions for the manufacture of an enzyme (a building block). For example, if you have brown eyes, it is because you have the enzyme which helps in the production of the brown pigment. This enzyme can only be made if you have this gene. So, you are a product of your genes! (See also the section on skin colouring, page 230.)

Global origins

Skin colouring also has its origins in where your ancestors were born. People living close to the equator, where the sun's rays are strongest, require more protection from the sun than those further north and south. Their bodies developed a natural defence against the intensity of the sun — a darker skin colouring. The darker the skin colouring, the more protection it offers from the sun's rays.

How the environment affects skin

After genetic influences, the second most powerful influence on the skin is the environment. The quality of the environment, both external and internal, affects the health of skin.

It is also affected by factors beyond our control:

- age and therefore the levels and influence of hormones
- the body's immune system and disease/illness.

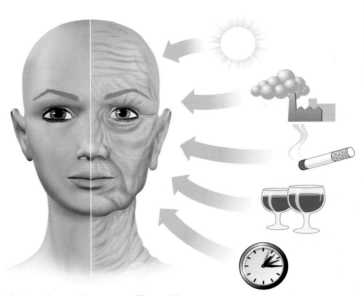

How the environment affects skin

> ### Think about it
>
> A healthy lifestyle does not only apply to the client you are treating; it applies to you too! How can you possibly recommend skincare treatments and give good home care advice, if your skin is suffering, because you do not follow your own advice?

Free radicals

The external environment is a major factor in the ageing process. It is widely recognised by leading dermatologists that up to 90 per cent of skin damage is caused by external environmental factors leading to ageing of the skin. The thickness of the skin can begin to decrease by the age of

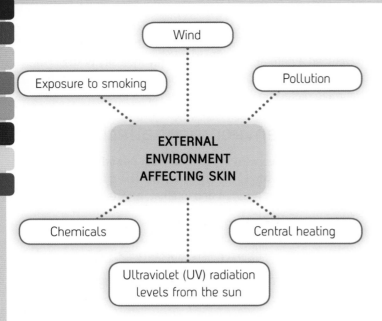

Wind

Exposure to smoking

Pollution

EXTERNAL ENVIRONMENT AFFECTING SKIN

Chemicals

Central heating

Ultraviolet (UV) radiation levels from the sun

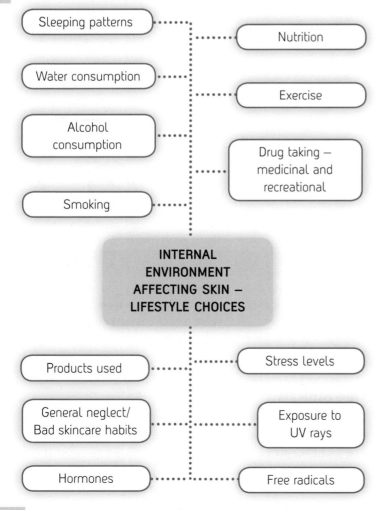

Sleeping patterns

Nutrition

Water consumption

Exercise

Alcohol consumption

Drug taking — medicinal and recreational

Smoking

INTERNAL ENVIRONMENT AFFECTING SKIN — LIFESTYLE CHOICES

Products used

Stress levels

General neglect/ Bad skincare habits

Exposure to UV rays

Hormones

Free radicals

twenty, so in biological terms if the cells are losing energy, they will also lose their ability to protect themselves against the environment.

Free radicals or oxidants are a big factor in the **ageing of the skin**, as they are harmful chemicals which can accumulate in the tissues. They are generated in the body as a reaction to the aggression of environmental invasion on the body including: sunlight, petrol fumes, chemicals used, smoking, wind, pollutions and internal factors such as stress and tiredness. A consequence of this attack on the skin is an acceleration of the skin's ageing process, resulting in the loss of radiance, elasticity and tone. Free radicals are controlled by enzymes, but should the production of the enzymes become poor, due to a poor lifestyle, lack of sufficient nutrition and so on, then chemicals and toxins will build up within the tissues.

Research is continuing into which chemicals within our environment stimulate free-radical production. Crop sprays, pesticides and household cleaning items are some of the products under investigation.

This explains why so many clients are coming to the salon for advanced facial and body skincare techniques — some bodies are just not coping.

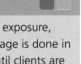

Think about it

People living in northern countries, with less UV exposure, have less skin damage. Although much UV damage is done in the early years, often the results are not seen until clients are in their forties and fifties. This is more of a problem now that international travel is so common and clients often travel in search of sunshine!

Key terms

Ageing skin – skin which is past its peak of maximum performance and is recognised by dryness, wrinkles, reduced elasticity and muscle tone, pigment changes and lack of elasticity. This is a natural process of cell deterioration as the body ages, but it can be accelerated by factors such as poor skincare, pollution, illness and insufficient nutrients.

Sleep and the skin

Research has shown that we sleep an average of 90 minutes less per night now than we did in the 1920s. Even so, doctors still recommend eight hours of good quality sleep, to recharge and replenish the body's systems.

While we sleep, growth hormone is released, and this, in turn, influences skin growth, even if the body has stopped growing in height. (Sleep is therefore very important in the very young – babies need nearly twice as much sleep as an adult for growth and development.) **Collagen** and **keratin** production within the dermis is increased, and the skin cells of the germinative layer (and therefore the rest of the epidermis) replicate faster than during the day.

Lack of sleep can affect other hormone production and is thought to be linked to adult **acne** and very dry skin conditions. As the body tries to cope with this lack of replenishment and the general fatigue that goes with sleep deprivation, the blood is diverted towards the major organs, draining away from the face. This causes the skin pallor and the dark under-eye shadows associated with poor sleeping habits.

Long-term sleep deprivation is bad for the body: the hormone cortisol is released by the adrenal cortex, which is important both for normal carbohydrate metabolism and for the response to any stress. When stress levels and glucose levels are not functioning normally, the changes in the body are similar to those which occur with age. It can lead to high blood pressure, obesity and the onset of diabetes. The good news is that the levels will return to normal once the individual has a regular pattern of eight hours' sleep.

Brain functioning and coordination are also affected by sleep deprivation, and account for a percentage of accidents at work, as well as poor performance generally in the workplace.

To encourage the client (and the therapist) to get good quality sleep, try the following.

- Avoid eating just before going to bed.
- Avoid stimulants such as tea, coffee and alcohol – alcohol may send you to sleep initially, but you will wake up in the night through dehydration.

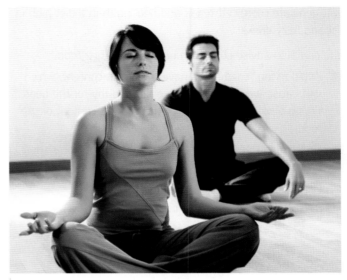

Physical disciplines such as yoga can be used to help relax body and mind

- Try a gentle walk for half an hour in the evening to use the muscles.
- Stick to the same time for going to bed, where possible.
- Relax and unwind in a warm bath with a pre-blended bath oil containing essential oils, for example jasmine or chamomile.
- Avoid over-stimulating the mind just before going to bed.
- If a particular worry is going around in your head, write it down and then list what you will do to tackle it in the morning. Prioritise what you can deal with: allow yourself time in the morning to get help with what you cannot deal with, and avoid wasting time worrying about the rest!
- Try relaxation tapes or soft music to help relax the mind and body.
- Visualisation can be a great help – imagine relaxing on a warm beach, with the sun shining, and drift off to sleep.

Nutrition and the skin

Good nutritional habits are not just about keeping the skin functioning well and looking good, they are also about maximising health potential for the whole body. A sensible mixture of all the food groups is essential for good health, and will provide the essential vitamins and minerals needed.

The food we eat = fuel for the body.

So, cell repair, energy and good health rely upon the fuel the body is given. It makes sense that a good diet, with a variety of foods rich in vitamins and minerals, with lots of water,

Key terms

Collagen – found naturally in the body, it is the main protein of connective tissue, providing strength. It is the main component of cartilage, ligaments, tendons, bone and teeth; it also strengthens blood vessels. In the skin it provides strength and elasticity. As the skin ages it breaks down so the skin is less supported and forms wrinkles.

Keratin – a group of fibrous proteins forming the main structural part of hair and nails.

Acne vulgaris – a common type of acne caused by an inflammation or infection of the sebaceous glands.

will generate more cell repair and healing than a diet high in fat and fizzy drinks!

You can also advise clients on how to cook their food:

- Avoid frying. Fried foods have a high fat content, which will cause weight gain and are not healthy for the heart. Frying also destroys much of the vitamin content of the food.

- Cook vegetables in a small amount of water for a short time, or preferably steam them, to retain their vitamin content. Some vitamins are fat soluble, but others such as vitamin C are water soluble, meaning the longer they are cooked in water the more of their goodness they lose.

- Grilling and steaming are an effective way of sealing in the nutritional content of the food.

- Eat some fruit and vegetables raw – the fibre content stays intact and is very good for the skin and the rest of the body.

Nutrient	Sources	Why it is needed
Protein	Red and white meat; dairy products; pulses and lentils; seeds and nuts	Maintains and supports body growth – vital for the repair of skin cells
Iron	Red meat; liver; egg yolk; dried fruits, e.g. apricots, raisins; dried pulses	With protein, it forms haemoglobin to carry oxygen through the body. Vitamin C taken simultaneously helps absorption; tannin and antacid medication limit absorption. Deficiency causes anaemia resulting in fatigue – so iron is essential for oxygen levels in the skin
Calcium	Dairy products; whole fish (sardines); sunflower and sesame seeds	With other minerals and vitamin D, helps strengthen teeth and bones
Vitamin A (retinol)	Animal fats; fish liver oils; egg yolk; carrots; margarine; fortified dairy products; liver; green vegetables	An anti-infective vitamin necessary for growth, reproduction, the maintenance of a healthy skin and mucous membranes. If applied in cream form on the skin it can help stimulate natural **collagen** production
Vitamin B1 (thiamine)	Wheatgerm; liver; whole grains; nuts; offal; unrefined cereals and pulses; yeast and yeast extracts; fruit; milk; egg yolks; pork meat; legumes; leafy vegetables	Aids digestion and utilisation of energy. Essential for carbohydrate metabolism and fats and nutrition on nerve cells. It also increases fatty acids in the skin – providing firmness – and aids in natural exfoliation
Vitamin B2 (riboflavin)	Milk; eggs; yoghurt; cottage cheese; liver; kidney; whole grains; green vegetables; whole-grain and enriched flour	Essential for growth and good vision. Aids in digestion and carbohydrate metabolism
Vitamin B3 (niacin)	Oily fish; whole grains; liver; fortified breakfast cereals; peanuts	Aids digestion and normal appetite needs. Promotes fatty acid production
Vitamin B6 (pyridoxine)	Meat; bananas; dried vegetables; molasses; brewer's yeast; whole grains; offal; fish liver	Helps to regulate body's use of fatty acids to fight infection
Vitamin B12 (cyanocobalamin)	Milk; eggs; meat; dairy food; liver and kidney; fish	Essential for the maintenance of red blood cells and nervous system, the metabolism of fats, proteins and carbohydrates. No vegetable source sufficient for daily needs. Vegans should see their doctor about synthetic forms

Nutrient	Sources	Why it is needed
Folic acid (folacin)	Green leafy vegetables; nuts; dried vegetables; whole grains; liver and kidney	Essential for blood formation within the bone marrow bringing oxygen and nutrients to the skin. Vital in early pregnancy as a lack of it is thought to lead to defects in babies
Vitamin C (ascorbic acid)	Broccoli; oranges and most citrus fruits; red, green and yellow vegetables; sweet potato, tomatoes, peppers	Helps build strong teeth and bones, for strengthening small blood vessels, muscles and connective tissue – for formation of the intercellular cement. Important in combating infections and prevention of scurvy. Increases resistance to infection, enables blood coagulation and iron absorption. More required during illness. This is the building block for collagen which provides the skin with its structure, tone and elasticity
Vitamin D	Fortified milk; oily fish; liver; eggs; butter. Also sunshine on the skin	Helps in absorption of calcium and builds calcium and phosphorus into bones and strengthens them. Also essential for the development of skin cells
Vitamin E	Vegetable oil; green leafy vegetables; wheat germ; egg yolk; whole grains	Protects fatty acids from destruction. This is an antioxidant helping to build and maintain good skin cells
Vitamin K	Fish liver; animal liver; alfalfa; cabbage; spinach; tomatoes; all leafy vegetables; green vegetables; soybean oil; fats; pork; cheese; egg yolk	Essential for the formation of prothrombin and the clotting of blood. Absorbed only in the presence of bile
Phosphorus	Milk products; meat; fish; whole grains; beans	Combines with calcium to strengthen bones and teeth
Iodine	Seafood; fortified salt	Regulates energy use in the body
Zinc	Lean meat; seafood; whole grains; dried beans	Makes up some enzymes and releases vitamin A from liver

Sources of nutrients and their importance to the body

Vitamin	Problems caused by deficiency
A *Special properties*: fat soluble; can be manufactured by the body and from carotene	Stunted growth; over-keratinisation of the skin and mucus membranes; skin infections; likelihood of bladder and bronchial infections because of altered epithelial membranes; lowered resistance to infection; disorders of the conjunctiva and retina (night blindness)
B1 (aneurine hydrochloride/thiamine)	Loss of appetite; fatigue; mental apathy; impaired functioning of the nervous, digestive, muscular, circulatory and endocrine systems; and if long term, beri-beri. (The symptoms of beri-beri are neuritis, paralysis, muscular wasting, chronic constipation, progressive oedema, mental deterioration, and finally heart failure)
B2 (riboflavin)	Inadequate functioning of cell enzymes; lowered resistance and vitality; cracks at the corner of the mouth and lesions on the lips; glossitis (inflammation of the tongue); anaemia; retarded growth; photophobia; cataracts
B3 (niacin)	Affects carbohydrate metabolism; pellagra – leading to glossitis; dermatitis; spinal cord changes
B6 (pyridoxine)	Symptoms of nervousness; can cause convulsions in infants; dermatitis; nausea; vomiting; affects protein metabolism

Continued

You and the skin

Vitamin	Problems caused by deficiency
BI2 (cyanocobalamin) *Special properties*: absorbed by villi of small intestine and stored in liver	Pernicious anaemia and other types of anaemia
Folic acid	Has anti-anaemic properties, so is useful to prevent all types of anaemia. Vital during pregnancy as lack leads to higher incidence of neural tube defects in babies
C (ascorbic acid) *Special properties*: water soluble; readily destroyed by heat	Sore and bleeding gums; dental caries; sore joints; tendency to bruise easily; fragility of capillary wall; lowered resistance to infection; retards tissue repair and wound healing; scurvy
D *Special properties*: can be made in the skin by action of sunlight (UV rays) on ergo sterols present; fat soluble	Inadequate development of bones and teeth; rickets; osteoporosis. Overdose is possible which causes vomiting, diarrhoea, headaches and drowsiness, high blood calcium and calcium deposits in walls of blood vessels, heart and kidney tissues
E *Special properties*: fat soluble	Rarely deficient in humans
K *Special properties*: fat soluble	Tendency to haemorrhage

Problems caused by vitamin deficiency

Water and the skin

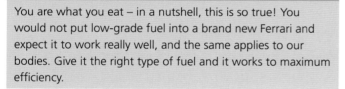

Think about it

You are what you eat – in a nutshell, this is so true! You would not put low-grade fuel into a brand new Ferrari and expect it to work really well, and the same applies to our bodies. Give it the right type of fuel and it works to maximum efficiency.

Water is essential to good health and makes up a large percentage of the body. It is lost from the body through the sweat glands at the rate of approximately 100–150 ml every 24 hours, during respiration and through the digestive processes. Blood should flow with a consistency of skimmed milk, light and liquid – but with low water content it becomes like thick clotted cream, congested and thick, and doesn't flow at all well. This is not good as blood is the transportation of vital oxygen and nutrients to all of the body's cells, from hair follicles on the head to the little toe. If it doesn't flow properly, then the cells don't get fed and watered either!

Ideally, the body's water balance should be maintained – the intake of water should equal the output. Drinking six to eight glasses of water daily is recommended and it is very beneficial to the skin and the digestive process, along with cell metabolism.

Body dehydration usually results in the sensation of thirst, and drinking to relieve it. However, clients often make the mistake of drinking stimulants, such as alcohol, tea and coffee, which may moisten the dry mouth, but are not as beneficial as water.

Clients also misinterpret the sensation of thirst as hunger, or

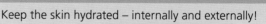

Think about it

Keep the skin hydrated – internally and externally!

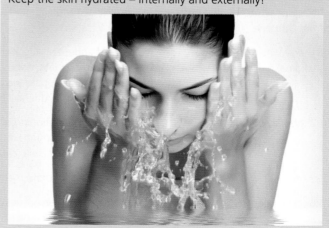

develop a headache, so take a painkiller instead of drinking a glass of water. Drinking a glass of water prior to and during a meal provides the body with adequate fluid to function properly, and prevents over-eating.

Skin dehydration is associated with clients who:

- do not drink enough water to replenish natural loss
- do not use the correct products to maintain the skin's hydro lipid (acid) mantle, so water is evaporated through the skin
- follow a completely fat-free diet, so are deficient in essential fatty acids, essential to the keratinocyte cell membrane, which results in low epidermal lipids, as well as reducing active and passive transfer of nutrients and oxygen within the cells
- work in a dry atmosphere, which also encourages water loss
- have a high alcohol intake, which is a factor in dehydration.

It is important to encourage clients (and yourself, as the therapist!) to maintain a good intake of water, daily. It can be in the form of water with added flavourings, or a low-sugar squash. The client should see the difference in a matter of days. Also check that clients are using the correct products for their skin type, so that water is not being lost unnecessarily through the skin's surface.

Exercise

Regular exercise which increases the heart rate and gives the lungs a good workout (cardiovascular exercise) is good for the whole body. It stimulates blood flow, strengthens the immune system, reduces stress levels and strengthens heart function – and the results show up in a healthy, glowing skin. Walking, running and swimming are all good energy-boosting activities. Try and encourage your client to fit exercise in two or three times a week – and do some yourself and see how well you feel, with higher energy levels and the ability to cope better with your studies.

Smoking

The health risks associated with smoking are well publicised and the new law banning smoking in public places (see 'You and the law' in Professional basics, page 74) means cutting down the risk of passive smoking – inhaling other people's smoke. Smoking not only diminishes the lungs' capacity to function well, it affects the oxygen levels in the bloodstream, showing up externally as a sallow, dull complexion. Smokers are depriving their skin of oxygen: they are prone

to fine lines and often age prematurely. Nicotine impairs the blood vessels, so the supply of nutrients and oxygen, and the ability to remove waste products from the cells, slows down. Over time skin may look pale yellow and grey, loose its elasticity and become wrinkled. Smokers also find that fingers and eyebrows become stained with a build-up of nicotine, if the cigarettes are untipped and rolled without a filter. Not a good look for the skin!

Alcohol

Continuous alcohol intake can have an adverse effect on the skin as alcohol stops the absorption of essential vitamins by the body, as well as being 'empty' calories with no nutritional goodness. This may lead to weight gain, which puts extra pressure on the skin. It can act as an appetite suppressant, so food is not desired and this can cause malnutrition in the long term. There is also an **allergic** potential to alcohol, as it contains both salicylates and yeast, which can cause hives and rashes. Yeast also feeds conditions such as thrush, irritable bowel syndrome (IBS) and general irritability in the nerve endings in the skin. If a client has rashes after eating Marmite, berries, bananas, almonds, apples or drinking wine, it may be they are having an allergic reaction. Cutting out these foods and avoiding alcohol will allow the allergy to calm down and the body functions to return to normal.

Stress

Key terms

Allergic – causing an allergy, where the body is sensitive to ingredients, products or substances which cause a physical irritation or reaction.

We all need a little stress in our lives to function fully and get the adrenaline flowing. However, long-term or constant stress on the body can cause ill health, mental function impairment and hormonal fluctuations, which show up in the skin. Adult acne and poor skin maintenance can be the result of long-term stress. It is important for your client to deal with the underlying causes of anxiety and stress and manage them – and to take care of the body, to allow it to function fully. Exercise is a good stress buster, and good nutrition is essential when the body is under duress. Regular beauty treatments are very therapeutic and regular massage will help with relaxation and improve skin function, as well as encouraging the client to maintain the skin with good product advice.

Drugs and medicines

You and the skin

Long-term use of drugs or medicine, either for an existing medical condition or for recreational use, is bound to have an effect on the whole body and be reflected in the skin's condition. The effects will depend upon the type and strength of the drug, the existing medical condition and how well the body copes with it.

All drugs have to be broken down: digested and synthesised by the liver and then delivered to the part that requires the medicine – even it is just a paracetamol taken for a headache. Some drugs are extremely strong and even toxic to the body, cancer treatment for example, and can have distressing side effects. Of course, some drugs are given to treat the skin and infections, such as roactane for acne or antibiotics for infections.

Antibiotics are notorious for upsetting the delicate flora in the gut and they can cause diarrhoea or general lethargy – all reflected in the skin looking tired and listless. Often clients will not remember which medication they are taking – you ask in consultation if they have any medical problems and they say no – then give you a list of tablets they take, when you get to the part in the consultation which asks about medicines!

Always seek medical advice before treating a client on high doses of medication – and remember that thinning skin can be a side-effect and, if it is, the client is not suitable for treatment.

Products used

The skin is remarkably resilient and will bounce back from many factors it has to deal with – thank goodness. However, don't be fooled – you have to be a bit of a detective to uncover misleading skin conditions, often caused by using the wrong products. The skin may be overly dry, because the products used have a high alcohol content and are stripping the skin of its **acid mantle**. Skincare products can be over-used, which dries out an oily skin, and dry skin can be over-moisturised, which makes it look as though it is greasy.

Key terms

Acid mantle – often termed the hydro lipid film. Hydro = water, lipid = fat, so it is the thin coating of the skin made up of sebum and sweat. Its job is to help prevent bacterial growth. It has a pH value of 4.5–5.5.

pH – potential hydrogen. This is the degree of alkalinity and acidity measured on the pH scale of 1–14, where 1 is a strong acid, 7 is neutral and 14 is a strong alkali. The pH of the skin is 4.5–5.5.

Redness and irritation may be a minor allergic reaction to products and medication can alter the skin's surface, too. The key here is a correct diagnosis, and balancing the skin's acid mantle in a gentle way, with the most suitable skincare.

Hormones

It is impossible to think of the skin and not think of hormone levels. Hormones are chemical messengers found in the bloodstream, produced by the glands to act on and regulate the functions of the body. (See Related anatomy and physiology, page 207, for a complete breakdown of the endocrine system.)

Therapists who treat mainly female clients will need to think about their client's age and the stage of hormone production – namely, puberty, pregnancy and the menopause. All fluctuation of hormone production during these key times will affect the skin. However, this may be in a positive, not necessarily negative, way. it is important to remember, however, that it is not just the female sex hormones which affect the skin, or just female clients that are affected by hormonal changes. The pancreas, the pituitary gland and the adrenal glands all produce hormones – as do our fat deposits, and any imbalance of hormone production can cause disease or disturbance to the body.

It's also not just hormones which can affect the body and your mood – they work in conjunction with chemicals called neurotransmitters, which send messages to and from cells. Endorphins are released in response to stress and pain, serotonin is a feel-good chemical (so low levels can lead to depression) and dopamine is part of the reward and pleasure system of the brain. If these are unbalanced, it can lead to lots of problems. Leptin is a hormone made in the fat cells, helping to regulate body weight, ghrelin is produced in the stomach and goes up when you are hungry and down when you have eaten, and PYY is a satiety hormone produced in the gut which tells the brain when you have had enough to eat. Any imbalance of these hormones can affect appetite, which ultimately reflects upon body function and the skin.

Skin colouring

The skin owes its colouring to:

- the carotene pigments within subcutaneous fat
- the concentration and state of oxygenation of the red haemoglobin found within the blood vessels
- the existence of other pigments such as blood bile pigments, reflected in the colour of the skin

- the amount of melanin present in the skin
- the general health and circulation of the client.

Various degrees of pigmentation are present in the different ethnic groups, but the differences are in the amount of melanin produced and are not dependent upon the number of **melanocytes** present.

Certain areas of skin are very rich in pigment, such as the genital area and the nipples, while practically no pigment is present in the palms of the hands and the soles of the feet. Pigment is stored as fine granules within the cells of the germinative layer, although some granules may also be deposited between the cells. In lighter skin types the granules occur only in the deepest cell layers and mainly in the cylinder-shaped cells of the basal row. In darker skin types pigment is found throughout the entire layer and even in the stratum granulosum.

All melanin is synthesised in cells called melanocytes from an amino acid (tyrosine) by a complex chemical reaction, which makes pigment granules called melanosomes. When the melanosomes are full of pigment they are then distributed to the epithelial cells, spreading the pigment throughout the skin. The melanocytes are scattered in the basal layers of the epidermis and mature as the embryo is developing in the womb – influenced by the units of inheritance in the gene code, so determining skin colour.

Melanin is the skin's main defence against acute effects of exposure to UV light, both occurring naturally through sunlight and through artificial tanning, using any form of sunbed. It acts as a density filter, reducing the harmful effects of UV radiation. The protective property of melanin is its ability to absorb and disperse radiation.

Key terms

Melanocyte – a pigment cell in the epidermis (basal layer) which produces melanin to protect the skin from ultraviolet radiation.

Albino – a person with no pigmentation in eyes, hair, or skin, so the eyes appear pink and the skin is translucent.

Macule – a pigmented area of the skin that is not raised.

Additional knowledge

Albinism

Some people are born without the ability to produce melanin within their skins and no hair pigment, a condition known as albinism. They have white hair, white skin and pink eyes.

Additional knowledge

Glabrous skin

The palms of the hands and the soles of the feet are often referred to as 'glabrous' skin, which lacks hair follicles and sebaceous glands and has a thicker epidermis.

Black skin and pigmentation

In general, black skin has more evenly distributed melanocytes, which are larger and more active than in white/Caucasian skin. Black skin is also more robust: it has greater elasticity and strength of collagen fibres, giving support to the skin, so there is less possibility of dropped contours of the face. Sebaceous glands are larger and denser, giving good lubrication and moisture to prevent the formation of wrinkles and making it less prone to premature wrinkles. This also means the ageing process is slower in black skin, with less cell deterioration, and because black skin flakes and is shed more quickly than white/Caucasian skin, cell renewal is faster.

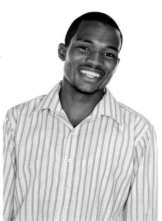

Each client's skin should be considered individually

Think about it

Some black skins are quite sensitive to skincare products, and care should be taken to avoid harsh, **abrasive** products, or strong alcohol-based toners. These types of product are often used to treat an oily skin. Do not always judge black skin as oily, as there is often a sheen or glow on black skin which is actually a reflection of the light, especially under a spotlight or facial examination lamp.

Key terms

Abrasives – beads in facial or body products to remove or break up the surface of the skin. They improve texture and aid desquamation (exfoliation) of the epidermis.

Malignant melanoma – a cancer of the melanocytes (pigment-producing cells) in the epidermis.

A condition called 'dermatosis papulosa nigra' occurs almost exclusively in black skin, usually on the cheeks. It consists of brown or raised dark spots. Do not treat if infected – ask the client to seek medical advice.

Skin cancer is not as common in black skin, due to its protection from the harmful UVC rays of the sun. Also, the epidermis is considerably thicker than in its white counterpart, and it is therefore less reactive, and not prone to allergies or infection. For example, warts are rarely found on black skin.

Due to the epidermis being thicker, black skin easily forms scars, which can turn into keloid tissue – seen as an over-thickening of the skin, in a pink/beige colour, which is more noticeable against a darker background.

Obviously each black skin should be considered individually, as skin reactions are a very personal thing. During the consultation, ask questions about product use and sensitivity, and the client will guide you by his or her own experiences about what works for his or her skin.

The pH of skin

The pH stands for potential hydrogen — or if it is easier to remember — parts hydrogen (i.e. the number of hydrogen parts in the substance).

The pH is a number that describes whether a substance or solution is acid, neutral or alkaline. A pH of 7 is neutral, 0–7 indicates acidity and above 7 indicates an alkaline is present. Chemicals applied to the skin should have a pH that is neither too high nor too low, to avoid skin irritation.

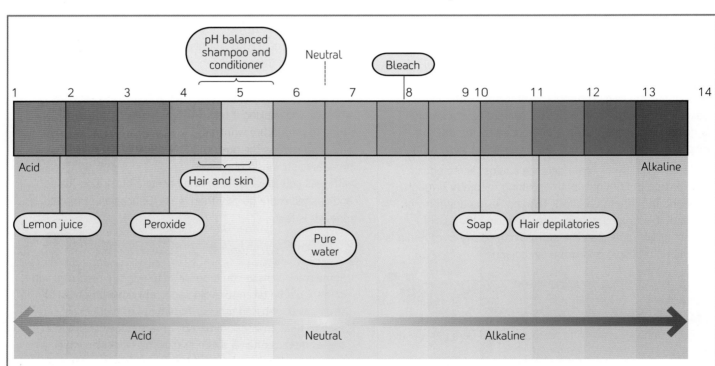

The pH scale

The skin acts as a defence against infection and has a protective barrier over the surface of the epidermis, which is often referred to as the acid mantle, or the hydro-lipidic mantle (see Related anatomy and physiology, page 168). The term comes from *hydro*, referring to the water from the sweat glands, and *lipid*, as in fat or sebum from the sebaceous glands. The acid mantle is a mixture of both of these gland secretions. This is a kind of water-in-oil emulsion on the skin's surface, which also contains minerals, urea, lactic acid and amino acids, and it is this combination which

gives the skin its acid pH of between 4.5 and 5.5 in a normal, healthy skin.

The average skin pH is about 5.4, and this inhibits the growth of bacteria. Fungi are controlled by sebum, which inhibits their growth, so it makes sense to maintain a steady pH balance in the skin, to help fight infection. Using products which are too harsh and strip the skin of its protective pH acid mantle will allow infections in and cause damage.

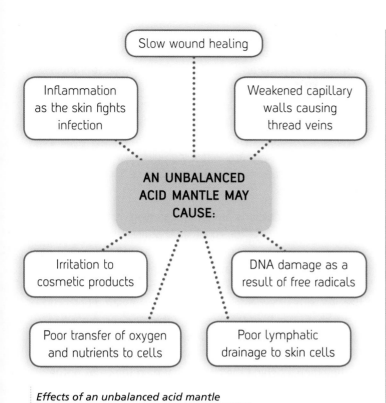

Slow wound healing

Inflammation as the skin fights infection

Weakened capillary walls causing thread veins

AN UNBALANCED ACID MANTLE MAY CAUSE:

Irritation to cosmetic products

DNA damage as a result of free radicals

Poor transfer of oxygen and nutrients to cells

Poor lymphatic drainage to skin cells

Effects of an unbalanced acid mantle

Think about it

An impaired acid mantle is often caused by lack of essential fatty acids (EFA) in the diet – ask your client about crash dieting, fat-free diets and restricted eating – it could be the cause of their skin problems.

Desquamation

The epidermis is continually renewing itself – the lower layers are continually growing and dividing, pushing cells upward until they reach the surface, and then they are rubbed away. Friction within everyday movements, such as using a towel, getting dressed and scratching the skin will be enough to shed thousands of dead skin cells. This process is called desquamation or exfoliation. Getting rid of the old cells allows the new ones to come up to the surface, keeping the skin healthy and able to fight infection. This goes on daily and is not normally visible to the naked eye. Desquamation can only

Key terms

Desquamation – also called exfoliation, the removal of dead skin cells from the epidermis using techniques that may include loofah scrub, dry brushing, salt glow, enzyme masks or abrasive scrubs.

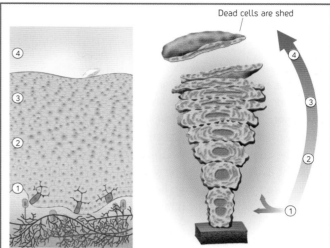

Dead cells are shed

The process of **desquamation**, or exfoliation, enables the skin to rid itself of old cells and allow new ones to come up to the surface, keeping the skin healthy and able to fight infection. (For more information on desquamation and keratinisation, see Related anatomy and physiology, page 170.)

Exfoliant products and brush cleansing are excellent methods of desquamation prior to other treatments, especially if the client does not have the time for a steam treatment or the full microdermabrasion process. Exfoliation both cleanses the skin and creates an erythema within the dermis, so the blood vessels are receptive to carrying absorbed substances further into the body. Avoid creating too much of an erythema, however, as another stimulating treatment may cause a skin reaction, and become a contra-action to treatment.

Desquamation is painless. Even controlled microdermabrasion (MDA), which is a skin peeling process for the treatment of skin problems such as scar tissue, pigmentation abnormalities and acne, is not felt, as the intensity of the peeling depth is firmly controlled by the therapist, and only restores the balance of healthy, well-functioning epidermal cells.

really be seen when a suntan is going and the skin becomes dry and peels off in visible sheets.

The life cycle of a cell from the germinative layer to the top horny layer takes about 28 days and the cells go through a process called keratinisation. Keratin is a form of protein, and the cells get harder, flatter and eventually die. As the dead cells have no nucleus and no nerve endings, you don't feel your skin shedding itself.

Disorders and conditions linked to skin shedding

Psoriasis

Psoriasis is a common skin condition. The life cycle of the cells drops to only five days from the germinative layer to the top horny layer, and as this happens so fast in the cells only the nuclei are retained. This forms itchy, red, scaly patches, most common on the elbows, knees, legs and scalp. The cause is not known, but it is a very common skin complaint and is thought to be stress-related. Sunlight or UV exposure from a sunbed often helps the condition and there are creams available to help too.

Ichthyosis (pronounced ik-the-osis)

This is a chronic condition, usually from birth, where the skin becomes rough and scaly because of the over-formation of keratin and the lack of natural exfoliation. The skin is rough and dry, and the hair is limp and lustreless. In cold weather the skin can become extremely itchy. In severe forms the scales can be all over the body.

Allergic reactions and sensitivity testing

Both in the European Union and the United States of America the law requires that cosmetic companies conduct very strict safety tests on materials they use to formulate products. Nevertheless, there will always be some people who are allergic to a substance which other people can tolerate without a problem.

This is a method of defence – the skin produces histamine, a compound derived from the amino acid histidine, found in **mast cells** in nearly all tissues of the body. Histamine causes dilation of blood vessels and contraction of smooth muscle: it is an important moderator of inflammation and is released in large amounts after skin damage. It produces flushing of the skin, irritation, itchiness of the area and often a wheal is seen. Pain may be experienced and/or swelling if a substance irritates the skin and the tissues release histamine. This is not a common reaction, but can occur if clients are allergic to any active ingredients within a product used, or other common substances such as nickel, food allergies or nuts.

Some allergic reactions are life-threatening as the throat closes up and swells too much so that breathing is inhibited. Adrenalin needs to be administered in the form of an **epi-pen** injection, and clients who suffer with this normally carry emergency medication to literally save their lives. This can happen with strawberries, shellfish or even with a bee or wasp sting. It is therefore essential that you complete a sensitivity test if you are concerned that the client may react to a product. This can be done by testing a small sample of the product behind the client's ear or in the crook of the elbow. If a reaction occurs within 24 hours the product should not be used.

A reaction could include:

- redness (erythema)
- swelling
- irritation to the area
- pain or itching in the area.

Stop the treatment and treat with calamine lotion and a cold compress as necessary. Always make a note on the record card so that the product is not used again on the client.

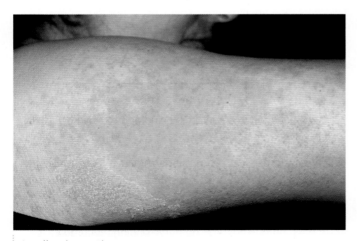

An allergic reaction

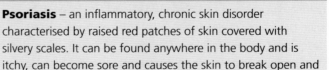

Key terms

Psoriasis – an inflammatory, chronic skin disorder characterised by raised red patches of skin covered with silvery scales. It can be found anywhere in the body and is itchy, can become sore and causes the skin to break open and become infected.

Mast cells – these specialist cells are part of the immune system. Originally from bone marrow, they settle in connective tissue and are part of the body's inflammatory process. When activated, they release histamine and heparin if the body is under attack from an irritant such as pollen, or during injury. Histamine causes swelling and itching of the affected tissue.

Epi-pen – a form of injection which delivers a dose of adrenaline via the muscles to counteract a reaction.

You and the skin

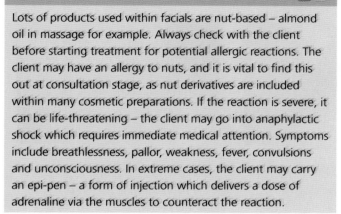

Think about it

Lots of products used within facials are nut-based – almond oil in massage for example. Always check with the client before starting treatment for potential allergic reactions. The client may have an allergy to nuts, and it is vital to find this out at consultation stage, as nut derivatives are included within many cosmetic preparations. If the reaction is severe, it can be life-threatening – the client may go into anaphylactic shock which requires immediate medical attention. Symptoms include breathlessness, pallor, weakness, fever, convulsions and unconsciousness. In extreme cases, the client may carry an epi-pen – a form of injection which delivers a dose of adrenaline via the muscles to counteract the reaction.

Product labelling

By law, ingredients which are known to be irritants (or sensitisers) must be listed on the packaging, together with the precautions for use. Some facial and make-up products contain substances which cause allergic reactions in people who are hypersensitive. For example:

- lanolin – a fatty substance used as a softening agent in skin creams and lipsticks
- eosin – a red dye found in some lipsticks

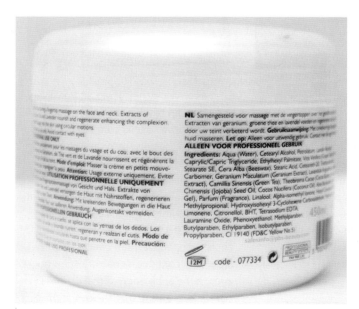

Beauty products must carry details of potential irritants in their ingredient lists

- perfumes – particularly those containing bergamot, lavender and cedarwood
- alcohol – a grease solvent and astringent used in cosmetics and skincare products
- cobalt blue – a pigment used to produce eye make-up colours
- pearlising agents – ingredients which give products a shimmering effect
- gums – adhesives and binding agents in cosmetics.

Eye irritation

Although products used around the eye area are very strictly tested, and only safe pigments are used, some can still cause irritation to some clients.

Hypo-allergenic products

If your client has sensitive or allergic skin you should use this type of product, which contains no perfume as well as fewer pigments and preservatives. Organic facial products are also freely available now, and are preferred by many clients – the only drawback may be that they may not last as long, as a result of removing the preservatives. Most large cosmetic and product companies recognise the need to produce quality products which are neither **comedogenic** nor allergy-causing, and use food grade preservatives.

Products are now also more environment friendly, with packaging that is recyclable and biodegradable, and many companies refuse animal testing on their products.

Key terms

Allergen – any substance which causes an allergic reaction. It can be through skin contact, eating, or inhaling.

Comedogenic – any product which may cause blackheads, block pores or aggravate acne.

Skin conditions and pigmentation disorders

Specific contra-indications to each treatment are covered within the relevant section of this book. These should be discussed during the consultation for whichever treatment you are considering for your client.

Skin conditions

The following conditions are contra-indications that will not necessarily stop the treatment from taking place, but treatment may need to be adapted to avoid the contra-indicated area.

Cuts, abrasions, broken skin	Bruises or swelling	Scar tissue

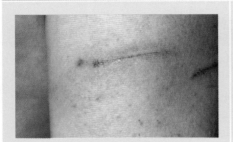
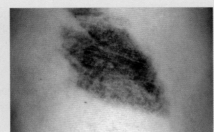
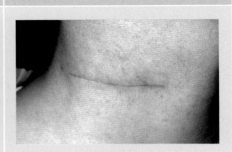

If recent, a scab will be forming, the skin may be tender and swollen in the area, and bruising may be seen. If cuts and abrasions are recent, avoid the area altogether. If the area has healed over, and is not too recent, get the client's agreement that gentle application can take place, with careful consideration of hygiene.

Easily recognised as a swelling, with discoloration in varying shades. Avoid altogether if recent or painful to the touch. If healing has taken place, a gentle application of make-up will help to blend in the colour differences to the client's normal shade. Always ask for the client's agreement.

Usually a different colour from the rest of the skin, following the line of injury. If the scar is recent, raised or angry-looking, then avoid the area altogether. If the area is healing and not very large, gentle application is possible with the client's permission. Scar tissue less than six months old, or over a large area, should not be touched with make-up.

Eczema	Dermatitis	Psoriasis

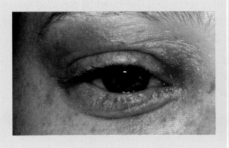
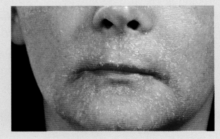
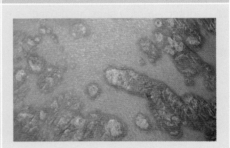

Very dry skin, often scaly and flaky, can be red and very itchy. If the eczema covers a large area, and is inflamed with broken skin, then leave it alone and suggest a visit to the GP. You may make it worse. If the eczema has irritated the eye area, it is unlikely the client would want make-up application. If it is only a small patch of eczema, and not angry, just exclude the area from treatment. The use of hypo-allergenic products is recommended and a patch test if the client is very sensitive.

This is similar to eczema in appearance, but the cause is not the same. A reaction or allergy to something in contact with the skin usually causes dermatitis.
Skin allergies may result in a contra-action so if the client's skin tends to react, do a skin patch test 24 hours prior to the make-up application. It may be wise to use hypo-allergenic make-up, and ask the client to bring in her own make-up if she knows she is safe using it.

Seen as scaly patches of red and/or silvery skin. This can break open and become sore. The cause is unknown but is thought to relate to the nervous system. A contra-indication would be if the psoriasis is open or bleeding. One of the common sites for psoriasis is the scalp, so the client may have a little patch visible along the hairline. If the client agrees to make-up application, and it is not directly over the area, then continue. A patch test 24 hours prior to the application of make–up is advisable to ensure that the condition is not aggravated.

Acne vulgaris

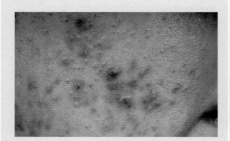

Inflamed whiteheads, blackheads and pustules in various degrees of congestion. Mostly associated with hormones – and the presence of bacteria can make the condition infected.

Infected inflamed acne is a contra-indication. However, a client with mild acne can be treated in the salon, and a light water-based foundation applied. There may be a tendency to greasy skin, and therefore a light application of powder keeps the skin looking matt.

Acne rosacea

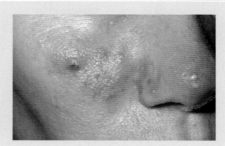

Seen as a flush of red over the nose and cheeks with a raised feel to the skin. Often those who have suffered acne vulgaris in youth are prone to rosacea in later life. If the skin is not tender and the client agrees, application of make-up can tone down the redness and therefore lessen the angry look of the skin.

Skin tags

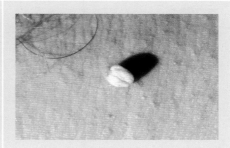

These are usually found on the eye area or lids and/or on the side of the neck. They resemble little 'mushrooms' of skin on a stalk, which move when touched. As these are not painful or dangerous, make-up application can take place. If they become enlarged and irritating to the client they can be removed under local anaesthetic, usually at the GP's surgery.

Milia

These are small white pearls under the skin, often around the eyes or on the side of the cheek, caused by a build-up of sebum. Make-up application can take place over **milia**, as they are not infectious.

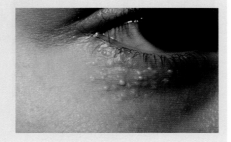

You should also refer to the Professional basics unit, page 44, to refresh your knowledge of types of skin conditions which are caused by bacterial, fungal or viral infections, and which may contra-indicate treatment.

Pigmentation disorders

These disorders are caused by irregularities in the skin's melanin production. They are not infectious and are not a contra-indication to facial or make-up treatments. Pigmentation disorders do affect the client's appearance, however, and may make the client feel embarrassed and self-conscious; as a therapist, you therefore need to treat them sensitively. The use of camouflage cosmetics may help more effectively with the matching of the pigmentation than ordinary foundations and concealers.

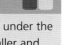

Key terms

Milia – tiny white or yellowish lumps which sit just under the skin's surface and look like whiteheads, but are smaller and do not contain pus. They are made up of sebum from the sebaceous gland which is blocked by the skin cells covering the mouth of the follicle

Papules – small solid round lumps rising from the skin. They do not contain pus, usually appear in clusters and may be caused by infection, inflammation, or abrasions.

Melanoderma

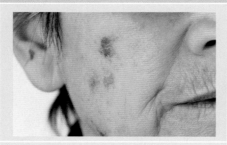

This is a general term used to describe patchy pigmentation.

This is usually an increase in melanin caused by applying cosmetics or perfume which contains light-sensitive ingredients (e.g. bergamot oil used in the perfume industry) – the skin becomes extra-sensitive to UV light. Some drugs have a similar effect. This can also follow inflammation and is sometimes the cause of brown patches following sunburn.

Vitiligo

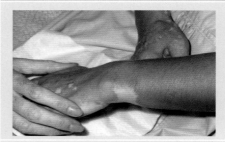

This is also called **hypopigmentation**. It is a condition in which small patches of skin have lost their pigmentation, and appear a lighter colour than the rest of the skin. These lighter areas burn easily in the sun and need to be protected. It is not raised or painful to the touch.

Chloasma

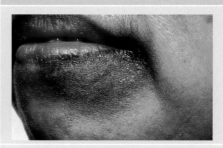

This is also called **hyperpigmentation**. It consists of irregular patches of brown pigment caused by the over-production of melanocytes. This often appears on the face during pregnancy and is sometimes linked to the contraceptive pill. The discoloration usually disappears when the hormone balance is restored.

Freckles

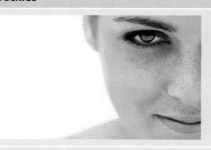

These are tiny, flat irregular patches of pigment on white/Caucasian-skinned people, particularly blonds and redheads. They are due to the uneven distribution of melanin, and this becomes more noticeable on exposure to strong sunlight. The freckles often increase in size and join together. The skin between the freckles contains little or no melanin so burns easily. As a therapist you should recommend a good sunscreen to the client.

Lentigo

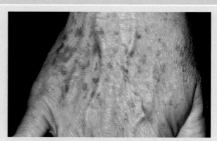

Larger and more distinctive than a freckle, and may be slightly raised. This pigmentation does not increase in number or darken on exposure to UV light.

Haemangioma

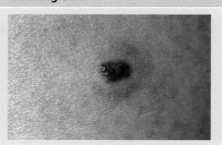

This consists of various conditions caused by the permanent dilation of superficial blood vessels. Stimulating treatments will therefore be contra-indicated, but camouflage cosmetics can be used.

Key terms

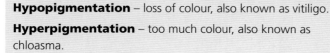

Hypopigmentation – loss of colour, also known as vitiligo.

Hyperpigmentation – too much colour, also known as chloasma.

Post-inflammatory hyperpigmentation – this is the discoloration of the skin remaining after a skin disease or disorder has healed. It is commonly seen in skins recovering from acne vulgaris, allergies, injury or dermatitis. The areas affected can become darker if exposed to sunlight.

You and the skin

Dilated capillaries

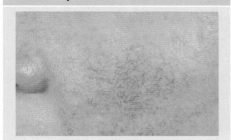

This is the result of loss of elasticity in the walls of the blood capillaries – the cheeks and the nose are often most affected. Exposure to weather, harsh handling and lack of protection, along with spicy hot foods and alcohol, can also be contributing factors. Clients with dry/sensitive skin types are most likely to be affected.

Split capillaries

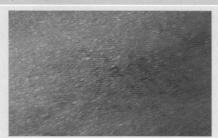

Weakening and rupturing of capillary walls – clients should avoid stimulating treatments. This condition can be treated using diathermy – the production of heat in body tissues using a high frequency current. (For more on diathermy see chapter B29 Provide electrical epilation treatments, page 510.)

Strawberry naevus

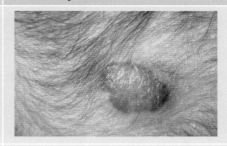

This is a raised and distorted area, often on the face, bright pink or red. It appears a few days or weeks after birth and usually clears up completely by the age of eight.

Spider naevus

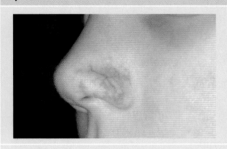

A central dilated vessel with leg-like projections of capillaries. The face and cheeks tend to be most affected and this often occurs during pregnancy due to the increase in oestrogen levels.

Port wine stain

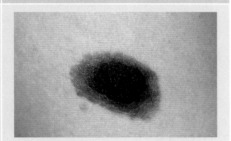

This is a bright purple, irregular shaped flat birthmark that can vary in size. These birthmarks are thought to be due to damage by pressure during foetal development. These birthmarks grow with the body and can be quite disfiguring to the client. As a therapist you should always treat such marks sensitively with good cosmetic camouflage make-up.

Different pigmentation disorders

The best way of caring for the skin is to:

- avoid skin damage, picking, bruising or scratching it
- take care of the skin internally with good nutritional habits/a balanced diet
- drink plenty of water
- avoid smoking
- limit alcohol and caffeine intake
- avoid crash diets or excluding fats from the diet
- use correct skincare products
- have regular facials from an expert
- always use sun protection on the skin when in the sun
- have a good work/life balance – avoid unnecessary stress
- take regular exercise
- limit medication or drug use where possible
- try and keep hormones regular and constant.

Reasons for skin damage	Recognition of signs and symptoms
Excessive exposure to the sun, artificial sunlight (sunbeds), excessive lines and wrinkles from alcohol intake and smoking	The skin ages prematurely, causing a breakdown in collagen and **elastin**, which supports the skin; uneven pigmentation can also occur
Pollution from chemicals, traffic and thinning of the protective ozone layer	Contamination of the skin leads to clogged and blocked pores, irritation occurs and a tendency to comedones and allergic reactions. This causes dehydration and over-activity of the sebaceous glands; loss of oxygen causes skin to look sallow and tired
Heat and steam	Overstretching of the skin, causing damage: pores enlarge and become congested; damage to capillaries seen as thread veins on the cheeks and chin
Incorrect use of skincare products	Inappropriate products can cause comedones to form or lead to an over-sensitive skin, dryness, flaky skin and congestion, if using product too rich for the skin
Excessive heat	Chapped and dehydrated skin, damaged capillaries and vascular flushness on the skin, spider naevus present on cheeks
Poor diet, insufficient nutrients, lack of fatty acids or a fat-free diet, and crash dieting	Sluggish and yellow or sallow-looking skin, with oxygen loss and slow healing and repair of skin; poor formation of the acid mantle
Impaired acid mantle due to poor products or ill health	Increased inflammation and sensitisation, poor healing and infection

The signs and symptoms of skin damage

Contra-indications to treatments on the skin

Although most advanced Level 3 mechanical or electrical treatments for the face and body are penetrating and work on a sub-dermal level, the first contact (and largest benefit) is to the skin. However, if the skin is already under duress from infection or an existing skin condition, or in poor health it is best to avoid treatment and refer the client to the doctor as a safeguard against making the condition worse. So, always do a full consultation with visual and manual checks of the skin – in the area to be treated: either the face or the body. It is important that any facial or body treatment is not carried out if a contra-indication is present.

Contra-indications include:

- infections – bacterial, viral and fungal infections of eyes, lips or face
- open cuts and abrasions
- bruising
- acute acne
- severe eczema or psoriasis
- immediately after a chemical or medical peel – glycolic acid or AHA
- immediately after waxing
- if client is taking certain medication – Retin A, Renova, and Accutane used to treat topical acne
- after Botox injections
- after collagen or other filler injections in the face
- if the client is having treatment for cancer
- recent dental work.

Please refer to the Professional basics section (page 42) for details of micro-organisms and the diseases they cause and

Key terms

Elastin – a protein similar to collagen, it is the main component of elastic fibres in the skin and other areas of the body which need to be able to stretch.

Key terms

Collagen therapy – the injection of collagen into the skin folds on the face which fills out lines, wrinkles and pitted scars. Clients can develop a reaction to it, and it may be rejected by the body or stay rigid. If this happens in the lips it may form a 'trout pout' as the media have named a condition of permanently swollen and angry-looking lips.

Aesthetic medicine – often termed Cosmo ceuticals (as in cosmetics and drugs), any use of specialised products, such as collagen or Botox, and equipment, such as laser and IPL (Intense Pulsed Light).

also how to minimise the risk of infection, and individual instructions for each piece of equipment for specific contra-indications.

Sensitivity testing

Failure of thermal and sensitivity tests will indicate a malfunction of the skin, and would be classed as a contra-indication (see Professional basics, pages 38–40).

Skin diagnosis tools

There are lots of good diagnosistic aids for salon use, but that is what they are – *aids* rather than a full and definitive answer. There is no substitute for a therapist's hands, experienced eye and a full consultation with lots of questions to determine skin type.

The magi lamp

A good magnification lamp with a surrounding light is the ideal tool for really examining the skin surface. The magnification glass allows you to get a really clear picture of

blemishes, and problems. Always check the lamp is working prior to putting it over the client's face, check the light bulb and the screws and joints so that it is safe, and not likely to drop suddenly.

Skin scanners and black light equipment

There are some very effective diagnostic tools for use in salons to give an in-depth analysis of skins and for measuring the acid mantle, pH, melanin and water content of the skin, as well as density and strength of the dermis. These machines have been use by dermatologists for years and salons are finding them very useful to support the other diagnostic and consultation techniques used.

Woods lamp (often called black light)

The woods lamp was originally devised by Robert William Wood in 1903 for producing a source of ultraviolet light – hence its name. It was used in hospitals for detecting fungal infections, bacteria and parasites and its clinical use in salons is to detect skin conditions. A woods lamp produces deep ultraviolet rays and it makes the skin glow, denoting different conditions and problems. There are both hand-held ones and a box type. The hand-held ones are difficult to get a true reading from because ideally the face needs to be in darkness, and it is difficult to operate the machine unless you black out the salon! With a box machine the client is seated, and the face is placed on a chin rest, rather like having an eye examination at the optician, and a curtain is pulled around the head so that the face is in darkness. The UV light can then be turned onto the skin. Certain colours will appear in patches, which is the sign of the skin's condition.

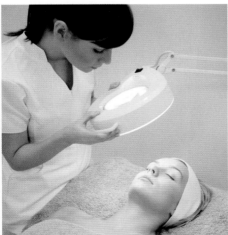

The magi lamp

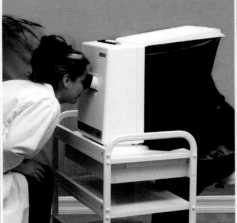

Skin scanner and black light equipment

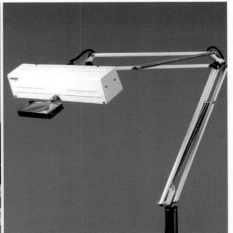

Woods lamp

Colour of fluorescence	Skin type or problem
Blue	A normal balanced skin
Weak violet/ light purple	Dry skin or patches of dehydration
Dark purple	Sensitive thin, fragile areas
Coral pink	Hydrated skin
Strong white	Thickened stratum corneum and the presence of dead skin cells
Orange	Oily skin or patches of over-productive sebaceous glands
Brown spots	Over-pigmentation/sun damage
Light yellow	Acne, comedones
Green	This shows the presence of pathogen pseudomonas – bacterial infection

These areas can be noted down on the consultation card and the appropriate treatment and products recommended to the client.

Think about it

These colours will vary depending upon the maker of woods lamp so please always follow manufacturers' instructions.

Skin scanners and hydration levels

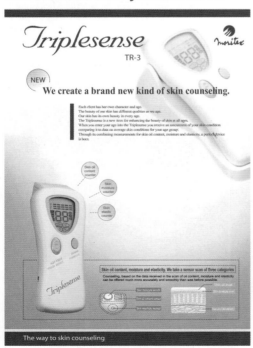

Skin scanner to measure the moisture content of the skin

A German electrical engineering company has devised a set of skin scanners – one of which measures the skin's moisture content. It looks rather like a pen, with a flat end, which is placed on the skin's surface. It is attached to a machine called a corneometer, which is where the reading is displayed.

This is a good tool for measuring the amount of water the skin is holding, and it will indicate whether the acid mantle is still intact and if the skin has enough of a defence barrier. It also shows the enzyme action of the epidermis. It is used in hospitals to measure patient intake of fluid and dispersion of fluid intake.

Skin lipid levels

The sebumeter determines the amount of sebum being excreted by the sebaceous glands onto the skin's surface, again to see if the acid mantle protection is in good condition. The sebum of the skin or hair is taken by a film on the cassette's measuring head. Its transparency changes according to the sebum content on the film and is then analysed.

Recognising skin types

You will be expected to treat all of the skin types within your treatment ranges, and you may need to refresh your previous training on how to recognise them (see 'Facial treatments', pages 263–264, for a full example of a facial record card and questions to ask the client).

The skin types are:

- normal
- oily
- dry
- combination
- sensitive
- mature
- dehydrated
- blemished/congested
- male skin.

The true skin type may not be easy to diagnose at first, as all skins react to the environment, products used and the lifestyle of the client. Some investigation is required and a patient approach within the consultation will help you identify the correct skin type.

Think about it

It is rare that a client falls into one category of skin type – they will likely have a combination of the skin types; they may have dry, mature, sensitive skin – or they may have oily blemished male skin, or any variation! It is also easy to misdiagnose skin types if clients are using the wrong products.

Normal skin

This supposedly does not exist, as a 'perfect' skin is only found in teenagers unaffected by hormonal influences, when the oil and sweat glands are working in harmony. However, many clients who look after their skin, or who were born with good skin, would class their skin as normal in its behaviour and properties.

This type of skin has a good balance of moisture content and oil to keep the skin soft, supple and flexible, so this is the ideal skin type to aspire to, even if rarely found. The skin is finely textured with no visible pores and smooth to the touch; it is plump, clear and has a healthy glow. It should feel warm to the touch, and heals well if damaged. This type of skin has a good hydro-lipidic (acid) mantle, so control of bacteria and protection against germs are good, as is the moisture content, which is well contained within the skin. This skin type would be considered to be the most balanced.

Dry skin

A dry skin is deficient in both oil and moisture, leaving the skin dry to the touch, and there may be some loss of elasticity depending upon the client's age, and a tendency to flakiness. All skins tend to dry out as they get older, because of reduced functioning of the sebaceous and sweat glands. However, a dry skin can be looked after and responds well to treatments.

Dry skin problems

The texture of the skin is usually fine and dry skin can often be thin, with small red veins (dilated capillaries) present on the cheek areas. Pores and follicles are often closed and inactive. Skin chaps easily and is inclined to be sensitive.

Lines and wrinkles may form early with dry skin, especially around the eyes. This can be inherited, and this skin type has a predisposition towards eczema and dermatitis.

This skin type is hard to judge, as it is possible the client is drying out the top layers of the epidermis by using the wrong products, and the skin is actually not a dry skin at all. Environmental factors could be influencing the hydro-lipidic (acid) mantle and the skin could be dehydrated.

If a dry flaky skin has pustules and comedones present, then the oil production is very much in evidence, and the client may have used a harsh retail preparation to dry out the comedones, but has dried out the epidermis too much. To be certain of this skin type, a very gentle exfoliant should be used on the skin, to remove the dry flaky skin cells which have accumulated on the epidermis and look at the underlying skin.

Oily skin

This type of skin is the easiest to recognise if there are problems, but be careful with this skin category. It also suffers from poor product use, along with over-stimulation of the sebaceous glands, leading to misdiagnosis of the true skin condition.

True oily, or greasy, skin is caused by an over-production of sebum from the sebaceous glands. It looks shiny; it can be slightly thicker in consistency than normal skin, sallow, coarse and have problems associated with it. This skin is often referred to as seborrhoeic.

Oily skin problems

Enlarged pores, congested pores, comedones and infection may occur on greasy skins, so care must be taken. A greasy

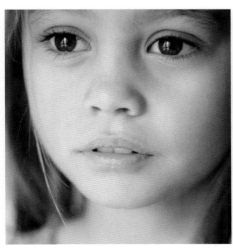

Normal skin

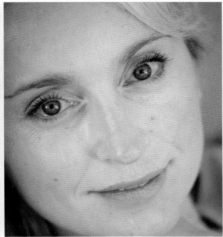

Dry skin

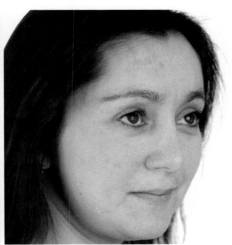

Oily skin

skin often develops during puberty, when there is a surge of hormonal activity under the influence of the sex hormones, as the teenager reaches sexual maturity. It often corrects itself when the hormone levels settle, and the use of the correct skin preparations can certainly help. Clients with an oily skin often use harsh, drying products as they feel they need to keep the skin 'clean' and oil-free.

What they are doing is:

- Stripping the hydro-lipidic (acid) mantle from the skin, risking infection and water loss, through lack of protection in the epidermis.

- Over-stimulating the sebaceous glands to produce more sebum, to replace the lost sebum contributing to the hydro-lipidic (acid) mantle. With vigorous pressure on the skin, the glandular activity becomes even more erratic.

Oil-based products will be inappropriate for this skin, as they interfere with the delicate hydro-lipidic (acid) mantle, so you will need to advise the client how to break the vicious circle of drying out the top of the epidermis, and trying to compensate by putting oil-based moisturisers on after a rigorous cleanse.

Unfortunately, acne can scar the skin quite badly and although the infection may be cleared up by the use of prescribed medication, the scarring left can be quite noticeable and make the client self-conscious. Microdermabrasion is very successful in minimising the effect of scarring, through normalising the stratum corneum, increasing the number of living cells and helping to restore good function to the cells, so salon treatments can make a difference to this skin type.

The advantage to having an oily skin in youth is that although there may be skin problems caused by too much sebum production, as the skin ages, the sebum production slows down but still keeps the skin soft. An oily skin does not dry out as much as a dry skin, and wrinkles are less noticeable.

Combination skin

Some skins are a combination of two or more skin types. The most common one is a greasy T-zone along the forehead and nose, with normal or dry skin on the cheek area. This is because there are more sebaceous glands along the T-zone which may therefore show all the characteristics of a greasy skin. This skin is very easy to recognise in youth — the nose may have comedones and the cheeks are noticeably drier than the rest of the face. As the skin gets older, and the sebum production slows down, the T-zone will become less oily. The cheek areas, if looked after well, should be stable and the skin looks more even and is not quite as easy to identify.

Sensitive skin

All skin needs to be sensitive for good health, but in beauty therapy a sensitive skin is one that is actually super-sensitive, that is, it reacts to even mild stimulus. Sensitive skins are often associated with pale skins or a dry skin that lacks the protection of enough sebum. They have a highly flushed look, with a tendency to colour easily, and may react to beauty products or chemicals used within the salon (see Allergic reactions and sensitivity testing, page 234). A sensitive skin will certainly react with some of the active ingredients within galvanic gels, so a range for sensitive skins should be suggested.

You and the skin

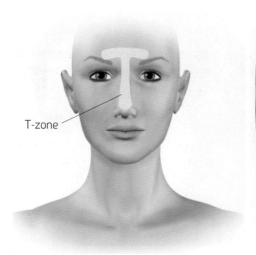

T-zone

Combination skin

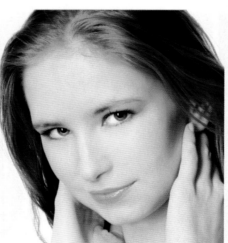

Sensitive skin

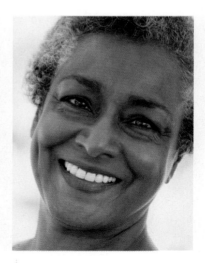

Mature skin

Mature skin

In a fine-textured, older skin the slower rate of the sebaceous secretions accompanied by loss of elasticity are contributory factors to the skin's appearance through the ageing process (see page 246). Wrinkles begin to form; the epidermis may become thinner, with a lack of springiness and loss of support from underlying muscles. Collagen becomes degraded and thinned out and the skin sags. Lack of oestrogen production in menopausal clients is a problem, as oestrogen helps maintain good levels of fat in the lower dermis, so fine lines and dryness are a result. Collagen and elastin fibre production is not as prolific as in youth, and this can produce a loss of firmness and slack contours to the face. Smoking, environmental influences and poor diet will be reflected in a mature skin which is sallow and dry.

However, a mature skin, when looked after, and when a good lifestyle promotes good health, can look very radiant. Although some maintenance is required, a mature skin is rewarding to treat within the salon as it responds so well to electrical, rehydrating treatments. Many salons find that the mature skin is the most frequent skin type treated: the client wants to minimise the signs of a mature skin, and older clients often have more time to spend in the salon and more disposable income to pay for treatment courses. While a programme of facials will mean the client sees a dramatic improvement in this skin type, a mature skin still needs a high degree of care at home to sustain the effects of salon treatments, especially night care products. Mature skin also suffers from dryness.

Dehydrated skin

Skin may have the normal sebaceous secretions and still suffer from flaking and tightness due to loss of surface moisture — a condition of dehydration. Any skin can suffer temporary dehydration, which may be caused through using harsh products on the skin or exposure to extreme temperatures, central heating or excessive dieting. Encourage the client to drink 6 to 8 glasses of water per day (see page 228).

Congested skin

Congestion occurs because the pores become blocked and sweat and sebum cannot escape onto the skin's surface. It can be seen and felt as lumpy and coarse. Whiteheads and blackheads can build up and the epidermis may harden. Poor removal of make-up, using the wrong products and excess sweat building up all contribute to this skin condition. Congested skin will need a course of treatments to help with the deep cleansing and balancing of the glands' production. Often, several sessions of exfoliation and galvanic desincrustation can return a congested skin to normal, as long as the salon treatments are supported by good home product use combined with a healthy diet and an exercise programme. Bad habits of not cleansing, or not cleansing sufficiently, and poor diet, along with a sluggish lifestyle, need to be rectified, so that all factors contribute to the healing of the skin.

Male skin

When looking at skin types and colours, it is important to include the male skin, as men are becoming big spenders in the skincare market. One of the fastest growing areas within the beauty industry is the demand for specific men's salon treatments and related care products.

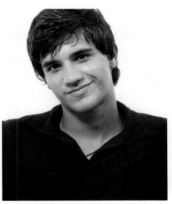

Products designed for men have been developed to reflect the fact that the skin is more resistant, but conversely may also be more fragile, through neglect, misuse or total lack of protective products such as moisturisers and sun blocks.

Male skin is approximately 25 per cent thicker than female skin, due to the influence of the male hormones testosterone and androgens, so is it therefore more resistant but becomes thinner more quickly when ageing. Because of testosterone influences, male skin tends to be oilier than female skin, so men prefer lighter moisturising products and products which solve their particular problems — healing and soothing products, creams that reduce razor bumps, products which reduce the possibility of ingrown hairs and anti-ageing creams are popular.

Men who shave daily are automatically exfoliating the upper epidermal cells, so the skin stays healthy looking and clear. There are many products available for sensitive skins, both for dry and wet shaving, to avoid shaving rash, which can be very sore and unsightly.

Anti-ageing creams (a misleading term as nothing can stop the ageing process) are a fast-selling line because, although the signs of ageing appear later on a male face, when they do arrive the wrinkles are more intense and visible – men have fewer small lines, but more deep wrinkles.

Most men's basic product needs are for the daily routine of washing, shaving and moisturising, unless calming products are needed for the specific treatment of blocked pores, irritation from shaving and razor burn or folliculitis (inflammation of the hair follicle in the skin, commonly caused by an infection). Some men use salon treatments to enhance their natural good points – eyelash tinting and the application of tinted moisturiser are very common, and manicures and pedicures are also a favourite with male clients.

Ageing of the skin

Along with the skin type clients inherit, the care they take of it and their general health, age is the other largest influence on the skin, not only because of the hormonal impact. Ageing is a natural part of the life cycle of a human being – it cannot be stopped or reversed, and skin cells begin to age from the age of 20 onwards.

Unfortunately, western culture is geared up to the young and growing older is not seen as a desirable trait – unlike eastern cultures where age is equated with wisdom and knowledge. Western society tries to push back the ageing process – there has been a marked rise in the demand for face lifts and extreme beauty treatments, such as Botox injections, to delay the ageing process.

Ageing happens to us all – and at generally the same rate, unless we are unfortunate enough to have a disease that interrupts these natural processes. The inherited factor comes into play again, with the ageing process – if your parents age well, enjoy good health and have good skin, the chances are that you will too.

The ageing process affects the skin for the following reasons.

- Cell renewal is always faster in youth; the older we get, the slower the renewal process becomes, until it stops altogether.

Think about it

There is an old saying – 'You get the face you deserve', and this is partly true because if you lead a healthy lifestyle, follow a good skincare routine and protect against ultraviolet exposure, this will minimise the risk of skin damage and premature ageing.

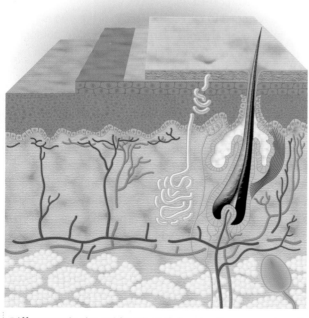
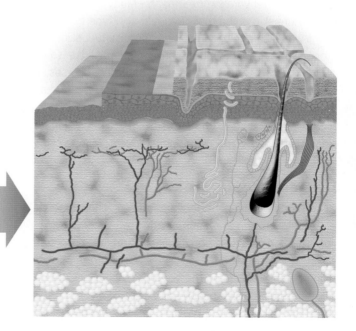

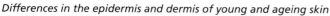
Differences in the epidermis and dermis of young and ageing skin

You and the skin

- The genetic information in each cell gets a little diluted every time the cell reproduces, so the cells of an 80-year-old do not have the same information as a young baby's.

- Hormone production in both sexes varies with age and contributes to the skin's development, health and deterioration.

- Fewer skin cells are being reproduced.

- The underlying structures supporting the skin begin to offer less support — the collagen and elastin fibres in the skin degenerate, muscular tension diminishes and wrinkles appear.

- The adipose tissue supporting the skin diminishes and the skin starts to sag — the skin can no longer fight the gravitational pull.

- Sun damage and pigmentation disorders become more noticeable as the melanin production within the skin lessens, along with **age** or **liver spots** on the surface of the epidermis.

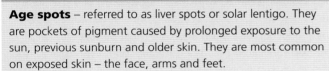

Key terms

Age spots – referred to as liver spots or solar lentigo. They are pockets of pigment caused by prolonged exposure to the sun, previous sunburn and older skin. They are most common on exposed skin – the face, arms and feet.

Age grouping of the skin

The teenage years: 14–20 years

Just as the body is changing with puberty, in preparation for the reproductive part of the human life cycle, so emotional development also begins, making teenagers acutely aware of themselves and their relationships with their peers. In females, the onset of puberty usually starts around the age of 10 or 12. Hormonal activity dictates the development of the body, changing both the sexual physical development and the emotional highs and lows that accompany this dramatic change.

At this age, the skin should be firm and compact, with a good supporting structure of collagen and elastin to give a firm, smooth feeling to the touch. Unfortunately, the hormone levels can be unbalanced and the sebaceous glands produce too much sebum, leading to blackheads and congested skin. Acne is common in this age group and may be directly related to high testosterone levels, so is more common in boys than girls.

Teenage boys may also cause skin problems by neglect — regular skin cleaning with the correct products can diminish skin problems but may be perceived as not a masculine pastime. However, with males taking a larger proportion of retail skincare sales than ever before, there is no reason for a male not to use a foaming facial cleanser designed for the male skin to help keep the skin clear.

A proportion of late-teen skins are not as clear as they could be, for self-inflicted reasons. Poor diet and an excessive alcohol intake, combined with the introduction of smoking, do little to enhance the skin. The only advantage is that this age group has youth on its side to recover more easily!

Early adulthood: 20–30 years

This is when the chubbiness of the teenage years disappears and hormonal activity settles down, so the skin is at its peak. It looks fresh, radiant and glowing. The underlying structure is good; there are no fine lines developing yet, and providing good health is enjoyed, and a healthy diet gives the body the correct nutrients, the skin is good.

In pregnancy, hormonal changes may affect the pigmentation of the skin and darker patches, called chloasma, may appear — commonly found along the hairline and on the neck or hands. Also, tiredness in young parents, poor lifestyle choices and simply 'burning the candle at both ends' will take its toll on this generation, if care is not taken. Good choices in the appropriate skincare range and protection with a moisturiser, along with correct use of sunscreens, will be an investment for the future.

Adulthood: 30–40 years

The skin begins to dry out and its reproduction slows down, with fine lines appearing, usually on the neck area first. The jaw line is firmly defined at the beginning of the decade but can shows signs of change. It may lose its definition or, if the client puts on weight, it will fill out and a double chin may form. Puffiness may be found in the cheeks — any weight gain in the face or body is instantly ageing.

The facial tissues begin to lose their fatty layer and tiredness can creep into the eye area. Creases and wrinkles remain after the depressions that form them have disappeared. Correct use of skincare products and protection against UV damage is essential in this generation, as prevention is better than cure! A neck and hand cream will prevent dehydration. Many clients forget this — they concentrate on their faces, forgetting that hands and neck areas are the true age reflector.

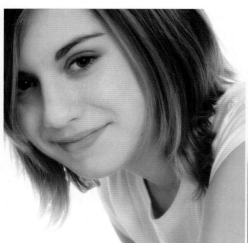

Teenage skin is firm and compact

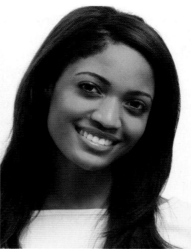

Skin is at its peak in early adulthood

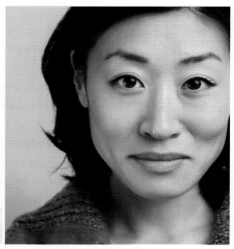

Skin in adulthood begins to show signs of ageing

Middle adulthood: 40–50 years

There is still a good clear definition of features, but 'temporary' double chins and wrinkles developed in the late thirties become a permanent fixture. Elasticity and the supporting structures of collagen and elastin fibres are diminishing, especially if the client is undergoing the menopause, which may start towards the fifties. Oestrogen levels start to fall and this affects bone density, elasticity in the tissues and skin thickness. The skin has begun to become thinner and more prone to damage from UV radiation and the environment. Blemishes, broken capillaries and pigmentation changes begin to occur.

Later adulthood: 50–60 years

All women will have begun, or completed, the menopause in this generation, and the skin will be loose and thin. It may feel coarse to the touch, and the eyes are lined and puffy. The muscle tissues around the eye and mouth develop depressions, seen as wrinkles around them, and the lip line loses definition. The sebaceous glands have slowed down the production of sebum and care must be taken to keep the skin lubricated and free from infection. With ageing, the skin loses some of its ability to fight infection and heal itself quickly. Facial hair growth may start to be obvious around the mouth and chin, and the hair is coarse and thick because of the influence of the male hormone testosterone, which is not being balanced by oestrogen.

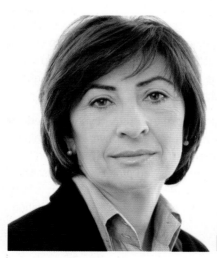

Elasticity diminishes during middle adulthood

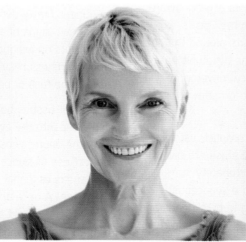

Skin will often be loose and thin in later adulthood

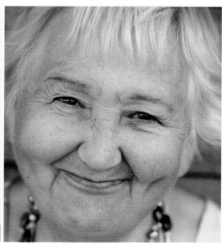

Skin can look soft and paper thin in late adulthood

Think about it

Age and the skin is very relative – some people will defy their age and have great skin, others will look older than their years.

Late adulthood: 60–70 years

At this stage, the skin has the appearance of being soft, paper thin and pappy. There is very little underlying fat to support the facial structure, and deeper furrows appear from the corner of the nose towards the lips and from the outer mouth down to the chin. Darkened patches may appear, or loss of pigment can be seen, especially on the hands and arms. The throat, neck and chest are very lined and like tissue paper, with very little sebum to lubricate the skin.

Maintaining the skin

Evidence suggests that the chances of living a long life are affected by your genes – long life seems to run in families. It is also known that cells have a programmed maximum number of divisions before they die off, so your life span is, to some degree, predetermined. However, there are some sensible precautions that clients should take.

- Eat healthily – people on lower-calorie diets tend to live longer, and meeting the body's additional demands as you age is important. A female who has heavy periods throughout her life will need more iron, but a menopausal client will need more calcium to help keep bones healthy.

- Keep physically active – three half-hour aerobic sessions a week helps keep circulation and metabolism going and stimulates the body to repair itself (this means a brisk walk or swim to get the cardiovascular system working).

- Get enough sleep or rest – rest allows the body to repair and heal itself and for the brain activity to slow and sift through all the stimulation it has received through the day. Sleep deprivation is very harmful to the body in the long term.

- Remain mentally active – the more you use your brain, the better it works, and the longer you remain alert. Doing a crossword, mental arithmetic, music and learning poetry are ideal brain activities as you get older.

- Remember good health maintenance – smoking ages the skin; a high alcohol intake is also damaging.

Anti-ageing treatments

The key here is 'prevention is better than cure'. In other words, encourage clients to look after their skin as early as possible, rather than waiting until the signs of ageing have begun to show. Anti-ageing treatments cannot turn back years of poor skincare and neglect, nor can they stop the ageing process. Some can significantly enhance the skin's appearance, but not on a long-term basis or without continuous treatments.

Scientific research into the different types of ageing is enabling cosmetic houses and beauty product manufacturers to develop anti-ageing treatments which target the symptoms of ageing more accurately than ever before.

Moisturisers

Contrary to popular belief, moisturisers do not add moisture to the skin, but rather they prevent moisture from being lost. This is achieved with the use of non-irritating oils and emollients such as lanolin and vegetable- or petroleum-based oils, which form a thin layer on top of the epidermis and stop water from literally evaporating out of the body. The result is that the outermost layers of skin absorb the water being released by the deeper layers, and so small wrinkles are filled out, and the skin looks and feels a lot softer. Moisturising the skin also helps protect it from air pollution, harsh weather conditions and the drying effect of heating and air conditioners. Most importantly, the majority of moisturisers contain ingredients that provide UV protection, which can affect the skin throughout the year, not just in the summer months.

Salon treatments

Any treatment which helps the desquamation process is going to help the skin look clean and fresh looking. Combine

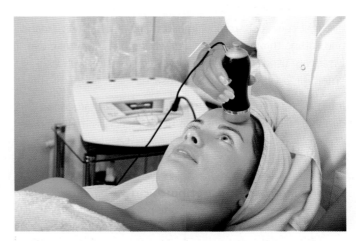

Facial treatments can help reduce the effects of ageing

a treatment that deep cleanses and then rehydrates the skin using an electrical current, such as in a galvanic facial, and the result is instant – the skin looks plump and refreshed, and very clean. However, salon treatments will only last as long as the treatments are carried out regularly.

Scrubs, face masks and electrical treatments work on the outer layers of the epidermis, and will improve the look and feel of the skin, but under the Trade Descriptions Act a salon would be liable to prosecution if advertising these treatments as anti-ageing.

Alpha-hydroxy acids/skin peels

These treatments work by applying to the skin a chemical agent/acid (for example **alpha-hydroxy acids** (AHAs) or retinoic acid/vitamin A) which dissolves the outer layers, thus temporarily reducing fine lines and other superficial signs of ageing. However, adverse reactions can occur, particularly if the concentration of the active ingredient is quite high, or if the product is left on the skin for too long. Peels also leave the skin far more susceptible to damage from UV rays and so sun protection is essential following treatment. You must space out the treatments for the client and make sure they are spread out over a period of time – the skin is quite vulnerable after a peel.

Laser skin resurfacing

Laser therapy for the skin is becoming a very popular salon treatment. Laser treatment can be used for skin ageing and wrinkles, as the light stimulates the capillary level, so improving the circulation. Acne and cellulite also respond well to laser treatment, as do pigmented lesions and the removal of tattoos. The pigment is broken down into minute particles and removed through the lymphatic system. Laser or intense pulsed light (IPL) treatments cross over from the beauty therapy field into medicine – lasers are used in eyesight correction, removing birthmarks and tattoos, treating and cutting through cancers and wound healing. Pulse dye lasers are used for targeting port wine stains as well as smaller red vessels, scars and rosacea.

Intense pulsed light systems are very good at targeting dilated capillaries by causing a heat reaction in the blood, causing coagulation and therefore destroying the protein in the wall of the vessel. The vessel breaks down and is absorbed by the body's natural removal through the lymphatic system and bloodstream.

Within beauty therapy, lasers can be used for treating active acne, improving acne scarring and hair removal. Full training and a certificate of competence are required for insurance, as laser work is very specialised and has many contra-indications.

Collagen treatments

The protein collagen is the principal ingredient of white fibrous connective tissue found within tendons, skin, bone, cartilage and ligaments. Despite any claims made for collagen-containing products, the skin cannot absorb artificial collagen.

However, one collagen treatment that is temporarily effective and growing in popularity is collagen replacement therapy (CRT). This involves collagen being injected directly into the dermis to improve the appearance of fine lines and pockmarks. Collagen injections to the lips to create a 'bee sting' pout to the lip shape are common, but can go wrong if the client has an allergic reaction to the injection, leaving the lips very swollen and sore.

There are also treatments available where the patient's own collagen-producing cells – called fibroblasts – are collected using a biopsy from an unnoticeable area, say from behind the ear. These cells are then cultivated within the laboratory and mixed with nutrients to help them grow. They are then injected back into the patient, along the facial expression lines. The theory is that as they are the patient's own cells, there is likely to be no rejection reaction, as there is with some bulk-filling injections. The new cells stimulate growth in the existing collagen cells and within 4–6 months lines appear softer and acne scars are said to be practically invisible. This is not a salon practice, as it has to be carried out under local anaesthetic to harvest the biopsy, and can be expensive.

Key terms

Alpha hydroxy acids/retinoic acid – chemical compounds widely used in skincare products, to reduce the signs of ageing by loosening and dissolving dead skin cells, which allows the newer cells to come through.

For your portfolio

A protocol treatment plan is set out by most Awarding Bodies. Check what yours says regarding laser treatments. Is there a specialist salon offering laser treatments near you? Do a price comparison with normal facial treatments. What training did the therapists have to undergo? Does this appeal to you? Would you like to specialise in this area?

Botox treatments

Botox works by paralysing muscles located at the site where it is injected, thus reducing lines and wrinkles in that area. It is often used to treat frown lines and crow's feet around the eyes. Once again, the effects are temporary, and the treatments are required on a regular basis. The long-term effects of this botulinum-based treatment are not yet known. A recent report in the *Journal of Cosmetic Dermatology* suggested that people using Botox to defeat the signs of ageing may simply be developing more wrinkles in nearby areas, as neighbouring muscles try to compensate for those that are paralysed.

Cosmetic surgery

Surgery is an invasive treatment and carries all the risks of any other medical operation. It is, however, considered an affordable treatment by many, and it can be very successful. Correcting sagging contours and removing wrinkles, by tightening the eye area, chin or a complete face-lift, will reduce the signs of ageing. However, there is a danger of the skin looking too tight and not in keeping with the rest of the body — many film stars may look good facially, but their necks and hands reflect their true age. There is also a risk of the facial contours looking pulled and taut, which will look odd.

Cosmetic surgery should only be considered after a great deal of research and through a recognised medical referral. In some cases, corrective surgery can be very successful and most beneficial, especially if the physical problem causes psychological distress, too. The correction of a hare lip, reshaping of a broken nose or pinning back ears which protrude can give back confidence to clients and improve their perception of themselves.

Think about it

As a beauty therapist, it is not within your job role to give medical advice or pass any judgment about medical matters, including cosmetic surgery. You may only recommend that the client seek medical advice, and nothing else.

Ageing and the sun

The effects of ultraviolet rays on the skin are well documented. Clients like a tanned, toned skin, which is usually associated with holidays and relaxation. An artificial tanning unit, in the form of sunbeds and showers, and fake tan application are very lucrative for salons. The government has now introduced a law banning under-16s from having

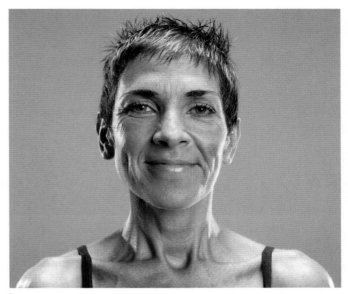

Too much sun damage results in the skin having a leathery, coarse appearance

sunbed treatments as many tanning shops are completely unsupervised and very few, if any, checks are performed to see if the skin is suited to the treatment.

Apart from helping to relieve certain conditions like asthma, aching joints and psoriasis, along with aiding vitamin D production, the sun's health benefits are primarily psychological. The truth is: too much sun can be positively harmful.

The immediate result of too much sun is sunburn, and many of us have experienced the painful blisters, fever and swelling that come from too much sun, too fast. Another result of sun exposure is prematurely aged skin. The sun causes the skin to thicken and gives a leathery, coarse appearance. With enough time, the sun weakens the skin's elasticity by cross-linking the collagen fibres in the dermis. This results in sagging and wrinkles on all sun-exposed areas.

The sun also causes dark pigmentation patches and scaly grey growths known as keratoses, which are often pre-cancerous. Sunburn and prematurely aged skin are not the worst results of constant exposure to the sun — skin cancer is. Almost all of the 300 000 cases of this disease developed annually are considered to be sun-related. Some people are more at risk than others of skin damage. Britain is fast catching up with Australia for numbers of skin cancer patients. In fact, the promotion of skin cancer awareness in hotter countries is bringing down their skin cancer patient numbers, as ours are growing.

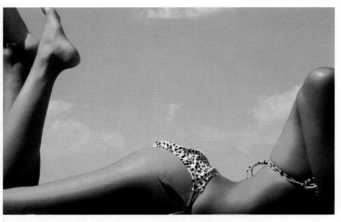

Advise clients to always use suitable sun protection

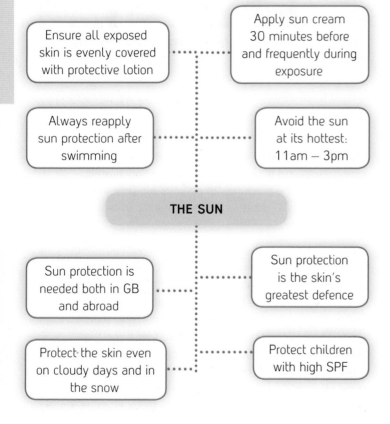

Ensure all exposed skin is evenly covered with protective lotion

Apply sun cream 30 minutes before and frequently during exposure

Always reapply sun protection after swimming

Avoid the sun at its hottest: 11am – 3pm

THE SUN

Sun protection is needed both in GB and abroad

Sun protection is the skin's greatest defence

Protect the skin even on cloudy days and in the snow

Protect children with high SPF

Black skins are relatively safe because the darker tone provides good protection from ultraviolet light. White/Caucasian skins, notably in redheads and blonds, are at the greatest risk due to less melanin in the skin.

Certain drugs such as antibiotics, medicated soaps and creams, and even barbiturates and birth control pills can make the skin more susceptible to damage. The best cover-up of all is a chemical one, in the form of sunscreens and sun blocks. All clients concerned about premature ageing

should be advised of the dangers of sun exposure, and recommended a sunscreen or sun block. Those clients who are sun worshippers should be educated to understand the relationship between the sun and skin cancer.

Once the ultraviolet light has caused cross-linking and thickening in the dermis and has predisposed the skin to premature ageing, no reversal of the damage is possible. Plastic surgery techniques can help disguise the sagging by re-draping the skin, but this does not compensate for the damage that has occurred. It is, therefore, the first topic that must be discussed with the client who expresses concern about ageing, and advice on sun protection should be given verbally and in a written fact sheet. Indeed, the only cosmetic product that can legally be labelled 'anti-ageing' is a sunscreen or sun block preparation.

Additional knowledge

The Fitzpatrick skin type classification

Not only can skin be classified by ethnic origins and environmental factors, some cosmetic houses base their product ranges — especially sun protection creams — around the Fitzpatrick system of categorising skin into six different types. This is especially popular in America. It is based upon melanin content in the skin and how quickly the skin burns.

It was developed in 1975 by Harvard University's Dr Thomas Fitzpatrick, and is still used by dermatologists using laser and light therapy, as it can help highlight risks of poor reactions to treatment. There are six varieties of Fitzpatrick skin types, ranging from extremely pale-skinned people who are highly likely to burn, to extremely dark-skinned people who may suffer serious discoloration from laser or light treatment, or other pigment altering therapies or conditions.

A variety of questions are asked about genetic history, physical attributes such as eye colour, hair colour, and freckling, and your personal observations of your skin's reaction to sunlight. Depending on the answers to the determination questions, most people fit into one of the six skin categories, usually labelled with roman numerals I–VI.

Skin type	Typical features	Tanning ability
I Celtic, English, Northern European	Pale white, fair skin Blond or red hair Blue or hazel eyes	Always burns, freckles, does not tan
II Nordic, North American	White, fair skin Sandy to brown hair Green, brown or blue eyes	Burns easily, tans poorly and with difficulty, freckles
III Central Eastern European, Mediterranean, Maori New Zealand	Darker or olive-white skin Brown hair Green or brown eyes	Tans after initial burn
IV Chinese, Korean, Japanese, Thai, South American, Indian, Filipino	Olive to light brown skin Brown hair Brown eyes	Burns minimally, tans easily
V East African, Ethiopian, Northern African, Middle Eastern Arabic	Dark brown skin Black hair Dark brown eyes	Rarely burns, tans darkly easily
VI African Caribbean, African American	Dark brown or black skin Dark brown or black hair Dark brown-black eyes	Never burns, always tans darkly

The Fitzpatrick skin type categories

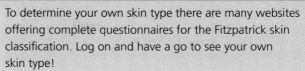

For your portfolio

To determine your own skin type there are many websites offering complete questionnaires for the Fitzpatrick skin classification. Log on and have a go to see your own skin type!

Products and the skin

Mechanical and electrical treatments for the skin are excellent at penetrating products into the skin, for various beneficial purposes. Most professional suppliers have their range of supporting products to be used with their own machine, and it is very important that you follow the manufacturer's instructions. What works with one machine might not be suitable or give the same benefits to the client as another. The active ingredients react with the various polarities and frequencies used (see Unit B14, Improve face and skin condition using electro-therapy, for a full explanation of how the machines work).

During most professional training for new equipment and products there will be a practical test of competency and then a written paper on the benefits and effects of each product. Don't think that as you have left college, gaining knowledge and then testing that knowledge stops!

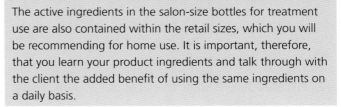

Think about it

The active ingredients in the salon-size bottles for treatment use are also contained within the retail sizes, which you will be recommending for home use. It is important, therefore, that you learn your product ingredients and talk through with the client the added benefit of using the same ingredients on a daily basis.

Massage or mask – which comes first?

Product knowledge and research are advancing all the time, and professional suppliers will have their own procedures for performing the treatment. This may contradict the application knowledge you gained within Level 2 treatments. Some cosmetic houses would argue that you always apply a mask first, to cleanse and exfoliate the skin, in preparation for the massage and electrical treatments to follow. After all, why dry out the skin after all the benefits of a massage cream have been absorbed by the skin?

Another product house would state that their mask content has the same active ingredients as the massage cream, and reinforces the treatment performed, and needs to be applied

Think about it

This system should be used as a guideline rather than a definitive analysis for determining skincare. You must do a full consultation, a manual and a visual examination and use all diagnostic tools available to you as a therapist.

Think about it

You are not medically trained and cannot recommend treatment of a medical nature. Always refer your client to their GP and do not pass comment on any skin irregularity. You are not trained to do so.

You and the skin

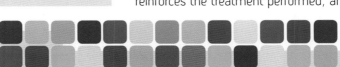

after the skin has been warmed and softened by massage. Who is right? They both are! As long as you use the procedure recommended for the product, then the benefits are not going to be diluted. It is only when you ignore the manufacturer's recommendations that problems occur.

Think about it

Always use the correct product with its correct machine – the client deserves to have the treatment she is paying for, and the effects on the skin may not be as good if you cut corners. It may also invalidate your insurance if you have not followed the manufacturer's procedures.

Think about it

When you qualify and start work at a salon, it may sponsor your training with a particular make of machine and product. In return, the salon will expect a period of loyal employment from you. What you learn in product knowledge may not be the same as the products you used at college, so be flexible – there are several procedures available for different machines. Be open to new training, which is the way to learn new skills and techniques.

Check your knowledge

1 The acid mantle of the skin should have a pH of between:
   a) 2.5 – 3.5
   b) 4.5 – 5.5
   c) 5.5 – 6.5
   d) 6.5 – 7.5.

2 The Fitzpatrick skin category tells:
   a) the age of the skin
   b) the tanning ability of the skin
   c) the products used on the skin
   d) the oiliness of the skin.

3 A woods lamp is often referred to as a:
   a) white light
   b) green light
   c) violet light
   d) black light.

4 The phrase *intrinsic factors of the skin* refers to:
   a) the external factors influencing skin health
   b) the skin type of the client
   c) the internal factors influencing skin health
   d) the products the client should be using.

5 The function of protein in the diet is to:
   a) maintain and support body growth
   b) aid digestion
   c) regulate fatty acids
   d) help you see in the dark.

6 Folic acid is found in:
   a) milk
   b) liver
   c) meat
   d) green leafy vegetables.

7 Impetigo is what type of infection?
   a) Viral
   b) Bacterial
   c) Fungal
   d) Skin disorder.

8 Vitiligo is a skin condition recognised by:
   a) hypopigmentation
   b) hyperpigmentation
   c) infection and pus
   d) dry skin and flakes.

9 The special property of vitamin E is that it is:
   a) fat soluble
   b) water soluble
   c) olive oil based
   d) collagen based.

10 Which of these is NOT a contra-indication to a treatment?
   a) Cancer
   b) Impetigo
   c) Lentigo
   d) Dermatitis.

4

Facial treatments

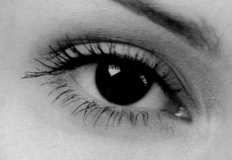
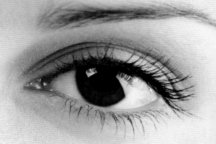

Facial treatments

What you will learn:

Facial treatments – theory and consultation

- The benefits and effects of electrical treatments
- Choice of equipment
- Properties of electricity
- The facial consultation
- Equipment used in facial treatments

Facial treatments — theory and consultation

Electrical treatments are a large source of revenue for salons, and are very popular with clients. While therapists may argue that nothing is more relaxing than manual massage, electrical treatments are more effective for treating skin problems, figure problems and for deeper penetration of products into the skin.

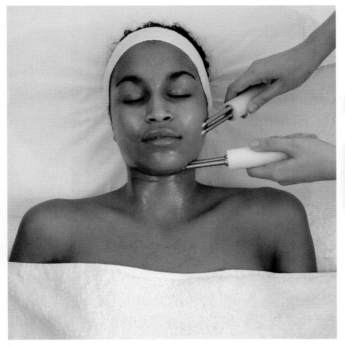

Non-surgical face-lifting

Key terms

Current – the rate of flow of electricity around a circuit. It is measured in amps (named after French physicist and mathematician, André-Marie Ampere).

Think about it

Any treatment using an electrical current, adapted to any of the machinery used with beauty therapy, will be more effective than manual treatments alone. Do remember though that although there are a wide variety of treatments available, not all treatments are suitable for all clients.

The benefits and effects of electrical treatments

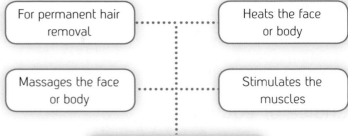

For permanent hair removal ··· Heats the face or body

Massages the face or body ··· Stimulates the muscles

WHY WE USE ELECTRICAL CURRENT IN TREATMENTS

Deep cleanses the skin ··· Helps products penetrate into the skin

Stimulates the circulation, lymphatic flow and glandular functions ··· Improves cellular functions

Supports the treatment of the ageing process

Effects of electrical current for beauty therapy treatments

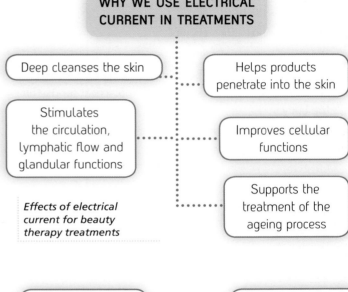

Visible results in the skin's condition ··· More effective than manual treatments

BENEFITS TO THE CLIENT OF USING ELECTRICAL CURRENT IN TREATMENTS

Long-term benefits with a long-term treatment programme ··· Better results on specific areas and conditions

Instant results can be felt and seen by the client e.g. relaxation, hair removal

Benefits to the client of using electrical treatments

Choice of equipment

This will depend on:

- the client's needs
- any contra-indications present
- the client's personal preferences – likes and dislikes
- the area of the body to be treated – some equipment is suitable for the face, but would be impractical for use on the body
- the cost of a treatment or course of treatments
- the time constraints for a course, i.e. fitting into a client's lifestyle
- the skin type
- the body condition/shape and fat type
- the type of business the salon caters for, and the clientele's requirements.

Be informed about all the latest reports in the media about new electrical treatments within the beauty industry. You could be missing an opportunity to expand your business and offer clients something new and innovative. Talk to the clients about the benefits of the new treatments, and be specific about the benefits for the client's skin. Take extra training to learn new equipment usage and increase your client base by having the latest treatments available.

Electrical therapies

Electrical therapies use a range of different currents and frequencies. To understand the differences in equipment, you will need to know:

- the type of current used and how it behaves
- how each piece of equipment works
- its benefits to the client
- its risk assessment and hazard potential
- how to use it most effectively for the client's needs.

To appreciate these topics, you first need to understand the properties of electricity.

Properties of electricity

The atom

All matter, whether solid, gas or liquid, is composed of units called **atoms**. Every atom has a nucleus and an external or outer layer.

- The nucleus contains positively charged particles, or **protons.**
- The nucleus also contains **neutrons**, which have no charge.
- The outer layer contains negatively charged particles called **electrons.**

Each electron rotates continuously around the nucleus, always in the same orbit.

An atom has one of the following three characteristics:

1 Atom without electrical charge – when the number of electrons and protons is equal, the atom therefore has no charge.
2 Negative ion or **anion** – if the atom gains an electron, the number of electrons will be greater than the protons, so the atom takes on a negative charge. The atom becomes a negative ion or anion.
3 Positive ion or **cation** – if the atom loses an electron, the number of protons is higher, and the atom becomes a positive ion or cation.

All ions relate to each other according to the physical **laws of electricity**: the same charged ions repel each other, while opposite charged ions are attracted to each other. Therefore, two negatives repel one another and so do two positives. A positive is only attracted to a negative, and vice versa.

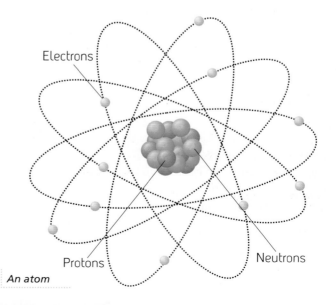

An atom

Key terms

Atom – basic block of all matter; can be solid, liquid or gas.

Protons – positively charged particles.

Electrons – negatively charge particles.

Neutrons – no charge, found in the nucleus of an atom.

Anion – an atom with a negative charge.

Cation – an atom with a positive charge.

Laws of electricity – opposite charge attracts, same charge repels.

This theory of opposites attracting is very important in galvanic work, when the active ingredients in the gels and solutions used have active ions, and they are used to aid skin penetration.

Electricity and electrical circuits

An electric current is a flow of electrons passing through a fixed point in an electrical circuit per second, measured in amps. Electrons flow from negative to positive as they are negatively charged. The pressure required to drive the electric current around a circuit in measured in volts. So, the voltage is the force produced by a generator (or battery) to 'push' the electrical current around the circuit — sometimes referred to as the potential difference.

The amount of electricity an appliance uses depends upon how much work it is designed to do — called the power rating. This is measured in **watts** or kilowatts.

Resistance is anything in the circuit that slows down the flow of electricity. There is a balance — the voltage is trying to push the current around the circuit and the resistance is opposing it. The relative sizes of voltage and resistance indicate how big the current will be.

- If you increase the voltage, more current will flow.
- If you increase the resistance, less current will flow.

Key terms

Voltage – the force produced by a generator to push the electricity around a circuit. It is measured in volts (named after Alessandro Volta, the Italian inventor of the battery).

Ohms – the resistance to the flow of electricity, seen as a calculation.

Ohm's law – ohms = volts ÷ amps.

Watts – units that measure the power of an appliance. Watts = volts × amps.

Resistance is measured in units called ohms, but they cannot be measured directly. They need to be calculated from the volts and amps. The relationship between volts, amps and ohms is called Ohm's law:

ohms = volts ÷ amps

For example, if the voltage of a lamp is 12 volts and the current flowing is 2 amps, the number of ohms would be calculated as:

12 volts ÷ 2 amps = 6 Ω or ohms

Power rating

How much electricity a piece of equipment or an appliance uses depends on how much work it is designed to do — called its power rating. The power of equipment is measured in watts. 1000 watts (W) = 1 kilowatt (kW).

Watts cannot be measured with any electricity meter. They need to be calculated from the appliance's volts and amps — by multiplying them together.

watts = volts × amps

For example, if the voltage of a lamp is 12 volts and the current flowing is 2 amps, the number of watts would be calculated as:

12 volts x 2 amps = 24 W

Electrical circuits can be seen as:

- a voltage pushing the current round with resistance opposing the flow
- energy transfer.

Anything which supplies electricity is also supplying energy. Electricity comes from different sources:

- cells
- batteries
- generators
- solar cells.

Key terms

Abbreviations for electrical terms:

V – volts

A – amps

Ω – omega (for ohms)

W – watts

The most practical source of electricity is from the generators at power stations via the National Grid. Cells and battery-operated equipment will need recharging and are not suitable for small portable pieces of equipment such as blood pressure machines. Solar energy is unreliable in countries that do not have a regular supply of strong sunlight.

An electrical circuit transfers the energy to components such as lamps, resistors, bells, motors, and so on. These components perform their own energy transfer and convert the electrical energy into other forms of energy, such as:

- heat, for example hairdryers, kettles
- light, for example light bulbs
- sound, for example speakers
- movement, for example motors.

Series or parallel circuits

Circuits are classified as either series or parallel.

A series circuit is all or nothing – the components are connected in a line, end to end, and they all share the electrical current going through them, so once one part is broken the whole series breaks down. Think about the lights on a Christmas tree. If one bulb blows, the whole line of bulbs goes out, and it is a process of elimination to find out which one has gone. This is not very practical and, generally, few things are connected in series.

In a parallel circuit, each component is separately connected to the supply. This type of circuit is sensible to work with, as removing or disconnecting one component of the circuit will not disrupt the whole circuit. Household electrics are run this way, so you can switch everything on or off separately.

Think about it

A complete circuit is needed for the current to flow. If the circuit is broken, there will be no current flow and no transfer of energy. This is important during electrical treatments when you think your machine is not working properly. Often you have not completed the circuit by giving the client the saturator, or passive electrode, to hold (and sometimes you have just not switched it on at the plug socket!).

Where does electricity come from?

Electricity is generated in power stations throughout the country and is distributed through the National Grid to local electricity substations, where the electricity is converted to a lower voltage for use in factories, businesses and homes. Factories require very high voltages (33,000 volts), whereas small businesses such as your salon will receive a 240-volt supply. In urban areas, the 240-volt supply comes into individual premises through underground cables beneath the street. The supply cable enters the building underground and arrives at the meter, fuse board, or circuit breaker, where usage is measured, and once the meter is read, electricity bills can be calculated.

Most electrical equipment in a beauty salon runs from the 240 volts coming through the wall sockets (**mains electricity supply**), and the machine will convert it into the type of current it is built to provide, e.g. faradic, high frequency or galvanic. The exceptions to this are the bigger electrical units, which require a higher voltage, such as saunas and steam cabinets. They require a greater supply than 240 volts and have to be connected using a special consumer unit, by the installation company. The local electricity supplier will have to be informed and special rates of payment will be required – a sauna, shower unit and spa may need more than double the amps/volts normally available.

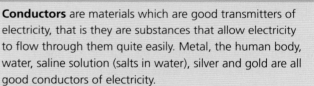

Think about it

Conductors are materials which are good transmitters of electricity, that is they are substances that allow electricity to flow through them quite easily. Metal, the human body, water, saline solution (salts in water), silver and gold are all good conductors of electricity.

Insulators are materials which are not good transmitters of electricity, that is they do not allow electricity to flow through them easily. They are used as protection from an electrical current. Examples include glass, oil, plastic, rubber and wood, and they either inhibit or prevent the flow.

Key terms

Mains electricity supply – a normal domestic supply of electricity is 240 volts.

Maximum current – from a power socket, this is 13 amps.

Conductors – good transmitters of electricity, e.g. the human body.

Insulators – poor transmitters of electricity, e.g. rubber.

Direct current (DC) – flows in one direction only.

Alternating current (AC) – alternates its directional flow.

Topic	Measured in	Symbol used	Information
Electric current – a flow of electrical charges called electrons	Amps, using an ampmeter	A	Named after the French electrical pioneer André-Marie Ampère
Pressure needed to drive current (driving force)	Volts, using a voltmeter	V	Named after Alessandro Volta, the Italian inventor of the battery
Power used to run equipment	Watts and kilowatts	W and kW	Named after James Watt, who invented the steam engine (1000 watts = 1 kilowatt)
Resistance, which slows the current down	Ohms	Ω	Named after Georg Ohm, another electrical pioneer. Often referred to as potential difference
Alternating current (AC) – flows in one direction, then in the reverse direction in the circuit. One complete back and forth is called a cycle	Hertz (one Hertz = one alternation per second)	Hz	Named after a pioneer in sending and receiving radio waves, Heinrich Hertz

Summary of electricity terms

Effects of an electrical current

An electrical current is able to produce:

- chemical change
- heat
- light rays
- mechanical movements (kinetic effects)
- sound waves
- magnetic fields
- changes of matter from one state to another, for example water to steam through heating.

Effects of electricity	Type of equipment	Effect on the body
Heating	Sauna, steam units, infrared heat lamps, spa pool, foam baths, showers, paraffin wax heaters	Relaxes the muscle fibres and raises body temperature; induces perspiration and therefore cleanses the skin; rehydrates the skin
Chemical	Galvanic treatments to the face, galvanic body treatments, galvanic hair removal	Deep cleanses the skin; forces substances into the skin; treats cellulite; removes hair
Magnetic	Mechanical massage units such as G5 vibro mat and Pifco units for facial massage. (The coil within the motor makes the head cause a circuit break and so the head taps the skin)	Stimulating massage movements encourage the skin's functions, glandular activity and desquamation of the dead epidermal cells; also helps soften and relax the muscle fibres
Light waves	Electro-magnetic waves used in infrared lamps and ultraviolet lamps	Warms the tissues, preparing them for other treatments such as massage or used as a counter-irritant – soothes the nerve endings; encourages production of melanin within the skin to produce a tanned skin, healing and helping with vitamin D production
Kinetic effects	Kinetic refers to movement, so muscular contractions caused by a faradic machine are classed as kinetic	Helps build tone and strength within the muscle fibres. May also have other benefits such as improvement in posture and confidence
Sound	Audio-sonic machine	Sound waves penetrate deep into the tissue, relaxing the muscle fibres

Effects of electricity

All of this is put to good use within the beauty salon equipment for the benefit of the client. An electrical current adapted for use on or through the body is able to:

- help improve skin function and appearance
- stimulate glandular and cellular activity in the region being worked upon
- improve the tone, functioning and appearance of the muscles
- provide relaxation to the tissues through heating them
- stimulate the systems of the body to encourage better functioning, that is the lymphatic system, circulation, cell reproduction and growth and repair.

Within beauty therapy, these electrical currents can be further broken down into categories of pattern, and the equipment can be adapted to alter the pattern to suit the client's needs, especially if it is a course of treatments and the body is getting used to the pattern and needs a little extra stimulation.

Additional knowledge

Vacuum suction and microdermabrasion

These machines do not require an adaptive current. Both a vacuum and microdermabrasion machine use a pump driven by an electric motor to create a negative pressure vacuum. So, although they are electrical equipment, that is, attached to the mains, they are classed as mechanical equipment.

Types of electrical current

Type of current	Description	Wave form
Galvanic Used for: • iontophoresis • desincrustation • epilation	Constant and direct (DC) – has no break in the flow of electrons	

Type of current	Description	Wave form
Faradic Used for: • muscle toning • passive exercise	Surged and interrupted – alternating and low frequency. The current and wave formations can be adjusted on the machine to suit the client's need	

High frequency Used for: • direct application • indirect application	Oscillating, high in frequency, higher in voltage with lower amps. Alternates rapidly at more than 50 times per second. Can be applied directly or indirectly to the body	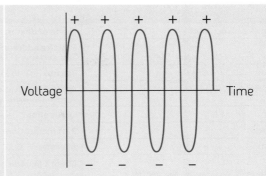
Microcurrent Used for: • uplifting facial contours • uplifting body contours	Modified direct currents (DC) – a galvanic current which can be altered on the machine for the client's needs and differing stages of treatment	Various microcurrent waveforms 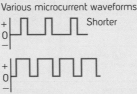 A basic interrupted direct current shows as a square wave 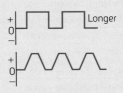 The 'square wave' can be made more gradual  The waveform can either attack or decay more gradually 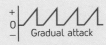

Types of current

The facial consultation

As you work through this section refer closely to all the information you learned in the Professional basics unit, for a really professional consultation.

Facial record card

The facial consultation begins with you and the client talking through the record card. Page 264 shows a typical completed card.

Once you have filled out the client's record card, place it on the trolley for additions during the treatment and you will be ready to begin the facial observation. You should note any adaptation of treatment necessary, should the client have a small contra-indication that is not a barrier to treatment.

The client may also have questions for you, for example 'What can I do about my open pores?' or 'What will I gain from an electrical treatment?' This will open up the consultation and you will have created a trusting atmosphere in which the client feels able to say exactly what their concerns are and what they are most conscious about, allowing you to give professional advice.

Think about it

If you are worried about discussing personal details with the client and don't know how to phrase the topics, turn them into questions. For example:

• *How much water do you drink during the day, Mrs Jones?*
• *Do you burn easily in sunlight?*
• *Do you have a tendency to redness if you get hot?*
• *Do you ever have breakouts/spots? Is that linked to your menstrual cycle?*
• *Do you ever experience claustrophobia?*
• *What type of massage do you prefer?*

Then, record all of the answers on the record card – you will find that most clients are very happy to talk about themselves, given the right questions, and you get a full and round picture of their skin and lifestyle. Your skin analysis is then complete and you will be able to recommend the perfect treatment plan to suit the individual needs of your client.

Personal details	Medical details
Name of client: Mrs Jane Jones	**Name of doctor:** Michael Springfield
Address: 2 The Farthings, Faith Hill, Canley, Oxford OX19 7PQ	**Practice address:** The Surgery, 1 Sale Avenue, Canley, Oxford OX19 3XY
Daytime tel. no: 01234 567890	**Tel. no:** 09183 923456
Home tel. no: 09183 456784	**Present medication:** Anti-inflammatory for IBS; anti-histamines for allergies
Date of birth: 13/10/56	**Occupation:** Nursery teacher
No. of pregnancies: 3	**Past medication:** Contraceptive pill 20 yrs
No. of children: 2 (16 + 18 years)	**Allergies:** Dogs, cats, most animal fur, eggs
Lifestyle: Quite busy with work and family, husband in a demanding job	**Client's general health:**
Sleeping pattern: Not always good	Eating habits healthy, weight loss slow but good. Likes to unwind with a glass of wine in the evening. Gym twice a week. Job quite stressful – paperwork is heavy, currently undergoing OFSTED inspection. Client feels it is disturbing her sleep pattern. Feels need for more relaxation.
Smoker (yes/no)/no. per day: No	
Alcohol units per week: 0–10	
Diet: Client trying to lose weight on Weightwatchers programme – recording food/drink intake which is healthy. Lots of fruit/veg/water.	

Facial condition – please (✓) if present and use comments box	**Comments box:**
Muscle tone scale (1 = poor; 3 = good) For: Chest area 2 Neck 2 Jaw line 2 Cheek area 2 Eye area 2 Forehead 2	Client's muscle tone good for age (54). Chest, neck and jaw would benefit from facial faradic stimulation + home exercises. Facial contours are good, eye + cheek area is lovely – great cheekbones! Elasticity good – skin springs back quickly.
Skin colour and tone	Warm, pink + healthy looking, no yellow present. In good condition. Colouring: blonde w/pale, fair skin.
Skin texture (lines present)	Fine – soft and smooth, with no obvious problems, only fine lines visible around eyes.
Skin damage (broken capillaries, etc.)	Small, dilated capillary on left nostril – client would like to have it cauterised – refer to electrologist.
Pigmentation areas (any sun damage or loss of pigmentation)	Small pigmentation around the hairline – v.faint, due to pregnancy/hormonal changes. Client has hair in a fringe – hardly noticeable.
Pores (fine, large, comedones, blocked, pustules, etc.)	Fine and clear. No shine, matt and dry to the touch.
Skin type and any skin problems (oily, dry patches, etc.)	Skin fairly dry, but in good condition with correct products. Some dry patches, due to menopause. Client prone to dry, chapped lips in winter.
Other (skin tags, scarring, superfluous hair, etc.)	Client has soft downy hair on the cheek + upper lip areas, v.fair but client quite conscious of it.
Skin exfoliation history and products used: Has client had chemical peels, used accutane from GP, or other prescribed medical skin products?	No – client has not been prescribed anything, or had AHA treatment or any resurfacing treatments in the last three months.
Products used and type preferred	Cream cleanser, toner and rich cream moisturiser. No exfoliant products used.
Hormonal influences: (Pregnancy, breastfeeding, trying to become pregnant, hormonal supplements, HRT, oral contraception, etc.)	Client going through menopause – started a couple of years ago. Occasional periods, hot flushes when hot, sleeping patterns disturbed, hot at night. Taking black gohosh as recommended by practice nurse after routine check up/ smear. Client feels menopause has made skin drier.

Overall comments: Client has taken care of skin: not a smoker, drinks plenty of water. Her general health is reflected in her healthy skin, with no obvious signs of any problems, except her concerns about going through the menopause. Not keen on sunbathing as she is fair, and has always worn a hat when abroad.

Client's previous treatments/results: Mrs Jones has had no electrical facials with this salon, but did enjoy the paraffin mask and would like to have more moisturising masks.

Recommendations:
* Course of facial faradic treatments and galvanic facials to keep skin exfoliated and rehydrated
* Warm oil mask would be enjoyed
* Galvanic facial would rehydrate the skin
* Recommended microdermabrasion treatment to deeply exfoliate the skin
* Speak to Elaine regarding removal of capillary damage around the nostrils
* Upper lip wax as client is aware of hair on the upper lip

Client signature: J. Jones	**Date:** 12/9/10
Therapist signature: T. Sumera	**Date:** 12/9/10

A typical facial record card

The facial observation

When you are confident that no contra-indications prevent the client from having the treatment, you should invite the client to lie on to the couch in readiness for the skin analysis. The positioning of the client is the same as for manual facial treatments. The client should be cocooned within the bedding, with only the face showing, turban on, and jewellery on the trolley in a bowl. The client should feel warm and secure.

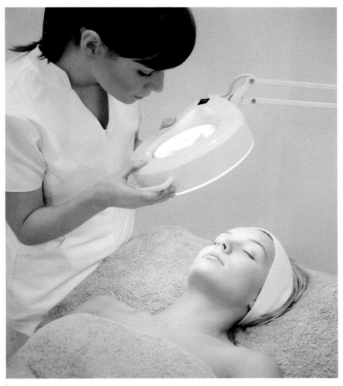

Facial observation

An electrical facial consultation is very similar to a Level 2 consultation/observation, except that your treatment recommendations will involve electrical equipment, so try to be meticulous and thorough. You will need to see the skin in its natural state, that is without make-up — if a client is adept at make-up application, then the true condition of the skin could be hidden.

Think about it

Ask your client if he or she is wearing contact lenses. The client may be happy to keep them in, or might prefer to remove them. For steaming and electrical treatments, the client may prefer to take out the lenses.

Client modesty

For the female client:

- Tights and half-slip may be kept on, but shoes should be removed.

- Bra straps may get oily and should be dropped off the shoulder, or the bra may be taken off altogether, especially if it has metallic strap adjusters. Metal is a good conductor of electricity, and the client may find there is an accumulation of current, and a stronger sensation under the metal, if she keeps her bra on.

- If the client chooses to push her straps down on to the top of the arm, there is still a danger they will get massage medium on them, as you will be going halfway down the upper arm with your movements. Encourage the client to remain topless, but with a small modesty towel around the bust area, which she may wish to keep with her at all times.

For the male client:

- Since facial massage includes the upper back and shoulders, the shirt or T-shirt should be removed, and the client's chest covered with towels and/or blankets to prevent his upper body getting cold.

- Most male clients are not as sensitive to current as a female, as their skin is slightly thicker, but the current is attracted to the moisture in hairs, so if the client is hairy, he may transmit the current quite well.

- Metal facial piercings should be removed, and if the body has any piercings, cover them with a plaster, where appropriate.

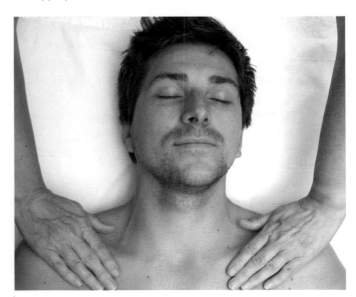

Male facials are big business and increasingly popular

Skin analysis

Once the client is comfortably positioned on the couch, and you have washed your hands, you will be ready to begin skin analysis (for information about the skin, see page 222).

Ask the client if they would prefer to have their eyes covered with cotton wool rounds, or if they would just like to close their eyes. If the client is prone to migraines, fold over a small towel to block out the light, to make it more comfortable for them, or use eye goggles for extra protection.

Look closely when doing a skin analysis. Use a magnifying lamp to illuminate the face, and study the facial contours, jaw line, chin, nose, cheeks and forehead. You are looking for:

- the skin's general condition
- texture, colour and secretions on the skin
- pore size
- any area of shininess
- dry flaky patches
- comedones or blocked pores or papules
- skin problems, for example acne rosacea or acne vulgaris
- the contours of the face — any loss of elasticity or dropped contours
- dilated capillaries
- build-up of dead skin cells, seen as uneven and dull-looking skin
- horizontal lines in forehead and lines appearing in the nasolabia folds of the mouth
- dehydration
- areas of pigmentation.

What you see is very important, and you need to use your consultation skills to confirm verbally with the client exactly what you have seen and how this may affect the client and the treatment plan. Questions such as 'How long have you had a broken capillary on your nose?' will lead into a discussion as to whether the client regards it as a problem, if she is conscious of it and would like to have it treated, or if it does not bother her, perhaps because she can hide it with make-up.

When looking at the skin, you can also talk about the client's current skin care range, and how happy the client is with the results.

For example:

- Are they using a regular exfoliant to help slough off the dead skin cells?
- Does the colour look a little flat and dull?
- Would the skin benefit from having the circulation stimulated, bringing oxygen and nutrients to the cells?
- Are the current products drying out the top layers of the skin?
- Does the skin look plump and full of moisture, or dehydrated and dry, with lines?
- How firm is the jaw line? Is the client developing a double chin?
- How much water is the client drinking every day to keep the skin clear and healthy?

Manual examination of the face

Most of the information gathered on the record card is from questioning the client and observation of the facial skin condition, but you will also need to feel the skin's texture, warmth and contours. This will be done when carrying out the superficial and deep cleansing routine — your fingertips will alert you to rough patches of skin, moles and raised areas of skin, which may not be visible but can be felt.

A cold face will often indicate poor circulation, or a hot face may be a sign of the client's age, and the onset of the menopause, which often affects body temperature regulation. In fact, hormones are one of the key factors in the skin's behaviour, along with diet, water intake and environmental aspects and product use. (To refresh your knowledge of factors that influence the skin, see You and the skin and Related anatomy and physiology.)

Be aware that the client may be very adept at applying make-up, so the skin might look flawless and there may be no visible problems. However, with make-up removed, your light massage technique during cleansing may tell a different story. Feel for cysts, raised moles and indentations. You are also feeling the firmness of the tissue, whether there is good muscular support and the skin feels firm to the touch, easily springing back when manipulated. Older skins are less springy because the supporting collagen fibres begin to weaken, resulting in the skin and underlying tissue feeling a little slack. (For a full breakdown of skin types see You and the skin, page 242.)

Think about it

Another factor affecting the contours of the face is if the client has had extensive dental work done, or has recently had dentures fitted – this affects the gums, cheek muscles and jaw line, especially if the client is not yet comfortable with their new teeth. If this is the case, avoid any heavy pressure along the lower face, as it will be uncomfortable for the client.

Once you have completed the facial examination, you are ready to discuss and then carry out facial treatments with the client's permission.

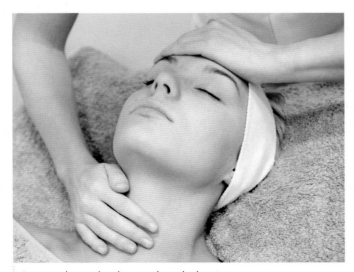

A manual examination can be relaxing too

Equipment used in facial treatments

On the following pages is a brief rundown of the equipment used in facial treatments, their benefits to the client and the client type most suited to the equipment. For a list of the equipment used in body treatments, see pages 354–361.

Although most equipment used would be classed as electrical because it works from mains electricity, in beauty therapy equipment is also grouped according to the effect it has on the body.

- Electrical treatments such as galvanic current, microcurrent, high-frequency and faradic treatments are those which send an adapted electrical current through the body.

- Mechanical treatments are those using equipment that has only an external effect on the body. These include G5, vacuum suction, microdermabrasion and small massage equipment such as audio-sonic.

Think about it

Refer to Unit B14 Provide facial electrical treatments, for a full explanation and procedure of use for all equipment in facial procedures.

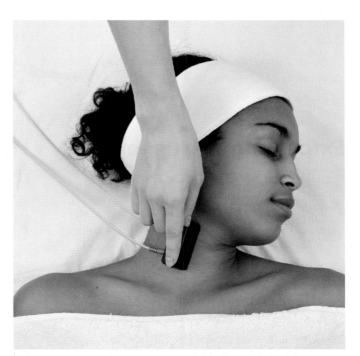

There is a range of equipment available for use in facial treatments

Pre-warming treatments

STEAMING (facial unit or the wet area cabinet or steam room)

Uses and client needs	Suitable skin type/body type	
Moist heat – a heating element boils the water, which creates a jet of steam from a nozzle or outlet. Can be used to warm the tissues of the face, upper chest or back when using a facial steaming unit. The whole body is immersed in a steam room. A steam cabinet treats the body only; the face is outside the cabinet Helps open the pores and cleanse the skin Warms the muscle fibres and relaxes them, making other treatments after steaming very effective Very good prior to comedone extraction, but be careful to time the treatment, as if erythema occurs too strongly it may contra-indicate other treatments	Most skin types, except where contra-indications are present Timing of treatment can be adjusted to suit skin types	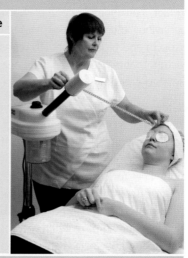

INFRARED LAMP

Uses and client needs	Suitable skin type/body type	
An infrared light bulb is fixed into a fitting with a swivel arm on a stand, making it easy to place the lamp into a suitable position Used to create extra blood flow, which generates heat for the skin and underlying tissue. Muscle fibres will soften and it can be used effectively on any part of the body Can only treat small areas at a time, due to the limited arc of light from the lamp. Can be used on the face, chest or upper back Time the treatment, as if an erythema occurs too strongly, it may contra-indicate other treatments Can also be used on the face with a hot oil mask	Most skin types, except where contra-indications are present Timing of treatment can be adjusted to suit skin type. Where used with hot oil mask, dry skin only	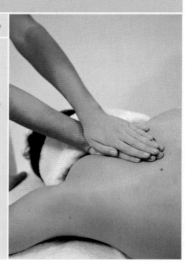

Exfoliating treatments

FACIAL SCRUB

Uses and client needs	Suitable skin type/body type	
An exfoliant can be applied prior to most facial electrical treatments and is convenient if the client does not have the time to have a steam treatment The product is applied using the hands, in small circular motions, and then removed with sponges and warm water, once the entire face and neck have been covered Some manufacturers provide mitts or facial sponges with a rough surface to enhance the exfoliation, so always follow manufacturer's instructions	Most skin types, except where contra-indications are present Timing of treatment can be adjusted to suit skin types. Can be used on acne-prone skin on the body as well	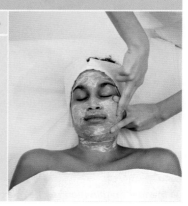

BRUSH CLEANSING

Uses and client needs	Suitable skin type/body type	
A brush-cleansing machine has a motor, which rotates a hand-held head that can have a variety of brushes inserted into it. The speed of the rotations is adjustable to suit the client's needs and preference, as is the direction of the revolution – clockwise or anti-clockwise. Brushes of various thickness and stiffness will alter the treatment effect, as will the accompanying products used with the machine Most water-based products are suitable, from basic foaming facial wash used to cleanse the face, back or congested chest area, to cleansing grains and specialist creams for particular skin problems The effect of the treatment is one of exfoliation and stimulation to the skin and circulation. Can also be a useful tool in the removal of peels or masks from the face	Most skin types, except where contra-indications are present. Product use will be determined by skin type or problem Timing of treatment can be adjusted to suit skin type	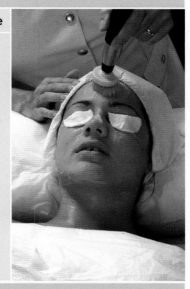

MICRODERMABRASION

Uses and client needs	Suitable skin type/body type	
Microdermabrasion works using a controlled flow of ultra-clean aluminium oxide crystals set in motion by vacuum-created low pressure. The crystals are applied to the skin with a special hand piece that allows for the controlled and gentle removal of dead cells from the stratum corneum of the epidermis. The same hand piece removes the used crystals and skin particles in a single process and deposits them in a separate container There is no risk of crystal-related side effects as they are completely inert The flow of crystals and the depth of peeling is perfectly controllable, and the treatment also allows deep penetration of hydrating products into the clean skin	All skin types except where contra-indications are present. Excellent as a rejuvenating treatment before a special event such as a wedding, or for a course of treatments to help clear acne or reduce the appearance of scarring or stretch marks	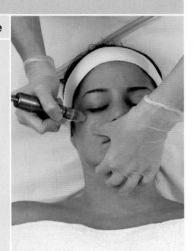

Manual massage treatments

SWEDISH MASSAGE

Uses and client needs	Suitable skin type/body type	
Using the hands, the tissue is manipulated in a series of movements for the neck, upper back, head and face Can be stimulating or relaxing, depending upon the movements used, but the most sought-after treatment outcome is for removal of tension nodules within the muscle fibres and total relaxation of the mind and body	Most skin types, except where contra-indications are present Timing and product use will be determined by skin type or problem	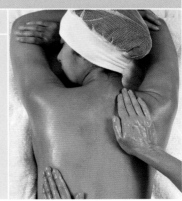

AROMATHERAPY MASSAGE

Uses and client needs	Suitable skin type/body type	
Massage to the head, face and body using pre-blended aromatherapy oils Offers the benefits of massage with the addition of the relaxing, uplifting and stimulating effects of the blends of oils Oils are personally chosen by the therapist to suit the client's emotional and physical needs and the effects required	All skin types except where contra-indications are present	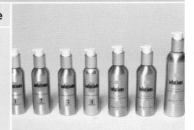

INDIAN HEAD MASSAGE

Uses and client needs	Suitable skin type/body type	
Indian head massage is an Eastern technique based on Ayurvedic philosophies, which date back 5000 years. It includes massage of the shoulders, neck, face and scalp Offers the benefits associated with massage, but also rebalancing of the chakras of the body and restoration of the emotional wellbeing of the client Various oils are used to further enhance the effectiveness of the massage – for stimulation, relaxation or the improvement of the hair and scalp condition	All skin types except where contra-indications are present	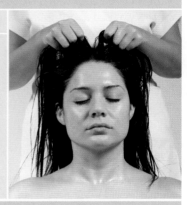

HOT STONE MASSAGE

Uses and client needs	Suitable skin type/body type	
The use of hot stone massage is an ancient tradition in countries with volcanic geology. The hot basalt stones serve as an extension of the therapist's hands to enhance the effects of massage and also to reduce the possibility of repetitive strain injury for the therapist Warming effects of hot stones on the tissue help deepen the effects of the massage and can rebalance and neutralise negative energy Cold stones can also be used in conjunction with hot for a stimulating effect and the vibration energy of the stones also helps balance the seven chakras in the body	All skin types except where contra-indications are present	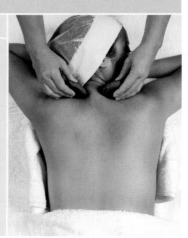

Mechanical massage treatments

AUDIO SONIC

Uses and client needs	Suitable skin type/body type
Deep penetrating sound-wave emissions can be used on any condition where deep massage helps, e.g. fibrocystic nodules, or tense muscle fibres of the upper back	Most skin types, except where contra-indications are present
This is a small hand-held device and therefore only suitable to treat small areas in one treatment: not suitable for a whole body massage, as it would be too time-consuming and not cost-effective	Not suitable/comfortable for fine-featured clients with very delicate facial contours or bony clients with very little body muscle bulk
When using on the face, it is most comfortably applied over the therapist's fingers, so they absorb some of the sound waves. The facial structure does not have the depth of muscle tissue to absorb the sound waves that the body has, and it is not as relaxing directly on the skin	

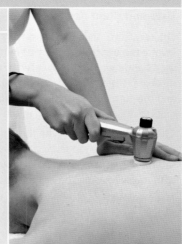

VACUUM SUCTION

Uses and client needs	Suitable skin type/body type
This machine uses a pump to create a vacuum within an attached cup, which picks up the tissue Can be used either: • to glide to the lymphatic nodes, in a single movement, or • to create a pulse within the vacuum, for extra stimulation	Check for contra-indications, as treatment will not be suitable for all skin types, especially thin or fine skin with a tendency to bruise easily
Vacuum suction promotes the face's lymphatic and circulatory systems, thus helping the removal of toxins from the area	Also, will not be comfortable on thin, bony clients or clients with older, crêpey skin
It is desquamating; it stimulates glandular activity and improves the general skin texture	
Very relaxing facial treatment, and can replace manual massage as part of a routine: many clients find it very soothing and drop off to sleep!	
There is also a multi-cup static vacuum suction machine for use with up to six cups at a time, but the cups remain static on the body, rather than used with a gliding movement. This is suitable for treating larger areas in one treatment such as the buttocks and upper thighs	

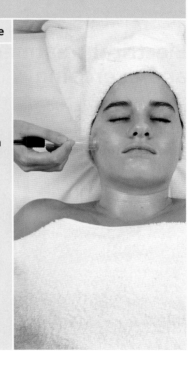

Electrical massage treatment

INDIRECT HIGH FREQUENCY

Uses and client needs	Suitable skin type/body type
Often called a 'Viennese massage', indirect high frequency involves creating a circuit of current, flowing through the client via a hand-held glass rod, called a saturator, connected to the machine. The therapist's hands make contact with the client and the current is discharged through her fingertips, as she is massaging, creating warmth in the area Can be used in place of the facial massage routine, although if clients become too relaxed, they will lose contact with the saturator which they should be holding. Avoid losing contact with the skin, as this breaks the circuit This deep massage will improve a dry skin, relax the tissues and help increase a poor or sluggish circulation to the area Creates warmth in the lower legs and feet, so could be incorporated into a pedicure	Most commonly used on dry or fine skins. The medium used is oil, which helps the glide of the treatment and lubricates the skin 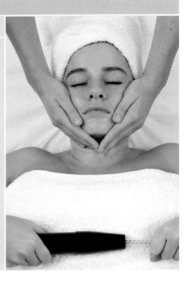

Electrical treatments for cleansing, healing, moisturising and exercising

DIRECT HIGH FREQUENCY

Uses and client needs	Suitable skin type/body type
Using a high-frequency machine, the current is transmitted into a glass electrode, which is in direct contact with the skin. Light circular motions then disperse the current This is a drying germicidal treatment, ideal for a seborrhoeic skin, one that is congested or has blemishes	Most commonly used on oily, congested or acne skin types, to the face, back or chest area 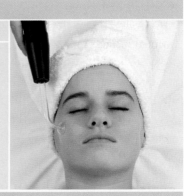

GALVANIC

Uses and client needs	Suitable skin type/body type
A galvanic machine uses a direct constant current for both face and body work, and the results depend upon the method of use and the gels and products used. The current has to create a circuit flowing through the client, either by using rollers with a connection in the client's hand or a pad under the shoulder, or by the use of body pads, to complete the circuit Can be used in two ways: • Desincrustation – removes the incrustation, i.e. the excess sebum, and gives a deep cleansing to the skin • Iontophoresis – introduces beneficial substances into the skin, to rebalance and rehydrate the skin, or to get active substances to stimulate the body's systems, which aids lymphatic drainage	Most skin types, except where contra-indications are present Desincrustation for oily skins or skins in need of a deep cleanse; iontophoresis for a dry skin or to rebalance the skin, to improve the skin texture or as an anti-cellulite treatment 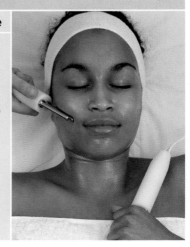

MICROCURRENT

Uses and client needs	Suitable skin type/body type	
A modified direct, low-frequency current which is used on its own for lifting of the facial or body contours and in conjunction with a galvanic current for skin improvement Can help with fine line reduction, stretch mark minimising and scar reduction, and deep cleansing	Most skin types, except where contra-indications are present	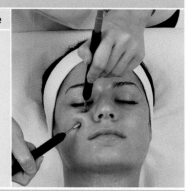

FARADIC

Uses and client needs	Suitable skin type/body type	
Using a surged and interrupted current, a faradic machine can stimulate muscular contractions on both the face and body Often referred to as passive exercise, you can actually see the muscles contracting under the pads whilst the client lies motionless on the couch The pads for the face are smaller than those used in body work, so it is possible to target specific muscle groups for improvement in tone and suppleness Treatment is ideal for double chins, dropped jaw line and cheekbone definition	Most skin types, except where contra-indications are present	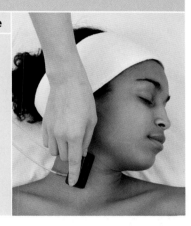

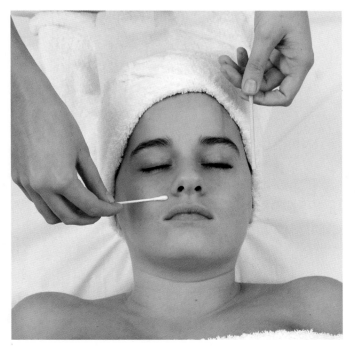

Always carry out thermal and sensitivity tests before any electrical treatment

Think about it

Whichever pieces of equipment you choose as the most suitable for the client's treatment plan, always follow the five golden rules:

1 Complete a full consultation.
2 Complete a contra-indication checklist.
3 Carry out thermal and sensitivity tests.
4 Follow the manufacturer's instructions.
5 Test the equipment on yourself before using it on the client.

Check your knowledge

What am I?

1 I improve muscle tone and facial contours, improve circulation and increase metabolism.

2 I stimulate circulation and increase metabolism, improve skin condition, alter the pH of the skin and help with absorption of products.

3 I am deep cleansing, open the pores, soften sebaceous plugs or comedones, improve the appearance of the skin and alter the pH of the skin.

4 I improve muscle tone and facial contours, lift and tone, improve the skin's condition and relax the client.

5 I dilate lymph and blood capillaries so increasing circulation and metabolic rate, removing lymph and waste, and improving the skin's appearance.

6 I heat the skin, increase vasodilation, speed up metabolism, dry the skin out slightly and am germicidal.

7 I am warming, soothing, relaxing and soften fine lines. I also improve the skin and stimulate the skin's functions whilst aiding the penetration of products.

8 I am an alternating, oscillating current.

9 I am a direct current with negative and positive polarity.

10 I am interrupted direct current low frequency surged and intermitted with biphasic or monophasic pulses.

11 I could be epilepsy, a pace maker, undiagnosed lumps and swellings, dysfunction of the nervous system, or failure of a thermal or sensitivity test.

12 I could be a galvanic burn, bruising, irritation, excessive erythema, muscle fatigue or fainting.

13 I filter toxins, produce antibodies and become swollen when infection is present in the body. You always work towards me.

14 I cause dropped contours, loss of muscle tone and often dryness, or dehydration.

15 I cause hot flushes and pigment changes, or oiliness and blackheads.

16 I cause redness of the skin and vasodilation of the surface capillaries.

Unit B14

Provide facial electrical treatments

What you will learn

- Maintain safe and effective methods of working when providing facial electrical treatments
- Consult, plan and prepare for treatments with clients
- Carry out facial electrical treatments and provide aftercare advice
- High frequency
- Lymphatic drainage (vacuum suction)
- Galvanism
- EMS – electro muscle stimulation (faradism)
- Microcurrent
- Microdermabrasion
- Micro-lance

Introduction

Choosing the right pieces of equipment for the client and then using them in a safe and appropriate manner will ensure the client receives a first-class treatment, with instant results. All of the electrical treatments used on the face perform several functions and offer a combination of the following benefits.

- They improve the skin condition.
- They improve muscle condition and the contours of the face.
- They improve lymphatic drainage to the face.
- They aid relaxation, both physical and mental.

In this section you will learn how to achieve all of this using:

- a high-frequency unit
- lymphatic drainage equipment (vacuum suction)
- a galvanic unit
- an electro muscle stimulator (a faradic unit)
- a microcurrent unit
- a microdermabrasion unit
- a micro-lance.

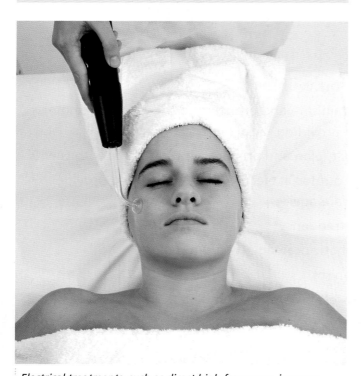

Electrical treatments, such as direct high frequency, improve skin condition and lymphatic drainage

The Standards set out detailed performance criteria regarding:

- maintaining safe and effective methods of working when providing facial electrical treatments
- consulting, planning and preparing for treatments with clients.

The majority of these requirements apply to all beauty therapy treatments and are therefore covered in detail in the Professional basics unit, the Facial consultation section and G22 Monitor procedures to safely control work operations. You should also refer back to the units on You and the skin and Related anatomy and physiology, as required.

Treatment-specific requirements for facial electrical treatments are covered within this unit in the individual treatment sections.

Carry out facial electrical treatments and provide aftercare advice

Using equipment safely

Using equipment safely and with confidence is essential, and it is very important that you follow the manufacturer's instructions for the machine you are using, since these will vary. Products used, treatment times and the dials showing strength of current will differ from one make of machine to another. The only way to be totally safe and competent for your assessments is to understand each machine thoroughly and know its capabilities. This will provide you with the confidence to treat clients in a professional manner, which in turn will give the client confidence in your abilities.

Before beginning a facial electrical treatment, you will need to refer closely to all the information you have learned so far – see Professional basics (page 2) and Facial treatments – theory and consultation (page 256).

Think about it

When learning how to use a new piece of equipment, gain dexterity skills by using it without current for a few sessions. This will help you gain confidence in using the rollers, prongs or pads, without the fear of breaking contact with the skin, or worrying about hurting the client. Once you feel comfortable and able to control the application of the equipment onto the skin, then use current.

Preparing the skin for treatment

Let's assume that the facial consultation has gone smoothly: the client has no contra-indications, the client is in a suitable

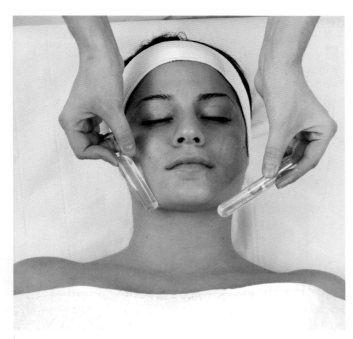

Carry out thermal sensitivity testing before beginning a facial electrical treatment

abrasion and the skin would be too red and irritated to have further treatments. These are massaged into the skin and then removed with warm sponges and water, or flannel mitts, which leave the skin softened and receptive. This form of pre-treatment is especially ideal for those clients who do not have the time for a full facial steam or brush-cleanse treatment.

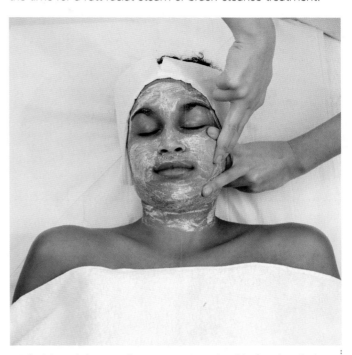

A facial scrub is a good way to prepare the skin for electrical treatments

position for treatment and you are ready to use your chosen electrical equipment (refer to Facial consultation, page 256, and You and the skin, page 222). The skin has been cleansed and is grease-free. It is still essential to further prepare the skin so it is receptive to the electrical treatment you are about to perform.

Also remember any electrical current is attracted to the moisture content in the hair shaft, therefore the hair needs to be well covered either in a towelling turban or a headband with net body. This should encase all of the hair to ensure the current stays concentrated on the skin.

Cleansing/exfoliants

Most commercial companies have a complementary pre-treatment cleanser, which differs from a make-up removal cleanser. Usually, it is an exfoliant containing micro beads to slough off any remaining dead skin cells from the surface of the epidermis, which may hinder the benefits of the treatment. Within the products, plant extracts and essential oils such as lavender, coconut, apricot kernels and aloe extracts ensure that the skin is gently exfoliated — too harsh an

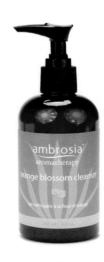

A pre-treatment cleanser

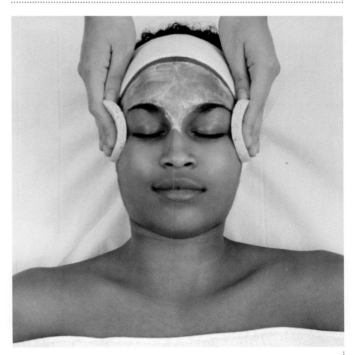

Remove the scrub with sponges and warm water

Facial cleanse and exfoliation – a step-by-step guide

1 Apply a cleanser and emulsify with a little water to make it wash over the skin easily.

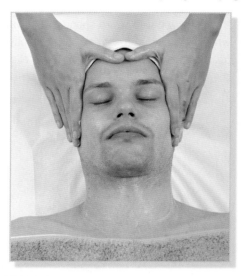

2 Remove cleanser with sponges and warm water.

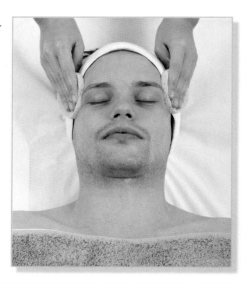

3 Apply a scrub or facial mask for a second deeper cleanse.

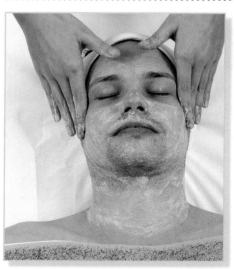

4 Remove scrub with sponges and warm water.

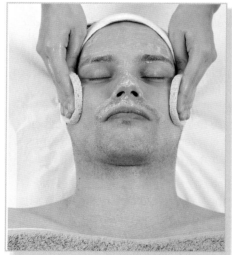

5 Blot the skin so it is dry and grease-free.

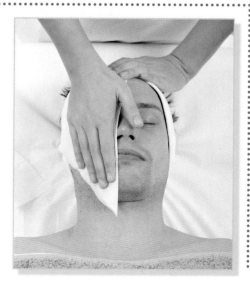

6 Skin is now fully prepared for further electrical treatments.

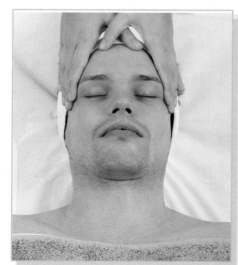

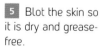

The different types of electrical currents have various effects on the body. Most of them will warm the skin and muscles through the increase in circulation to the area, lymphatic drainage will be stimulated by using the equipment in the direction of the nodes, and the nerve endings will be soothed by the heat generated. Only the faradic current is used to cause muscular contractions, and no electrical current has any effect on the skeleton.

High frequency

High frequency is a very useful multi-purpose machine: it can be used both directly and indirectly on most skin types and gives excellent results. However, the nature of the frequency means the machine is quite noisy to use, and some therapists are put off by this. However, use the machine often and, with practice, you will hardly notice the noise!

The high-frequency current

This is an alternating, oscillating, high-voltage, low-amperage current. A high-frequency machine produces a frequency of 100,000–250,000 Hertz (cycles per second).

Most beauty therapy equipment has a transformer within it, to alter the AC current but not the frequency (see Facial treatments – theory and consultation, page 260). This 'special transformer' in the high-frequency machine is an **induction coil** called an Oudin coil. The high-voltage, high-frequency current is not easy to confine with the insulation of a wire, so the Oudin coil is inside the hand piece which holds the **electrode**. This is why the electrode holder is round and fat. (Some manufacturers' instructions refer to the hand piece as the **Oudin resonator**.)

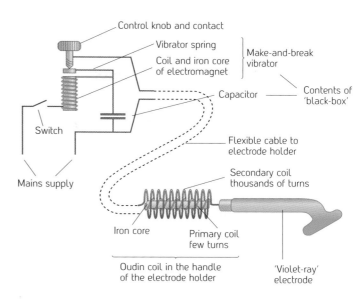

How a high-frequency unit works

The cabinet of the machine contains the **capacitor** and the 'make-and-break' vibrator to recharge it repeatedly. In most modern machines an electronic 'make-and-break' is used and this contributes to the buzzing noise when the machine is working.

As it alternates so rapidly, at more than 50 times per second, the current does not stimulate motor or sensory nerve endings. It is also the alternation that produces the high-pitched sound that is the characteristic of high frequency. High frequency is one of the few machines that does not require two connections to make a full circuit – the current is carried through the client's body, creating warmth by increasing the circulation.

It is very important that you are confident in the use of the machine, as the noise level can be disturbing to the nervous client, especially if applied on the face. A thorough explanation should be given during consultation.

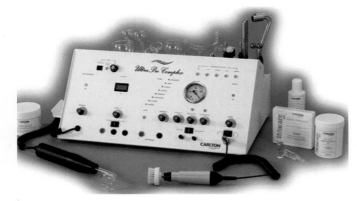

A high-frequency unit

Application

High frequency can be used in two ways:

- *Indirect* — the current flows through the client's body using the therapist's hands to perform massage which conducts the current. The client holds the intensified saturator electrode (called saturation).

- *Direct* — application is made directly onto the skin using an Oudin resonator (glass electrode).

High-frequency equipment may vary in general appearance between manufacturers, but the basic operations of the equipment will be similar. There are generally two main control switches — the on/off switch and the intensity control. A mains lead connects the unit to the power supply. A flex leads from the unit to the handle, which is used to house the glass electrodes. There are a variety of electrodes that the therapist can select to use, depending upon the method of application and the area to be treated and the desired effects. You will need to refer to individual manufacturer's instructions.

Think about it

Clean the heads with warm soapy water and dry thoroughly, or wipe with surgical spirit or Hibitane. The heads are made of glass, so be careful when handling them and store them correctly. They are easily broken and costly to replace!

Within each electrode a small quantity of inert gas is sealed, usually argon. As the current flows through the gas, a coloured glow is produced. The electrodes glow either blue/violet if they contain argon, or red/orange if they contain neon.

Contra-indications to high-frequency treatments

- Cuts or abrasions to the skin in the area to be treated
- Skin diseases or disorders
- Vascular conditions
- Sensitive skin
- Highly nervous clients
- Excessive metal in the area
- Swellings in the area
- Very hairy areas
- Sinus blockages
- Heart conditions
- Epilepsy or diabetes*
- Circulatory problems*
- Pregnancy*
- Asthmatics*

* Only to be carried out with medical approval.

Indirect high frequency

This method of applying the high-frequency current involves creating a circuit of current which flows from the saturator to charge the client. The therapist massages the client, which allows the current to discharge from the client's face or body to the therapist's massaging fingers or hand. This provides heat in the fingertips and creates a really deep, warming massage.

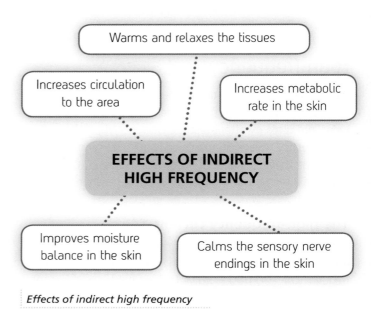

Warms and relaxes the tissues

Increases circulation to the area

Increases metabolic rate in the skin

EFFECTS OF INDIRECT HIGH FREQUENCY

Improves moisture balance in the skin

Calms the sensory nerve endings in the skin

Effects of indirect high frequency

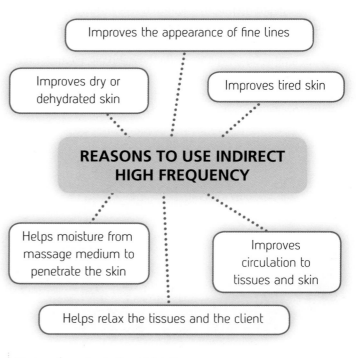

Improves the appearance of fine lines

Improves dry or dehydrated skin

Improves tired skin

REASONS TO USE INDIRECT HIGH FREQUENCY

Helps moisture from massage medium to penetrate the skin

Improves circulation to tissues and skin

Helps relax the tissues and the client

Reasons for using indirect high frequency

Indirect high frequency preparation and method – a step-by-step guide

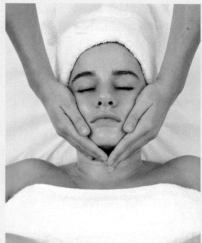

1. Observe general safety precautions for using electrical equipment.
2. Place the machine on a stable trolley.
3. Select the products required for treatment and place them on the trolley.
4. Check the machine and test to ensure it is working correctly.
5. Greet the client at reception and escort him/her to the treatment area.
6. Ensure a full consultation is carried out, contra-indications are checked, and the treatment is explained.
7. Help the client onto the couch, and protect hair and clothing in the usual manner.
8. Ask the client to remove all jewellery. Clean and prepare the skin with suitable products.
9. Carry out skin sensitivity testing.
10. Select a suitable medium and apply it to the client's face – a massage oil or nourishing cream is ideal – to feed the skin.
11. Ensure the mains lead is plugged into the mains supply and that all switches are off and all dials are at zero.
12. Test the machine in front of the client and reassure him/her where necessary about the buzzing noise that can be heard.
13. Apply talcum powder to the client's hands to absorb any perspiration; wipe the saturator with disinfectant and place it firmly in the holder. The client's talced hand makes good contact with the glass saturator. The other hand holds the black rubber handle.
14. Place one hand to make contact with the client's skin, using small circular effleurage movements, while with the other hand turning the intensity dial slowly to suit the client's tolerance. Always ask the client if he/she is comfortable with the intensity.
15. Place the other hand on to the skin by sliding over the first hand and begin your usual massage movements, ensuring that contact is not broken, i.e. no tapotement-type movements are used, as they would break contact and make the sensation of current uncomfortable.
16. The treatment time will vary between 8 and 12 minutes, depending upon the client's skin condition, skin reaction and the manufacturer's recommendations.
17. At the end of treatment, reverse the procedure of hands by taking one hand off, reducing and then turning off the current and then removing the other hand.
18. Remove the massage medium and continue with facial procedures most beneficial to the client, i.e. tone and moisturise.

Precautions during indirect high-frequency treatment

● Care should be taken around the hairline as sensation will be increased because hair is a good conductor.

● Contact must not be broken.

● Rings must not be worn by the client on the hand that holds the saturator.

● The client and therapist must not touch any metal conducting material while giving the treatment.

● The intensity of the current in the tissues will be increased when lifting one hand off.

● Care must also be taken with any belts that have metallic buckles that the therapist may be wearing as part of her uniform, or worn by the client if clothing is kept on.

● Try to avoid contact with the couch.

Think about it

Your normal massage routine can be followed, but you must not break contact with the skin, so avoid all tapotement-type (tapping, slapping) movements and concentrate on giving a relaxing, deep, penetrating, warm massage to those tense muscles.

Important note:

Indirect high-frequency application is the same for the face and body.

Used on dry skin with a suitable massage medium, in place of a normal manual massage.

Indirect contact – client holds saturator in their hand which is covered with talc.

Make contact with the skin before turning on the machine.

Ensure all dials at zero to start.

No tapotement movements.

After massage is completed, remove one hand and turn off machine before removing other hand.

Indirect high frequency at a glance

Wide comb electrode – some machines have a comb-like electrode which hairdressers can use over the scalp to stimulate blood circulation to the hair follicles. All the same procedures should be followed during treatment

Large facial bulb – used for direct high frequency facial and body work. Particularly useful for larger areas such as the chest and back

Roller electrode – this versatile roller can be used on any large area, especially the back, and is ideal for the nervous client as it does not spark because you shouldn't break contact with the skin. This glides easily and does not require any gauze or sliding agent

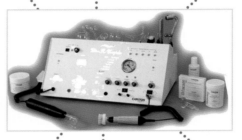

Neck electrode – specifically contoured to work on the neck area but equally versatile for any curved area, such as arms and legs

Small facial bulb – smaller bulb for use on the nose and around the ears – or if you have a client with a small face where the large facial bulb would be too big

Saturator – this electrode is used for indirect high frequency application only. The metal spiral inside the Pyrex or glass tubing ensures that only a gentle current is required for maximum effect

High-frequency electrodes

Think about it

After each treatment, wipe the electrode with an antiseptic solution, dry it and store it safely.

Direct high frequency

This method of application uses glass electrodes which are placed in direct contact with the client's skin. The current is dispersed at the point of contact with the client and as the effects are concentrated around the electrode, they are superficial but very beneficial to the skin.

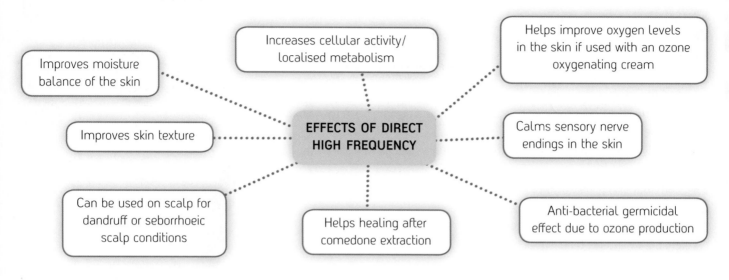

- Improves moisture balance of the skin
- Increases cellular activity/localised metabolism
- Helps improve oxygen levels in the skin if used with an ozone oxygenating cream
- Improves skin texture
- **EFFECTS OF DIRECT HIGH FREQUENCY**
- Calms sensory nerve endings in the skin
- Can be used on scalp for dandruff or seborrhoeic scalp conditions
- Helps healing after comedone extraction
- Anti-bacterial germicidal effect due to ozone production

Effects of direct high frequency

- Helps dry out a seborrhoeic or oily skin
- Helps destroy any bacteria present through the production of ozone
- **REASONS TO USE DIRECT HIGH FREQUENCY**
- Helps heal a problem scalp
- Improves condition of oily areas such as the T-zone or blemishes on the neck, chest or back

Reasons for using direct high frequency

Think about it

High-frequency currents should not be used on areas of skin that have been in contact with flammable liquids, such as alcohol toners, as there is a small risk that if sparking occurs they could ignite and cause burns.

Precautions during direct high frequency application

- Some manufacturers recommend the use of an oxygenating cream with direct high frequency, and because of the loose consistency of some creams (like beaten egg white), a gauze mask may be put over the skin to hold the product in place.

- Always use eye pads. Cut a nose hole for the client, to prevent the client feeling claustrophobic, and follow manufacturer's instructions.

- Sparking may occur when the electrode is lifted away from the skin. The spark produces ultraviolet rays which destroy bacteria. The germicidal effect is created by the ionisation of the oxygen in the air, which creates ozone. Controlled qualities of ozone help to promote the healing process; however, there are risks involved. The distance between skin and electrode should be only a few millimetres, causing the current to jump across the gap in an attempt to maintain contact. *Check with your individual Awarding Body regarding use of ozone and the practice of sparking.*

Direct high frequency preparation and method – a step-by-step guide

1. Observe general safety precautions for using electrical equipment.
2. Place the machine on a stable trolley.
3. Select the products required for treatment and place them on the trolley.
4. Check the machine and test to ensure it is working correctly.
5. Greet the client at reception and escort him or her to the treatment area.
6. Ensure a full consultation is carried out, contra-indications are checked, and the treatment is explained.
7. Help the client onto the couch, and protect hair and clothing in the usual manner.
8. Ask the client to remove all jewellery. Clean and prepare the skin with suitable products.
9. Carry out skin sensitivity testing.
10. Select a suitable medium and apply it to the client's face and neck – refined talc or ozone cream is ideal – to dry the skin.
11. Ensure the mains lead is plugged into the mains supply and that all switches are off and all dials are at zero.
12. Test the machine in front of the client and reassure the client where necessary about the buzzing noise that can be heard.
13. Apply the electrode in one of two ways. Either place the electrode in contact with the client's skin and move it around using small circular movements while turning up the intensity to suit the client's tolerance, or place the finger in contact with the electrode before turning the machine on, then turn the intensity dial up and place both finger and electrode in contact with the client's skin before removing the finger.
14. The treatment time will vary depending upon the client's skin condition, for example oily skin 8–15 minutes, but follow manufacturer's instructions and recommendations.
15. The facial can then continue in the normal way with appropriate products.

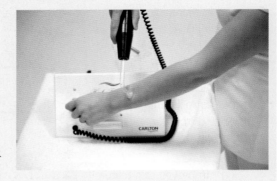

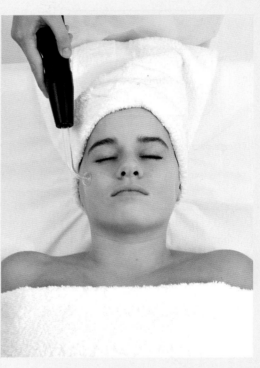

● Always follow the procedure recommended for the machine you are using. Some companies recommend finishing with oxygenating cream and direct high frequency, especially after a galvanic facial, so the client's skin benefits from the oxygenating cream as the final product; others continue with a mask and massage. This is especially true of companies whose products all contain the same active ingredients and therefore the mask and massage continue to bring benefits to the skin. Both of these methods are acceptable, so ensure you follow the product specifications fully.

● In the past, talcum powder was used as a medium for good conductivity, but its drying effects are not beneficial for a dry or dehydrated skin. Contact your own professional association for recommendations. Large quantities of talc should not be used as it is believed to have carcinogenic effects on some people, and its use is not recommended near the nose or mouth in case of accidental inhalation, especially if the client has a history of asthma or respiratory problems.

Think about it

The application of the direct high-frequency electrode creates warmth on the skin and converts the stable oxygen molecules in the oxygenating cream to unstable ozone molecules which may have a germicidal effect.

Drying, germicidal effect, often used with oxygenating cream or talc.

Place saturator on to the skin before switching on.

Use small, circular movements — avoid breaking contact.

Switch off before removing the saturator from the skin.

Often carried out after galvanic to finish treatment.

Direct high frequency at a glance

The following table gives a risk assessment for high-frequency treatments.

Identify the hazard	What is the risk?
Danger from electric shock	Low
Risk of sparking the client	High
Risk of small burn to the area	Low
Talc inhalation	Low
Postural problems for the therapist	Low

What should I do to prevent the hazard from becoming a risk?

- Follow manufacturers' instructions
- Make sure the saturator or bulb is firmly inserted into the handle
- Test on yourself before treatment
- Ensure no jewellery is worn by the client or therapist, especially using the indirect method, as current can be attracted to the metal and the client may experience a burn in the area
- Avoid inhalation of talc – especially if the client has respiratory problems
- Make sure the machine is positioned close to you, so that you have full control over the intensity dials and the saturator/electrodes – do not lean over the client or make contact with the couch
- Ensure correct posture and chair height to allow you to be in control of equipment
- Do not make sparks by breaking contact with the skin, especially around the eyes and mouth
- Not recommended for use with any flammable liquid, such as alcohol toner, as there is a small risk that if sparking occurs, they could ignite and cause burns
- The electrode should always be in contact with the client's skin before turning on the current and machine should be turned off before removal of electrode

Risk assessment for high frequency

Aftercare and homecare for high frequency

- Discuss the client's normal product use – this is often the cause of recurring skin problems, where clients are not using the correct product type for their skin's needs.

- Often the skin is so completely clean and has a germicidal finish (with direct high frequency) that no other care, such as cleansing or toning, and moisturiser are required for 24 hours after treatment.

- Advise the client to avoid picking or touching the skin, especially with unclean hands.

- See You and the skin, page 222, for other skin recommendations.

Lymphatic drainage (vacuum suction)

When used properly, vacuum suction is a gentle and effective treatment, and so relaxing that the client should fall asleep when this treatment is being carried out! The only rule of thumb with vacuum is that you should work towards the lymph nodes, to reinforce the natural draining ability of the lymphatic system. Vacuum suction is effective when used in conjunction with other treatments, or it can be offered on its own, and good results will be seen in the skin's appearance after a course of treatments. It is equally effective on the body: the principle being the same, just with bigger cups.

Think about it

In the United States this technique is referred to as non-invasive sub-dermal therapy (NIST).

The vacuum suction current

A vacuum therapy treatment to either the face or body is classed as a mechanical treatment performed with the aid of a compressor, as there is no electrical current flowing through the body.

A vacuum suction machine works using a pump action which creates a vacuum in the various cups attached to the tubing. A cup is referred to as a ventouse, and they come in a variety of shapes, depending upon the client's needs.

Most vacuum suction machines are very straightforward and have an on/off switch, an intensity control to adjust the vacuum pressure within the cup and a pulsation switch to alter the vacuum, which creates a mini pressure within the cup.

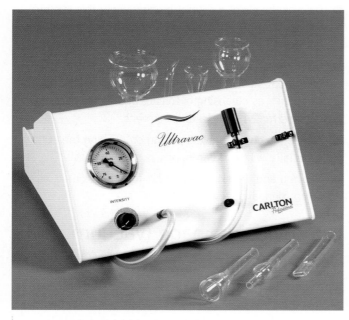

A vacuum suction machine

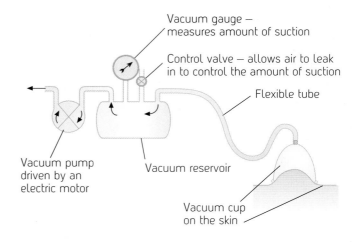

Vacuum gauge — measures amount of suction

Control valve — allows air to leak in to control the amount of suction

Flexible tube

Vacuum pump driven by an electric motor

Vacuum reservoir

Vacuum cup on the skin

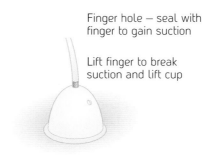

Finger hole — seal with finger to gain suction

Lift finger to break suction and lift cup

How a vacuum suction machine works

Application

By compressing the tissue into a cup and using a gliding and/or pulsation method of application, you will be aiding the body to move the lymph fluid nearer to the nodes to be filtered and improve the skin's condition.

Care must be taken not to have too great a vacuum within the cup as this compresses the tissue and capillaries may burst, causing bruising. However, facial cups are quite small, and testing on yourself prior to application should prevent this.

To ease application and removal, most cups have a small inlet hole, which needs to be covered with the finger so that the tube is sealed to create the vacuum. This means that when you want to break the vacuum and lift the cup away from the skin to go on to the next movement, you can do so easily, without having to flick the cup off the skin, so giving a smoother sensation and preventing possible damage.

Application is always carried out over a lubricating product, usually oil-based, to prevent dragging of the skin. Always glide the ventouse towards the nearest lymph nodes. Avoid pressure on the skin; instead try to create a little lift away from the skin, while keeping the vacuum inside steady, to avoid bruising and to make the gliding action pleasant for the client.

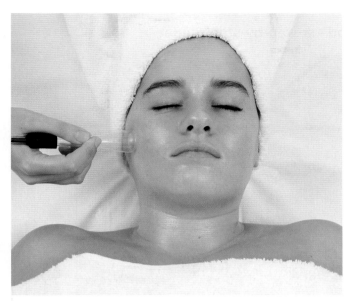

A vacuum suction treatment

Think about it

If you are unsure whether the client is suitable for a facial vacuum treatment, try to pick up on the facial tissue around the jaw line. If you cannot pick up any tissue, the client's skin is too thin for a vacuum treatment; offer an alternative treatment.

Contra-indications to vacuum treatments

- Delicate, sensitive skins
- Broken capillaries or thread veins
- Couperus conditions
- Loose, older skin with little underlying tissue
- Infected skin sites
- Acne with the presence of pustules
- Recent scar tissue
- Cuts, bruises and abrasions
- Sunburn
- Thin, bony areas
- Undiagnosed swelling
- Fine skin texture, for example found in diabetics
- Epilepsy
- Herpes simplex
- Any glandular swelling
- Very hairy areas, while not strictly a contra-indication, may not be very comfortable for the client. This may apply to facial hair, as well as body treatments.

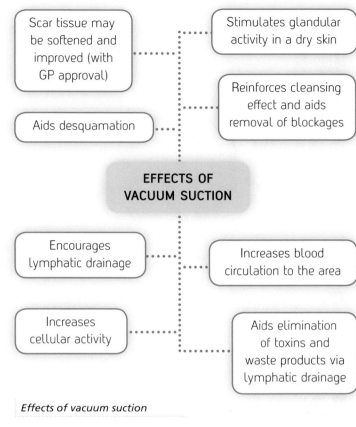

Scar tissue may be softened and improved (with GP approval)

Stimulates glandular activity in a dry skin

Aids desquamation

Reinforces cleansing effect and aids removal of blockages

EFFECTS OF VACUUM SUCTION

Encourages lymphatic drainage

Increases blood circulation to the area

Increases cellular activity

Aids elimination of toxins and waste products via lymphatic drainage

Effects of vacuum suction

Removes oily and cellular matter

General skin cleansing on normal, dry or combination skins

REASONS FOR USING VACUUM SUCTION

For dry, dehydrated or sluggish mature skins in need of stimulation for circulation, lymphatic drainage and cellular functioning

Removes skin blockages caused by incorrect cleansing of a seborrhoeic skin

Reasons for using vacuum suction

Vacuum suction treatment preparation and method – a step-by-step guide

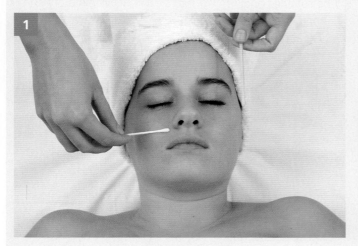

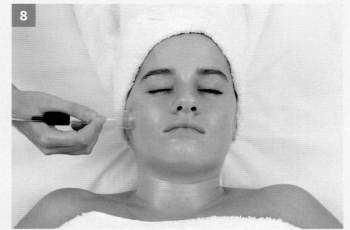

1 Ensure the skin is thoroughly cleansed. Carry out sensitivity testing on the face.

2 Carefully insert the selected ventouse into the black coupling connector at the end of the tubing (often referred to as a universal fitting, as it should house all sizes of ventouse).

3 Set switch to 'on' and check that intensity dial is at zero.

4 Test machine on yourself in front of the client by turning up the intensity control clockwise until sufficient suction is obtained to glide on the skin, while maintaining a vacuum.

5 Turn off, then apply the massage medium to the face and neck with a mask brush or manual massage strokes.

6 Apply the applicator on the chest below the clavicle in an easy flowing stroke over the surface – adjust the intensity to the skin's reaction and resistance. The lift into the applicator should not exceed 20 per cent.

7 Follow the diagram for the pattern of strokes. The duration of the treatment may vary from 3 to 5 minutes for general cleansing to 10 to 12 minutes for massage and lymphatic drainage.

8 Always follow in the direction of the nodes.

9 Check client's skin for reaction. If a strong erythema occurs, this would be a contra-action to treatment – do not continue with the treatment.

10 The size and shape of the applicators used depends on the skin's sensitivity and the effect required, for example general cleansing, toning or removal of skin blockage.

11 Turn off the machine with one hand, or break contact by releasing the air hole in the side of the ventouse.

12 The treatment concludes with the removal of the oil followed by a cleansing mask or further manual application, according to the routine chosen.

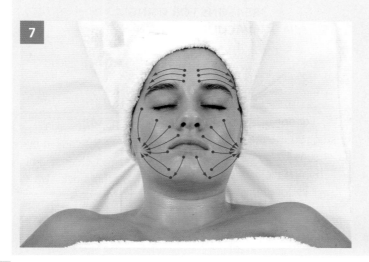

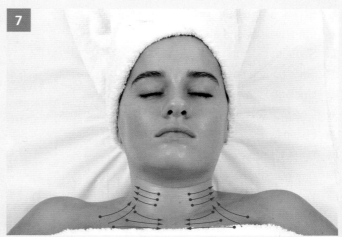

The table below describes the use of glass vacuum applicators.

Pore blockage – used to remove specific areas of blockage which group together and need intensive treatment, e.g. on the chin area. Also used in anti-wrinkle treatment

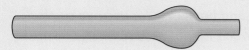

Comedone – the small round opening is placed over the comedone, ensuring that the pressure is exerted evenly on the surrounding tissue, to avoid scarring

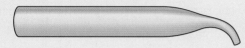

Lymph drainage – the flat-head ventouse can be used for most vacuum therapy treatments; it will cleanse the pores while ensuring that the skin is not over-pressurised. It can also be used to work in the facial lines or give a lymph drainage massage

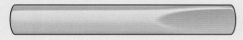

Facial cups (small = 21mm; medium = 27mm) – used for lymph drainage massage or general cleansing, lifting and stimulation of the area, depending upon the facial contours of the client

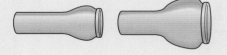

Glass vacuum applicators/ventouse

Each glass ventouse, except the comedone extractor, has an air hole on the side, which when covered creates the vacuum. This provides easy release and prevents skin drag or bruising.

Think about it

When using the pulsating programme of the machine, always start and finish with gliding only to help waste materials drain into the lymph nodes.

Always work towards the lymph nodes in the area.

Remove the ventouse by breaking the vacuum – release the finger from the hole.

Never flick or pull the ventouse from the skin.

Vacuum suction at a glance

Precautions during vacuum suction

- Choose the most appropriate-shaped ventouse and cup size.
- Cover the hole at the side of the ventouse to create the vacuum.
- Always test on yourself, even when changing the ventouse for a different-shaped one. When testing on yourself, only fill to 20 per cent of cup.
- Place ventouse on client before turning up intensity.
- The lift into the applicator should not exceed 20 per cent of the cup's volume.
- Put on plenty of product to lubricate the gliding movements.
- Always work towards the lymph nodes in the area.
- Always remove the ventouse by breaking the vacuum, by releasing the finger from the hole.
- Never flick or pull the ventouse from the skin.
- Keep a hand towel on the trolley and remove all oil from your hands before attempting to change the ventouse. With slippery hands, the ventouse can easily break and become a hazard. Always change the ventouse over the trolley, and not near the client.
- After each treatment, place glass applicators into warm soapy water with a little antiseptic solution, and clean thoroughly, then dry, to leave the glass clean and oil-free, or follow the manufacturer's recommendations. Be careful, the applicators are very delicate and can easily be broken.
- Place applicators in the back of the machine for safe storage, or wrap them up in cotton wool or similar, to prevent damage when not in use.

The following table gives a risk assessment for vacuum suction.

Identify the hazard	What is the risk?
Danger from electric shock	Low
Bruising to the area	High
Dragging on the skin resulting in pain for the client	High
Spreading of infection	High
Skin damage from broken ventouse	Low
Postural problems for the therapist	Low

What should I do to prevent the hazard from becoming a risk?

- Follow manufacturers' instructions
- Test on yourself before treatment to ensure less than 20 per cent tissue in the cup
- The ventouse should always be in contact with the client's skin before turning on the vacuum and the machine should be turned off before removal of ventouse
- Always start on zero intensity
- Always have sufficient product on the skin to keep it well lubricated
- Constantly monitor for any developing contra-actions
- Choose the correct size of ventouse for the area
- Always carry out a consultation and never treat a client who has an infection present
- Never flick or pull the ventouse from the skin; always use the hole in the tube to release the pressure
- Always change the ventouse over the trolley top and not near the client, and always remove oil from your fingers when attempting to pull the ventouse from the nozzle, to avoid slippery fingers dropping the glass ventouse
- Always clean and sterilise the ventouse thoroughly after each treatment
- Ensure correct posture and chair height to allow you to be in control of equipment

Risk assessment for vacuum suction

Recommended course of treatment

This treatment should be appropriate for most skin types.

- Dry, mature skin – within the normal treatment course.
- Oily, seborrhoeic skin – used in conjunction with steam treatment, desincrustation or specialised cleansing masks. Course of six to ten treatments or until desired effects achieved; once a week.
- Normal skin – within the normal treatment course.

Salon treatment

Vacuum suction can be used with any appropriate treatment or electrical therapy suitable for the client's skin type. It is especially beneficial after facial faradic treatment to aid with the elimination of lactic acid build-up in the muscles.

Aftercare and homecare for vacuum suction

- Recommend suitable skin preparations and masks.
- Suggest a regular skin cleansing routine and regular salon treatments.
- Stress the need for regular use of a good moisturiser and night cream.
- If skin is congested and comedone extraction is required in the salon, recommend an exfoliant suitable for the skin type.
- Advise the client to avoid picking and touching the skin after treatment.
- See You and the skin, page 222, for other skin recommendations.

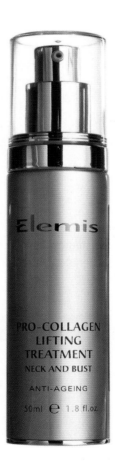
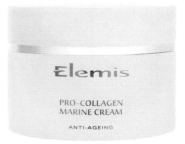

Suggest appropriate aftercare products

Galvanism

Most commercial companies offer treatments using a galvanic current, and although the products and names may be slightly different, the underlying principles are the same. Once you understand the theory of how a galvanic current is used, any other external training you receive should make sense.

Larger salons are offered training when they initially invest in a branded galvanic system such as Rene Guinot, Perfector or Carlton, and they also purchase a stock of products for retail and salon use. The financial outlay may be quite high, but the training of staff is often included within the price and in return for training, the therapist is expected to be loyal to the salon for a period of time (anything from 1—3 years, depending upon the contract of employment).

Along with understanding how to use a particular machine, the therapist receives very thorough product knowledge, which supports the salon treatments, and also becomes certificated and insured for that machine. The therapist also receives a badge stating that she has trained with the company. So, although your NVQ Level 3 training will be sufficient to operate a machine, you will still be expected to undergo further commercial training for galvanic use when you join a salon.

The galvanic current

The galvanic current is a direct, constant current, with low voltage, which can be used in two ways on the face and body. It is measured in milliamps. This is shown on the front on the machine in either a window with a metal arm moving along a series of numbers, or a digital reading, or crystal display unit. (Refer to Unit B13 Provide body electrical treatments for information on galvanic body treatments.)

A galvanic machine contains:

- a rectifier, to change the alternating mains current into a direct one
- a capacitor, which smoothes any irregularities within the constant stream of electrons
- a transformer, to reduce the voltage from the mains supply.

Think about it

A galvanic current is an electric current produced by a chemical action, and can be used for hair removal (electrolysis), and the penetration of substances into the skin for deep cleansing and hydration.

Application

A galvanic current can be used in two ways:

- Desincrustation — deep cleansing of the skin, usually to prepare the skin for iontophoresis, but it can also be used on its own.
- Iontophoresis — used to penetrate beneficial creams, ampoules or solutions into the skin for a specific treatment depending on the client's needs. It is also used in cellulite treatments on the body to penetrate diuretic-based gels into the skin to stimulate lymphatic drainage.

Both methods have two fundamental principles for correct use:

- the polarity of the product used on the skin
- the polarity setting of the machine.

Penetration of products into the skin is only successful because of the action of the **ions**, when forced into action by the current. According to the basic laws of polarity, the same poles repel each other but opposite poles are attracted to each other, because the atoms want to hook up and be complete in their formation.

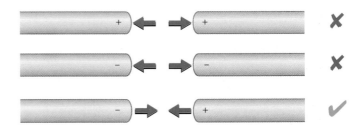

Like poles repel; unlike poles attract

The client forms a circuit by holding a covered **electrode** in the hand, which is linked to the machine. The rollers are also linked to the machine and when placed on the face, a circuit is formed through which the current can flow. If the polarity of the rollers is the same as the cream, then they

Key terms

Ions – atoms, or group of atoms, which have a positive or negative charge.

Anion – a negatively charged ion.

Cation – a positively charged ion.

Electrodes – the conductors of the electrolytes in contact with the skin.

Provide facial electrical treatments **Unit B14**

will not attract one another – and the ions in the cream will be attracted to the electrode in the hand, therefore going through the skin to get there. (If the polarity is set wrongly, and the cream is negative and the rollers are positive, or vice versa, then the cream is attracted to the rollers, and the client's skin receives no benefit at all!)

That is the basis of any galvanic treatment, regardless of which system you are using.

Manufacturers produce many differing creams, ampoules and gels with **electrolytes** (or ions) in them, so you will always have to check which polarity to use, but as long as the rollers and the gels are the same polarity, they will not be attracted and as the client has an opposite electrode in the hand, the cream/gel will penetrate.

On some machines, the current will not work if you insert the coloured leads into the other coloured socket, for example the **black lead** into the red socket. Also be careful that you do not put one of the rollers into the red socket and the other one in the black – this will not work either, as you are not completing a circuit. *The rollers must be of the same polarity* – usually, they come out of the red socket, and the hand-held electrode is out of the black. Confusion occurs because the rollers are a pair, but often have a linking wire into the **red lead**, so check to make sure they are not plugged into the different sockets.

Key terms

Electrolysis – the chemical decomposition of a substance by passage of an electric current through it. Also used in the destruction and permanent removal of hairs, moles, spider naevi, etc.

Polarity switch – dial found on the machine. It can reverse the polarity of the electrodes, without having to remove them from the body – although on most machines you have to turn off the current before you reverse the polarity. If you were doing desincrustation only, you might want to reverse the polarity for just a minute to reduce the erythema on the skin. For anti-cellulite treatments, you may find you do the same thing for the same reason – check with individual manufacturer's instructions

Electrolytes – atoms dissolved in a liquid or gel.

Black lead – inserted into the black socket on the machine, and usually negative so tends to be the electrode that the client holds or is placed under the shoulder.

Red lead – often referred to as a jack lead. Some machines are colour coded – the red lead is inserted into the red socket. Usually positive, and is mostly used for roller or prong insertion, but check with individual machines and manufacturer's instructions.

Contra-indications to galvanic treatments

- Failure to respond to thermal and sensitivity testing, which would indicate a loss of skin sensation
- Very sensitive skin
- Recent sunburn/windburn
- The presence of skin infection or diseases
- Broken skin, such as cuts, abrasions or acne with open pustules
- Pregnancy
- Epilepsy
- Metal plates in the head
- Metallic pins or bridge work or excessive amalgam fillings in the mouth
- Heart conditions, pacemakers fitted or any heart condition requiring medication
- Headache or migraine sufferers
- High or low blood pressure
- Highly nervous clients
- Contact lenses should be removed

If in doubt, always seek the client's doctor's approval before treatment.

Think about it

Some manufacturers state that pregnancy, extensive dental work and bridge work are not contra-indications as the current is low. Never assume this is the case, however – always follow specific instructions.

Some manufacturers recommend the client waits at least 12 hours before and after any heat treatments, including facial waxing, electrolysis, sauna, sunbeds, hood hair dryers and swimming.

After collagen injections, galvanic facials should be avoided until the consultant's approval is gained (approximately two weeks).

Contra-actions to galvanic treatment

- Clients may experience a metallic taste and a tingling sensation in the mouth, as the current is drawn towards the metal in amalgam fillings.
- Some clients will feel the current quite strongly; others may have quite a high tolerance to it, and not feel very much at all. It is important not to turn the intensity up higher than is recommended, as a galvanic burn can occur. Always reassure clients that even if they cannot feel it, the treatment is working.

It is rare, but some clients have been known to develop a heat rash and irritation in response to galvanic preparations, so if this happens, turn off the machine, remove the rollers and then remove the product and place a cool water compress over the face. Allow the skin to calm down, and recommend the client uses a calamine-based lotion at home if the sensitivity continues, and avoids any other products which would cause further irritation. Remember to put this on the client record card for future reference.

Think about it

Desincrustation is usually carried out using the negative polarity, but always check because some manufacturers have changed their desincrustation gel for use under positive polarity. It is a good idea to write the polarity required on the lid of the gel for future reference, both for yourself and for colleagues.

If the polarity is not stated on the box or in the instructions, look for the pH value of the product:
- If it states it is acidic and below a pH reading of 7, use the positive polarity.
- If it states it is alkaline and above a pH reading of 7 – use the negative polarity.

(For more information on the pH scale, see You and the skin, page 232.)

Think about it

When testing galvanic equipment on yourself, you have to form the circuit and should be holding the neutral (covered) electrode in one hand, and make contact with the roller on your arm. Gradually turn up the current until sensation is felt. If you have the roller on your arm and the client is holding the neutral electrode, you will not form the circuit and will feel nothing.

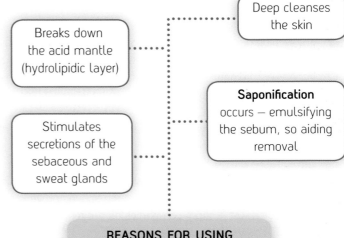

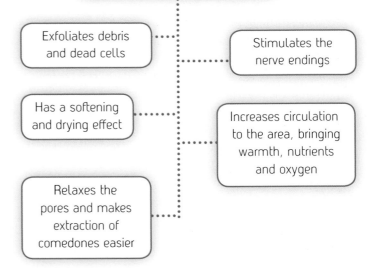

Reasons for using galvanic desincrustation

Using the negative pole rollers as the active electrode changes the gel which contains sodium carbonate

Sodium carbonate interacts by electrolysis with the moisture in the skin – the moisture is turned into sodium hydroxide, which is alkali

This saponifies – forms a soap

Results in a deep cleansing effect which softens the skin

Effects of galvanic desincrustation

Key terms

Saponification – conversion into soap or a soap substance so sebum becomes emulsified and is easy to remove.

Unit B14 Provide facial electrical treatments

Galvanic desincrustation treatment preparation and method – a step-by-step guide

1. Set up machinery with all appropriate equipment required. Check polarity of the desincrustation gel and set machine accordingly.
2. Carry out a full consultation.
3. Prepare client on the couch, with turban in place to keep hair away from the current, and remove eye make-up, then cleanse the skin thoroughly – twice is ideal to remove both make-up and perform a deep cleanse. Remove cleanser and blot, so the skin is clean and grease-free.
4. Carry out thermal and sensitivity testing on the face.
5. If steaming or pre-warming of the skin is required, it should be carried out now, but remember not to over-stimulate the face and adjust timings accordingly – some manufacturers do not recommend steaming, but prefer a mild exfoliant to be used in place of the second cleanse.
6. Test the machine on yourself and in front of the client – if required, test it on the client, too – so the client feels the sensation and is comfortable with it.
7. Give the client the covered, neutral electrode (bar) to hold in a hand without jewellery on, and make sure the sponge glove is damp, but not wringing wet – some companies do not require the bar to be covered (always check).
8. Decant desincrustation gel into a bowl, and apply to the face with either massage movements or a mask brush.
9. Make contact with the roller on the skin, and turn up the current gradually, until the client feels a tingling sensation; turn down the intensity slightly and introduce the other roller to the face.
10. Use slow, even, rhythmic movements all over the face, but do not allow the rollers to come into contact with one another.
11. Follow the directions of the arrows (see the next page) and work all over the face and neck area – approximately 5–7 minutes depending upon skin type and reaction, etc.
12. When roller use is completed, remove one roller; keep the one in contact with the skin moving and turn current down and then off. Remove other roller.
13. Change to ball or double-pronged electrode and start machine again, with electrodes in contact with the skin, working around the crevice of the nose and chin area.
14. Turn off the current, remove the electrode and thoroughly remove all the product with damp sponges.
15. Comedone extraction with sterile probe or covered fingers can now be completed.

There are various methods of performing galvanic treatment. A: commonly, the client holds the passive electrode and active roller(s) are applied to the face. B: two probes are used; one active on the face, one passive on the neck. C: two sponge heads are used; one active on the face, one passive on the neck.

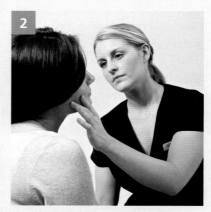
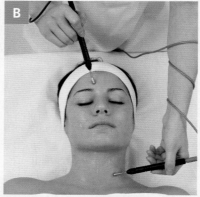
Roller
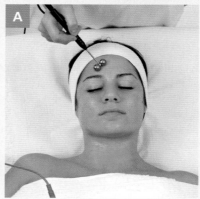
Probes
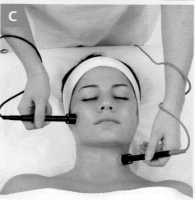
Sponge heads

Think about it

Recommend that a male client has a very close shave prior to galvanic treatment as the current is attracted to the moisture content in the hair and may cause a concentration of current in one area.

Think about it

The client never makes contact with the uncovered neutral electrode bar. It should always be covered by a dampened sponge glove or sleeve. It is important to check it thoroughly before every use to ensure there are no cracks or damaged areas. This will prevent the client sustaining a galvanic burn through a concentration of current at a weakened area.

If you are not continuing with iontophoresis, then some companies recommend reversing polarity for the last minute of desincrustation to calm the skin down. If you are moving on to iontophoresis, then carry straight on to that procedure.

Type of skin	Setting
Dry/sensitive	0.15 milliamps
Normal/combination	0.20 milliamps
Oily/problem	0.25 milliamps

Suggested galvanic settings for desincrustation. Always check individual manufacturer's instructions

Ingredient	Description
Sodium chloride (10%)	Common table salt; astringent and antiseptic properties
Sodium carbonate (5%)	Soda ash found in sea water and lakes
Sodium bicarbonate (10%)	Baking soda; alkali
Reasons for use	

Used under the negative (–) polarity for saponification of fatty acids and desincrustation; especially effective on an oilier skin

Common ingredients in desincrustation gels

Think about it

Before the treatment, rub the rollers in the palm of your hands (with no current on) for a few minutes to pre-warm them and discharge any ions sticking to them from a previous treatment. This also helps the flow of the ions once in contact with the face. Some manufacturers recommend soaking the rollers in surgical spirit after treatment, both to clean them and to discharge any residue of cream/gel.

Think about it

Initially, the skin has a natural resistance to the current and the client may have little or no sensation. However, once the skin's resistance has been broken down, through the warming of the tissue, there may be a rise in the sensation felt – in which case the intensity will need to be turned down slightly.

Think about it

Always adjust the intensity of the current and the duration of the treatment to suit the client's needs – some skins will need, and respond to, more current than others and the ratio of time spent on desincrustation and iontophoresis is proportional to the skin type and the client's needs.

Recommended course of treatment

If the skin type is normal, the client would benefit from desincrustation at least once a week for three weeks. Oily or congested skins would require slightly more treatments. A rest of two weeks should be suggested, to avoid over-stimulation of the sebaceous glands, which may worsen the condition — this will depend upon individual reactions and the manufacturer's recommendation for the particular system used.

Key terms

Active electrode – the 'working' electrode at the skin site where the electrolytes are penetrating into the skin. This can be in the form of rollers, a single ball probe, a double-pronged probe or covered pads for the body.

Passive electrode (sometimes called neutral, inactive, indifferent) – the electrode held in the hand to complete the circuit. On new machines, it can be a covered pad which sits under the shoulder or strapped to the upper arm.

Unit B14 Provide facial electrical treatments

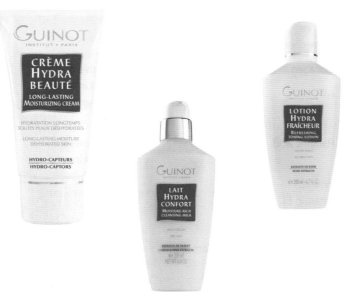

Use suitable skincare products for client's skin type

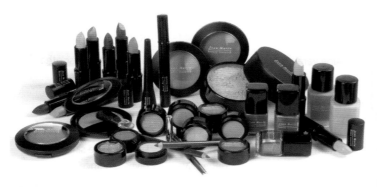

Advise client that skin may be sensitive to make-up

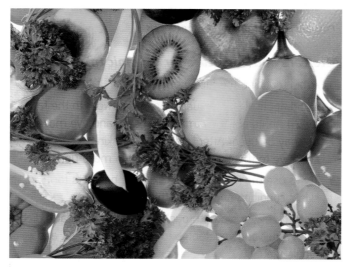

A diet rich in fruit and vegetables helps keep the skin healthy

For a full programme of steps the client should follow for skin improvement, see You and the skin, page 249.

Identify the hazard	What is the risk?
Danger from electric shock	Low
Galvanic burns	High
Postural problems for the therapist	High
Allergic/sensitive reaction	High

What should I do to prevent the hazard from becoming a risk?

- Follow manufacturers' instructions
- Carry out thermal and sensitivity tests
- Test on yourself before treatment
- Always have sufficient product on the skin to keep it well lubricated
- Constantly monitor for any developing contra-actions
- Remove all jewellery
- Never exceed recommended current intensity
- Always start on a zero current intensity and confirm that the client is comfortable
- Always carry out a full consultation and never treat a client who has an infection present
- Never use a broken spontex cover for the neutral electrode cover
- Always break the ampoule over the trolley top, using a tissue, and not near the client, and dispose of the broken glass safely
- Always clean and sterilise the rollers/equipment thoroughly after each treatment
- Make sure the machine is positioned close to you, so that you have full control over the intensity dials and the rollers/electrodes – do not lean over the client or make contact with the couch
- Ensure correct posture and chair to allow you to be in control of equipment

Risk assessment for galvanic unit

EMS – electro muscle stimulation (faradism)

The faradic current

Modern beauty therapy equipment combines various types of medium- to low-frequency currents. The type of current used is an alternating, low-frequency, surged and interrupted current. The source of electricity can be either the mains or a battery.

Application

The aim of facial faradic treatment is to intensively exercise the individual muscles, or groups of muscles, in the face to firm and tone them, which produces a firmer look to the contours of the face. Most modern faradic machines have both face and body outlets on them. (For information on body procedures see B13 Provide body electrical treatments.)

The faradic unit

The faradic unit is named after Michael Faraday, who studied the nature of electricity, but it is in fact an electrical muscular stimulation (EMS) unit, often referred to as neuro-muscular electrical stimulation (NMES). Some beauty therapists simply call the unit by its trade name such as Ultratone, Slendertone or Slim Master. (In the United States, faradic current is known as excitomotor current.)

Whatever the name, a faradic unit is a machine which induces the muscles to contract and relax through stimulation of the motor nerves within the belly of the muscle. As the client has no control of this muscular contraction and there is no physical movement of the body from A to B, it is called passive exercise, and as there is no movement of the joints or limbs it is a form of isometric exercise. It is extremely effective on both the smaller facial muscles and on the larger muscle groups within the body. (For information about the muscles, see Related anatomy and physiology, page 187.)

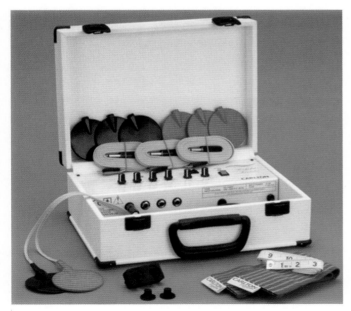

A faradic unit

At first, the machine may seem daunting to understand because of the range of settings available – the machine is designed to personalise treatment by altering the time, strength and pattern of the contractions. It may take some time for you to become familiar with it, but the more you use it, the more knowledgeable and confident you will become.

Detailed information on machine settings and the underpinning knowledge of faradiasm can be found in B13 Provide Body electrical treatments.

Dial settings

The machine has three dial settings that must be switched on and active for the equipment to work:

- A *master on/off switch* – some machines also have a timer that has to be set, and the machine will not light up ready for use unless the timer has been activated.

- A *reset button* at the back of the machine, which will not allow the machine to work unless the outlets where the pads go in are set to zero – this prevents the therapist from switching on the machine and giving the client a very strong initial contraction.

- A *'panic button'*, which is a switch on a lead plugged in at the back of the machine for the client to hold. Should the current be too strong or any discomfort be felt, the client can cut out the current and stop the treatment. This is very reassuring for the client, but as the therapist would never leave a client unattended, it should not be necessary to use it.

Some machines make a loud whining noise to alert the therapist to incorrectly set dials. The reset button needs to be pressed and the dials set at zero, and the noise alert will stop.

The other dials control the contraction patterns.

> **Think about it**
>
> Muscle contraction can be controlled by the strength, speed and variation of current, impulse duration, direction of the current (polarity) and frequency. All contribute to the duration and strength of contraction.

> **Think about it**
>
> To help you understand the dials, it may help to study how a muscle contracts, its origins and insertions, in Related anatomy and physiology, page 187.

Pulse sequence

This is the wave form, or phasic control, of which there are four types.

- *Bi-phasic regular* pulse. The electrical impulses pass in both directions between the pads, giving a good firming, toning and strengthening treatment to the muscles. In normal body treatments, the pads should ideally be bi-phasic for comfort and to work the muscles to their full potential. The lights above this dial alternate to show that the current is alternating between the pads.

- *Mono-phasic regular* pulse. The electrical impulses pass in only one direction, helping to lift the muscles being treated. When a mono-phasic pulse sequence is selected, the black (negative) pad should always be placed on the insertion of the muscle and the red (positive) on to the origin (remember this as BIRO – Black Insertion Red Origin – so that the black pad is below the red). The muscle fibres are then lifted towards the origin. This is recommended for use on face and neck muscles, and also indicated for physiotherapy work. When the mono-phasic pulse sequence is in operation, only the positive (+) light will illuminate on the unit. Although not usually used on the body, this setting is sometimes used by body builders who require more muscular definition for shows and competition work. After several courses of treatment, the muscles get used to the contractions and may even begin to anticipate them – this does not work the muscle to its full capacity and the machine has the facility to change the pattern sequences to an irregular pattern to keep the muscle working. Always start on the regular phase settings, but introduce irregular pulses during the course of treatment.

- *Bi-phasic irregular* pulse. This adds variety and is useful for the nervous client who clenches the muscles in anticipation of the current – neither the client nor the therapist knows the pattern. This would only apply in body treatments.

- *Mono-phasic irregular* pulse. The irregular pulse sequence is designed to aid in the treatment of nervous or tense clients. The pulses come in groups of three and five, and due to the irregularity of the impulses, the client cannot anticipate the muscle contraction, thereby avoiding discomfort during treatment. This would apply in facial faradic work and can be used half-way through the course of treatment to keep the muscles working hard.

Contraction and relaxation settings

This setting may be altered to give a longer or shorter length of muscle contraction, and will vary according to the client's muscle tone. Weak muscle should be exercised on a lower setting, that is 1.5 seconds on and 1.5 seconds off, with the setting increased as muscle tone improves.

You will need to adjust the timings of the contraction and relaxation so that the relaxation time is never less than the contraction time.

Type of work	Setting
Normal body	80–100 Hz
Facial	120 Hz
Deep muscle	60 Hz

Suggested frequency settings

Type of work	Setting
Normal body	160 µs
Facial	90 µs
Deep muscle	240 µs

Suggested pulse width settings in microseconds

The frequency and pulse width settings can be altered to ensure the impulse penetrates to the correct depth of the muscle being contracted, ensuring the maximum comfort is achieved for the client.

Think about it

For facial faradic work, the setting should be: Mono-phasic regular pulse, 120 Hz, 90 µs.

Think about it

Contract each muscle 10–15 times before moving on to the next muscle, and up to 20 contractions on a mature client with poor muscle tone.

Precautions during facial faradic work

- Just like normal exercising, the muscles work more efficiently after some form of warm-up – for a facial treatment, this could be a steam treatment, infrared application, hot towels or manual massage. This will prevent muscle damage.

- After treatment, lymphatic drainage should be carried out for a few minutes as lactic acid will have accumulated in the muscles as a by-product of oxygen and nutrient exchange.

- Ensure surge speed is not too slow as this would make the muscle contraction too long, which would be uncomfortable for the client.

- Never exercise a muscle to the point of no reaction, as that is muscle fatigue. Always reduce the current around the eye area, bony areas, or where there are fillings or dentures.

- Never give treatment over areas where metal has replaced tissue, or around a mouth with extensive fillings.

- Always re-adjust the placement point if the client experiences discomfort or the required exercise is not being produced.

- Keep pads dampened with **saline solution** throughout the treatment – this breaks down the skin's resistance to the current.

- Ensure the amount of current flowing is minimal at the beginning.

- Always have the machine facing you, so you can constantly check the dials.

Key terms

Saline solution – a solution of water and salt (one teaspoon of salt in one pint of water) often used in desincrustation because it is a good conductor and contains sodium chloride. Most of the liquid in our body tissue is saline, so humans are good conductors of electricity

Contra-indications to facial faradic treatments

There are not many contra-indications to faradism because it is an action very similar to natural movement, but there are instances where it should not be applied or where medical guidance should be sought before treatment.

If clients are unaware of the state of their health, then it is advisable to ask them to check with their doctor before treatment, especially as a facial treatment plan will probably include other treatments and factors (for example vacuum suction, preheating treatments, microcurrent or galvanic treatments). Contra-indications include the following:

- Failure of the sensitivity or thermal tests

- Muscle disease or spastic, paralysed muscles

- A history of strokes, facial paralysis or Bell's palsy (which responds well to EMS but should only be carried out in a medical/physiotherapy context)

- Skin cuts, grazes, inflammation, sunburn, etc. Small breaks in the skin may be protected by a small piece of plaster. With certain minor skin complaints, wet a sponge disc and position it between the pad and the body. Sponge discs should also be used for anyone found to be allergic to the rubber surface of the pad.

- Pregnancy (especially the early stages) and after birth until a doctor's clearance is given (usually six weeks)

- After operations

- Old scars in the treatment area can cause discomfort if the skin has underlying adhesions or is taut or puckered

- Epilepsy

- Asthma – only with a doctor's approval

- High blood pressure or heart conditions (particularly in the obese client) – only with a doctor's approval

- Metal plates or pins in bones adjacent to treatment area

- Implanted electronic devices, for example pacemaker

- High temperature.

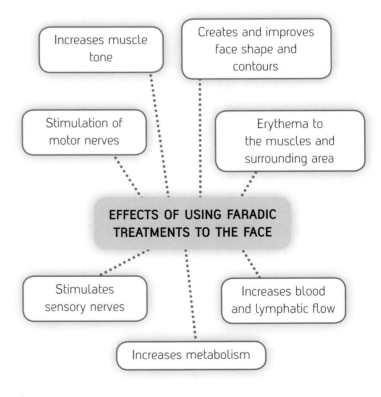

Effects of faradic treatments to the face

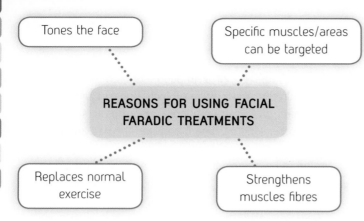

Reasons for using facial faradic treatments

Stimulation of sensory nerves

The primary reaction is one of a mild prickling sensation underneath the pads. This is due to the stimulation of sensory nerves and ceases as soon as sufficient intensity of current is applied and muscle contraction is brought about. This sensory stimulation causes reflex vasodilation of the superficial blood vessels producing a slight erythema in the area. Sensation may be increased once the skin's resistance has been broken down, and the current is able to penetrate further into the skin.

Think about it

Although muscle has a good blood and fluid supply, so conducts current well, adipose tissue does not, and a larger client will have less sensation and may require a higher intensity than a thinner one.

Stimulation of motor nerves

A faradic-type current stimulates the motor nerves, and provided the current is of sufficient intensity, causes contraction of the muscles which they supply. To avoid tetanic contractions, the current is surged. To avoid muscle fatigue developing, the current is also interrupted to allow the muscle to rest between contractions.

Think about it

Tetanic contractions get their name from the medical condition tetanus, which causes muscles to go into spasm, as in lockjaw. Tetanic contractions are muscular spasms or stiffness. The current is surged gradually to increase stimulation in a smooth contraction, to avoid such spasms.

Increased blood and lymphatic flow

As the muscles contract and relax, they exert a pumping action on the veins and lymphatic vessels lying in and around them.

Increased metabolism

There is an increase in demands for oxygen and nutrients and an increase in waste products.

Erythema

A mild erythema is produced under the pads due to dilation of the superficial blood vessels.

Increased muscle tone

When a muscle is exercised it increases in 'tone', i.e. it responds more readily to a stimulus and becomes firmer. It becomes stronger and more able to hold the contours of the body more firmly and effectively without strain.

Increased muscle bulk

In order to increase the bulk of a muscle, it is necessary for it to contract an adequate number of times against the resistance of a suitable load. When a muscle is very weak, the weight of the part of the body that it moves forms an adequate load and therefore electrical stimulation can be of assistance in restoring muscle bulk.

Facial faradic treatment preparation and method

For facial faradic work, there are three types of electrode:

- Facial block electrode
- Mushroom electrode
- Faradic mask electrode.

Facial block electrode

The facial block electrode is most widely used. It is easy to hold in the hand, has both the **anode** and **cathode** in its casing, which is made of rubber for insulation, and both red and black wires go into one outlet on the machine. Some of facial block electrodes have an intensity built in to them, but most commonly, the block is held in one hand, placed on the face and the current turned up on the machine by the other hand.

Key terms

Anode – the positive electrode; if the ions are negative, they will be drawn to this.

Cathode – the negative electrode; if the ions are positive, they will be drawn to this.

Remove all make-up and jewellery.

Test on yourself in front of the client

Insert lead into facial applicator.

Adjust pulse sequence, frequency and pulse width settings.

Check all intensity dials are in the 'off' position.

Switch on minute timer and press reset button.

Dampen facial electrodes and place on muscle.

Turn up intensity control and contract ten times (this can increase with subsequent treatments). Pulse width settings may be increased if required until the most comfortable contraction is obtained.

Turn down intensity control, move electrode to next muscle and repeat.

Continue until all required facial muscles have been treated.

Facial faradic at a glance

Think about it

Faradic treatments are like any exercise – a regular course of treatments, say twice a week for six weeks, is far more effective than just one treatment. Results will be even better if the client also does the homecare exercises and has a good skincare regime.

Mushroom electrode

A mushroom, or disc, electrode is not widely used, but some companies still provide them. The mushroom needs another pad to complete the circuit. The electrode is the active pad, making contact with the muscle motor nerve, and the indifferent pad is either under the shoulder or strapped to the upper arm. The mushroom and the indifferent pad need to be covered with several layers of lint to prevent the client coming into contact with the metal, which could cause a burn. The advantage of the mushroom electrode is that as a single application, rather than the dual application of the block, the individual muscle can be easily isolated, and contracted.

Face mask electrode

The face mask electrode has the advantage of several points of contact and so multi-application of the current is easy. It consists of a facial mask as the active electrode and a covered arm pad that goes either under the shoulder or strapped to the arm. Its drawback is that it would not be suitable for claustrophobic clients and the therapist cannot actually see the contractions taking place to monitor them and therefore control them for client comfort.

Think about it

Only turn up the contraction intensity when the block is in contact with the skin, and the contraction light is on. This will ensure you do not exceed the client's tolerance. If turned up in a relaxation phase, the client may have too strong a sensation – it will be uncomfortable and may hurt.

Aftercare and homecare for facial faradic treatment

See You and the skin, page 249, for suitable skincare recommendations.

The best form of homecare for muscular development is some simple facial exercises which the client can carry out several times a day, to continue the work done in the salon.

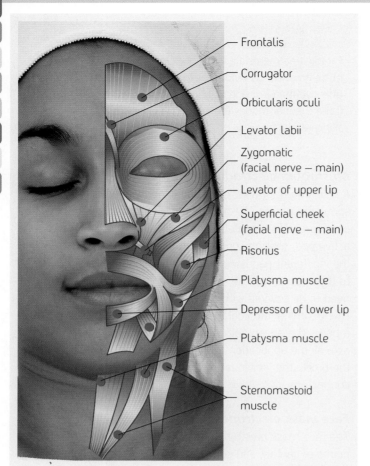

Frontalis

Corrugator

Orbicularis oculi

Levator labii

Zygomatic
(facial nerve – main)

Levator of upper lip

Superficial cheek
(facial nerve – main)

Risorius

Platysma muscle

Depressor of lower lip

Platysma muscle

Sternomastoid
muscle

The hotspots on this diagram indicate placement points on the muscles for the pads during facial faradic treatment

9 Try to reach your nose with your lower lip. Hold for 30 seconds.

10 Turn the lower lip down, stretching neck and jaw muscles.

Also recommend neck rolling for relaxation.

Sit straight in a chair. Drop the head onto your chest, then slowly swing your head up to the right shoulder, following through the back and down to the left shoulder, then back on to the chest. (*Do not roll the head right around over the back – this is not recommended.*) Repeat six times clockwise and six anti-clockwise.

Identify the hazard	What is the risk?
Danger from electric shock	Low
Minor shock from current sensation	High
Muscle fatigue from over-exercising the muscles	High
Allergy to the pads	High
Postural problems for the therapist	Low
Allergic/sensitive reaction	High

What should I do to prevent the hazard from becoming a risk?

- Follow manufacturers' instructions
- Carry out thermal and sensitivity tests
- Test on yourself before treatment
- Always have sufficient product on the skin to keep it well lubricated
- Constantly monitor for any developing contra-actions
- Remove all jewellery
- Never exceed the recommended current intensity
- Always start on a zero current intensity and confirm that the client is comfortable
- Never over-exercise the muscle – count the contractions and never exceed client tolerance
- Make sure the machine is positioned close to you, so that you have full control over the intensity dials and electrodes – do not lean over the client or make contact with the couch
- Only turn up the intensity in a contraction phase
- Use damaged sponges as a barrier between the skin and the pad
- Ensure correct posture and chair height to allow you to be in control of equipment

Risk assessment for faradic unit

1 In a sitting position, tilt the head back, keeping teeth together. Contract neck and chin muscles for 30 seconds.

2 Repeat exercise 1 – with teeth slightly apart when head is tilted back, close the teeth. Repeat and hold for 30 seconds.

3 Say the word 'cue' pushing your lips forward.

4 Say the word 'ex' pulling the muscles back towards the ears. Repeat 20 times.

5 Open the eyes wide and drop the mouth open, stretching all the muscles as far as possible for 30 seconds.

6 Repeat exercise 5, but stick out your tongue as far as possible for 30 seconds.

7 Close your eyes and screw your face into a ball for 30 seconds.

8 Tilt head slightly, push lower jaw and teeth forward.

Facial faradic treatment – a step-by-step guide

1 Carry out a full consultation to check for contra-indications.

2 Prepare the client and ensure comfort.

3 Remove all make-up, jewellery and accessories.

4 Carry out thermal and sensitivity tests. Ensure the area is clean and grease-free and that the muscles are relaxed by some form of heat treatment or good massage.

5 Place the client in a semi-reclining position to enable you to see the contours of the face quite clearly (when the client is in a supine position, the contours of the face are distorted slightly by the forces of gravity). Check the machine, ensure all dials are at zero and set up ready for treatment.

6 Position the machine so that all dials are useable by the therapist without restricting movement and without wires causing discomfort. Prepare a warm saline solution — one teaspoon of salt to one pint of water. Wash hands.

7 Test the equipment on yourself in front of the client, by holding the pad in the palm of your hand. Switch on slowly until the current causes a mild contraction. Turn machine off. Briefly describe what the treatment will do, and the sensations felt as treatment begins and is built up. Warn the client of any noises and flashes which may cause alarm.

8 When the client is confident, position the surge and interval periods for one second each, dampen the electrodes with a warm saline solution and ensure the output dial is still at zero. Place electrodes on to the lower part of the sides of the neck, locating the motor point for the sternocleidomastoid and platysma muscles, turn on the output switch to release the current and slowly increase during surge periods only until exercise can be seen. Ensure that the client is not experiencing discomfort and never apply the current beyond tolerance level. As the muscle becomes more relaxed, an increase in surge and discomfort may become apparent. It is most important to watch the client's face throughout the treatment to make sure no pain is experienced. It may be necessary to reduce the current once the muscles increase their reaction to the current and this should be done during an interval period. Discomfort may also be experienced if the motor point has not been located accurately — a slight alteration in placement should solve the problem. Never remove the electrodes from the skin during a contraction period, and then reapply! Having stimulated this point for the required number of contractions (usually 10–15 for a general toning treatment) turn down the intensity control and move the electrode to the upper part of the neck (great oracular point of cervical nerve).

9 Work upwards, exercising all of the main facial muscles.

10 When treatment is completed, carry out lymphatic drainage, either manually or with vacuum suction to the face, to help the lymphatic system drain the build-up of lactic acid within the muscles.

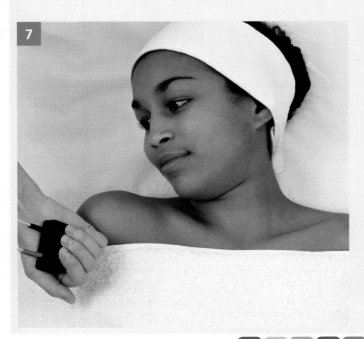

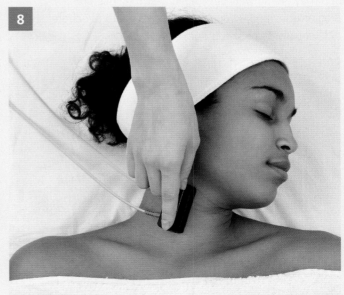

Microcurrent

Microcurrent has been used for about 25 years in medicine. Good results have been achieved in the treatment of Bell's palsy, facial paralysis, stroke, wound healing and pain control. The 'MENS' and 'TENS' systems for pain management utilise microcurrent.

Microcurrent mimics the body's own natural bio-electrical impulses. Our brain is continuously sending out impulses through the spinal column to muscles and soft tissues. As we get older, the body slows down, the muscles start to age and the skin begins to deteriorate (for the effects of ageing on the skin and the contributory factors for healthy skin, see You and the skin, page 222).

Microcurrent has the ability to speed up the whole metabolism of the tissue and cellular activity. It works in two ways – preventative and corrective. It heals the tissues so that a visible result will be seen after only one treatment. The skin will tighten, and lines and wrinkles will be softened because of the cellular activity being stimulated. In addition, because the muscle and tissue is then in a better state of repair to receive the body's own natural bio-electrical impulses, there is preventative care as well. The ageing process is being delayed and a healing effect is produced.

Most progressive salons offer microcurrent treatments for both face and body treatments and incorporate it into skin enhancement programmes as well as facial lifting.

Application

There are many microcurrent machines on the market, and they are so well developed that they use pre-set programmes and a variety of wave forms to penetrate different levels of skin tissue.

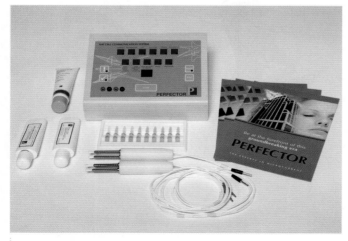

A microcurrent unit

The more advanced machines are also self-calibrating to compensate for varying conductivity levels among individuals and this ensures constant results. The current is applied by dual-tipped probes, using cotton bud heads, rollers or pads, depending upon the manufacturer. Some microcurrent treatments also combine the galvanic current for iontophoresis treatments and the combination is very effective in treating the skin; a course is highly recommended, rather than just one treatment.

About the current

Microcurrent is a thousand times smaller than a milliamp and a million times smaller than an amp – that's how tiny it is!

We measure microcurrent in Hertz (Hz) – the frequency or speed of the current. Medical research has shown:

- 600 Hz touches the skin and bounces off
- 500 Hz penetrates just below the skin level
- 300 Hz stimulates lymphatic drainage
- 20 Hz stimulates circulation
- 10 Hz lifts superficial facial muscles
- 0.8 Hz gives a lift to deep facial muscles.

Microcurrent uses four wave forms:

1. synergenic
2. ramp
3. square
4. rectangular.

Synergenic wave form – used in face-lifting programmes 1,5,6. Superficial effects

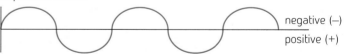

negative (–)

positive (+)

Ramp wave form – used in face-lifting programme 2. Pumping effect

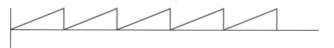

Square wave form – used in face-lifting programme 3. Lifting effect

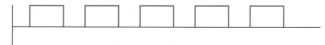

Rectangular wave form – used in face-lifting programme 4. Lifting effect with a longer hold

Microcurrent wave forms

These allow penetration through different levels of the tissue. So, for instance, if working on a muscle, the most suitable form is the square wave — this builds the current up quickly, holds it, then drops it off very quickly. If working on the skin, a very gentle wave form is required as no depth is required, so the synergenic, which is a wavy, very mild form, is used.

Microcurrent uses the different combinations of current, frequency and wave form to penetrate through different levels of the tissue.

Contra-indications to microcurrent treatments

- Recent operations with general anaesthetic — within nine months add two more treatments to course, as it can act as a barrier to microcurrent
- Anti-depressants — add two more treatments to course, as they can act as a barrier to microcurrent
- Heart conditions — do not treat
- Collagen injections — avoid area for 6—8 weeks
- Botox injections — avoid area totally as microcurrent will stimulate the area
- Pregnancy — do not treat
- Epilepsy — do not treat
- Metal implants — do not treat if the metal implants are in the head or neck area
- Diabetes — be aware of any skin reaction during treatment
- Smokers — due to the thickening of the skin and premature ageing, the advice is to add a further six treatments to the course
- Chemotherapy/radiology — client must be totally clear of cancer for four years before starting
- Retin A or Ro-Accuntaine — this medication used in the treatment of acne can cause thinning of the skin, so avoid treating for one year

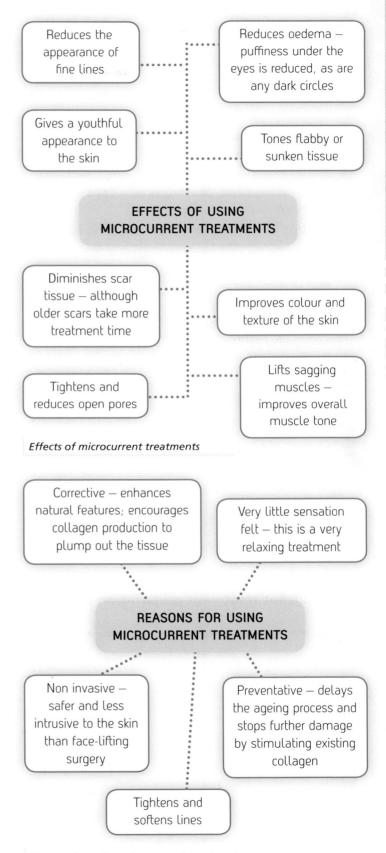

Effects of microcurrent treatments

Reasons for using microcurrent treatments

Effects of non-surgical face-lifting treatment

Circulation

This part of the treatment stimulates the epidermal and dermal blood circulation. It also has an activating effect on the lymph circulation.

Drainage/relaxation

This part of the treatment:

- increases circulation of the upper arm and lower layers of the connective tissue, providing increased nourishment of the epidermis
- detoxifies by activating the lymphatic system, ridding the tissue of waste, so reducing puffiness and fluid retention
- increases mitotic activity within the basal layer of the skin, so improving texture.

Lifting – short and long

This part of the treatment reprogrammes the muscles. Each muscle is stretched or relaxed, that is, the muscle length is modified, which results in:

- reduction of deeper wrinkles – has a long-term lasting effect
- general firming up of loose tissue, for example jowls
- general toning of the dermis and reduction in the size of pores.

Firming

This part of the treatment concentrates on the epidermis and dermis. The probes follow the weft of the skin. It results in:

- stimulating and speeding up the rate at which the skin produces its own corrective tissue fibres (collagen and elastin), so increasing the supportive framework of the dermis
- reducing large pores
- softening scar tissue
- refining the texture of the skin
- reducing fine lines and wrinkles
- increased local circulation causing increased nourishment, thereby increasing the regenerative process, and so firming up the tissue
- increased detoxification which improves the general colour of the skin and gives a more refined texture.

Ionisation

This part of the treatment allows ionised substances, in this case collagen and elastin, to pass into the epidermis of the skin with the aid of a galvanic current. Collagen and elastin promote the natural regenerative process of the skin and give added tone and elasticity to the tissue. Other ionisable products may be used.

Think about it

Not all microcurrent machines are the same – always follow the manufacturer's recommendations for timing and settings.

Microcurrent treatment preparation and method

Programme	Current (in micro amperes)	Wave form	Duration (in minutes)	Frequency (in Hz)	Polarity
1	300	Synergenic	2	20	Alternating
2	50	Ramp	10	300	Alternating
3	160	Square	16	10	Alternating
4	80	Rectangular	8	0.8	Alternating
5	500	Synergenic	10	500	Alternating
6	200	Synergenic	3	30	Direct

Treatment programmes for face-lifting

Face-lifting – setting up the machine

1 Plug machine into mains using the lead provided.
2 Switch on machine at rear.
3 All indicator lights will light up and a single audio signal will be heard. The lights stay on for a few seconds while the machine checks all circuits.
4 The **LED** will go to zero indicated by two lines (- -) and the on indicator (represented by a tick) will stay lit up.
5 Plug the probe leads into one channel: positive (+) and negative (−).
6 When ready, press the panel switch to start programme 1 (2 minutes). Then press start. The LED will begin counting down and the audio signal will sound every eight seconds.
7 At the end of the programme, the LED will return to zero (- -) and the light on the programme 1 button will go out. A single lower-toned beep will sound at the end of each programme.
8 Proceed through the remaining five programmes.

The programme you are working in can be paused or stopped at any time using the appropriate button on the right of the display panel.

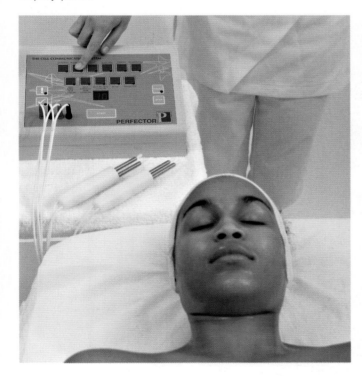

Think about it

If the (!) light comes on, you do not have conductivity. Check all leads and ensure you are using sufficient gel.

Key terms

Moving coil meter – the window at the front of the machine with a metal arm moving along the milliamp readings.

LED – light emitting diode, for reading milliamps on the front of the machine.

LCD – liquid crystal display, for milliamp registering.

Face-lifting procedure – a step-by-step guide using a Perfector machine

1 Cleanse, tone and apply the conductive gel of choice. Apply a thick layer all over the face, including eyebrows and upper lip, and apply gel to electrodes.
2 *Programme 1:* Oxygenation (2 minutes). Sine waveform/low-frequency microcurrent (do not follow beep). Movements should be quick and covering the whole of the face.
3 *Programme 2:* Regeneration (10 minutes). Nano range/rectangular waveform (follow beep). Follow face-lifting movement for whole face (×1).
4 *Programme 3:* Lifting (10 minutes). Nano range/square waveform (follow beep). Follow face-lifting movements for the top half of the face (×2). This programme is best suited for the eye lifts, cheek lifts etc.
5 *Programme 4:* Sculpting (10 minutes). Square waveform (follow beep). Follow face-lifting movements for the bottom half of the face (×2). This programme is best suited for sculpting and adding definition to the face, for example, the jaw line.
6 *Programme 5:* Firming (10 minutes). Sine waveform/high frequency microcurrent (follow beep). Follow lymphatic drainage movements over the whole face (×2).
7 *Programme 6:* Rejuvenation (10 minutes). Nano range rectangular waveform. Concentrate on areas of concern using a flat probe. Repeat movements on the areas of choice.
8 *Programme 11:* On the next row down, using last button (3 minutes). High absorption microcurrent/sine waveform. Hold the negative probes (black ends on cable); the client holds the positive probe (red end on cable). Use a tissue to break the ampoule. Apply the ampoule as quickly as possible; proceed to saturate the client's whole face using cupping movements. It may be necessary to add a touch of water to the client's skin beforehand to stop complete absorption. Mentally divide the clients face into six sections, being careful to cover each section thoroughly with the negative probe. Use butterfly-light pressing movements.

Provide facial electrical treatments **Unit B14**

Face-lifting

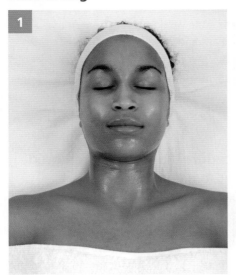

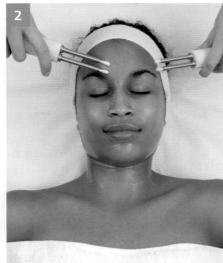

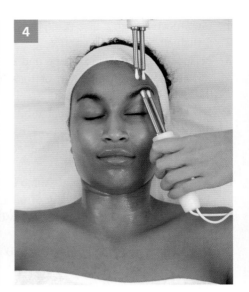

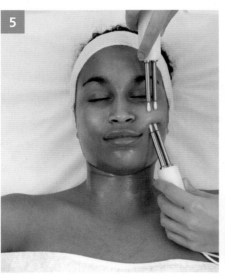

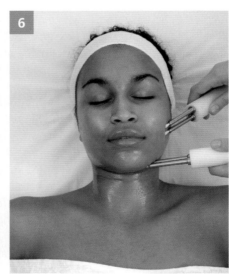

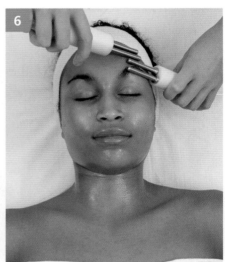

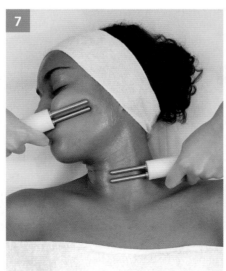

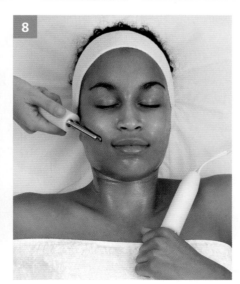

Remove make up and jewellery.

⬇

Insert cotton buds into facial electrodes.

⬇

Set machine to appropriate setting.

⬇

Programme 1: oxygenation.

⬇

Programme 2: regeneration.

⬇

Programme 3: lifting.

⬇

Programme 4: sculpting.

⬇

Apply more gel.

⬇

Programme 5: firming.

⬇

Programme 6: rejuvenation.

⬇

Remove all gel thoroughly.

⬇

Change cotton bud and attach bar electrode to +.

⬇

Choose correct ampoule.

⬇

Programme 11: high absorption.

⬇

Apply moisturiser and eye balm.

Microcurrent at a glance

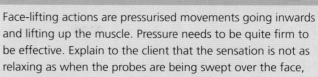

Think about it

Face-lifting actions are pressurised movements going inwards and lifting up the muscle. Pressure needs to be quite firm to be effective. Explain to the client that the sensation is not as relaxing as when the probes are being swept over the face, but the firmness is essential to the results.

Remember the five golden rules. See Facial treatments – theory and consultation, page 273.

Aftercare and homecare for microcurrent treatment

● Help to continue the effectiveness of the salon treatment by using the complementary correct skincare routine at home.

● Complete the facial exercise routine that is included in the aftercare for faradic treatments to keep the muscles active and toned.

● Drink plenty of water to keep the skin rehydrated and replenish the moisture lost through perspiration and through the respiration process.

See You and the skin, page 222, for all aspects of promoting a healthy skin and the correct products to use.

Risk assessment for microcurrent

As the microcurrent is such a low-frequency current, it is a very low-risk treatment – however, the last part of the treatment uses a galvanic current, which is direct and constant, so you will need to refer also to the galvanic risk assessment for the potential hazards in that part of the treatment (see page 298).

Identify the hazard	What is the risk?
Danger from electric shock	Low
Allergy to the cotton buds	High
Bruising of the skin by too firm lifting movements	High
Postural problems for the therapist	High
Allergic/sensitive reaction to conductive gel	High

What should I do to prevent the hazard from becoming a risk?

- Follow manufacturers' instructions
- Carry out thermal and sensitivity testing
- Test on yourself before treatment
- Always have sufficient product on the skin to keep it well lubricated
- Constantly monitor for any developing contra-actions
- Remove all jewellery
- Never exceed the recommended current intensity
- Never push the probes too heavily into the skin before lifting the muscle
- Make sure the machine is positioned close to you, so that you have full control over the intensity dials and electrodes – do not lean over the client or make contact with the couch
- Ensure correct posture and chair height to allow you to be in control of equipment

Risk assessment for microcurrent

Microdermabrasion

Microdermabrasion (MDA) has been used to great effect in the medical field over the last twenty years. Plastic surgeons and dermatologists have been able to improve the skin's condition and to stimulate its own regenerative processes. Controlled microdermabrasion is a modern technique of a gentle mechanical peeling process. It restores the delicate balance of healthy functioning skin cells needed for a clear and radiant skin, and the dead corneocytes required for the protection of the skin from the environment.

Think about it

micro = small particles

derm = skin

abrasion = removal by friction

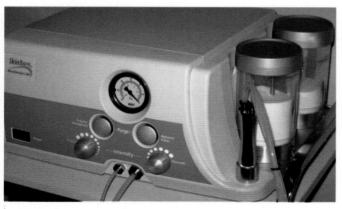

A microdermabrasion unit

How it works

Microdermabrasion works by providing a gentle, consistent flow of ultra clean aluminium oxide crystals, in a one-way flow over the skin, from a hand unit, using a low-pressure negative vacuum. The crystals are pumped over the skin's surface through compression flow and then sucked back into the hand unit and stored in a separate, sealed container from the fresh crystals, so there is never any contamination from used crystals to the new ones.

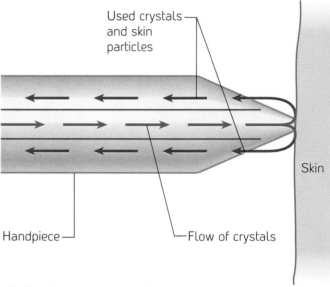

Used crystals and skin particles

Skin

Handpiece

Flow of crystals

The hand unit showing the flow of crystals

The feeling of crystals flowing over the skin is a little like being licked by a cat – slightly rough, but not unpleasant, and your client may drift off to sleep during the course of the facial.

Microdermabrasion is a controlled exfoliation: the thorough removal of the stratum corneum cells leaves the skin able to renew itself faster and look, and feel, healthier.

The skin

Refer back to You and the skin, page 222, and Related anatomy and physiology, page 153, to refresh your learning of the layers of the epidermis.

In a healthy skin there should be a ratio of 65–70 per cent living epidermal cells with 25–30 per cent dead corneocytes, sitting on the top, waiting to be sloughed off through friction in the course of the day. However, in older skins, damaged skins with scarring and the ageing process, this ratio can change and the dead corneocytes can be up to 50 per cent of the skin's surface. This leaves the skin looking dull and flat, with poor healing qualities, because the newer cells are not able to come through.

The epidermal layers also become tougher and thick with the exposure to too much ultra violet (UV) light and weather-beaten. Unprotected skin becomes coarse and thick, trying to protect itself against the elements.

UV light, cold, heat, wind and environmental pollution combined with poor diet, alcohol, negative stress and hormonal fluctuations can leave the skin prematurely aged in appearance and the acid mantle disturbed and unable to function properly .

Healthy skin has a renewal cycle of approximately 28 days, but this turnover can be slowed down by up to four months through a poor lifestyle and poor skincare routine. The microdermabrasion system of exfoliation can stimulate the skin to heal and repair itself through the removal of the dead skin cells and this then allows the active, moisturising and boosting products to penetrate and soothe the skin. The results are instantaneous – the client is very happy with the results and you will find that they want to book a course of treatments!

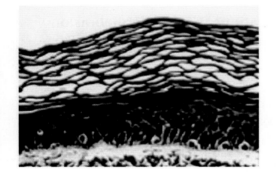

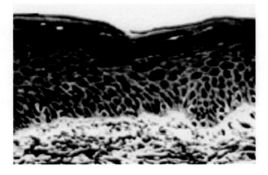

Cross-section of skin before and after microdermabrasion
(Source: Picture courtesy of Carlton Professional)

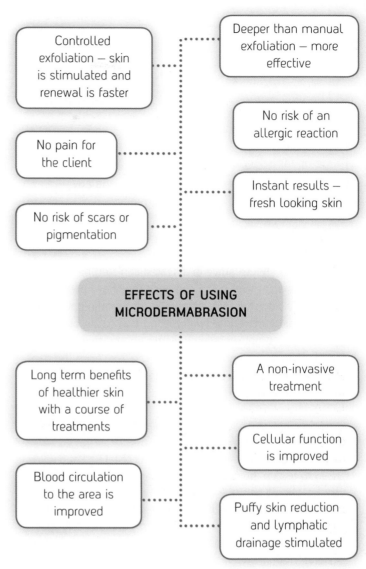

Effects of microdermabrasion

About the crystals

Not all crystals for microdermabrasion are equal in size, but they should all be made from aluminium oxide (A1203). The quality of the crystals is vital to success of the treatment and the performance of the machine – poor quality crystals or crystals that are too big will just clog the pump up and render the machine inoperable. Always buy the crystals from the supplier of your machine – they are designed to suit. You should look for correct:

- size
- distribution
- shape/form
- cleanliness.

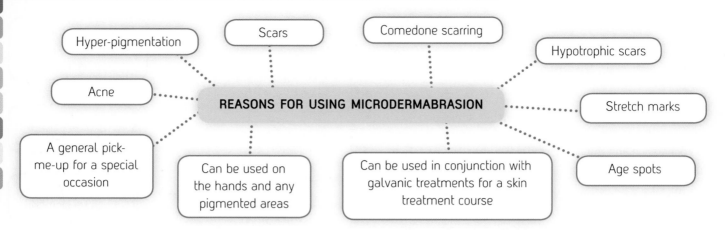

REASONS FOR USING MICRODERMABRASION

- Hyper-pigmentation
- Scars
- Comedone scarring
- Hypotrophic scars
- Acne
- Stretch marks
- A general pick-me-up for a special occasion
- Can be used on the hands and any pigmented areas
- Can be used in conjunction with galvanic treatments for a skin treatment course
- Age spots

Reasons for using microdermabrasion

Your crystals should arrive in a sealed canister, be 100 per cent sterile and never be reused once they have passed over the skin. The crystals are mined and refined and polished so that they are formed into two types: a ball for smoothness and one with slightly sharp edges for an abrasive effect. The combination of the two ensures that the flow from the hand unit is even and controllable and that the abrasive qualities are to the right degree.

Think about it

If your machine does not have a sealed crystal unit and you need to top up the crystals into the canister manually, the crystals should be dry and fresh – once crystals get damp they will clump together and be unusable, and could potentially damage the unit, so always store in a dry area. Because of this, always wipe your machine over with a fine cloth and not a damp cloth or wet wipes.

Peeling depth according to treatment indications

The more sensitive the skin, the less pressure should be applied. Too much pressure makes it uncomfortable to the client and you may go deeper into the epidermis than required. Obviously the most sensitive areas of the skin are around the eyes and the neck region.

So, a working pressure of −3Hg vacuum is suggested – but always follow the manufacturer's instructions, as each machine may differ. The rest of the skin on the face is less sensitive so a working pressure of −5Hg vacuum is adequate.

Key terms

Hg – a measurement of pressure.

Think about it

All skin types are suitable for treatment, but the intensity of the vacuum and crystal flow is determined by the treatment to be given, tone and texture of the client's skin and client comfort. All client needs will be slightly different.

Contra-indications to microdermabrasion (MDA)

- Any skin infection or disorder – you risk cross-contamination of the infection
- Any recent cosmetic procedure performed under a dermatologist such as a chemical peel or laser surgery. The skin is already weak and thin and needs sufficient healing time, agreed with a doctor
- Keloid scarring – MDA could make the condition worse
- Roactane medication for acne – MDA treatment should be avoided for six months after a course of roactane has been completed to avoid damage to the tissues
- Failure of skin sensitivity or thermal testing – this would indicate nerve damage and needs further investigation by the client's GP. Treatment should be postponed until underlying causes have been established
- Auto immune diseases – if the client has any healing problems MDA is not a suitable treatment
- Blood disorders such as hepatitis B, AIDs and the HIV virus as there is a danger of cross-infection
- Do not use MDA immediately after a wax depilation treatment
- Recent sunburn
- Highly vascular or super-sensitive skins

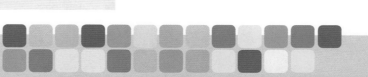

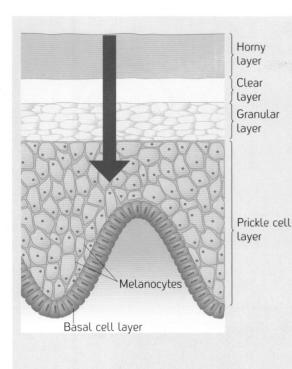

Horny layer

Clear layer

Granular layer

Prickle cell layer

Melanocytes

Basal cell layer

Layers of the epidermis and suggested depths of peeling

Stratum corneum peel
This is the top layer of the epidermis and its removal is all that is required to trigger an impulse to the base layer to start to create new cells. This superficial peel can be used to great effect for a general regeneration treatment in skins with no major problems but just needs a boost – i.e. before a special occasion, big night out or a wedding. With a smooth surface make-up application is enhanced.

Stratum granulosum peel
The layer of cells directly underneath the corneum are in the process of flattening out and dying off. Peeling at this layer is necessary to combat acne (especially in young adults) as this layer is affected by hormonal changes. This level of peel is also effective for treating sun-damaged skin.

Stratum spinosum
The deeper the peel, the stronger the message is that the skin needs to reproduce more healthy cells from the basal layer. So a peel at this level is most suitable for deeper skin problems such as stretch marks, cellulite, scars and aggressive deep-rooted adult acne.

Stratum basal
As this is the source of all new regenerated cells this level of MDA is essential for the effective use of scar treatment. The body's natural wound-healing mechanisms are stimulated and scar tissue can be greatly reduced.

Critical peeling depth
This is the point at which irreversible scarring would be caused with any kind of peeling. Even the deepest peeling should stop at the basement membrane of the epidermis – this means no pain and no blood as you are not penetrating the dermis where the nerve endings and blood supply are found.

- Neuro dermatitis – an allergy to milk and protein. This skin looks brittle and dry and abrasion of the skin type will make the condition worse

- Psoriasis – as the cell renewal rate is already faster than normal, MDA would increase the cellular production and make the condition worse

Microdermabrasion hand treatment

- Prepare the client's hands by washing them in warm, soapy water so they are grease-free.

- Apply pre-peel to dry cotton wool and wipe over the back of the hands.

- Next apply a thin layer of enzyme peeling paste to the back of the hand only. Leave for a *maximum* of 5 minutes and then remove with a dry gauze disk.

- Re-apply the pre-peel lotion, making sure the back of the hands are totally dry and free from enzyme peeling paste residue.

- Set the microdermabrasion vacuum/crystal flow to the correct level, start near the thumb and stroke all over the back of the hand. If hands are very lined, pull the skin slightly with your free hand to smooth the surface, for better application.

- Perform stroking movements along the fingers and repeat the procedure on the other hand. Once completed remove excess crystals with the soft goat-hair brush.

- Apply post-peel lotion to dry cotton wool and wipe over the back of the hands.

- Brush vitamin C cream gel mask on the back of hands.

- Leave mask for 5–10 minutes to soak in. Any residue can be massaged in to aid penetration.

- To finish, give a relaxing hand and arm massage with a regenerating cream designed to heal and soothe.

Recommend to the client that they look after their hands by using a sun factor cream of a good quality and a high SPF, wearing gloves when doing domestic chores and putting a good quality hand cream on every night before bed.

Microdermabrasion treatment – a step-by-step guide

1 Carry out a manual cleanse.

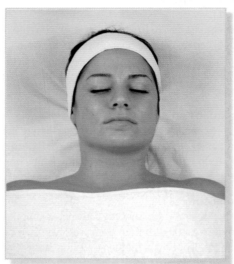

2 Apply a pre-peel mask.

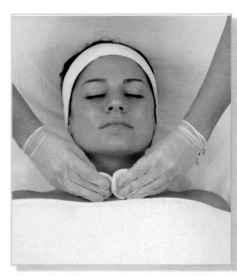

3 Apply an enzymatic mask.

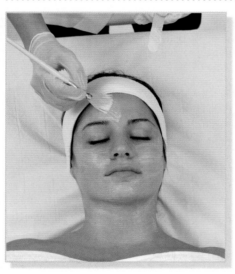

4 Remove mask with gauze disk.

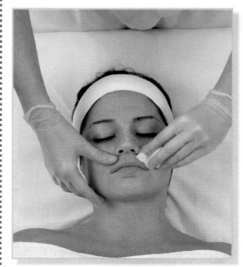

5 Carry out the process of microdermabrasion.

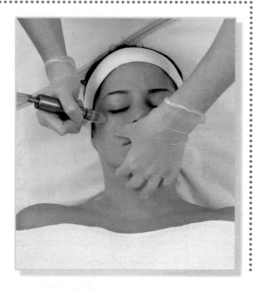

6 Remove with soft goat-hair brush.

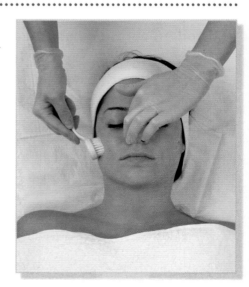

7 Apply post-peel to calm the skin.

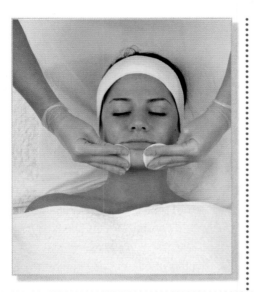

8 Apply oxygen moisturiser.

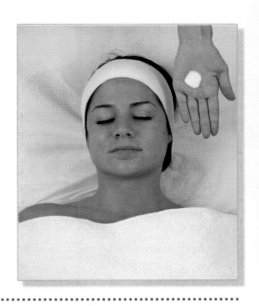

9 Apply vitamin C cream gel.

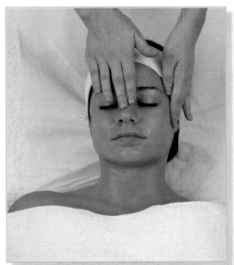

10 Apply OPC cream.

11 Finish the treatment, leaving skin cool and glowing.

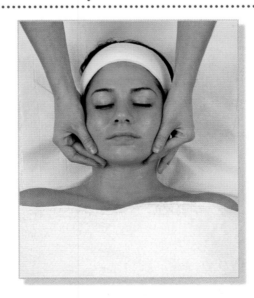

Aftercare and homecare for microdermabrasion

- Avoid further skin treatments to allow the skin to settle and regenerate.
- Avoid make-up application for 24 hours if a deep peel has taken place.
- Avoid UV exposure and always use a sun block cream for protection (you must wait 24 hours before applying creams, so take extra care during this time).
- Use the correct retail homecare products to suit skin type.
- Avoid heat treatments to the area.
- Avoid self-tanning applications to the area for 24 hours.
- Avoid scratching the skin and apply soothing cream if the skin is slightly irritated.
- Recommend other suitable electrical treatment to suit the client's needs in the future, such as galvanic and microcurrent.

Risk assessment for microdermabrasion

Identify the hazard	What is the risk?
Danger from electric shock	Low
Allergy to the enzyme masks or other products	High
Bruising of the skin by too high vacuum pressure	Med
Postural problems for the therapist	High
Allergic/sensitive reaction to crystals	Low

What should I do to prevent the hazard from becoming a risk?

- Follow manufacturers' instructions
- Carry out thermal and sensitivity testing
- Test on yourself before treatment
- Always have sufficient product on the skin to keep it well lubricated
- Constantly monitor for any developing contra-actions
- Remove all jewellery
- Never exceed the recommended vacuum pressure
- Never go too deeply into the dermis level
- Make sure the machine is positioned close to you, so that you have full control over the intensity dials
- Ensure correct posture and chair height to allow you to be in control of equipment

Maintenance of the machine

Check the filter – blocked filters lead to a loss of working pressure and therefore the peeling effect.

- Unscrew the clear plastic canister counter-clockwise.
- Remove the white filter and any micro crystals by wiping with a dry cloth, or tap the filter element gently to dislodge any beads.
- Replace the filter and tighten the canister, making sure it is sealed properly.
- Do not wash the machine or allow any dampness to get in, as this will clog the crystals.

Regularly test the cartridge by turning it on to maximum and covering the hand piece with your finger – then ensure the gauge measures the maximum reading of 15Hg. This will make the crystals vibrate or bounce in the container – you then know the flow and vacuum are working fine. Always follow the manufacturer's instructions for maintenance of each piece of equipment.

Micro-lance

A micro-lance is a sterile probe with a sharp edge for piercing the skin when removing foreign objects from under the skin, such as splinters, milia extraction or in-growing hairs.

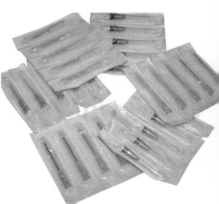

A micro-lance

How to use them:

- Check the area of skin to be treated. Do not treat any infected skin or go too near the eyes.
- If possible soften the skin with steaming to the area for five minutes or use an exfoliant to remove any dead skin cells before you break the skin's surface.
- Always use gloves and keep the micro-lance in its sterile packet until you need it.
- Wipe over the area to be treated with antiseptic lotion.

- Remove the probe from the packet.
- For milia extraction – pull the skin taught between the fingers and break the skin to one side of the milia, only going as deep as the edge of the milia is. You may draw blood, which can be wiped away with clean cotton wool. The milia should then be extracted by gentle pressure from the therapist's fingers (which are covered with tissue) and it will pop out of the small incision made. Milia are hard and white and made up of a plug of sebum – they will not burst as an infected pus spot would. You should be able to get the milia on a cotton wool round to show the client.
- Apply gentle pressure to the area, until the bleeding has stopped. Apply a weak antiseptic lotion or cream and carry on with the rest of the facial, avoiding the area.
- For an in-growing hair, follow the stages for milia extraction but go along the direction of the hair shaft, if you can see it underneath the epidermis. Break the skin – if you do not make contact with the dermis, there will be no contact with the blood vessels.
- For foreign objects such as a splinter, follow the same procedure.

Aftercare and homecare for micro-lance

You must dispose of the needle, with its lid on, into a yellow sharps box (needle bin), so that it can be taken away with your clinical waste. A company will come and remove all yellow bins with body-fluid contaminated waste on a regular basis. Please refer to the epilation unit for further information on removal of needles from salon premises.

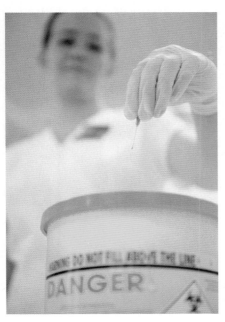

Always dispose of sharps correctly

Encourage your client to be extra careful with the area around the extraction and not to pick at it if a scab does form – they should allow it to heal naturally and not rub it off. Suggest the use of an antiseptic cream, keeping the area dry and clean and the use of an exfoliant to prevent the build up of milia again.

The treatment – high frequency

Skin type	Benefits and effects	Treatment time
Dry, flaky skin	Indirect HF applied as for manual massage (avoid tapotement) Moisturises and warms the tissues, stimulates sweat and sebaceous glands	10–15 minutes
Mature, dry skin	Indirect HF applied as for manual massage (avoid tapotement) Moisturises and warms the tissues, stimulates sweat and sebaceous glands	10–15 minutes
Oily skins	Direct HF using mushroom electrodes over gauze dries skin, and increases oxygen to skin if oxygenating cream is used	5–10 minutes
Oily skins, mild acne or congestion	Direct HF using mushroom electrodes over gauze dries skin and is germicidal, which aids healing	8–15 minutes

The treatment – lymphatic drainage (vacuum suction)

Skin type	Benefits and effects	Treatment time
All clients (Not contra-indicated)	Aids lymphatic drainage and helps with removal of waste and improves circulation in the area Can last as per manual massage routine	10–15 minutes
Dry, flaky skin	As above and stimulates gland activity, both sebaceous and sweat	10–12 minutes
Dull, sluggish skins	As above and stimulates gland activity, both sebaceous and sweat Circulation is increased therefore appearance is improved	5–10 minutes
Oily skins, comedones	Loosens comedones for extraction Avoid over-application of oil on an already oily skin	3–5 minutes

Salon life

Selina's story

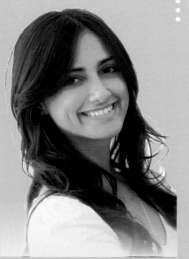

My name is Selina and I have worked for a large beauty salon for four years. We specialise in skincare and facials. I had a client in her forties who had woken up with Bell's palsy down the left-hand side of her face. She had been through a real ordeal; her son was killed in a car crash and her doctor thought it was probably stress that caused her muscles to go into paralysis. After surgery and extensive physiotherapy, she was still not quite right and feeling very self-conscious about her slightly lopsided features. When she came to see me, her partner had recently proposed and she wanted to find out about treatments to help her look good on her wedding day. I knew that microcurrent was originally developed within hospitals for muscular rehabilitation so I wrote to her doctor explaining the currents and treatment and he gave consent for a course of treatments. I also did a thorough skin diagnosis and we felt she would benefit from a galvanic treatment to deep cleanse and rehydrate her slightly dry skin, as well as a course of non-surgical face-lifting, targeting the muscles stimulated by the seventh cranial nerve, and specifically more lifting works on the poorer side of her face. After ten treatments, her eye had opened up, her face looked more even and her skin looked lovely. Best of all, her confidence was back! The treatments really helped both physically and psychologically and she was able to move forward with her life.

Effects for the therapist:

- Thorough knowledge of currents and the effect of treatments gives the therapist the ability to offer an effective course of treatments, targeting the client's specific needs

- Being able to link treatments enhances the effectiveness and shows the client that a combination of treatments can be beneficial

- The therapeutic benefit of being able to substantially help a client is very rewarding and offers great job satisfaction

- Good word-of-mouth advertising from a satisfied client who believes in the treatments.

Effects for the client:

- Physical changes in the skin and muscle tone are evident and will make the client feel that the treatment is effective and that something can be done to help — a positive effect

- Muscle tone can be increased and healing promoted within the collagen and elastin fibres

- Being able to help the client physically empowers them to feel better, instilling confidence and boosting morale — this helps with their emotional stability and creates a feeling of wellbeing.

The treatment – galvanic

Skin type	Benefits and effects	Treatment time
Mature skins	Desincrustation softens and reduces skin's resistance Deep cleanse iontophoresis improves and rehydrates the skin according to products used	Desincrustation 2–5 minutes Iontophoresis 10–15 minutes
Dry, dehydrated skins	Desincrustation softens and reduces skin's resistance Deep cleanse iontophoresis improves and rehydrates the skin according to products used	Desincrustation 2–5 minutes Iontophoresis 10–15 minutes
Oily skin	Desincrustation deep cleanses skin Iontophoresis rebalances the acid mantle according to products used	Desincrustation 5–10 minutes Iontophoresis 3–5 minutes
Congested, sluggish skin	Desincrustation deep cleanses and makes extraction easier Iontophoresis rebalances the acid mantle according to products used	Desincrustation 5–10 minutes Iontophoresis 2–3 minutes
Normal skin	Desincrustation deep cleanses Iontophoresis rebalances the acid mantle according to products used	Desincrustation 3–8 minutes Iontophoresis 3–5 minutes

The treatment – EMS (faradic)

Skin type	Benefits and effects	Treatment time
All skin types	Increases circulation to area Stimulates muscle contraction to aid dropped contours Stimulates sensory nerve endings Temporary reduction of puffiness	6–8 contractions per muscle No more than 10–15 minutes in total

The treatment – microcurrent

Skin type	Benefits and effects	Treatment time
All skin types for non-surgical face lifting	Programme 1 – Circulation Stimulates the blood circulation in the dermis and activates the lymph circulation. Programme 2 – Lymph drainage Increases the lymphatic drainage, ridding the tissue of toxic waste Programme 3 – Lifting The muscles are shortened or lengthened to firm the contours of the face Programme 4 – Lifting Same as programme 3 but uses a lower frequency to create deeper lift Programme 5 – Firming Improves the weft of the skin and underlying structure Programme 6 – Iontophoresis Introduction of collagen and elastin into the skin promotes the skin's natural regenerative process	Circulation – 2 minutes Lymph drainage – 10 minutes Lifting – 16 minutes Lifting – 8 minutes Firming – 10 minutes Iontophoresis – 3 minutes

The treatment – microdermabrasion (MDA)

Skin type	Benefits and effects	Treatment time
Aged or mature skin	Deep exfoliation stimulates cellular renewal for wrinkles, loss of elasticity, age spots, hyperkeratosis and sun damage	60 mins facial time for complete treatment
Other skin problems	Deep exfoliation stimulates cellular renewal for impure completion, acne scars, pigmentation, cellulite, stretch marks and enlarged pores	50–60 mins facial time for complete treatment
Hand treatments	Deep exfoliation stimulates cellular renewal for pigmentation, loss of elasticity	5–10 minutes of MDA whole treatment with massage 30 mins

Provide facial electrical treatments **Unit B14**

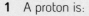

Check your knowledge

1 A proton is:
- **a)** a positively charged particle
- **b)** a negativity charged particle
- **c)** an atom
- **d)** a neutron.

2 The outer layer of an atom which contains negatively charged particles is called:
- **a)** a proton
- **b)** a neutron
- **c)** an electron
- **d)** a compressor.

3 Volts measures the ... of electricity.
- **a)** flow per second
- **b)** pressure
- **c)** power rating
- **d)** insulation

4 A conductor is something which:
- **a)** allows electricity to flow through it
- **b)** allows electricity to be stored in it
- **c)** stops electricity flowing through it
- **d)** stops you getting an electrical shock.

5 A galvanic current is:
- **a)** oscillating, alternating
- **b)** constant and direct
- **c)** surged and interrupted
- **d)** intermittent.

6 High-frequency current is:
- **a)** oscillating, alternating
- **b)** constant and direct
- **c)** surged and interrupted
- **d)** intermittent.

7 Direct high frequency is used for:
- **a)** dry skin
- **b)** older, mature skin
- **c)** oily or combination skin
- **d)** skin with fine lines.

8 Microcurrent is:
- **a)** a modified high-frequency current
- **b)** a modified low-frequency current
- **c)** a negative low pressure
- **d)** a vibrating pressure.

9 A make-and-break circuit is found in:
- **a)** a vacuum suction machine
- **b)** a percussion vibrator
- **c)** a microcurrent unit
- **d)** a high-frequency machine.

10 Vacuum suction is always carried out towards the:
- **a)** heart
- **b)** limbs
- **c)** lymph nodes
- **d)** hair follicles.

Getting ready for assessment

The evidence for your facial electrical unit will grow as you become more confident with the use of the equipment, and you will need a longer period of time to ensure that you cover all the ranges required. You will be directly observed by your assessor on at least five separate occasions and on at least three different clients, but you may do many more assessments than this — this is just the minimum requirement. Although this seems a lot, it will occur quite naturally as you take on clients with differing ages, skin types and treatment requirements, enabling you to use a variety of the electrical equipment. At this stage, your massage and cleansing techniques, choice of masks and so on are not assessable; you are already competent in those areas. This unit is about showing confidence with the machinery, choosing the most appropriate treatment for the client's needs and carrying out the treatment with assurance. You do need to use all of the equipment in your ranges and be able to discuss with your clients the other options available in the treatment objectives, so that your assessor gets a good overview of your knowledge and understanding of how to plan and link treatments, including all types of advice for aftercare, homecare and further treatments.

5

Body treatments

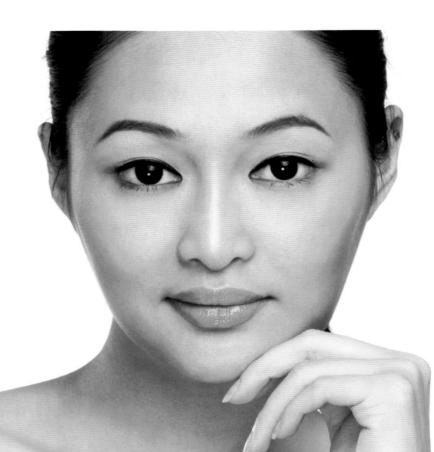

Body treatments

What you will learn

Body treatments – theory and consultation

- Consultation techniques
- Body consultation record card
- Posture
- Body types, classification and conditions
- Manual examination
- Skin conditions
- Fat and fat stores
- Weight problems, obesity and fluid retention
- Equipment used in body treatments

Body treatments — theory and consultation

A client's body image is linked to their self-confidence, so a body consultation requires tact and careful handling. To undergo a body consultation — opening up to a therapist and allowing your body to be scrutinised — takes a great deal of courage. Even clients with a 'model figure' have insecurities about their bodies. The average client comes to you because they believe you will be able to improve their body shape. It may take a couple of sessions before clients feel sufficiently comfortable with you to discuss their body image. To make your client entirely comfortable you need to maintain a positive, polite and reassuring manner. You also need to maintain client modesty, privacy and comfort at all times — in fact, treat the client as you would wish to be treated: lavished with care and attention.

Consultation techniques

Consultation techniques include a variety of methods to determine the best course of treatment to meet the client's needs. These include:

- questioning
- visual observation
- manual examination
- reference to client records.

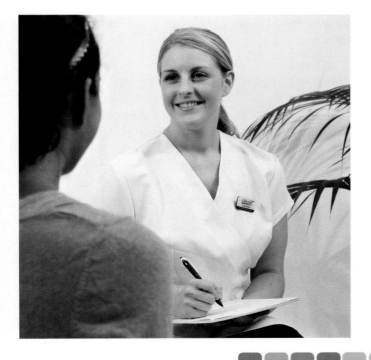

Think about it

There are common threads running through the consultation for all body treatments. To refresh your knowledge of consultation techniques, refer to Professional basics, pages 34–36.

The initial assessment of the figure and **posture** of the client is a visual one. The next part involves the client removing clothing as far as underwear, to allow a thorough physical and manual assessment. The client needs to be informed *prior* to the appointment that this will happen, to allow them to be prepared to be undressed in front of you — both for the practical reason of wearing the right underwear, and also mentally. This should be discussed when they make the appointment.

Individual needs

Remember to be aware and mindful of the client's cultural and religious beliefs, age, disabilities and gender — this needs consideration, as all clients bring their own special needs into a consultation. You should reassure the client that their cultural and religious beliefs will be upheld and they will not be forced to reveal too much when undressing or do anything that conflicts with their beliefs. This needs to be discussed with the client in a private and confidential manner prior to the treatments taking place.

The age of the client needs consideration — an older client may be more hesitant about taking clothes off, and may not be used to having their body touched, as you would do during manual examination. Older clients may also have physical or mobility restrictions to consider, or impairments such as limited hearing. Clients with disabilities need a full discussion about their capabilities and how you can best help them — talk about what you would normally do and how you may be able to adapt the treatment to suit them. Remember it may not be a physical disability.

The gender of the client should also be considered, as males and females will have different needs. Male clients tend to be concerned more with loss of **muscle tone** and

Key terms

Posture – the position of the human body when standing, sitting, or lying down. Good posture keeps the bones and joints in correct alignment so that the muscles are used properly and it contributes to a good appearance.

Muscle tone – the ability of muscles to respond to a stretch or a state of permanent partial contraction of the muscles. Muscle tone helps the body maintain its posture.

sport-related muscle damage, therefore require massage and G5 treatments. Weight distribution and fat deposits are also different. However, it is wrong to generalise and assume a client wants a certain treatment because of their gender. Men are also concerned about weight loss and ageing, just as women are — and men get acne, wrinkles and sluggish circulation and require just the same treatments!

Observation

Although you will be looking at the skin in the area to be treated for visible signs of damage, correction required and possible contra-indications, you will first observe the whole client in order to see:

- any posture/postural problems
- weight and height ratio
- mobility problems or a disability requiring treatment adaptation
- general body language reflecting confidence or self-esteem.

Your observation will need to begin before the client is aware of you, as this is when you will be able to see the client's unconscious body language and posture. How is the client carrying him- or herself? Do they look weighed down with worry, or are they confident, with a spring in the step? This will indicate not only self-confidence, but also energy levels. Store your first impressions for when you complete the physical examination — only then will you see the true state of posture, with the client undressed, when you can observe the spine and balance of the shoulders and hips, and the distribution of body weight (see Posture on page 331).

Questioning

Personal details and medical records will be recorded in the same way as for facial consultation (see Facial treatments — theory and consultation, page 256, to refresh your memory). These details will only need updating or revising if, for example, the client moves home or changes doctor. See the example of a personal details record card on page 327.

Think about it

A client who has poor self-esteem will not easily make eye contact. It might be that the client's visit to the salon is because of a facial or body problem that is causing negative feelings. This will be reflected in the individual's posture, demeanour and lack of enthusiasm. You will need to observe this and handle the client with care.

Think about it

At this stage, the client should be sitting with outdoor clothing removed to discuss his or her lifestyle and treatment requirements.

However, on every visit you will need to check for contra-indications and allergies, medication taken and any lifestyle changes. Any or all of these can change on a weekly basis, and a client can develop an allergy to a product he or she has been using for years.

Body consultation record card

Use the body consultation card to guide you through your questioning. This is often printed on the reverse of the facial record card. Pages 328–330 show a typical body consultation card, completed for a body massage treatment.

Lifestyle and eating patterns should be discussed as well as sleeping patterns, stress levels and the client's perceptions, goals and wishes, as well as your professional advice. The client's physical wellbeing is only one part of the whole picture; discuss the client's relaxation choices, hobbies and family commitments and physical recreation. All of these play a part in how the body behaves and reacts. For example, repetitive muscle movements can cause tension and problems in the muscle fibres, such as fibrositis, and a simple chat about using a wrist support when typing, or changing the height of the chair in relation to the screen, may be enough to prevent the problem, along with heat treatments and plenty of massage to release the muscular tension.

Think about it

You are asking very detailed personal questions within a consultation, and clients may not have thought in detail about their lifestyle and the contribution it makes to their health. For example, if you ask them if they consider themselves to generally enjoy good health, they may well say yes. But, when it comes to the medication section, they may list three or four medicines they are taking for various health problems!

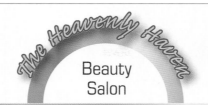

Personal Details Card – CONFIDENTIAL

(Keep in locked file after consultation)

Personal details:

Client name:	Title: Mr/Mrs/Ms/Dr/Other

Client unique reference number:

Client address:

Postcode:

Home telephone:	Mobile:

Work telephone:

Email: (for special offers)

Emergency contact number:

Emergency contact name:

Medical details:

Doctor name:

Surgery address:

Postcode:

Telephone number:

Within the last year have you been under the care of a health professional?   Yes/No

If yes – please state why:

Treatment details:

Therapist/Stylist	Treatment	Date

A personal details record card

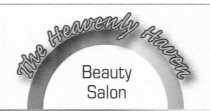

Beauty
Salon

Client Record Card

BODY TREATMENT SHEET: Body massage

Date: 30/6/10   **Client ref no.** 1245

Any factors which need to be considered today: Client feels low after family bereavement; generally tired + lethargic. Finding her sleep pattern is disturbed and it's hard to relax.

Client details: Please tick or circle the appropriate ranges covered within this treatment

Client: Male ——————————— Female ——————— ✓ ———————

Skin type: oily /(dry)/ combination / mature / young   Massage medium:(oil)/ cream / talc

Muscle tone: (good)/ average / poor

Age: under 21 / 30s /(40s)/ 50s / 60s / over 70

Body Type: ectomorph /(endomorph)/ mesomorph / combination

Postural faults: scoliosis / kyphosis / lordosis /(other) None

Frame size: small /(medium)/ large

Weight: 55 kg   underweight/(normal weight)/ overweight
Height: 5ft 4in

Actual body mass index: 23   Desirable body mass index for good health: Yes

Muscle tone: (good)/ average / poor   Posture: Quite good; slumped today as client is feeling low; tension in shoulders and upper back

Female hormone levels: At what stage in your monthly cycle are you?
Client about to start period – no stomach massage. Client feeling bloated, slight water retention. Hormonal fluctuation (combined with bereavement) could account for low mood.

Distribution of body fat:

Type of fat: hard / medium /(soft)/ cellulite   Where: tummy and hips

Circulation: (good)/ poor   Varicose veins present: Yes /(No)   Where:

Any other considerations: disabilities / impairment
N/A

Client Health:

Overall Health: (good)/ average / poor
Comments: Generally, client in good health / free of illness. Feels she may be coming down with a cold – autoimmune system may be low due to psychological state

Medication being taken:
Occasional paracetamol for period pains – only when required

Last visit to doctor: Date: Relating to what:
N/A Client doesn't remember the last visit she needed

Skin condition: good /(average)/ poor   specific problems/conditions to be avoided:
Client feels her skin is getting dryer as she gets older and wants to keep it nourished.

Lifestyle Analysis:

Sleep: Does the client sleep well? yes / no   Approx hours per night: 5-6

Is it disturbed sleeping patterns? Do they wake up a lot through the night? Why?

Yes, client is awake through the night and has worries that seem worse at night.

Profession: Doctor's receptionist   Sedentary/physical job: Sedentary

Although job quite sedentary, client enjoys using Wii fitness game at home and tries to walk to work as often as possible

Family life: Marital status / children: Married with two teenagers - both girls

Exercise taken: duration / type of / how regular / likes / dislikes:

See above

Energy levels: 1–10 rating (1 being lowest 10 being highest):

3 - low at present and a bit less enthusiastic than her usual self.

Relaxation: good / poor

Comments: Client finds it hard to switch off, especially at night. Now worried about her Mum being on her own after the death of her father.

Fluid intake: Eight glasses of water taken daily? No

Other drinks: Client not drinking enough water, drinking too much coffee - may contribute to poor sleep and dehydrated skin.

Other factors: regular meal times / shift work / eating in a hurry / supplements / allergies or food intolerances:

No real dietary concerns, has little appetite at the moment but is still cooking meals for family & tries to eat a varied diet.

Diet: varied / poor / good / average – give examples of types of food eaten:

Usually good but light at the moment. Takes packed lunches (roll/fruit), breakfast usually toast and coffee. Cooks full meals for her family in the evening w/plenty of veg. Feels it's important for her children to eat well and for them to eat together as a family.

Food allergies: N/A

Likes/dislikes: Most fruit except oranges, most veg. except Brussels sprouts. Client eats most food groups. Prefers an early evening meal.

Alcohol consumption: units per week: 3-4 glasses of wine at weekend

Smoking: per day/week Non-smoker

Fluid intake: per day x6 coffees, 2 glasses water

Drugs/other: Paracetamol for period pain

The treatment:

Reasons for treatment: Lot of tension in upper back and feeling low, due to bereavement. Recommend relaxing massage but avoid the tapotement movements and abdomen for this treatment. I/red would be very soothing.

Other:

Massage techniques: Effleurage / Petrissage / Tapotement / Vibrations

Treatment chosen: Galvanic / EMS / microcurrent / vacuum suction / microdermabrasion / Infra red / G5 / audio sonic / massage / aromatherapy / hot stones / other: please state:

Reason for this treatment: To warm the upper shoulders and soften the area, and bring blood flow to the trapezius muscle.

Treatment areas: Neck face and scalp massage / Chest and shoulders / Back and gluteals / Arms and hands / Abdomen / Full body / Legs and feet / Full body with scalp & face

Continued

Any further necessary action: No

Contra indication present: yes / no

Was client encouraged to seek medical advice?

Explain why treatment cannot be carried out

N/A

Does treatment need adapting due to minor contra-indication?: yes / no

Explain:

Environmental conditions: Lighting / Heating / Ventilation / General comfort / Suitable music / Sounds

All completed

Client preparation: Removal of appropriate clothing / Accessories removed / Covering of cuts / abrasions Covering client / Removal of makeup / Secure and protect hair

All completed

After treatment:

Aftercare/homecare advice given: Client should try and relax more and use a hot water bottle on the top of the back to ease tension.

Healthy eating and exercise advise given: Try and substitute herbal teas for coffee; avoid drinking coffee in the evening – it may be a contributory factor in the client not sleeping.

Suitable home care products and how to use them: Lavender essential oil in a carrier oil to add to the bath at night for a sleeping aid, and body moisturiser to be applied after the bath.

General notes: I let the client sleep on a little after the back massage as she dozed off and was so relaxed I didn't like to disturb her! I didn't have another client for half an hour so it was good that she did have a little relaxation. I would recommend my client try a hot stone massage for deep relaxation.

Client declaration:

I declare the information is true and correct and that as far as I am aware, I can undertake treatment with this establishment without any adverse effects. I am fully aware of the contra-indications: I am therefore willing to proceed and accept this treatment.

Client signature: M. Pearson   Date: 30/6/10

Therapist signature: Jodie T   Date: 30/6/10

Please note – without signature treatment is unable to proceed

Key terms

Body fat – produced in the body and stored when there is a high intake of calories. Essential body fat is required for normal physiological functioning and consists of fat stored in bone marrow, the heart, lungs, liver, spleen, kidneys, intestines and muscles. Stored fat is accumulated in adipose tissue, primarily beneath the skin, in the subcutaneous layer, where it provides insulation and cushions the body. There are two types: *white fat*, important in energy metabolism, heat insulation and cushioning; and *brown fat*, abundant in newborn babies and important for making heat (it decreases in amount as we age). Too much body fat is bad for the functioning of the body and may result in diseases such as diabetes.

Calorie – a food measure. Its full description is: a unit of heat, the amount required to raise the temperature of one gram of water by one degree. Food has the amount of calories displayed on the outer packaging.

Cellulite – a type of fatty tissue causing a dimpled or uneven appearance in the skin of certain parts of the body. It occurs when fat cells swell and the surrounding tissue changes in texture, causing a pulling on the tissues and giving the skin the characteristic dimpled effect.

Diet – although diet can refer to a person's or group's usual range of foods, its other – more commonly recognised – meaning is a restricted selection of food, chosen to (a) decrease a person's weight, (b) improve a person's physical condition, or (c) prevent/treat a disease.

Ectomorph – a lean and angular body shape, with narrow hips and shoulders and very little body fat or muscle.

Endomorph – a round body shape, with narrow shoulders; may have wide hips and can have a high proportion of body fat.

Mesomorph – a strong muscular body type, angular with broad shoulders and narrow hips; usually well muscled with little body fat.

Metabolism – the result of physical and chemical processes in the body, by which material substances are produced, maintained and destroyed. It is the rate at which the body burns fuel/food and transforms it into energy.

Varicose veins – distended veins occurring most commonly in the legs. The condition is often inherited or caused by obstruction to blood flow.

Consultation questions to ask the client	How this helps you, the therapist
What are you hoping to gain from this treatment?	You can assess whether this is achievable and realistic for the client (e.g. a G5 treatment is not going to make the client lose a stone in weight before a dinner dance on Saturday night!). It also stops you assuming you know what the client wants. You may think they need to lose weight but they may come to you for muscle toning – so never assume!
Have you had these treatments before? Were they successful? Did you enjoy them?	The client's likes and dislikes, how successful the treatment was, if it was a course of treatments, if the client was committed, if they contributed to the success of the plan and what the results were
How long ago were your previous treatments? Do you think the condition has got worse with time? Why did you stop the treatment?	This will give you some idea of the time and cost implications of the treatment, what their homecare and lifestyle contribution is to the condition being treated and how much support they will need to maintain a new course of action

Posture

A good posture is one in which the body is relaxed and balanced in an upright position, allowing the organs and systems of the body to work efficiently and effectively. This depends largely upon the tone of the muscles at the front and back of the trunk and legs working together, so that the body is balanced and not strained in any way – allowing muscles, ligaments and joints to move freely in their range of movement, without pain or injury. The muscles supporting posture are the anti-gravity muscles. They balance the front and the back of the body, using as little energy as possible.

Imagine there is an invisible thread or cord, holding the body upright (rather like a puppet on a string, but with one central string) from the centre of the top of the skull, through the middle of the body, shoulder and pelvic girdles, right to the ground. This is often referred to as a plumb line.

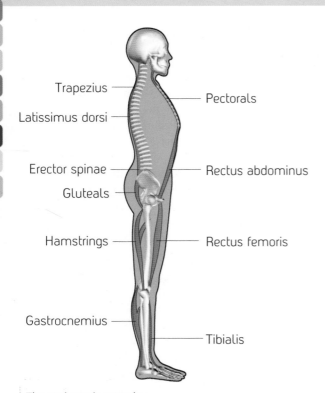

The anti-gravity muscles

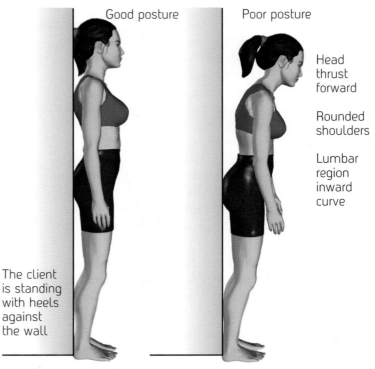

Good posture   Poor posture

Head thrust forward

Rounded shoulders

Lumbar region inward curve

The client is standing with heels against the wall

Standing posture

The benefits of good posture include the following:

- Breathing is easy as the lungs can be filled deeply when inhaling because they are not compressed or the chest contracted.

- The digestive tract has enough room to function correctly, without being cramped or restricted.

- An even distribution of body weight ensures that the body does not become too tired, nor is too much strain put on any one set of muscles.

- The bones, ligaments and joints are allowed to work fully, without undue effort or the risk of damage.

- The shape and figure looks at its best when the posture is correct, and this, in turn, gives a feeling of confidence and provides a positive mental outlook.

Poor posture results in the following:

- The lungs are not able to expand fully, as the chest may be restricting their capacity, resulting in poor oxygen levels in all the cells of the body, and lack of oxygen flow to the brain, causing dizziness or headaches.

- The digestive system suffers, ranging from indigestion pains or cramps, to wind and reflux, due to pressure on the sphincter muscle, which prevents food from coming back up from the stomach.

- The muscles become strained, causing lower back pain, or backache, because of poor distribution of weight.

- Tension headaches occur, caused by tension in the trapezius muscle, especially if the upper body is hunched over a keyboard or machine for long periods. This leads, for example, to poor blood and lymph flow to the restricted areas, leading to aches and pains, tiredness and pain in the joints and ligaments.

How to assess posture

Ask the client to remove the gown. The client will be in their underwear, or if going into the spa or sauna, may be in dry swimwear. Ask the client to stand in a normal, relaxed manner.

1 Observe the natural stance of the client from the front, side and then from the back.

2 Note the shape of the spine, the level of the shoulder blades and the level of the hips and pelvic tilt. Are they even on both sides? Place your hands on the hips and shoulders to gain a perspective of the balance. If one hip or shoulder is higher than the other, there may be a postural fault, pushing it out of alignment.

3 Mark the scapulae and measure the distance between the vertebral border and the spine — is it the same, or is one further away than the other?

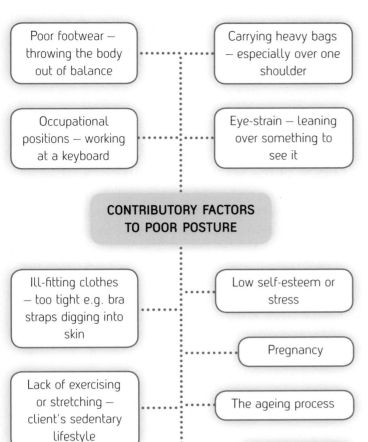

Poor footwear — throwing the body out of balance

Carrying heavy bags — especially over one shoulder

Occupational positions — working at a keyboard

Eye-strain — leaning over something to see it

CONTRIBUTORY FACTORS TO POOR POSTURE

Ill-fitting clothes — too tight e.g. bra straps digging into skin

Low self-esteem or stress

Pregnancy

Lack of exercising or stretching — client's sedentary lifestyle

The ageing process

Illness

4 Look at the shape of the vertebrae — you should be able to trace with your finger the shape of the spine, along the protruding spinal processes. This will enable you to see and feel if the spine is out of alignment — see below.

5 Fill out the record card accordingly.

What to look for

- The head sits comfortably on the top of the vertebrae, not too far forward or back, with no protruding jaw line or the head being more forward than the pelvis.

- The arms are relaxed at the sides and are even in position and length.

- The shoulders are even and neither shoulder droops or is over-extended.

- The scapulae are even and of equal distance away from the spine.

- The spine follows its natural curve and does not force the hips to lie sideways or one higher than the other.

- The abdomen is flat and the waist curves are even and level on both sides.

- The buttocks are sitting naturally, without protruding, and the pelvic tilt looks relaxed, not forced.

- The legs are straight, the knees point forward and are level, and both feet point forward — without the legs being forced into the position or looking unnatural.

- The client is free from any pain in the joints or muscles, and is easily able to maintain the position, while you observe body shape and posture.

Checking the spinal column

The spine is a very unstable structure because it consists of 33 small circular vertebrae, piled on top of one another, with discs of cartilage (acting as shock absorbers) in between. (For further information on the spine, see Related anatomy and physiology, page 153.)

The spinal cord runs through holes in the middle of the vertebrae, just behind the discs — a column of nerves connecting the brain to the body. To help us move and remain upright, the spine is held rigidly in position by numerous bands of tough muscle and ligament.

Good posture involves holding the body erect so that the concave curvatures of the vertebrae at the neck and the base of the back are not lost. The aim when sitting, walking, driving, standing and even sleeping should be to maintain these natural curves in the back. If the curves are allowed to become convex, the muscles are put under strain and the

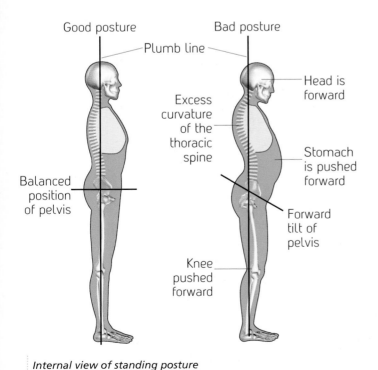

Good posture

Bad posture

Plumb line

Head is forward

Excess curvature of the thoracic spine

Stomach is pushed forward

Balanced position of pelvis

Forward tilt of pelvis

Knee pushed forward

Internal view of standing posture

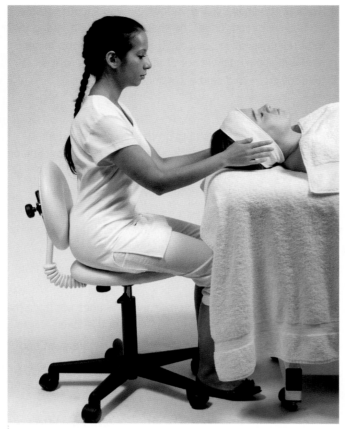

A good sitting posture

spine is weakened, leading to the possibility of a prolapsed intervertebral disc (a slipped disc), with severe backache, and sometimes **sciatica**.

Think about it

Good posture is as important to the therapist as it is to the client. Therapists can easily develop repetitive strain injury in the course of the working day, and can often suffer bad backs if they are not very careful about stance and spinal alignment during treatments. Go back and read the Manual Handling Operations Regulations 1992 in Professional basics, 'You, your client and the law', page 71, to ensure you are not over-straining and can pick up heavy objects in the correct manner.

Key terms

Sciatica – pain along the line of the sciatic nerve, i.e. through the buttock, back of the thigh, calf and down the foot. It may be caused by injury or damage to the lumbar vertebrae.

Main causes of spinal deformities

- Congenital – present at birth or arising as a direct result of hereditary factors.
- Traumatic – damage resulting from accidents, the most common being a whiplash injury.
- Environmental – resulting from bad posture, occupation, bad habits. Tall people may stoop to minimise their height.

Curves of the vertebral column

The primary curve is the first curve to form when the foetus is curled up in the womb. The head and knees are almost touching, because space is a little cramped as the baby develops. The secondary cervical curve develops after birth when the baby has developed sufficient skill and control over the neck muscles to pull the head upright, generally after three months. The secondary lumbar curve develops when the child learns to stand upright and to walk, any time after the first year. The thoracic and sacral primary curves are retained.

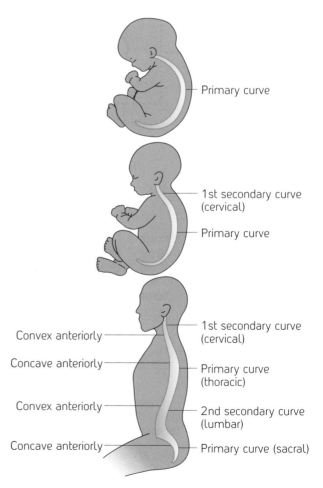

Curves of the spine

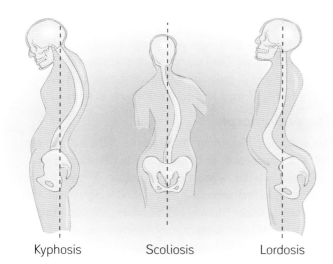

Kyphosis   Scoliosis   Lordosis

Common postural problems

This means that all healthy, normal babies have perfect posture, and that poor posture is due to external and environmental influences — poor footwear, diet, psychological factors, poorly fitting clothes or low self-esteem.

There are three types of abnormal curvature of the spine that you will need to check for:

- kyphosis
- lordosis
- scoliosis.

Kyphosis

- Seen as a rounded back and rounded shoulders.

- The pectoral muscles on the chest are short and constricted, which restricts breathing and the chest feels tight.

- The thoracic area of the back bows outward as the muscles are over-stretched.

- This results in the abdominal muscles becoming lazy — the abdomen tends to droop and the breasts may sag forwards, due to lack of support from the Cooper's ligaments and pectoral muscles.

- The condition is common in people who have jobs that cause them to lean forward for extended periods of time, for example if they have to drive for long periods, or office workers who lean over a keyboard. It also occurs in girls who try to hide large breasts, or are taller than average. Poor posture when carrying heavy loads also contributes to the development of this condition.

Think about it

Kyphosis, lordosis and scoliosis are recognised medical conditions and a doctor's referral is essential before treating a client — written permission should be sought, and these conditions should be treated as a contra-indication until that happens, even if the client insists you go ahead with treatment.

You can give treatments which release muscular tension and allow the muscles to relax, such as heat and massage — these are often very effective and therapeutic, but the client's doctor's approval is required.

Lordosis

- Seen as a hollow lower back, which becomes arched, tight and stiff.

- The muscles in the lower back become short and may cause back ache.

- The pelvis and abdomen are pushed forwards and the gluteal muscles tend to stick out.

- Quite common in the later stages of pregnancy, when the weight of the growing baby pushes out the abdomen, and in men who develop a 'beer belly'. It may also develop from wearing high heels, which alters the centre of gravity and forces the posture to compensate.

Scoliosis

- Seen as a sideways pull on the spine, resulting in the curve of the spine going left or right.

- This makes the shoulders uneven, as it unbalances the scapulae, and the leg length may differ on each side, depending upon where the lateral curve is.

- The waistline will be uneven, and a client with scoliosis may walk with a slight roll of the hips.

- Mothers carrying infants on one side at the hip can develop this condition, as can people carrying uneven loads, or standing for long periods of time with all the body weight on one side. It can also be hereditary.

Body types, classification and conditions

Before you can fully conduct your consultation, you will need to be able to recognise the most common body types and conditions, as this will influence your treatment planning.

The most common body conditions to look for are:

- cellulite
- poor muscle tone
- sluggish circulation
- blemished/congested skin.

You will need to look at the trunk (the torso) and the limbs.

There are three main body types:

- ectomorph
- endomorph
- mesomorph.

Some people are very typical of one body type and are easily classified; other clients are a mixture of types.

The ectomorph

The ectomorph tends to be long, lean and angular. This body type is often tall, as the long bones (the femur), which gives the legs their length, are well developed. Ectomorphs have very little fat, which gives a lack of curves, or breast tissue. They are quite narrow in the hips and shoulders and have small joints. They do not have much muscle bulk and often have a high metabolism, which means they can eat a high quantity of food and not lay it down as body fat.

The endomorph

The endomorph is almost the opposite of the ectomorph. This body type tends to be well-rounded, tending towards heaviness in build, with a high percentage of fat in relation to muscle bulk. Endomorphs easily put on weight, even though they may consider themselves as having a small appetite. Their general frame is solid and the limbs and neck tend to be short, with small hands and feet.

The mesomorph

The mesomorph is usually strong with an even distribution of weight, and is of an athletic build. There are well-developed shoulders, with a slim waist and hips, the muscles are well-defined and there is a low percentage of body fat. While active, this body type remains lean and strong with good muscle tone, but may develop more fat if the body does not exercise.

Other factors to check in figure diagnosis

After checking the body type, the spinal position and the general posture, work methodically down the body, noting all areas, as they may be relevant to the treatment plan.

Round shoulders

This problem may not be acute enough to cause kyphosis, but can be prominent enough to be noticeable. For example, people with chest problems such as asthma often hunch over and develop round shoulders. Correcting the condition may require heat and massage to release the muscular tension in the pectorals and trapezius muscles, along with stretching exercises and regular postural correction — you may need to physically move the shoulders back into the correct position. The Alexander Technique of realignment, Pilates and yoga, all of which stretch the muscles, are very good for this postural fault.

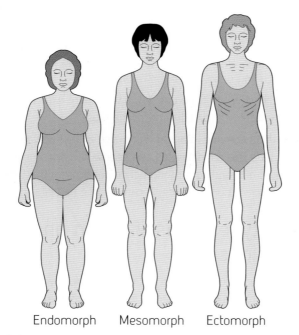

| Endomorph | Mesomorph | Ectomorph |

Body types

Winged scapulae

This is quite visible from the back, as the vertebral borders of the **scapulae** protrude outwards and can look a little like wings. This is common with students or backpackers who carry heavy rucksacks on their backs — the scapulae spread out trying to distribute the weight. It is also common if there is a combination of poor posture and a lack of fat to pad the contours, so it is more noticeable in thinner clients. This needs to be considered when giving massage and using electrical equipment on the back (such as G5 mechanical massage), as it can be quite uncomfortable for the client.

The rib cage

The position of the sternum and rib cage is important, as it tends to dictate the height and angle of the breast position. Thinner clients may have a more noticeably defined shape to the rib cage, and usually with this body type, the breasts have little fat, and are higher up on the rib cage. Note if the client has a slight boxy look to the rib cage or a 'pigeon' or hollow chest — an over-expanded rib cage becomes more obvious when the client is lying down, face upwards (supine position).

Key terms

Scapulae – shoulder blades. They are triangular-shaped bones that connect the humerus (arm bone) with the clavicle (collar bone).

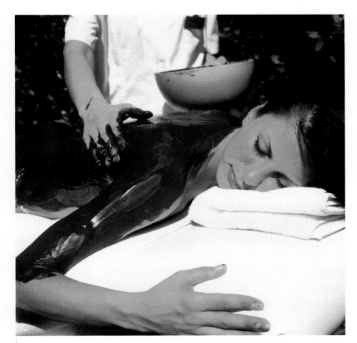

Body mask

The breasts

Breast treatments are very popular, and many cosmetic houses and product suppliers make creams especially for the delicate skin found on the breast. The breast has no muscle tissue of its own, and consists of fat and milk ducts, which are stimulated to produce milk by hormones after childbirth.

There are no exercises which affect the breast itself, but size and shape are dictated by weight loss or gain. Surgery can be performed to enhance the size of the breast by implants, or to reduce the fat content in the breast, also affecting its shape. (Males have also been known to have implants under the pectoral muscles to give a better definition to the shape of the chest.)

The breasts are held in place on top of the pectoral muscles by strong ligaments called Cooper's ligaments, and as long they remain attached to the breast, then exercise will strengthen the attachment and therefore improve the position of the breast.

To check if the Cooper's ligaments are still attached to the breast and the pectoral wall, ask the client to raise her arms from the side to over the head. If the nipples move higher, and the breast moves, then the Cooper's ligaments are attached and can be strengthened through exercise. Diet or surgery are the only two effective methods of altering the breast shape, although creams will help the skin's appearance and tone.

Think about it

Some clients may not wish to appear topless, and you should respect their privacy. Others will not mind and may ask if anything can be done to alter their breast shape.

If a client has had a full or partial mastectomy, they will be more self-conscious and may not wish for any treatments to be carried out in the area. Also remember that chemotherapy and radiotherapy are a contra-indication to all treatments.

The body is not symmetrical. One side is slightly larger than the other, the face is slightly lopsided with one eye slightly higher than the other and this lack of symmetry includes hands, feet and breasts! Reassure your client that it is natural to have one breast slightly higher or fuller than the other.

Underwear/clothing

Underwear and clothing, surprisingly perhaps, play a part in poor posture. If the client has gained weight, had a pregnancy or just changed shape, then her underwear size, especially bra size, will have changed too. Clients who develop permanent strap marks and indentations in the skin on top of the shoulder are wearing the wrong size bra, and may be constricting muscles as a result. Check to see if the back of the bra is digging into the flesh, or riding too high up over the shoulder blades. A correctly fitted and sized bra will support the breasts, leave no skin irritation or marks and sit very securely. The cups should encase the entire breast and not give a squashed appearance or large cleavage, where the breasts are pushed together. The same applies to pants and shoes. Some clients suffer because they would rather endure the pain than admit to being a larger size, or wear a slightly lower heel.

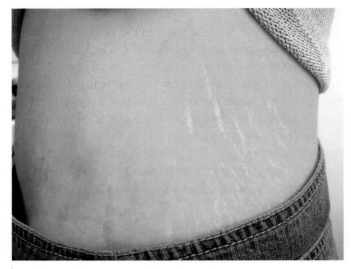
Abdominal stretch marks

Think about it

Tact and diplomacy are essential. You can only suggest to the client that she gets measured correctly, but when you develop a rapport with her, she may be prepared to take your advice. Salon treatments and expensive creams will not correct the problem if the underlying source of discomfort is not corrected.

Abdomen and hips

These tend to be the main areas of fat accumulation, and a number of treatments are aimed at the tummy, hips and thighs. Look for the amount and type of fat — hard, soft or with cellulite present (see the section on page 343).

Women tend to accumulate fat in the lower body and men to put weight on in the abdominal area. These figure types are often referred to by their hormonal influences — the male shape may be described as android **obesity** and the female pear shape can be called gynaecoid obesity.

Think about it

When discussing the abdomen, remember to ask about the client's general digestion and diet. Discuss any problems such as irritable bowel syndrome, constipation, diarrhoea etc. This will indicate the client's stress levels and whether digestion is affected by stress. This will help with treatment plan – you can offer relaxing treatments. Conditions such as gall stones or an inflamed gall bladder are helped with good nutrition and good posture – it relieves the pressure in the top of the abdomen under the diaphragm.

Stretch marks

Look for stretch marks, often called striations, on the abdomen and hips. Stretch marks appear on the skin as long, faint scars, or wiggly lines in the skin's surface. When they first appear, they can look quite red and angry, and then they diminish into pearly white lines after several years. On black skins, they will appear pink and stand out due to the contrast in skin tones. Stretch marks occur as a result of a breakdown of the skin's connective tissue, which occasionally ruptures. They are most commonly seen on the breasts, abdomen, upper arms, inner thighs and hips.

Stretch marks can be improved with treatments. They will diminish with microcurrent application and skin treatments to firm the collagen and elastin layers, along with the application of good quality, skin-firming creams or oils.

Not every client who is pregnant will develop stretch marks, but pregnant clients, clients with fine skin, or sun-damaged skin should be encouraged to keep the skin supple with regular application of skincare emollients. General massage to the area, in gentle circular motions, with high quality oils will stimulate the blood flow, bringing oxygen and nutrients to the skin, which in turn will help the collagen and elastin fibres become stronger. A healthy diet and drinking lots of water will also improve the general health of the skin.

Key terms

Obesity – the excessive accumulation of fat in the body.

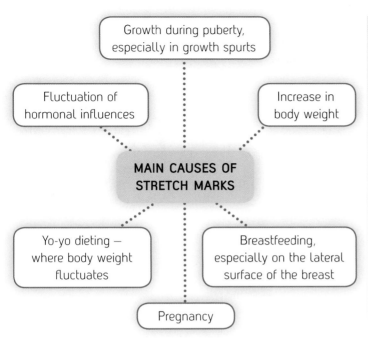

Growth during puberty, especially in growth spurts

Fluctuation of hormonal influences

Increase in body weight

MAIN CAUSES OF STRETCH MARKS

Yo-yo dieting — where body weight fluctuates

Breastfeeding, especially on the lateral surface of the breast

Pregnancy

Stretch marks are a contra-indication to some treatments which may make the condition worse, for example vacuum suction and G5 mechanical massage, or even skin stretching massage movements.

Additional knowledge

The pregnant teenager

Pregnant teenagers, particularly those who are overweight before they get pregnant, are more susceptible to stretch marks because of their youth. Their bodies have not completed growing and the skin is put under tremendous pressure to stretch very quickly to accommodate the expanding womb.

Think about it

During toxic or infectious invasion of the body, the infection may alter the elastic tissue and makes it prone to rupture as a result of substantial protein loss affecting the connective tissue content. This will show up as stretch marks.

Key terms

Adipose tissue – loose connective tissue in which fat cells (adipocytes) accumulate. Its main role is to store energy in the form of fat. It is located beneath the skin in the subcutaneous layer and around internal organs, such as the kidney and eyes, to provide protective padding.

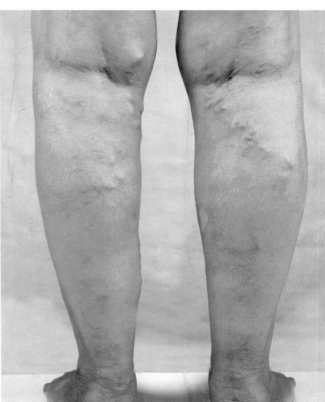

Varicose veins

Legs and feet

- Check the legs for the presence of cellulite and any surface distortion of the skin, such as varicose veins or inflamed varicose veins, a condition called phlebitis. Phlebitis is easily recognised as the vein becomes painful and tender, and the surrounding skin becomes hot and red. It is a contra-indication to treatment, but responds well to medical treatments, such as elastic support for the leg, and medication. Varicose veins commonly develop during pregnancy or with a considerable weight gain.

- Other contra-indications to treatment in this area include broken capillaries, seen as small thread veins on the skin's surface, and broken skin, or cuts on the lower leg caused by shaving rather than waxing the hairs. Small cuts could be covered over, or avoided during massage, but because of a cut's moisture content, an electrical current would be drawn to it. Therefore, it is a contra-indication to electrical treatment.

- Very thin, bony legs are a contra-indication to treatment, as there is little or no **adipose tissue** to work upon, and the client may bruise if massage movements or heavy mechanical massage were to be carried out.

Check the legs for knock knees, bow legs and hyper-extended knees:

- knock knees (genu valgum) is an abnormal in-curving of the legs, resulting in a gap between the feet when the knees are in contact
- bow legs (genu verum) is an abnormal out-curving of the legs, resulting in a gap between the knees when standing
- hyper-extended knees is an extensive and forceful extension of the knee joint which can affect balance and the ability to stand and may require surgery to correct the condition.

All of these conditions should only be treated after medical approval has been given, as the muscles involved are short and tight and may be damaged if massage or electrical treatments are attempted.

The ankles

The ankles should be clearly defined and the skin clear. If the ankle is swollen and puffy, there may be fluid retention (**oedema**). Oedema is an accumulation of tissue fluid, caused when the veins and capillaries become congested, and the fluid is not fully dispersed back via the lymphatic system. This is often caused by pregnancy, when the added weight of the baby puts pressure on the veins in the pelvis so fluid is not drained correctly, or by weight gain. It can also indicate there is a systemic problem in the kidneys. (For more information on the lymphatic system and the functions of the kidneys, see Related anatomy and physiology, page 201.)

Feet should be checked for any infections, especially if the client is going into the wet area, as bacteria thrive in warm, moist conditions. (For details of bacterial, viral and fungal infections, see Professional basics, pages 44–47.)

Key terms

Oedema – a build up of excess fluid in the body leading to swelling of the tissues, most commonly found in the ankles or legs. It occurs when the body's normal fluid balance is disturbed.

Think about it

It is not within your role to diagnose any medical condition, and you should refer the client to their doctor. Avoid mentioning any condition by name – you are not medically trained, and may be wrong!

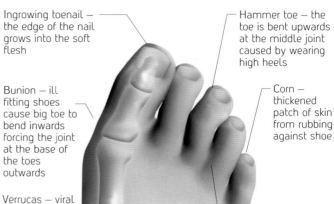

Ingrowing toenail – the edge of the nail grows into the soft flesh

Hammer toe – the toe is bent upwards at the middle joint caused by wearing high heels

Bunion – ill fitting shoes cause big toe to bend inwards forcing the joint at the base of the toes outwards

Corn – thickened patch of skin from rubbing against shoe

Verrucas – viral disease of the skin forms a wart on the sole of the foot

Athlete's foot – fungal disease usually starts between the toes

Complaints of the foot

Also check on any conditions which may have a bearing upon posture, such as **bunions** or **hallux vulgus**. A **bursa** often develops over the site and the big toe becomes displaced towards the others. Bunions are usually caused by ill-fitting shoes and may require surgical treatment. Hallux vulgus can be caused by pressure of footwear, if the client has a broad foot, and is usually associated with a bunion.

Key terms

Bunion – a swelling of the joint between the big toe and the first metatarsal bone.

Hallux vulgus – a displacement of the big toe, where it bends towards the other toes.

Bursa – a tiny fluid-filled sac. A bursa is found between tendon and bone, skin and bone, or muscle and muscle. Their function is to allow movement without creating friction. It looks like a swelling or bunion-type inflammation.

Manual examination

Manual assessment includes:

- weight
- height
- measuring the body (when carrying out reduction treatments which may not result in body weight loss, but cause a reduction of inches, i.e. faradic treatments and body wraps)

- **blood pressure**
- pulse rate
- muscular tone and strength testing
- skin conditions.

Key terms

Blood pressure – the measurement of the force applied to the walls of the arteries as the heart pumps blood through the body. *Systolic pressure* is the maximum pressure in an artery at the moment when the heart is beating and pumping blood through the body. *Diastolic pressure* is the minimum arterial pressure during relaxation and dilation of the heart.

Height to weight ratio

Height
Accurate height measurement is important – clients often do not know their height, and people can lose height as they get older through the ageing process and spinal shrinkage.

The best way to measure height is to have a fixed ruler on a permanent fixture such as a wall, and ask the client to stand against the wall. With the head held evenly, ask the client to look straight ahead, while the client's body maintains a good, relaxed postural stance. Using a flat surface, such as a book or ruler, lay it flat upon the head, and measure against the ruler on the wall.

Weight
To record the client's weight accurately, all salons should have a good quality set of calibrated digital scales, or traditional scales with weights sliding across a crossbar scale. Domestic scales with a dial and moving pointer are unreliable as well as being affected by the surface on which they are placed.

Think about it

Height and weight must be recorded together, to get a true reflection of the size and health of the client. A recording of 102 kilograms would be of concern if the client was only 1.5 metres tall, as this would be considered morbidly obese, but for a man 1.9 metres tall, it might be in the normal range for his body mass index.

Weight needs to be looked at objectively to take into account the client's:

- general build
- height
- body type
- 'spread' of the skeleton.

It is a myth that people can be 'heavy boned', but it is essential to note the client's general frame size. A small woman will have a smaller framework, and weigh less than a large, tall woman with larger feet and hands. So, the skeletal spread may vary – a six-foot man will have a heavier skeleton with longer long bones than a five-foot woman.

Think about it
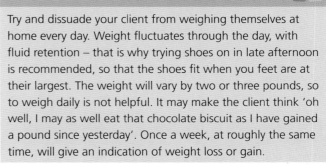

Try and dissuade your client from weighing themselves at home every day. Weight fluctuates through the day, with fluid retention – that is why trying shoes on in late afternoon is recommended, so that the shoes fit when you feet are at their largest. The weight will vary by two or three pounds, so to weigh daily is not helpful. It may make the client think 'oh well, I may as well eat that chocolate biscuit as I have gained a pound since yesterday'. Once a week, at roughly the same time, will give an indication of weight loss or gain.

Frame size guide
As a rough guide, measure the wrist at its slimmest point – just below the knob of bone:

- up to 14cm = small
- 14cm – 16.5cm = medium
- 16.5 or more = large.

Muscle tissue
Muscle tissue weighs more than fat, so a body builder with developed muscle bulk would appear to be obese on paper, whereas there will probably not be an ounce of fat on him or her! Clients who work out regularly and have a high proportion of muscle will also have a higher weight reading compared with a client of the same frame who does little exercise.

Body mass index

A body mass index (BMI) reading will enable you to discover if the client has a healthy height—weight ratio. This can be worked out as follows:

BMI = weight in kilograms ÷ height in metres^2

Now, check the BMI chart below to see if this is an acceptable reading.

You can also use a height : weight chart to see if your client has a healthy weight.

BMI reading	What the reading means
Less than 20	Below normal weight
20–24.9	Normal (grade 0)
25–29.9	Overweight (grade i)
30–40	Obese (grade ii)
More than 40	Morbidly obese (grade iii)

BMI readings

For your portfolio

To work out your own BMI:
- Find your weight in kilograms (e.g. 57.2kg).
- Find your height in metres (e.g. 1.64m).
- Multiply your height reading by itself (e.g. 1.64m × 1.64m = 2.69m).
- Your BMI is:
  57.2kg ÷ 2.69m = 21.26

Are you within the healthy BMI range of 20–25?

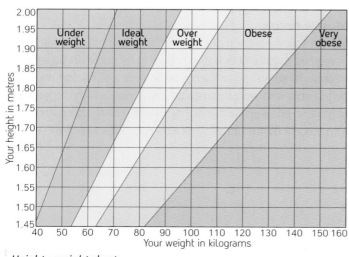

Height : weight chart

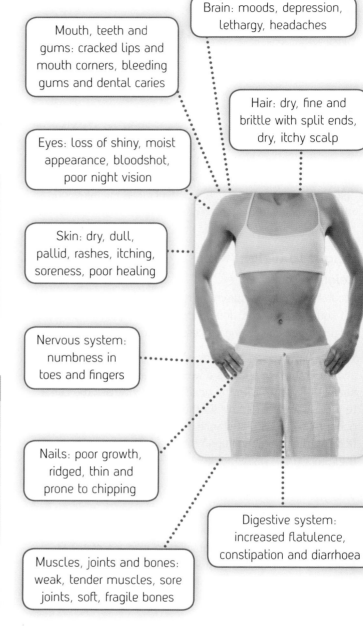

Mouth, teeth and gums: cracked lips and mouth corners, bleeding gums and dental caries

Brain: moods, depression, lethargy, headaches

Hair: dry, fine and brittle with split ends, dry, itchy scalp

Eyes: loss of shiny, moist appearance, bloodshot, poor night vision

Skin: dry, dull, pallid, rashes, itching, soreness, poor healing

Nervous system: numbness in toes and fingers

Nails: poor growth, ridged, thin and prone to chipping

Muscles, joints and bones: weak, tender muscles, sore joints, soft, fragile bones

Digestive system: increased flatulence, constipation and diarrhoea

The effects of being underweight

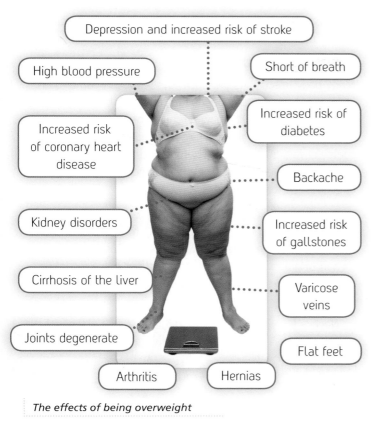

Depression and increased risk of stroke

High blood pressure

Short of breath

Increased risk of coronary heart disease

Increased risk of diabetes

Backache

Kidney disorders

Increased risk of gallstones

Cirrhosis of the liver

Varicose veins

Joints degenerate

Flat feet

Arthritis

Hernias

The effects of being overweight

Using body fat skin callipers

Some salons use fat callipers to measure body fat. This type of measurement is not as reliable as the body mass index, as it depends upon the client having enough soft fat to pick up. However, callipers still have a place in the consultation when used correctly.

Four sites of the body are measured, using the gauge:

- triceps
- sub-scapular
- biceps
- supra-iliac crest .

With the client facing away from you:

- Triceps — take the reading from about midway between the shoulder and the elbow joint at the back of the arm, gently pick up the body fat in the callipers, but try to leave out the muscle bulk.

- Sub-scapular — pick up the skin just below the inner angle of the scapula, just above the line of the bra strap.

With the client facing you:

- Supra-iliac — you are aiming to measure just above the line of the iliac crest of the pelvis, but inwards, slightly towards the navel. This is quite difficult to do, and if the client has little body fat, you may have to ask him or her to lean forwards while you pick up the body fat, and then the client can straighten up.

- Biceps — pick up midway between the shoulder and elbow joint on the front of the arm at a right angle to the muscle, rather than in the direction of the muscle. Try to measure with the elbow slightly bent to allow the muscle to soften, although be careful only to pick up body fat.

You should note the four readings, and then add them together to get a total figure in millimetres.

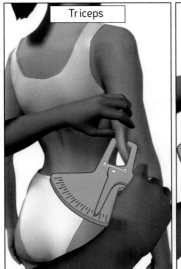
Triceps

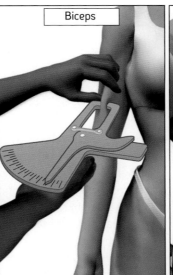
Biceps

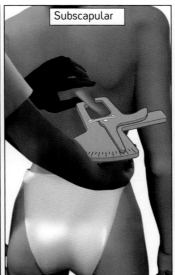
Subscapular

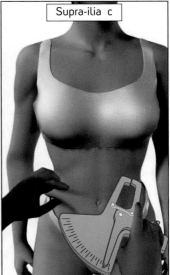
Supra-ilia c

How to use body fat skin callipers

Body fat measurements

Using the body fat measurements in the table below, check the percentage of body fat.

Total figure (mm)	% of fat	Total figure (mm)	% of fat
8	13	50	28
12	14	52	29
14	15	56	30
18	16	58	31
20	17	62	32
24	18	64	33
26	19	68	34
30	20	70	35
32	21	76	37
34	22	80	38
38	23	82	39
40	24	86	40
42	25	88	41
44	26	90	42
48	27		

Women – fat measurements

Total figure (mm)	% of fat	Total figure (mm)	% of fat	Total figure (mm)	% of fat
15	5	65	23	150	33
20	9	70	24	160	34
25	11	75	25	175	35
30	13	80	26	190	36
35	15	90	27	205	37
40	17	100	28	220	38
45	18	110	29	235	39
50	20	120	30	255	40
55	21	130	31	275	41
60	22	140	32	295	42

Men – fat measurements

You can then calculate the acceptability of the body fat percentage using the table below.

	Female	Male
Obese	35%+	32%+
Overweight	29–35%	26–32%
Average	24–29%	21–26%
Lean	19–24%	16–21%
Very lean	Less than 19%	Less than 16%

Body fat percentage

Finally, cross-check your readings against the BMI reading, for accuracy.

Why measure the body?

Many body treatments give inch-loss reduction, rather than weight loss, so it is a good idea to measure the client before and after treatment, to show a total inch-loss reading.

A client may simply want a firming treatment such as a course of faradic treatments to tone and firm the muscles, rather than a weight-loss treatment. A body wrap is also an effective inch-loss treatment.

Taking measurements at the beginning, middle and end of a course of treatment can be encouraging for the client, and if the treatments are combined with a weight-loss programme, a chart or graph can be drawn so the client has a record of how well he or she is doing.

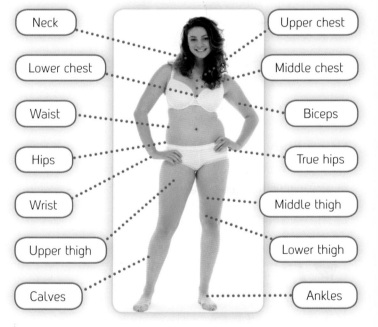

Measuring the body

Think about it

When measuring the body, take the readings from approximately the same area, to provide an accurate before and after comparison. Most record cards for body treatments have a little figure drawn on the back, which will help guide you to the right spot. Draw on the diagram exactly where you measured, for example 6 centimetres up from the elbow joint, when doing the bicep measurement. That way, you will know where to return to for the next measurement. Also, it may not be you taking the measurements next time, so a guide will be useful for the next therapist.

Blood pressure and the pulse

Accurately taking the client's blood pressure is important, as high or low blood pressure can be a contra-indication to treatment.

It is advisable to take the blood pressure and pulse reading of every client coming to the salon, regardless of the body treatment plan. It will indicate whether the client is suitable for treatment, especially if going into the wet area, as a client with high blood pressure is more likely to pass out in the heat.

What is blood pressure?

Blood pressure is the force or pressure which the blood exerts on the walls of the main arteries of the body. Pressure is highest during systole, when the ventricles of the heart are contracting (systolic pressure) and lowest during diastole, when the ventricles are relaxing and refilling (diastolic pressure).

Blood pressure is measured in millimetres of mercury using a sphygmomanometer at the brachial artery of the arm. This gives a true reading, as the blood pressure in the arteries is higher than in the veins.

Blood pressure is affected by and varies with:

- age
- weight
- activity levels
- stress levels
- emotional stability or anxiety
- diet
- smoking
- alcohol intake
- genetic factors
- the condition of the heart and vessels.

High blood pressure

The medical name for high blood pressure is **hypertension** and it is a common complaint. The most widespread form is associated with arteriosclerosis, a hardening of the arteries, and often leads to strokes and heart attacks. Excess weight, smoking and stress all contribute to a raised blood pressure.

Low blood pressure

People with low blood pressure or **hypotension** usually have poor circulation, with cold hands and feet. Low blood pressure is less serious than high blood pressure, but in hot weather, during exercise or in the wet area, the client may feel dizzy and need to rest.

This is also important if the client is lying down for a period of time, as in a body massage or an electrical facial treatment. The client will need to be brought back up to a vertical position slowly, to prevent dizziness.

Think about it

Both high and low blood pressure are contra-indications to some treatments, but with a medical clearance and adaptation of treatment, it is possible to treat the client.

Key terms

Hypertension – high blood pressure.

Hypotension – low blood pressure.

How to take blood pressure

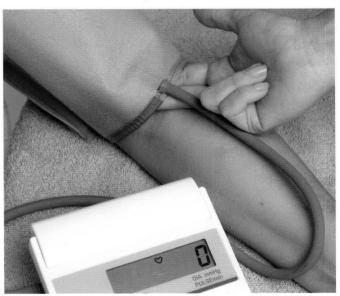

Measuring the cuff tightness

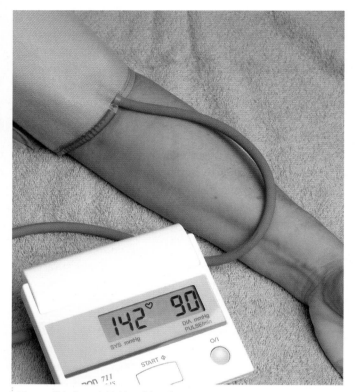

The cuff inflated. Taking blood pressure

The pulse

The pulse rate is the same as the heart rate, usually around 74 beats per minute. The pulse can be felt in arteries because of the expansion and recoil of their walls during each ventricular contraction. The pulse is strongest in the arteries closest to the heart. The pulse is usually taken on the radial artery in the wrist, but can also be taken at the carotid artery in the neck and the brachial artery in the arm.

Feel the pulse by using gentle pressure just to the right side of the wrist, in a direct line under the thumb. Using a watch with a second hand, count the pulse to a 30-second interval, and then multiply by two, to get a minute's reading.

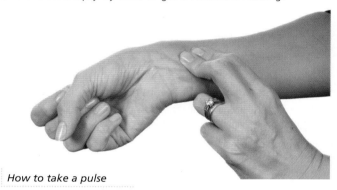

How to take a pulse

Before the reading it is advisable to ask the client to:

- visit the toilet to pass water, and then rest for 10 minutes
- refrain from eating or drinking
- refrain from exercise and try to relax.

Even in these ideal conditions, a person's blood pressure will vary depending on the time, day and season. In general, pressure readings are at their lowest when you are asleep and at their highest when you are at work. Refer back to the cardiovascular information in Related anatomy and physiology, pages 196–198, for further detail.

Blood pressure machines in most salons are automatic, although your salon may still use a manual machine. Always refer to the manufacturer's instructions for use.

Pressure	Reading
Systolic	High = 150+
	Average = 95–150
	Low = 95 or less
Diastolic	High = 95+
	Average = 60–95
	Low = 60 or less

Blood pressure guide

For your portfolio

What are your blood pressure reading and pulse rate? Are they in a healthy range for your age?

Muscular tone and strength testing

When a therapist talks of muscle tone she is discussing the muscle's ability to react and work quickly, how long it can work and how quickly it responds to stimuli from the nerves.

If the muscle:

- is firm to the touch
- is in a state of partial contraction
- contracts quickly
- looks firm and solid

then muscle tone is good.

If the muscle is:

- soft to the touch
- slow to contract
- flabby and loose

then muscle tone is poor.

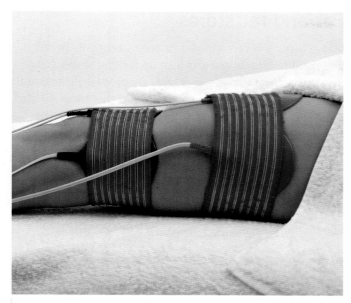

A faradic treatment will improve muscle tone

Some clients come to the salon for muscle toning treatments without needing to lose weight – they want more tone to the muscle to give better shape and definition, especially on the abdomen and hips, legs and arms. One excellent treatment for this is a body faradic treatment (see Unit B13 Provide body electrical treatments, page 367). As this is a form of passive exercise, because the body is not actually moving, the muscles need to be assessed for suitability for treatment, and the client's flexibility checked.

Flexibility is the ability of the joints to perform a maximum range of movement and the ability of the muscles to support required movement – to be agile and without stiffness. This can be checked by observing the client as he or she walks and gets onto the couch, and by a series of simple exercises, which will help gauge the client's existing muscle tone. The exercises can be performed on the couch, but it is safer to do them on a mat on the floor, with plenty of room for manoeuvre. Refer back to Related anatomy and physiology, pages 178–193, for muscle and joint information.

Think about it

If an elderly, rather stiff client comes into the salon, and has difficulty getting up onto the couch or getting undressed, then his or her flexibility and muscle tone would be so poor that it would be a contra-indication to treatment.

Area to check	Type of exercise
Back	Touching the toes with knees very soft
	How far the client gets will indicate flexibility
	Do not perform with the knees locked; movement must not be forced or jerked
Abdominal muscles	Ask the client to breathe in – if muscle tone is good, the abdomen should move upwards and inwards
	Perform a sit-up with knees bent and hands by the forehead
	Do not perform with the knees locked or hands behind the head
Legs	Leg raises: while lying on the back, ask the client to perform individual leg raises, slowly, and ask the client to hold the position in mid air. If the movement is smooth and fluid, muscle tone is good, as is hip mobility
Arms	A resistant movement: ask the client to try to place the right hand on to the right shoulder, while you try to prevent the movement by blocking at the forearm. If resistance is good, the biceps, triceps and deltoid muscles are in good condition

Exercises to gauge flexibility

Skin conditions

The skin on the body behaves very much like the skin on the face but does not always have the protection of products and make-up, or the pampering that a facial provides.

In most salons, body treatments and related skin problems tend to be seasonal. There is always an increase in demand for waxing, body exfoliation and toning treatments in the salon in the summer, for example. Dry skin tends to be a winter problem because the body is encased in winter clothing and application of nourishing creams tends to be less thorough. The chest and back tend to be the trouble areas for an oily skin, particularly during the winter months, with congestion or acne occurring just as it would on the face.

Treat the skin on the body as you would the face. An oily back benefits from exfoliation, steaming, comedone removal and suitable mask application, similar to the face. (See the treatment table on page 354 for suitable treatments and their benefits to the skin.)

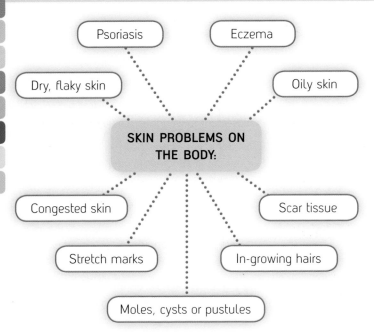

SKIN PROBLEMS ON THE BODY:

- Psoriasis
- Eczema
- Dry, flaky skin
- Oily skin
- Congested skin
- Scar tissue
- Stretch marks
- In-growing hairs
- Moles, cysts or pustules

Carry out a skin analysis and use the record card to note recommended treatments, which can be combined with the other body treatments of massage, toning or firming treatments. (For information on the skin and related problems refer to You and the skin, page 222.)

Fat and fat stores

Many clients will come to you for body treatments because they want to lose weight and burn up their fat stores, tone the muscles and improve their body shape. Many clients will be concerned about cosmetic appearances, but there are also health benefits to being the correct weight for your height. For example, losing just 10 per cent of total body weight increases mobility, eases pressure on the joints and reduces the risk of serious health problems.

To understand how to treat clients with excess fat deposits, you need to know why we have fat stores, and the best ways to treat this problem.

Think about it

You will need to emphasise to clients the importance of eating healthily and taking exercise, if they wish to benefit fully from salon treatments.

There are three types of fat stores within the body:

- essential fat
- non-essential fat
- brown fat.

My story

Shelly's story

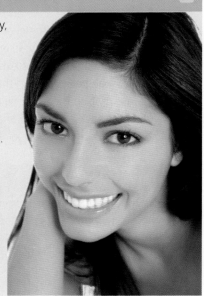

I had a regular client who enjoyed a full body massage and, as she was going on holiday, she had recently been in the salon for some toning treatments.

When my client returned, she booked in for a back massage and toning treatments on the legs. Although my client was tanned, she complained her skin was very dry and beginning to flake. Well, I began with her normal consultation and then prepared for the back massage, planning to use a rich oil to help with the dryness. I noticed a raised, angry-looking patch underneath the bra strap on the client's back. The area was weeping. I asked the client if she was aware of any irritation on her back, and she said she was. I explained that there was a patch of raised skin, and suggested she go to her doctor to have it checked. As the area was weeping, I decided the treatment was contra-indicated, and went on to the leg treatments.

The client took my advice and went to her GP. To her shock she was diagnosed with a skin cancer. Thankfully it was successfully treated over the following months. I was so relieved I had mentioned it — if I had ignored the problem the consequences could have been extremely serious.

Essential fat

Essential fat helps to protect vital organs, the central nervous system, the heart, lungs, intestines and even cushions the eyeballs. Essential fat is stored within bone marrow, and released when necessary.

Women have an extra supply of essential fat (four times that of men), which is sex specific. In other words, it creates the female shape – curvy with rounded breasts etc. The only women who burn off this essential fat are women with eating disorders, or those in heavy training schedules, such as top athletes. They tend to develop a boyish figure, with little or no breast tissue, and slim hips and shoulders.

Non-essential fat

This type of fat can be rapidly metabolised to produce heat and energy, and is stored in the adipose tissue of most animal species. Men and women alike have this fat, which can be easily shed. Men tend to accumulate fat around the abdomen and women below the waist and on the breasts. Every woman has her own particular pattern of fat deposits, usually governed by heredity, eating patterns and exercise.

Although a lot can be done with a client's basic shape, there is no diet or exercise plan that will enable the client to lose fat from one part of the body rather than another. It will be metabolised from all over the body, but in the long term the client can even lose stubborn fat deposits on, for example, the hips and thighs.

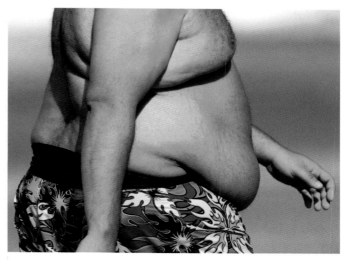
Men tend to accumulate non-essential fat around their stomachs – 'a beer belly'

Think about it

Under consumer protection law, it is illegal to make false claims regarding treatments and the results expected.

If you were to advertise that a course of faradic treatment guarantees a loss of a half a kilogram in weight, under which Act(s) would you be liable for prosecution? (To refresh your memory, turn to Professional basics, 'You, your client and the law', page 68.)

There are a number of variations in the fat cells, both in number and size. Gross obesity occurs when both increase. There can be an excessive number of fat cells, excessively large fat cells, or a combination of the two. Obesity due to an excessive number of fat cells is more difficult to control than obesity due to excessively large fat cells.

Non-essential fat categories

Non-essential fat can be divided into:

- hard fat
- soft fat
- cellulite.

Hard fat

Hard fat is usually found in the upper thighs, inner knees, upper arms and deltoid area. Hard fat cells are compact, that is they are firm to the touch and dense. These cells may also be trapped within the muscle fibres and this makes picking up and wringing movements very difficult to do, without picking up most of the muscle bulk. Although overweight on the scales and BMI index, the client with hard fat will be of stocky appearance, without necessarily looking very overweight.

Treatments that involve manipulation of the fat, such as vacuum suction, will not be suitable as the fat cells are not malleable (pliable), and these treatments may be uncomfortable for the client.

Think about it

Knowing which type of fat you are dealing with will help you to identify the correct treatment.

Soft fat

This fat is soft to the touch and can be manipulated with massage movements such as wringing and picking up.

Soft fat responds well to salon treatments, and diet and exercise. The fat cells are in the adipose tissue, and not within the muscle fibres. The female client will have soft fat visible in the lower body, hips, buttocks and abdomen, while the male client will have a spread of soft fat around the trunk. Males with a high proportion of soft fat often develop an increased chest size and a bosom shape, as well as a large double chin.

Cellulite

Cellulite is easily identified as an 'orange peel' effect seen under the skin. It is caused by interstitial oedema, initially reversible, attributed to abnormal capillary permeability. Adipose tissue is a network of fibres of connective tissue, known as reticular fibres. They form a delicate supportive meshwork around blood vessels, muscle fibres, glands, nerves and so on — everything in the dermal layer of the skin. Within the reticular fibres sit the fat cells.

If the fluid between the cells (interstitial fluid) is not drained properly, through the lymphatic system, fluid begins to accumulate between the cells, and over a period of time, will cloak the fat cells, and trap them, rather like a balloon caught in a net. This hinders the blood and lymphatic flow, which slows down, causing associated flooding or a pooling effect of the fluid.

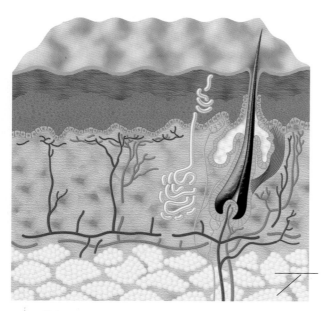

Cellulite positioned under the skin

As the blood flow slows, the blood balance becomes altered, and plasma, serum and electrolytes, especially sodium, seep into the subcutaneous tissue, further preventing proper functioning. This can cause pain because of pressure on the nerve endings and can reduce the skin's elasticity.

The reticular structure becomes thick and hard, and the mass of fat cells becomes nodular. If this happens to many cells, side by side, then the effect can be seen as irregular patterns on the surface of the skin, as dimples or 'orange peel'.

Cellulite treatments involve stimulating the body's lymphatic system to help internal drainage and include manual lymphatic drainage massage, mechanical massage, vacuum suction, microcurrent and anti-cellulite galvanic application.

As part of the cellulite treatment, the client needs to:

- take part in **aerobic** exercise
- drink plenty of water
- avoid processed and salty foods
- reduce consumption of alcohol, caffeine and other stimulants
- apply a good quality moisturiser in the area, using brisk massage movements.

Key terms

Aerobic – any exercise (walking, skipping, jogging, swimming or dancing) that uses the large muscle groups and increases the efficiency of the circulatory and respiratory systems, improving the body's utilisation of oxygen.

Brown fat

Brown fat occurs in the adipose tissue of many animal species and can be rapidly metabolised to produce heat energy. It is abundant in newborns but reduces significantly as we age.

Metabolism and fat stores

Metabolism is the collective term used for the chemical processes that take place in the body either to break down complex substances into simple ones (catabolism) or when a complex substance is built up from a simple

Think about it

Clients within their normal body weight range can develop cellulite. The most common areas are on the upper arms, thighs and buttocks.

one (anabolism). The thyroid gland in the neck produces hormones for controlling the body's metabolic rate.

The basal metabolic rate (BMR) is the minimum amount of energy used by the body to maintain the vital processes of respiration, circulation, digestion and so on, even when the body is at rest. Lifestyle and occupation also affect how much energy the body requires, for example a client in a heavy labouring job will require more energy than an office worker.

Using the body's fat stores

Both calorie reduction – dieting – and aerobic exercise, such as walking, cycling or swimming, are required to burn up the body's fat stores. To understand this process, you will need to know how food, or fuel, is stored.

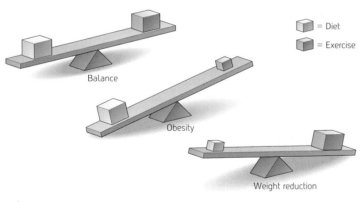

= Diet

= Exercise

Balance

Obesity

Weight reduction

A healthy balance of diet and exercise will burn up the body's extra fat

Weight problems, obesity and fluid retention

Obesity is now a serious problem in the western world. The latest research shows that obese children may be shortening their life expectancy by up to ten years because of the pressures put on the body's systems by being overweight. Obesity is the result of an over-dependence on high-fat and processed foods, which have become increasingly popular in western society, combined with a lack of exercise. Without physical activity, the body is unable to burn off the extra calories.

Besides the health risks, obesity is a burden to the client. It slows the person down physically and makes exercise difficult. The obese client often has very low self-esteem. The combination of these two factors can make the obese person prone to many illnesses and stress.

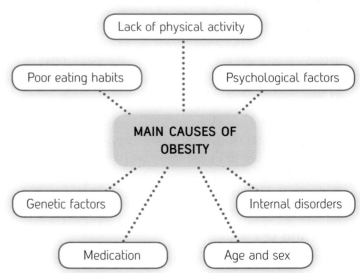

Lack of physical activity

Poor eating habits

Psychological factors

MAIN CAUSES OF OBESITY

Genetic factors

Internal disorders

Medication

Age and sex

Poor eating habits

The body needs the right balance of nutrients to keep it healthy and functioning properly. A diet of fast foods, take-away meals and processed foods, which generally have a very high salt and sugar content, will not provide those essential nutrients. Snacking between meals on high-carbohydrate foods such as crisps, chips and sweets also leads to poor health.

Changes in physical activity

A sudden drop in physical activity without readjustment of eating habits can easily lead to a weight gain, for example when a person retires or gives up a sporting activity.

Psychological factors

In times of crisis, many people turn to food, hence the term 'comfort eating'. This often becomes a vicious circle: the more overweight the person becomes the more they eat, in an attempt to find consolation. People who give up smoking often find they turn to food as a substitute — nicotine also acts as an appetite suppressant so the individual will naturally begin to experience food cravings.

Genetic factors

Obesity may run in families, although studies have yet to prove whether this is due to genetics or simply to family customs (poor eating habits, type of foods bought, lack of exercise, and so on).

Internal disorders

Obesity caused by internal disorders is rare. However, there are some genuine cases, particularly those associated with the endocrine system. If you suspect your client has an internal disorder, then you must refer them to a doctor, as further treatment could be harmful. In most cases, success is achieved with a combination of medical help and advice to the therapist, who may then devise treatments accordingly.

Medication

Certain drugs can cause weight gain, for example many women experience this when they start taking the contraceptive pill. Clients on medication should seek their doctor's advice before treatment is begun. Sometimes, the condition will be temporary.

Age and sex

This often has a bearing on weight gain, either due to hormonal influences, or changes in lifestyle that come with age. The older person is usually more susceptible to weight gain than the younger, more active person. Women are more affected than men, with pregnancy and menopause being two of the common times for weight gain.

Other factors

Research suggests that internal signals tell a person when he or she has eaten enough food. In an overweight person those signals do not work as well as they do in the slimmer person.

An obese person's fat cells have a greater capacity to store body fat and less is used in the body for energy or heat production.

Advice to overweight/obese clients

It is unlikely you will have a child in the salon for treatment, but check with your professional body regarding treating a minor, and always get a doctor's approval. Remember you do need written parental consent to treat a minor.

Adolescents should eat a diet rich in all the nutrients necessary for growth, but low in carbohydrates. Encourage participation in exercise (the client might be embarrassed to take part at school in group activities). It is good to recommend out-of-school solo activities until their confidence builds up, for example exercising to DVDs in the privacy of the client's own home, jogging/running to burn up extra calories.

After pregnancy, advice on diet, exercise and salon treatments will help the client to regain her figure. Skincare treatments and massage are also very therapeutic.

Think about it

When treating a client who has just had a baby, always wait until she has had her post-pregnancy check-up at six weeks and ask for a doctor's written approval before starting treatment — especially if the client is breastfeeding.

Many women experience fluctuations in weight when they reach the menopause, due to the reduction of female hormones. Once periods have stopped, the body's weight pattern tends to become more stable. Advise a suitable diet, exercise and salon treatments, as necessary. Correct nutrition is vital at this time to compensate for fluctuating hormone levels, which leave the body open to diseases such as osteoporosis. The skin may experience changes, just as it did in adolescence, so treatments can also be included for replenishing the moisture content or redressing the oil balance, depending upon the problem.

Some women may experience bouts of depression during the menopause, or 'empty nest syndrome' if their children have left home, and this may make them turn to food for comfort. It is important for you to be sympathetic, encouraging and understanding.

As people grow older and retire, they tend to use less energy, but often do not adapt their eating pattern. The basal metabolism decreases, so in order for excess weight not to be gained, they must decrease their food intake. However, it is essential for the correct foods to be eaten, ensuring variety and all necessary nutrients. The appetite does diminish, and the client just needs to ensure that the quality of the food taken is high and full of nutrients.

Too rigid an eating plan and the client will not stick with it. There is a school of thought which says that dieting doesn't work – for two reasons:

- The client sees this as something they do for a short time and not as a lifestyle change – so they diet for a special event, a holiday perhaps, and then revert back to their old, high-fat eating habits.

- When the diet is severely restricted the body thinks that there may not be any more food/nutrients available. It tries to protect itself by slowing down metabolism and conserving energy to lay down fat stores for the 'famine'. So dieting can make the body fatter – when food comes along the body stores everything it can!

Fluid retention

As previously mentioned, some clients suffer from fluid retention. This may be hormonal – the breasts feel full and heavy and the waistband may be tighter just before menstruation. After the period, the body returns to normal. If the client has a job which involves being on his or her feet for a long time, then fluid can accumulate around the ankles. Always seek a medical referral before treating a client with fluid retention, no matter how minor. (For more information on kidney and lymphatic drainage functions, see Related anatomy and physiology, page 201.)

Sluggish circulation

Some clients have very cold hands and feet, even on a warm day, and often the skin is very pale. During the consultation, the client should be asked if the condition is painful, especially as the extremities warm up – this could indicate a condition called Raynaud's disease, and will need a doctor's referral before treatment.

Find out more about Raynaud's disease.

Not all cold hands and feet are an indication of Raynaud's disease. It could be that the client simply has poor circulation. Once you have established that there is no medical basis for the condition, any stimulating and heating treatments would be beneficial for poor circulation, for example the wet area, massage, mechanical massage and paraffin wax application. The skin will suffer if the circulation is poor, so exfoliation treatments and massage are very good to bring blood to the area. The treatment objective is to create an erythema so that oxygen and nutrients are brought to the skin, and waste products are removed efficiently.

The underweight client

A severely underweight client may be suffering from an eating disorder, such as **anorexia** or bulimia, and should not be treated. Counselling and hospitalisation may be required and medical referral is essential – extreme low weight is a contra-indication to treatment.

However, a client who is perfectly healthy may still be fairly thin, with very little adipose tissue on the body. Careful choice of treatment plans and equipment is essential, as the client will bruise easily and the bony extremities may make some equipment painful. A client with very little underlying body fat may find the G5 mechanical massage too heavy, but will enjoy manual massage, or other skin pampering treatments. The client may have come to increase muscle bulk, and book a course of faradic sessions, which will tone and firm the muscles.

Treatment adaptation is essential on a slim client, and good communication throughout the treatment will ensure the client is comfortable and relaxed.

Equipment used in body treatments

On the following pages is a brief rundown of the equipment used in body treatments, their benefits to the client and the client type most suited to the equipment. For a list of the equipment used in facial treatments, see page 268.

For a list of the equipment used in facial treatments, see page 268.

Think about it

Whichever pieces of equipment you choose as the most suitable for the client's treatment plan, always follow the five golden rules:

1 Complete a full consultation.
2 Complete a contra-indication checklist.
3 Carry out thermal and sensitivity tests.
4 Follow the manufacturer's instructions.
5 Test the equipment on yourself before using it on the client.

Pre-warming treatments

HYDROTHERAPY

Uses and client needs	Suitable skin type/body type	
Any treatment involving water in any physical state, e.g. steam, liquid, water vapour or ice	Most skin types except where contra-indications are present Timing of treatment can be adjusted to suit skin type	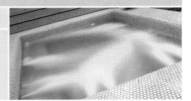

STEAMING   (facial unit or the wet area cabinet or steam room)

Uses and client needs	Suitable skin type/body type	
Moist heat – a heating element boils the water, which creates a jet of steam from a nozzle or outlet. Can be used to warm the tissues of the face, upper chest or back when using a facial steaming unit. The whole body is immersed in a steam room. A steam cabinet treats the body only; the face is outside the cabinet Helps open the pores and cleanse the skin Warms the muscle fibres and relaxes them, making other treatments after steaming very effective Very good prior to comedone extraction, but be careful to time the treatment, as if erythema occurs too strongly it may contra-indicate other treatments	Most skin types, except where contra-indications are present Timing of treatment can be adjusted to suit skin types	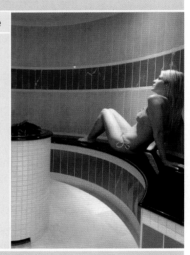

SAUNA

Uses and client needs	Suitable skin type/body type	
A pine log cabin, with coals heated over a powerful electric stove. The client adds water to the coals, which increases humidity, reducing the rate of evaporation of the sweat on the skin, felt as a dry heat, causing a rise in body temperature. A communal treatment The whole body is involved, and it prepares the body for other treatments by softening tissues, relaxing the muscles, cleansing the skin and stimulating glandular activity There are also individual vibration sauna units. The unit is self-contained, with a vibrating couch to massage the body as it is being heated. Fans and music make the treatment very comfortable for those who do not enjoy communal treatments	Most skin types, except where contra-indications are present Timing of treatment can be adjusted to suit skin types	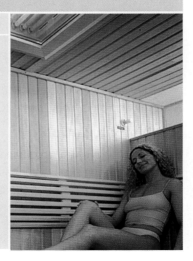

SPA

Uses and client needs	Suitable skin type/body type
A communal treatment – also called a hot tub or jacuzzi. Water is heated and pumped around a self-contained fibreglass tub, which can hold four, six or eight people, depending on size. Holes in the base of the tub send water jets and/or air bubbles on to the client to massage the tissues, as the body is being heated Skin is softened, muscles relax and a feeling of wellbeing is created	Most skin types, except where contra-indications are present Timing of treatment can be adjusted to suit skin types

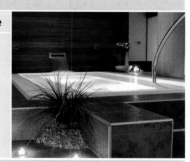

POWERJET SHOWER

Uses and client needs	Suitable skin type/body type
An impulse or power jet shower has a normal shower head for hot water, from above, and side bars for cold water. The unit is automatically set for alternative water jets onto the client. The cold spray may also have a pump action, which pulses the cold water in a set rhythm to massage the muscles The treatment is extremely stimulating for the skin and muscles and prepares the body for other treatments	Most skin types, except where contra-indications are present Timing of treatment can be adjusted to suit skin types

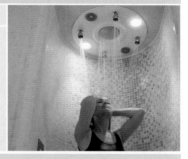

BATHS

Uses and client needs	Suitable skin type/body type
These can be pulsed, foam, wax or mud, with either all the body immersed, or partial immersion to treat a specific area such as the feet or arms. Pulsed and foam baths are rather like a normal domestic bath in shape, with holes in, for the air to be pumped through, creating foam and a massage effect. Products are added, such as seaweed or aromatherapy oils, to enhance the treatment Wax or mud baths involve heating up the product, changing it from a solid into a liquid state, and then pasting it onto the body area to be treated. Wrapping the body in plastic or tin foil and cocooning it in blankets keeps in the warmth of the product. The body temperature is then raised, the skin softened and the client is in a relaxed state	Most skin types, except where contra-indications are present Timing of treatment can be adjusted to suit skin types

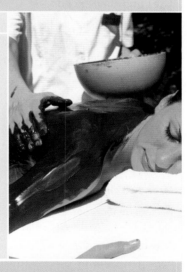

INFRARED LAMP

Uses and client needs	Suitable skin type/body type
An infrared light bulb is fixed into a fitting with a swivel arm on a stand, making it easy to place the lamp into a suitable position. Used to create extra blood flow, which generates heat for the skin and underlying tissue. Muscle fibres will soften and it can be used effectively on any part of the body Can only treat small areas at a time, due to the limited arc of light from the lamp. Can be used on the face, chest or upper back Time the treatment, as if an erythema occurs too strongly, it may contra-indicate other treatments Can also be used on the face with a hot oil mask	Most skin types except where contra-indications are present Timing of treatment can be adjusted to suit skin type. Where used with hot oil mask, dry skin only

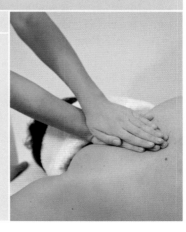

Exfoliating treatments

BRUSH CLEANSING

Uses and client needs	Suitable skin type/body type
A brush-cleansing machine has a motor, which rotates a hand-held head that can have a variety of brushes inserted into it. The speed of the rotations is adjustable to suit the client's needs and preference, as is the direction of the revolution – clockwise or anti-clockwise. Brushes of various thickness and stiffness will alter the treatment effect, as will the accompanying products used with the machine	Most skin types, except where contra-indications are present. Product use will be determined by skin type or problem
Most water-based products are suitable, from basic foaming facial wash used to cleanse the face, back or congested chest area, to cleansing grains and specialist creams for particular skin problems	Timing of treatment can be adjusted to suit skin type
The effect of the treatment is one of exfoliation and stimulation to the skin and circulation. Can also be a useful tool in the removal of peels or masks from the face	

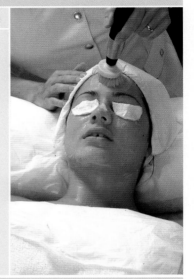

BODY SCRUB WITH MITTS

Uses and client needs	Suitable skin type/body type
An exfoliant can be used prior to a fake tan application – the product can be applied using just the hands, with buffer mitts worn, to accelerate the product use	Most skin types, except where contra-indications are present
	Timing of treatment can be adjusted to suit skin types

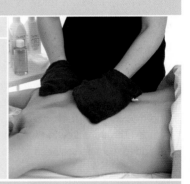

MICRODERMABRASION

Uses and client needs	Suitable skin type/body type
Microdermabrasion works using a controlled flow of ultra clean aluminium oxide crystals set in motion by vacuum-created low pressure. The crystals are applied to the skin with a special hand piece which allows the controlled and gentle removal of the dead cells from the stratum corneum of the epidermis. The same hand piece removes the used crystals and skin particles in a single process and deposits them in a separate container	All skin types except where contra-indications are present. Excellent as a rejuvenating treatment before a special event such as a wedding, or for a course of treatments to help clear acne or reduce the appearance of scarring or stretch marks
There is no risk of crystal-related side effects as they are completely inert	
The flow of crystals and the depth of peeling is perfectly controllable, and the treatment also allows deep penetration of hydrating products into the clean skin	

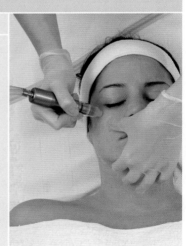

Although most equipment used would be classed as electrical because it works from mains electricity, in beauty therapy equipment is also grouped according to the effect it has on the body.

- Electrical treatments such as galvanic current, microcurrent, high-frequency and faradic treatments are those which send an adapted electrical current through the body.

- Mechanical treatments are those using equipment that has only an external effect on the body. These include G5, vacuum suction, microdermabrasion and small massage equipment such as audio-sonic.

Manual massage treatments

SWEDISH MASSAGE

Uses and client needs	Suitable skin type/body type	
Using the hands, the tissue is manipulated in a series of movements for the neck, upper back, head and face Can be stimulating or relaxing, depending upon the movements used, but the most sought-after treatment outcome is for removal of tension nodules within the muscle fibres and total relaxation of the mind and body	Most skin types, except where contra-indications are present Timing and product use will be determined by skin type or problem	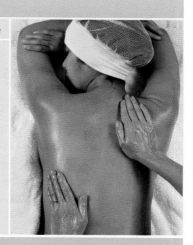

AROMATHERAPY MASSAGE

Uses and client needs	Suitable skin type/body type	
Massage to the head, face and body using pre-blended aromatherapy oils Offers the benefits of massage with the addition of the relaxing, uplifting and stimulating effects of the blends of oils Oils are personally chosen by the therapist to suit the client's emotional and physical needs and the effects required	All skin types except where contra-indications are present	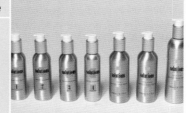

INDIAN HEAD MASSAGE

Uses and client needs	Suitable skin type/body type	
Indian head massage is an Eastern technique based on Ayurvedic philosophies, which date back 5000 years. It includes massage of the shoulders, neck, face and scalp Offers the benefits associated with massage, but also rebalancing of the chakras of the body and restoration of the emotional wellbeing of the client Various oils are used to further enhance the effectiveness of the massage – for stimulation, relaxation or the improvement of the hair and scalp condition	All skin types except where contra-indications are present	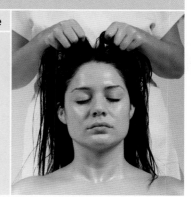

HOT STONE MASSAGE

Uses and client needs	Suitable skin type/body type	
The use of hot stone massage is an ancient tradition in countries with volcanic geology. The hot basalt stones serve as an extension of the therapist's hands to enhance the effects of massage and also to reduce the possibility of repetitive strain injury for the therapist Warming effects of hot stones on the tissue help deepen the effects of the massage and can rebalance and neutralise negative energy Cold stones can also be used in conjunction with hot for a stimulating effect and the vibration energy of the stones also helps balance the seven chakras in the body	All skin types except where contra-indications are present	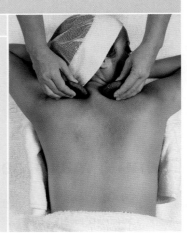

Mechanical massage treatments

AUDIO SONIC

Uses and client needs	Suitable skin type/body type	
Deep penetrating sound-wave emissions can be used on any condition where deep massage helps, e.g. fibrocystic nodules, or tense muscle fibres of the upper back This is a small hand-held device and therefore only suitable to treat small areas in one treatment: not suitable for a whole body massage, as it would be too time-consuming and not cost-effective When using on the face, it is most comfortably applied over the therapist's fingers, so they absorb some of the sound waves. The facial structure does not have the depth of muscle tissue to absorb the sound waves that the body has, and it is not as relaxing directly on the skin	Most skin types, except where contra-indications are present Not suitable/comfortable for fine-featured clients with very delicate facial contours or bony clients with very little body muscle bulk	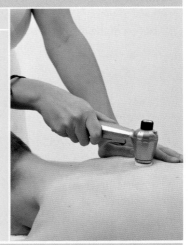

G5

Uses and client needs	Suitable skin type/body type	
An upright machine on a free-standing base, with a motor which makes a hand-held rubber head revolve. Various detachable heads are available, depending upon the effect required – ranging from a soft head for effleurage to a multi-pronged head for stimulating movements Gives a penetrating vibration massage, which is labour-saving for the therapist, and can be used on either the full body or just the back Creates a strong erythema and is useful for desquamation of the skin, stimulating for the muscle fibres and increased metabolic functions	Most skin types except where contra-indications are present Not suitable/comfortable for very thin, bony clients with very little muscle bulk Very suitable for large muscle bulk, and therefore large male clients	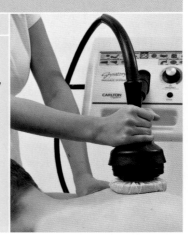

PERCUSSION VIBRATORS

Uses and client needs	**Suitable skin type/body type**
A hand-held smaller version of a G5 machine, with a smaller motor and therefore a less deep effect on the tissues	Most skin types, except where contra-indications are present
Has small detachable heads to provide a variety to the massage movements, but generally, the unit tends to produce a tapotement effect	
Only suitable on smaller areas, such as the shoulders and neck area. Some clients find it uncomfortable on the face, while others enjoy it	

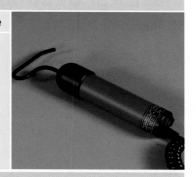

VACUUM SUCTION

Uses and client needs	**Suitable skin type/body type**
This machine uses a pump to create a vacuum within an attached cup, which picks up the tissue	Check for contra-indications, as treatment will not be suitable for all skin types, especially thin or fine skin with a tendency to bruise easily
Can be used either:	
• to glide to the lymphatic nodes, in a single movement, or	Also, will not be comfortable on thin, bony clients or clients with older, crêpey skin
• to create a pulse within the vacuum, for extra stimulation	
Vacuum suction promotes the face's lymphatic and circulatory systems, thus helping the removal of toxins from the area	
It is desquamating; it stimulates glandular activity and improves the general skin texture	
Very relaxing facial treatment, and can replace manual massage as part of a routine: many clients find it very soothing and drop off to sleep!	
There is also a multi-cup static vacuum suction machine for use with up to six cups at a time, but the cups remain static on the body, rather than used with a gliding movement. This is suitable for treating larger areas in one treatment such as the buttocks and upper thighs	

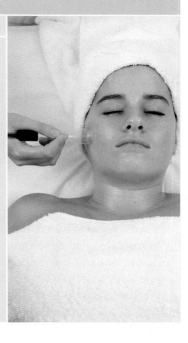

Electrical massage treatment

INDIRECT HIGH FREQUENCY

Uses and client needs	**Suitable skin type/body type**
Often called a 'Viennese massage', indirect high frequency involves creating a circuit of current, flowing through the client via a hand-held glass rod, called a saturator, connected to the machine. The therapist's hands make contact with the client and the current is discharged through her fingertips, as she is massaging, creating warmth in the area	Most commonly used on dry or fine skins. The medium used is oil, which helps the glide of the treatment and lubricates the skin
Can be used in place of the facial massage routine, although if clients become too relaxed, they will lose contact with the saturator which they should be holding. Avoid losing contact with the skin, as this breaks the circuit	
This deep massage will improve a dry skin, relax the tissues and help increase a poor or sluggish circulation to the area	
Creates warmth in the lower legs and feet, so could be incorporated into a pedicure	

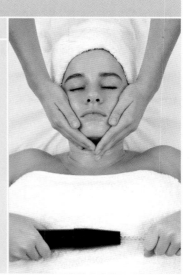

Electrical treatments for cleansing, healing, moisturising and exercising

DIRECT HIGH FREQUENCY

Uses and client needs	Suitable skin type/body type	
Using a high-frequency machine, the current is transmitted into a glass electrode, which is in direct contact with the skin. Light circular motions then disperse the current This is a drying germicidal treatment, ideal for a seborrhoeic skin, one that is congested or has blemishes	Most commonly used on oily, congested or acne skin types, to the face, back or chest area	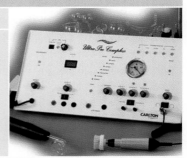

GALVANIC

Uses and client needs	Suitable skin type/body type	
A galvanic machine uses a direct constant current for both face and body work, and the results depend upon the method of use and the gels and products used. The current has to create a circuit flowing through the client, either by using rollers with a connection in the client's hand or a pad under the shoulder, or by the use of body pads, to complete the circuit Can be used in two ways: • Desincrustation – removes the incrustation, i.e. the excess sebum, and gives a deep cleansing to the skin • Iontophoresis – introduces beneficial substances into the skin, to rebalance and rehydrate the skin, or to get active substances to stimulate the body's systems, which aids lymphatic drainage	Most skin types, except where contra-indications are present Desincrustation for oily skins or skins in need of a deep cleanse; iontophoresis for a dry skin or to rebalance the skin, to improve the skin texture or as an anti-cellulite treatment	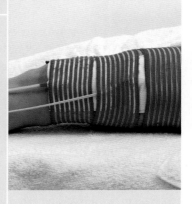

MICROCURRENT

Uses and client needs	Suitable skin type/body type	
A modified direct, low-frequency current which is used on its own for lifting of the facial or body contours and in conjunction with a galvanic current for skin improvement Can help with fine line reduction, stretch mark minimising and scar reduction, and deep cleansing	Most skin types, except where contra-indications are present	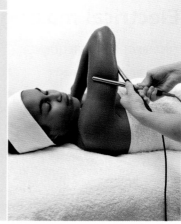

FARADIC

Uses and client needs	**Suitable skin type/body type**
Using a surged and interrupted current, a faradic machine can stimulate muscular contractions on both the face and body	Most skin types, except where contra-indications are present

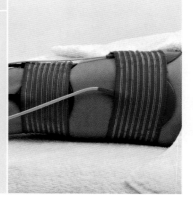

Often referred to as passive exercise, you can actually see the muscles contracting under the pads whilst the client lies motionless on the couch

The pads for the face are smaller than those used in body work, so it is possible to target specific muscle groups for improvement in tone and suppleness

Treatment is ideal for double chins, dropped jaw line and cheekbone definition

Check your knowledge

1 The primary curve of the spine is:
   a) the first curve to form in a baby
   b) the first curve to form in an adult
   c) the curve of the spine when sitting
   d) the curve in the lumber region.

2 Lordosis is recognised by:
   a) a rounded lower back
   b) a hollow lower back
   c) a sideways pull on the spine
   d) knock knees.

3 Scoliosis is recognised by:
   a) a rounded lower back
   b) a hollow lower back
   c) a sideways pull on the spine
   d) knock knees.

4 An ectomorph body type:
   a) is long, lean and angular
   b) has a solid frame with fat, and small hands
   c) has an athletic build
   d) is very overweight.

5 A mesomorph body type:
   a) is long, lean and angular
   b) has a solid frame with fat, and small hands
   c) has an athletic build
   d) is very overweight.

6 Winged scapulae are visible from:
   a) the top of the head
   b) the back
   c) the front
   d) the knees.

7 Phlebitis is a term for:
   a) a type of bunion
   b) a type of stretch mark
   c) a type of fat
   d) an inflamed varicose vein.

8 BMI stands for:
   a) British Medical Institute
   b) Body Mass Index
   c) Body Marking Ink
   d) Body Means Indicator.

9 Blood pressure is the force of the blood flowing in:
   a) the veins
   b) the skin
   c) the heart
   d) the arteries.

10 An average pulse rate is:
   a) 84
   b) 94
   c) 74
   d) 64.

Unit B13

Provide body electrical treatments

What you will learn

- Maintain safe and effective methods of working when providing body electrical treatments
- Consult, plan and prepare for treatments with clients
- Prepare the skin for a body treatment
- Carry out body electrical treatments
- Provide aftercare advice

You will learn how to achieve all of these outcomes using:

- a galvanic unit
- an EMS – electro-muscle stimulator (faradic unit)
- a microcurrent unit
- a microdermabrasion unit
- lymphatic drainage equipment (vacuum suction)

Introduction

Unlike facial electrical treatments, body treatments do not offer instant results although the skin will be improved almost immediately. Body treatments often require a course of six, eight or ten sessions alongside a commitment from clients to adjust their lifestyle, diet and exercise routines, which may contribute to their particular problem areas. Choosing a suitable treatment plan for the client and using the equipment in a safe and appropriate way are the focus of this unit.

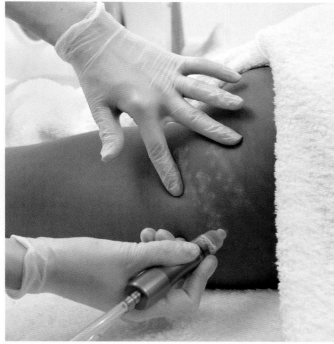

Microdermabrasion can help with stretch marks as well as scars on the body

Body treatments aim to:

- improve the skin and body condition
- improve muscle condition and the contours of the body
- improve lymphatic drainage of the body
- improve stretch marks or scars on the body
- aid in relaxation, both physically and mentally.

Using equipment safely and with confidence is essential, and it is very important that you follow the manufacturer's instructions for the machine you are using, since these will vary. Products used, treatment times and the dials showing strength of current will differ from one make of machine to another. The only way to be totally safe and competent in your assessments is to understand each machine thoroughly

and know its capabilities. This will provide you with the confidence to treat clients in a professional manner, which in turn will give the client confidence in your abilities.

The Standards set out detailed performance criteria regarding:

- maintaining safe and effective methods of working when providing body electrical treatments
- consulting, planning and preparing for treatments with clients.

The majority of these requirements apply to all beauty therapy treatments and are therefore covered in detail in Professional basics, Body treatments — theory and consultation, and G22 Monitor procedures to safely control work operations.

The details given in unit B14 Provide facial electrical treatments, are also pertinent and apply equally to body electrical treatments. You should also refer back to two earlier units — You and the skin and Related anatomy and physiology — as required.

Any treatment-specific requirements for body electrical treatments are covered within this unit.

Contra-indications

Contra-indications will be similar and common to all body electrical treatments, much as they are with facial electrical treatments. Always do a complete contra-indication and consultation session prior to treatment. Remember to ask whether the client has seen any other health care professionals recently and whether they have undergone any chemical peels, IPL (Intense Pulsed Light) or laser treatments or epilation in the area to be treated; this will always be a contra-indication to treatment.

Also remember that if clients are on medication which causes thinning or inflammation of the skin, for example steroids, Accutane or Retin A, this may occur on the body as well as the face. Thinned skin is a contra-indication. Refer to B14 Provide facial electrical treatments, for further detail.

Provide body electrical treatments B13

Think about it

When learning to use a piece of equipment, it is important that you, too, have experienced the treatment. You are then able to describe the sensation of the current to the client and can also fully understand the importance of client modesty. It makes you appreciate the apprehensions of the client when you become one!

> ### Think about it
>
> Always maintain client modesty when giving body treatments. Make sure you have plenty of big towels available, and only expose the part of the body to be worked upon. Keep the rest of the body warm, and then when you have finished on one particular area, keep that warm too. This will reinforce the relaxation of the muscle fibres and heat generated in the tissue.

Preparing the skin for a body treatment

Let's assume that the body consultation has gone smoothly, the client has no contra-indications, the chosen treatment can go ahead and the client is in a suitable position for treatment. You are ready to use your chosen electrical equipment. The skin has been cleansed and is grease-free. It is still essential to further prepare the skin to be receptive to the electrical treatment you are about to perform.

Ideally, before the treatment, the client should have taken a relaxing sauna, steam bath or jacuzzi treatment, finishing with a shower. This both prepares the skin and warms the tissues, making the body very receptive to the current and the treatment easier to perform.

The skin can be prepared for treatment by:

- cleansing
- exfoliation
- pre-heating treatments, such as infrared lamp.

Cleansing/exfoliants

If the client does not have time for a shower, using the wet area or an infrared treatment, the best way to prepare the skin is to use exfoliants, to slough off any remaining dead skin cells from the surface of the epidermis, which may hinder the benefits of the treatment. (For further information on exfoliation ingredients and their application and removal, see Unit B14 Provide facial electrical treatments, page 277.)

Pre-heating treatments

These include:

- infrared lamp (see Unit B20 Provide body massage treatments, page 420)
- sauna, steam cabinet or spa (see Unit S1 Assist with spa operations, on the website www.pearsonfe.co.uk/ BeautyTherapyLevel2UnitS1

- manual massage (see Unit B20 Provide body massage treatments, page 397)
- hot shower (see Unit S1 Assist with spa operations, on the website www.pearsonfe.co.uk/ BeautyTherapyLevel2UnitS1

These options require a certain amount of time in order to be effective, which the client may not have. If not, then treat the skin as if you were doing a facial treatment. Choose an appropriate cleanser, with a superficial and deep cleanse, using effleurage movements. This especially applies to a congested back, which can be treated exactly as the skin on the face, although you will need to use slightly more product, because of the larger surface area. Feet can be wiped over with an appropriate cleanser.

If the client has applied body lotion and you feel that the grease on the skin is going to interfere with the treatment, if no other treatment is available (and the client cannot shower), then wash the area to be treated with warm soapy water and pat dry with a towel.

> ### Think about it
>
> Whichever pieces of equipment you choose as the most suitable for the client's treatment plan always follow the five golden rules:
>
> 1 Always complete a full consultation.
> 2 Complete a contra-indication checklist.
> 3 Carry out thermal and sensitivity testing.
> 4 Always follow manufacturer's instructions.
> 5 Test the equipment on yourself and the client's hand before applying to the body.

> ### Think about it
>
> The different types of electrical currents have various effects on the body. Most of them will warm the skin and muscles through the increase in circulation to the area; lymphatic drainage is stimulated by using the equipment in the direction of the nodes; and the nerve endings are soothed by the heat generated. Only the faradic current is used to cause muscular contractions, and no electrical currents have an effect on the skeleton.

Carry out body electrical treatments

- how to safely use the equipment
- how to explain the sensation and the procedure to the client
- how to safely use the correct treatment settings, applicator and accessories for each piece of equipment
- the correct intensity and duration of treatment for each
- remedial action if required
- suitable post-treatment products
- how to ensure finished results meet with client expectations and to agreed treatment plans.

Galvanism

Refresh your memory of the theory of electrical treatments by referring to Unit B14 Provide facial electrical treatments.

What to tell the client

It can be used in two ways:

- Desincrustation – this removes the incrustation, i.e. the excess sebum, and gives a deep cleansing to the skin.

- Iontophoresis – this introduces beneficial substances into the skin, to rebalance and rehydrate the skin, or to get active substances to stimulate the body's systems, which aids lymphatic drainage.

The galvanic current – both desincrustation and iontophoresis – can be used on the body for:

- skin correction
- anti-cellulite treatment.

The sensation is rather like a warmth under the anti-cellulite pads and a tingling feeling – most clients go to sleep and find the treatment rather soothing, especially as the client is on the bed for half an hour!

Skin correction

If the client has skin problems on the back, then treat the area as you would for a facial treatment – using the rollers, complete a desincrustation to cleanse the area, with the client holding the indifferent electrode, and then perform iontophoresis to rebalance the skin. A back also benefits from a steam prior to treatment or a brush cleanse, and a face mask with direct high frequency to finish the treatment.

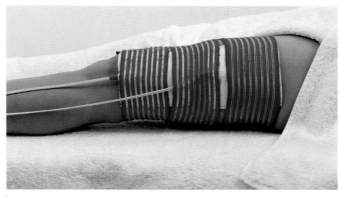

Pads are usually placed in pairs opposite each other. Adjust current to suit client's tolerance

Anti-cellulite treatment

This uses iontophoresis only. The galvanic unit for the body behaves exactly as in a facial treatment, but instead of rollers and an indifferent pad forming a circuit, the pads are the same size and go across the limbs, forming a circuit. The principle of iontophoresis is exactly the same – instead of using moisturising products to keep moisture in the skin, use diuretic anti-cellulite gels to help with the retention of fluids.

Galvanic padding

What to consider when using galvanic treatment

- The skin's resistance to the current is broken down more quickly if the area is pre-warmed by manual massage, a shower or infrared treatment.

- The skin must be grease-free and clean to allow the gels to penetrate the skin.

- The electrodes must be fully covered in damp sponges, otherwise a galvanic burn will result – refer to the manufacturer's instructions.

- Only place the anti-cellulite gel under the active electrode, that is where the treatment is taking place – paste it on like buttering a piece of bread to ensure even coverage.

- The pads are held in place with Velcro strips, so ensure the size is correct for the body part – too loose and the contact will be insufficient to penetrate the skin, and a galvanic burn may be the result of uneven contact with the skin; too tight and you will stop the circulation in the area (the Velcro strips act like a tourniquet) or the strips may come undone halfway through the treatment.

- Never exceed the recommended time or milliamps recommended by the instructions, usually a maximum of 3.0 mAs for no more than 20 minutes.

- Time the treatment and never leave the client unattended.

- Always turn the current off before removing the pads.

- There will be an obvious erythema under the active pad. This is perfectly normal, and shows the treatment has worked. Some manufacturers recommend reversing the polarity for 3–5 minutes of the treatment to reduce the erythema effect. Do this by turning down and then off, and then switch polarity on the machine – you do not have to adjust or swap over the pads.

- Finish with lymphatic drainage, either manually or with vacuum suction, but be careful not to over-stimulate the area, as it already has an erythema. Some manufacturers also recommend G5 massage or faradic after galvanic.

- A course of treatment is most beneficial and can be recommended for three times a week, up to 12 sessions. The treatment responds well to good homecare – diet and exercise play a big part in aiding the dispersal of pockets of cellulite.

Think about it

The cream/gel should be the same polarity as the active pad, so that they repel, and the ions in the cream are drawn towards the indifferent electrode opposite.

Think about it

It is vitally important to carry out a thermal sensitivity test for *each* area you are treating.

Think about it

The first treatment should not exceed 10 minutes and the maximum treatment time is 20 minutes.

Think about it

A diuretic substance causes an increase in the flow of urine, so one of the effects of using anti-cellulite gels is that for a day or so after treatment, the client will be urinating more frequently than usual. Reassure the client that this is part of the treatment working. Therefore, specific contra-indications to a body galvanic treatment are:

- kidney problems
- urinary tract infections
- fluid retention, which may indicate kidney problems (for information on how to spot fluid retention, see Body treatments – theory and consultation, page 353).

Think about it

Leave the equipment as you would wish to find it! Wash the sponge covers in warm, soapy water to remove any gel, and leave them to dry as naturally as possible – drying them over a heater or radiator will cause the sponges to dry out and crack, which causes uneven concentration of current and a galvanic burn.

Pairs of pads should be placed opposite or in line with one another. Never place pads diagonally opposite.

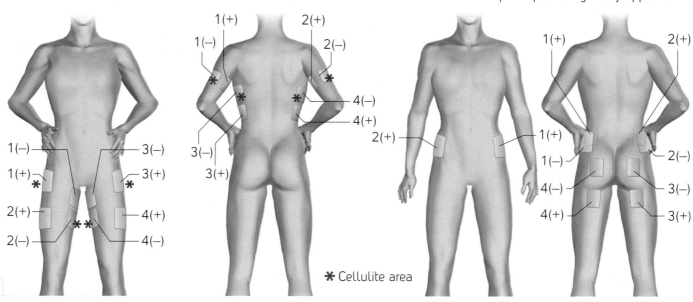

✱ Cellulite area

Check product polarity needed for anti-cellulite gel and choose the correct polarity.

⬇

Check electrodes are covered with damp sponge covers or sleeves.

⬇

Active pad and cream/gel must be the same — only place gel on the active sponge, not on both.

⬇

Check active electrode is over area of cellulite.

⬇

Turn up current gradually, and never exceed 3 mAs.

⬇

Time treatment and reverse polarity for final 3–5 minutes.

⬇

Turn current off, remove pads and remove any residue of the gel.

⬇

Carry out other treatments which encourage lymphatic drainage such as manual massage, G5 or vacuum suction.

Galvanic at a glance

Possible contra-actions

Explain to the client that there will be a slight itching sensation under the active pad, especially as the product/ current is beginning to break down the skin's resistance. If the itchiness is severe, or is accompanied by a burning sensation, then the client is having a reaction to the gel and the current should be turned off, the pads removed and the products removed at once. A cold compress should be sufficient to calm down the area.

Faradism

A faradic treatment to the body is carried out along the same principles as on the face, except that the settings are altered to be more suitable for larger muscle groups and the pads are bigger and come in pairs, rather than together in one unit as they do in the facial unit.

How does it work?

The machine is artificially contracting the muscles without any conscious effort on behalf of the client. In order to do this, an electrical circuit must be completed using an alternating current between two pads. (The technical term is electrodes but this is often a worrying term to use in front of a nervous client — pads will prevent any negative associations!)

Voluntary skeletal muscles contract by pulling on the tendons which attach the muscles to the bones. For stimulation to take place the impulses should make contact with the motor point of a muscle (or a group of muscles, as they rarely work in isolation), usually found in the 'belly' (widest part) of the muscle. However, it is important to know the origin and insertion of each muscle, if you are using mono-phasic settings (see settings on the machine on the next page).

The *origin* of a muscle is the fixed point that doesn't move and is where the muscle begins; the *insertion* is the other end of the muscle which moves when the muscle contracts — going towards its origin. For example, the large group of four muscles in the front of the thigh, quadriceps femoris, all originate on the pelvis and femur bone and insert in the lower leg on the tibia bone and patella. This allows movement at the knee joint. So to extend the leg and cause flexion at the knee, the origins are fixed and the insertions come up towards it. See the muscles section in the Related anatomy and Physiology unit (page 187) for a full breakdown of all the muscles.

We actually don't want to cause movement over a joint, so the padding would not go on the origin and insertion — as this would make the knee bend. We want to cause static contractions of the muscles, so the padding would be on the belly of the muscle, both pads on the upper thigh.

What to tell the client

Faradic, passive exercise of specific muscle groups is very effective in creating tone and muscle definition, and if used in conjunction with a healthy diet and regular exercise, can visibly reduce inches. Be careful about stating that a faradic treatment can help the client lose weight — if you are increasing the muscle bulk, then muscle weighs more than fat, so the client may find he or she gains a little weight, but it is lean muscle tissue rather than fat.

The sensation is a tingling feeling to start with, until the therapist gets the contractions going — and then the muscles contract without any help from the client. The client must relax and let the machine do the contracting — it will give a pulling sensation in the muscles if they try and fight the current or tense the muscle as it is being contracted. The muscles will tire easily at first, especially if they have not been exercised regularly. It is important that, just like regular exercise, you build up the muscle stamina in small bursts, increasing the duration as the muscle become fitter and able to sustain more exercise.

The effect of faradism

- The current stimulates the nerves and causes muscular contractions, which is classed as a form of passive exercise — meaning the body doesn't move, and there is no movement of joints, or of the skeleton. The muscles become firmed, toned and strengthened. When a therapist refers to muscles being toned this is not in a cosmetic, defined manner as in a body builder with a 'six pack' muscle torso, it really refers to the muscle's ability to work efficiently for longer periods without tiring.

- Muscles have a shift system of working within their bundles of fibres. Once one set of fibres have used up their energy store of glycogen and have contracted for as long as they can, they stop working to gain more oxygen and nutrients from the blood flow, and another set of fibres takes over. So muscles can be trained and built up, working longer and more powerfully and getting less tired. This is what a therapist would define as true muscle tone. This is what faradism does.

- Blood circulation and lymphatic flow are improved because of the pumping action of the muscular contractions — and lymph return is increased because the lymph relies on the pressure of the skeletal muscles to help it, as in any activity such as walking. This is why inactivity in less mobile people often results in oedema or swelling of the ankles and lower limbs.

- The metabolic rate of cellular activity is increased, so the condition of the muscles and growth and repair of tissue is stimulated.

- Erythema is produced in the area of exercise, so blood flow brings oxygen and nutrients more quickly and waste is effectively removed.

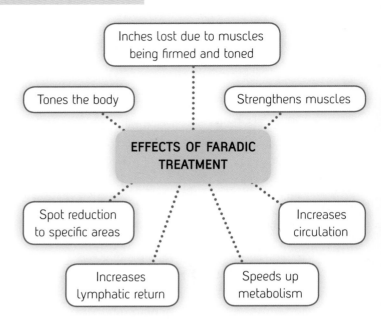

EFFECTS OF FARADIC TREATMENT
- Inches lost due to muscles being firmed and toned
- Tones the body
- Strengthens muscles
- Spot reduction to specific areas
- Increases circulation
- Increases lymphatic return
- Speeds up metabolism

What to consider when using faradic treatment

- Ensure that all leads are firmly inserted into the faradic unit.

- Black and red pads should be inserted into corresponding mini plugs.

- Ensure the unit is off and all intensity dials are in the off position.

Dial settings on most faradic machines

There are timing buttons, each set of leads has its own strength setting for contraction buttons and there is a pulse sequence setting.

Pulse sequence — one of four mode buttons

1 Bi-phasic regular pulse (red button) — the electrical impulses pass in both directions between the pads giving an even, firming, toning and strengthening treatment for the muscles. This is ideal for the beginner, who has done little exercise in the past and wants a gentle start to the exercise programme.

2 Mono-phasic regular pulse (blue button)* — the electrical impulses pass in one direction only, helping to lift the muscle being treated. This works the muscle harder than bi-phasic and is good for the client who regularly exercises and perhaps wants more definition to the muscle shape. (NB Facial treatments are always carried out in mono-phasic, as you only want an upward contraction and pull on the facial muscles.)

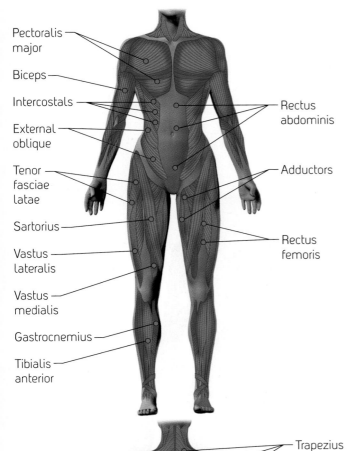

- Pectoralis major
- Biceps
- Intercostals
- External oblique
- Tenor fasciae latae
- Sartorius
- Vastus lateralis
- Vastus medialis
- Gastrocnemius
- Tibialis anterior
- Rectus abdominis
- Adductors
- Rectus femoris

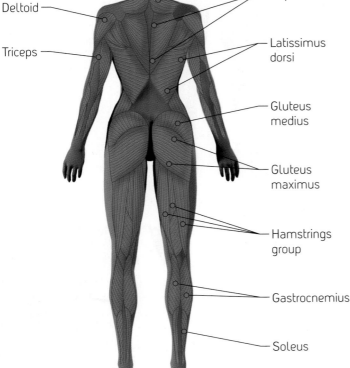

- Deltoid
- Triceps
- Trapezius
- Latissimus dorsi
- Gluteus medius
- Gluteus maximus
- Hamstrings group
- Gastrocnemius
- Soleus

Motor points for the front and back of the body

3 Bi-phasic irregular pulse (green button) — this is for clients who have been coming to the salon for faradic treatment for some time and are perhaps halfway through their treatment course of 8–10 sessions. Because the muscles get used to the rate and rhythm of the pattern of contractions, the muscles become lazy and almost anticipate the current. The irregular pulse setting changes the pace of the contraction, say one second intervals, then three, then two and so on. The muscle has to work hard again to respond to the irregular stimulation, and it doesn't know the pattern, as the machine does a random selection of contraction and rest phases.

4 Mono-phasic irregular pulse (yellow button) — this irregular pulse sequence is most suited to the nervous or tense client. The pulses come in groups of 2 and 5 and due to the irregularity of the pattern the client cannot anticipate the current flow and will avoid tensing the muscle in anticipation, therefore causing more discomfort.

Important padding information

If you are doing any bi-phasic setting work, the pulses are alternating between the two pads, so in theory the pads can go in either direction as long as they are near the motor points of the muscles. However, if you are in mono-phasic setting, the current is pulling in one direction only — and the pads must be placed with the black lead towards the insertion of the muscle and the red lead near the origin.

Remember BIRO = **B**lack lead near **I**nsertion, **R**ed lead near **O**rigin.

Contraction and relaxation settings

This setting can be altered to give a longer or shorter length of muscle contraction in seconds. This will be dependent upon the client's muscle tone and you can increase or decrease the timing to suit — if the client is halfway through a course of treatments, the muscles will be able to contract for longer than when they first start.

Weaker muscles should start on a lower time of 1.5 seconds on contraction and 1.5 seconds on relaxation. You can build the times up from there and also alter the times for a longer contraction and shorter relaxation, for example 2 seconds contraction, 1 second relaxation. This will work the muscles harder, but they will tire more quickly.

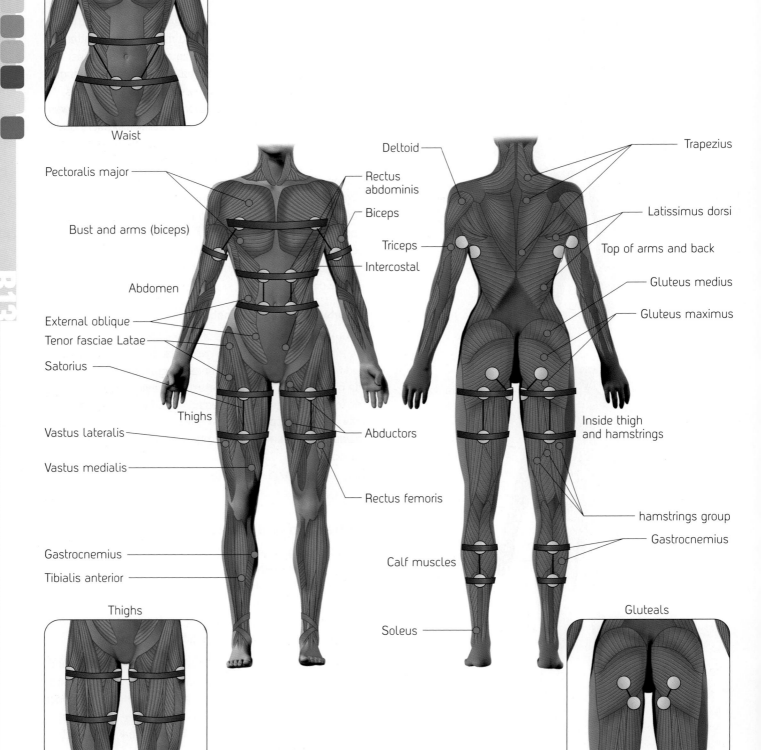

Waist

Pectoralis major

Bust and arms (biceps)

Abdomen

External oblique

Tenor fasciae Latae

Satorius

Thighs

Vastus lateralis

Vastus medialis

Gastrocnemius

Tibialis anterior

Thighs

Deltoid

Rectus abdominis

Biceps

Triceps

Intercostal

Abductors

Rectus femoris

Trapezius

Latissimus dorsi

Top of arms and back

Gluteus medius

Gluteus maximus

Inside thigh and hamstrings

hamstrings group

Gastrocnemius

Calf muscles

Soleus

Gluteals

Padding layouts and motor points for faradic treatment

	Frequency setting	Pulse width setting
Normal body work	80–100 Hz	160 µs
Deep muscle work	60 Hz	240 µs
Facial work	120 Hz	90 µs

The frequency and pulse width settings can be altered to ensure the impulses penetrate to exactly the right depth to the muscle being contracted, which provides maximum comfort for the client.

Reset facility

Most modern machines have a reset facility to ensure that no current can be accidentally passed through to the client when the unit is switched on. When switching on the reset button a little light at the front should be illuminated. To enable the machine to work, you need to turn the 'set time' knob clockwise to display a treatment time, for example thirty minutes. Press in the reset button and the light will change to show the machine is ready for use. If you have set up the machine and padded up your client, but the machine will not work, it is because you have not overridden this reset button. Also remember that when you do set the reset button the intensity dials should all be back to the off position or 0, as this too will prevent the machine from working. This is a safety device so that you do not give your client a high contraction, should another therapist leave the settings on from a previous treatment.

Treatment timer

This timing facility allows you to automatically set the exact time you decide upon for your treatment, and this will vary depending upon where the client is in the treatment plan, and how good the muscle tone is. The 'set time' dial will go from 0–99 minutes and can be moved both clockwise and anti-clockwise, which is perfectly normal. A time must be set before you can use the reset facility to start the machine – again, if the machine doesn't work, ensure that you have put the clock on!

Panic button

Most modern machines have a panic button which can be given to the client, which cuts out the current they should feel it is too much for them, or the muscles get cramp or they experience discomfort. The button plugs into a small jack at the back of the unit and the client can have the comfort of holding it. When pressed, the button turns off the machine, an alarm will sound and a light may flash. All dials must be set back to 0 before the machine can be reset.

Contra-indications to a faradic treatment

- Epilepsy, as the current may induce an attack
- Diabetes – unless with GP approval, due to poor circulation and thin skin
- Spastic muscles – although faradic work is carried out by physiotherapists for this condition, it should be under medical supervision
- Metal plates and pins – the current is attracted to the metal and impairs the treatment
- Pacemaker and heart conditions – the current may interfere with the electrical impulses to the heart and cause irregularity
- Pregnancy – but faradic treatments can help with muscle retraining after birth – post-natal after six weeks with GP approval
- Over cuts and abrasions – the current is drawn to the moisture content of blood and may cause a concentration of current in the area
- Directly over varicose veins, in case inflammation occurs and the blood is over-stimulated making the condition worse
- Very high blood pressure – due to over-stimulation

Safety precautions

- Always carry out a full consultation and check for contra-indications.
- Make sure pads are in direct contact with the skin so current is evenly distributed.
- Do not use pads that are damaged or cracked.
- Never operate the unit with wet hands.
- Do not place water or damp pads on the unit.
- Ensure all jewellery is removed prior to treatment as metal is a conductor of electricity and a concentration of current may occur.
- Do not use the equipment if you have not had sufficient training or do not understand the settings.
- Always follow manufacturer's instructions as machine settings vary.

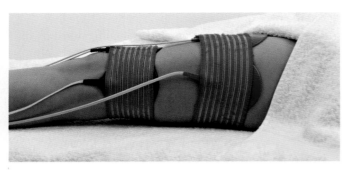

Faradic pad layout for the thighs, working all the muscle groups

Treatment procedure – order of work

- Carry out a thermal sensitivity test.

- Pre-warm muscles in the area with massage or infrared treatment.

- Dampen the rough side of the faradic pads with warm water and test on yourself prior to treatment (a saline solution of one teaspoon of salt in a pint of warm water will aid conductivity as salt is an electrolyte).

- Place the pads on to selected muscles. Secure into place with Velcro faradic straps ensuring good, firm contact with the skin. Select the required pulse sequence.

- Ensure that contraction and relaxation dials are at minimum.

- Select the required frequency and pulse width.

- Switch on the unit by turning the minute timer clockwise and press the yellow reset button. The alarm will sound until the reset button is pressed (alarm on/off switch) at the back of the unit.

- Turn up each individual intensity control slowly until the desired muscle contraction is obtained.

- Increase the contraction and relaxation settings as required.

- Turn the minute timer to the required treatment length, that is 30–40 minutes.

- Cover the client to ensure warmth and muscle relaxation.

- Give the client the panic button and instructions on its use. After 5–10 minutes, check the contraction intensity and increase as necessary. The pulse width may now be adjusted to ensure maximum comfort of the muscle contraction.

- After the treatment time has elapsed, the unit will automatically switch off. Turn all intensity controls to the off position and switch off the unit. Remove the straps and pads.

Preparation of pads

The pads must be clean. After every client, wash with warm, soapy water, or follow manufacturer's instructions to remove grease and wipe with a suitable antiseptic preparation. Any grease on the pads will act as a barrier to the current.

Ensure the pads are thoroughly wet with solution and warm on their working surface before applying them to the skin. This breaks down the skin resistance and allows the free flow of current. Lack of moisture on pads can cause a faradic burn.

Always make sure the pads are conductive side towards the skin – they have a slightly rough surface to them, rather than the shiny side which is the top. It is essential the pads are all held firmly against the body by the straps.

Client variations

A slim, well-toned person will produce contractions with very few pads and low levels of intensity as there is little resistance. A larger person presents more resistance: a larger load and padding must reflect this. Body fat is not a good conductor of current. Reinforced padding should be used when the load or resistance that the muscle has to carry is excessive and contractions will be difficult to get, for example a pair of pads on each thigh for the rectus femoris muscle will produce a good result – it needs more than one pair of pads as it is a big band of muscle.

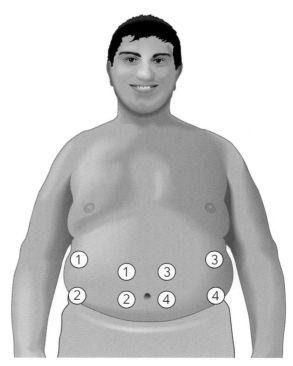

The size of the client will affect the number of pads required

Important considerations with faradic padding

The natural movements of the muscles should be considered and pads placed to copy these movements as much as possible. If the muscles of an area normally work together to produce a movement, they should be padded and exercised as a group. It is not natural for each segment to work independently, for example the quadriceps.

Muscles must never be made to work against each other. As natural antagonists, the back and front of the body should not be worked together, as the body cannot lean forwards and bend backwards at the same time, and should not be asked to do so artificially. Anything which does not produce a natural movement will not be helping the body back to natural strength and tone in its muscles. For example, it would be unnatural for the buttocks to contract one side at a time – they should always be artificially stimulated so both sides work evenly at the same time. The trapezius muscle works evenly along both sides of its spine attachments for most movements, and this is how it should be exercised. The quadriceps and hamstrings work as a group and not separately.

Think about it

Faradic treatments are like any exercise – a regular course of treatments, say twice a week for six weeks, is far more effective than just one treatment, and results will be increased if the client also does the homecare exercises and has a good diet

Types of padding

Longitudinal padding

Originally, the term longitudinal padding referred to the padding of the origin and insertion of a muscle where the current had to flow via the motor point to bring about a contraction. Modern longitudinal padding usually refers to the placing of the electrodes onto a muscle with two motor points.

Modern longitudinal padding involves placing the pads towards the top and bottom motor points of the same muscle, for example rectus abdominus, triceps, rectus fermoris, bringing about a smoother, even contraction. It is essential that there is no movement, so you must not place the pads right over the origin and insertion as these would run over joints, causing movement.

Dual or duplicate padding

This type of padding involves using a pair of pads on one or two muscles on one side of the body and then mirroring the placement of another pair on the adjacent muscle group, for example, the oblique muscles, rectus abdominus, adductors, abductors.

Split padding

With this type of padding, one pair of pads is split and placed on the same muscle group on opposite sides of the body, for example, gluteus maximus, pectorals.

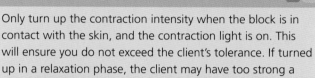

Think about it

Only turn up the contraction intensity when the block is in contact with the skin, and the contraction light is on. This will ensure you do not exceed the client's tolerance. If turned up in a relaxation phase, the client may have too strong a sensation, and it will be uncomfortable and may even hurt.

Think about it

If the client wishes, you could offer her another treatment while she is lying on the couch, for example a facial, eyebrow tidy, eyelash tint or similar, but make sure you do not have water near the machine. Some clients just prefer to rest quietly.

Treatment planning

Faradic body treatments can, in theory, be undertaken daily just like regular exercise, but you may realistically find your client is unable to commit enough time for a daily session. Like natural exercise, three times a week with a faradic machine soon begins to show effects and muscles will improve in tone and working capacity. The muscle can be exercised gently at first in ten-minute sessions, building up to a maximum of 40 minutes for well-toned clients.

After treatment ensure that the client is able to keep the muscles warm, to prevent cramp setting in, and also that the muscles are not overworked with regular exercise on top of a faradic treatment. Vacuum suction to the muscle will ensure that any build-up of lactic acid in the muscle is moved towards the lymph nodes and dispersed.

Microcurrent

Refresh your memory of microcurrent treatments from Unit B14 Provide facial electrical treatments, page 306.

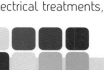

What to tell the client

This is a modified direct, low-frequency current which is used on its own for lifting of the body contours. The sensation is minimal as it is such a low current – you do not feel anything. The body-lifting effect of a microcurrent offers very good results for the client but requires the therapist to have a firm hand as the movements are firm and controlled. Body lifting works on the first four programs of the face-lifting routine. Instead of rollers, there are two bar electrodes to move along the skin. They do not need a sponge cover – as microcurrent is such a low frequency, there is no risk of a burn to the client.

A course of treatments is recommended. Most parts of the body can be lifted, but the treatment is especially popular for the thighs, abdomen, hips, buttocks and breasts. Older clients like to have their arms lifted, so that the biceps are firmer.

Contra-indications to microcurrent treatment

- Heart conditions
- Metal in the area to be treated – as it will gain a concentration of current; especially an IUD contraceptive coil if treating the abdominal area in a female
- Skin diseases and infections – cross-infection may occur
- Diabetes – due to very thin skin
- Very high blood pressure
- Pacemakers
- Hypersensitive skin
- Cuts, abrasions
- Bruises
- Epilepsy
- Spastic muscles

Treatment programmes for areas of the body

Thighs

Programme 1: Circulation
Light pressure. Hold one fixed electrode ① at the top of the thigh. Move the other probe ② from just above the knee slowly towards the fixed electrode. Move from one side of the thigh to the other, concentrating on the inner thigh.

Programme 2: Tightening
Firm pressure. With adductors stretched (knee straight), leg outwards, pinch the lateral edges of the muscle with the tips of the probes and hold, moving down each muscle on the thigh (quadriceps), concentrating on the inner thigh. Hold movements for 8 seconds.

Programme 3: Tightening
Firm pressure. Hold a fixed probe ① on the upper outer thigh. Push the other probe ② from the inner thigh, diagonally up to meet the fixed probe, slowly and firmly, and then hold. Work across the thigh.

Programme 4: Firming
Very firm pressure. The hip and knee should be bent. Allow the knee to fall outwards (approximately 45 degrees – the adductor magnus is then stretched). Active contraction is now needed to prevent the knee falling outwards. Place the probes at each end of the adductor magnus muscle and press as if to move them together but without slipping. Hold movements for 8 seconds.

Upper arms

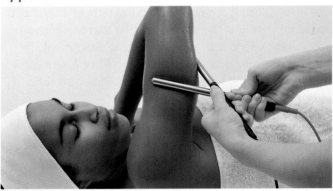

Programme 1: Circulation
Light pressure. Place one probe just under the shoulder ① (at the top of the biceps for the front or the triceps for the back). The other probe ② is pushed up over the front and back faces of the arm, from the elbow towards the fixed probe. (The flat edge or the tips of the probe may be used.)

Programme 2: Tightening
Firm pressure. Biceps stretched, elbow straight for the front. Triceps stretched, elbow bent for the back. The lateral edges of the muscle are pinched with the tips of the probes moving towards the shoulder. Hold movements for 8 seconds.

Programme 3: Tightening
Strong pressure. Repeat programme 1 but with more pressure.

Programme 4: Firming
Firm pressure. Biceps stretched, elbow straight for the front, with static contraction of the biceps. Triceps – stretched, elbow bent for the back, with static contraction of the triceps. The probes are placed at both ends of the muscle (biceps or triceps) and pressure is exerted as if together but without slipping. Hold movements for 8 seconds.

Breasts

There are three movements used when treating the breasts: grab, slide 1 and slide 2. Each movement needs to be applied in three positions on the breast and repeated three times.

Grab

Hold one probe (the red one) stationary with light pressure, hold the other probe (black lead) parallel to it on the other side of the breast. With a little pressure move this electrode towards the stationary one lifting and squeezing the breast between the two.

Hold this position for 10–15 seconds. Use this movement in the three positions shown on the right and repeat these three positions three times each (9 moves in all).

Slide 1

Probes are placed in the same position as for the grab movement, but both move towards each other, lifting the breast between the two probes, applying enough pressure to lift, but not to pinch the client. Only move the probes to either side of the nipple area. Each movement should take 10–15 seconds. Use this movement in the three positions shown and repeat these three positions three times each (9 moves in all).

Slide 2

Starting with the probes in an open V-shape position, gradually move upwards and outwards to the top of the breast, with medium to firm pressure. Each movement should be 10–15 seconds. Use this movement in the three positions shown below and repeat these three positions three times each (9 moves in all).

1 Cleanse area with a hot towel or cleansing milk.
2 Start with one breast at a time and avoid the nipple area.
3 Apply suitable ampoule (for example collagen) and massage lightly to help the penetration.
4 Also apply gel to the area to be worked upon.
5 With the client relaxed, arms by her side, perform the grab, slide 1 and slide 2 movements detailed above.
6 With the client's arm raised with the hand behind her head, repeat the sequence of grab, slide 1 and slide 2 movements but on the third repeat of each movement allow the muscle to contract by offering resistance to the client. This is performed by placing your upper arm (underside) into the arm of the client (her underside, too) and asking her to push against your arm, which is held stationary. The resistance automatically contracts the muscle – for 9 contractions during the treatment.

7 Return the client's arm to the relaxed position and repeat the sequence of grab, slide 1 and slide 2 movements. Apply more gel to the area as required which will help the ease of gliding.

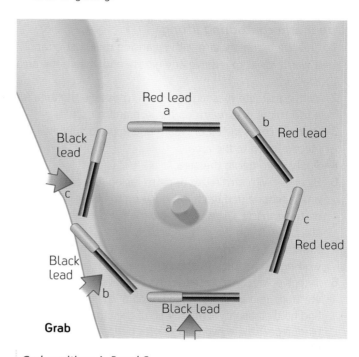

Grab positions A, B and C

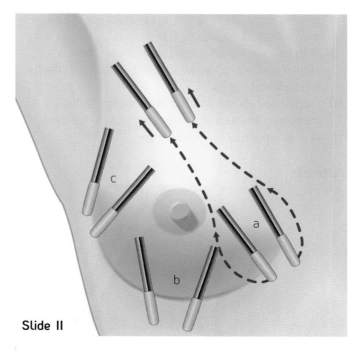

Slide positions A, B and C

8 Repeat the whole treatment to the other breast.

9 Remove the gel with hot towels

10 Apply bust firming cream and massage lightly to aid penetration.

Upper arm contouring lifting

1 Cleanse the upper arm with cleansing milk, gel or apply a warm towel to remove any grease and ensure the area is clean.

2 With a suitable massage medium, massage the area for a few minutes to warm up the skin and muscles.

3 Remove massage oil or cream and apply a suitable electro-lotion to the area.

4 Apply ionto-gel to the area.

5 Biceps – with arm relaxed, palm facing forward, place one electrode (red lead) flat edge on the base of the deltoid muscle just above the armpit. Hold this position stationary. With the other electrode (black lead) move toward the stationary electrode with medium pressure, working from elbow to shoulder. Repeat 6 times.

6 Triceps – with arm placed across the chest, place one electrode (red lead) flat edge on top of the deltoid base and hold stationary. With the tip of the other one (black lead) repeat the movements as for biceps above, 6 times.

7 Biceps – with arm relaxed, palm facing forward, place electrode flat either side of the muscle, apply pressure, lift and hold for 5 seconds. Working from the elbow to the shoulder, apply 5–6 lifts. Repeat 4–5 times.

8 Triceps – with arm relaxed and turned in (with palm of hand on couch) or across the chest apply the same movements as for biceps, 8 times.

9 With hand on hip offer resistance so you create a natural contraction, repeat moves 6–7 but with the flat electrode not the tip.

10 Remove excess gel and complete treatment by massaging the area with medium for 2–3 minutes.

11 Repeat procedure on the other arm.

Buttocks

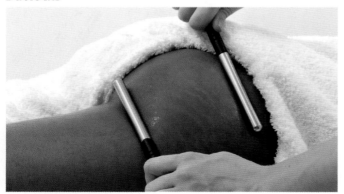

Programme 1: Circulation

Firm pressure. Place one fixed probe ① at the top of the gluteal muscles. Move the other probe ② from below the cheek up to meet the fixed probe. Cover the entire cheek.

Programme 2: Tightening

Very firm pressure. Hold the two probes approximately 12.5 centimetres apart. Slowly push them together to meet. Split the buttocks up into sections, depending on the size. Hold movements for 8 seconds.

Programme 3: Tightening

Very firm pressure. Repeat programme 2 but in diagonal sections.

Programme 4: Firming

Firm pressure. Repeat programme 1 but in diagonal sections.

Abdomen lifting

Programme 1: Circulation

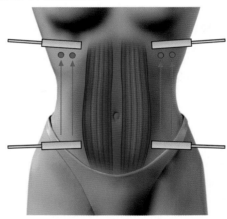

Firm pressure. Hold one probe fixed just below the ribs. Lift the other electrode up from the pubis over the whole surface of the abdomen. Move across in three or four sections.

Programme 2: Tightening

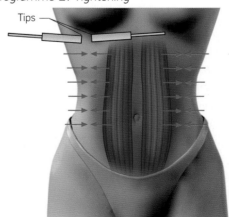

Very firm pressure. With the muscles stretched (arms lifted), move from the pubis to under the ribs. Pinch the lateral edges of the muscle with the tips of the probes. Move across the abdomen in sections. Hold movements for 8 seconds.

Programme 3: Tightening

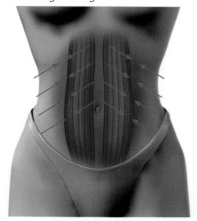

Very firm pressure. Repeat programme 2 but in diagonal sections.

Programme 4: Firming

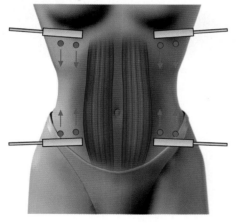

Firm pressure. Abdominal muscles stretched with active contraction (client must raise head and chin towards the sternum). Probes placed at both ends of the abdominal muscles and pressed as if together but without slipping. Hold movement for 8 seconds.

Microdermabrasion

A microdermabrasion facial routine can also be used on the body to improve skin condition, for example acne on back or chest, or as a stretch mark treatment. Refer back to B14 Provide facial electrical treatment, for application detail.

Scar tissue techniques

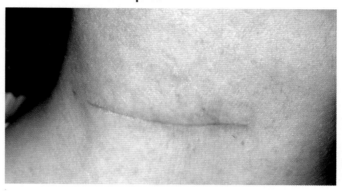

Microdermabrasion can be used to improve the appearance of scar tissue or stretch marks

Microdermabrasion stretch mark treatment

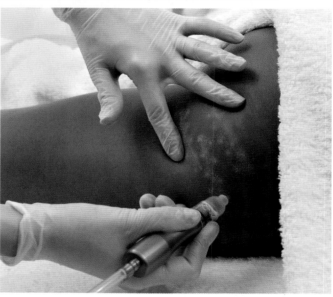

Products required:

- pre-peel lotion
- post-peel lotion
- post-abrasion soothing gel
- EGF repair cream.

1 Cleanse and prepare the area with pre-peel lotion.
2 Set the vacuum intensity to −6 to −8 and the crystal flow to 1 (low crystal setting).
3 Apply the hand piece to the specific area, work down the stretch marks and healthy tissue at a medium to slow pace. Do this only once.
4 Next apply the hand piece to the specific area, work across the stretch mark and healthy tissue by moving across and back in one stroke, slightly overlapping in a zig-zag pattern. Lift the hand piece off the skin and continue to

work in this pattern for the duration of the stretch marks. If no internal punctual bleeding appears, do this once more. If internal punctual bleeding does occur then only work the area once — you will see this as a bruise appearing.

5 Brush any excess crystals from the area.
6 Apply the post-peel lotion to the area.
7 Apply a thin layer of the post-abrasion soothing gel to the area and leave to dry.
8 Apply EGF cream to the area to promote healing.

Vacuum suction

The application of vacuum suction to the body is the same as the facial procedure except that the cups are bigger and the lymph nodes you work towards are positioned differently (for positioning of lymph nodes, see Related anatomy and physiology, page 201; and for the facial procedure, see Unit B14 Provide facial electrical treatments, page 288).

What to tell the client

Vacuum suction promotes the body's lymphatic and circulatory systems, thus helping the removal of toxins from the area. It is desquamating, stimulates glandular activity and improves the general skin texture. It is a very relaxing body treatment, and can replace manual massage as part of a routine: many clients find it very soothing and drop off to sleep!

Contra-indications to vacuum treatment

All contra-indications as for facial application, plus the following:

- Delicate sensitive skin or reduced skin elasticity — the pressure of the vacuum may make the condition worse
- Skin disease or infections — due to possible cross-contamination
- Loose skin — too uncomfortable for the client and may cause bruising
- Bony areas or lack of body fat — if you can perform manual massage, wringing movements and picking up, then there is enough body tissue to support vacuum suction. If not, do not treat
- Excessively hairy areas — may be uncomfortable for the client
- Recent sunburn ⎫
- Recent scar tissue ⎪ vacuum may make
- Stretch marks ⎬ these conditions worse
- Excessively crêpey areas of skin ⎭

Benefits and effect of treatment

- Aids natural desquamation of the skin, so improves texture and appearance
- The metabolism to the area is increased.
- Blood and lymphatic flow to the area is increased.
- The blood flow brings oxygen and nutrients to the area, and speeds up the removal of waste.
- Increases circulation, so is good for chilblains and related poor-circulation problems.

Treatment programme

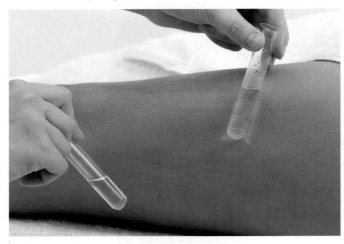

Thermal testing on the area to be treated

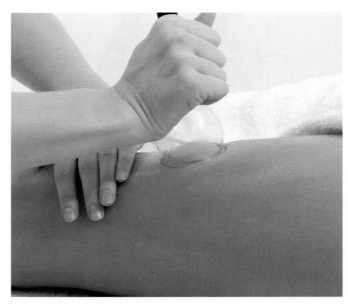

Only fill 20 percent of the cup

1 Apply a covering of oil to the area to be treated ensuring that the rest of the body is covered both for client modesty and also to keep the body warm.

2 Select a suitable body cup and insert into the connector – remember these are quite fragile and expensive to replace, so make sure your hands are oil-free when you do this.

3 Set switch to on and check intensity is at 0.

4 Test on yourself where there is enough tissue to fill 20% of the cup – usually on the inner upper arm.

5 Show the client how the machine works and be in a position so that they can see you testing the machine on yourself.

6 Place the vacuum cup onto the skin, ensuring a complete connection to the skin is made and cover the air hole with a finger so that a vacuum is created in the cup.

7 Glide to the nearest lymph gland and release by breaking the vacuum by removing your finger from the hole.

8 Work methodically over the area, slightly overlapping you strokes until the whole area or limb has been covered. This will be approximately 20 minutes for a complete body treatment; never work longer than 5 minutes over any single area. The strokes should be rhythmic and flow easily, almost replicating a manual massage sensation for the client.

9 After treatment, wipe the area clean of oil, cover and move on to the next area.

What to consider when using vacuum suction treatment

▪ Although very hairy areas on male clients are not contra-indicated, the treatment may not be very comfortable for the client – a lot more oil is required.

▪ Almond oil is fine oil, suitable for the face, but it is quite expensive so is not cost-effective for body treatments – use the usual massage oil instead.

▪ All contra-indications apply as for the facial application, but remember to avoid varicose veins on the legs.

▪ The treatment makes a very good deep lymphatic drainage massage, especially after body faradic treatments where there may be a build-up of lactic acid in the skin.

▪ If the client is using anti-cellulite treatments (galvanic, diet and exercise), then vacuum suction is very effective, but if the fat is solid and hard, there may not be enough tissue to get comfortably into the cup (20 per cent fill only). Avoid treatment if the legs have hard fat – the golden rule is that if you can do petrissage movements of wringing and picking up on the tissue, then there is enough soft fat to use a vacuum machine.

Think about it

Always work towards the major lymph nodes in the body.

Care of body glass applicators

After each treatment, place the glass applicator into warm, soapy water with a little antiseptic solution, clean thoroughly and dry. Place in a sanitiser or store in the facility provided in the back of the machine.

Think about it

Never force the cup into the tubing as it is made of glass and will break. However, most companies manufacture a set of four plexiglass body cups together with an adaptor handle vacuum tube as an option.

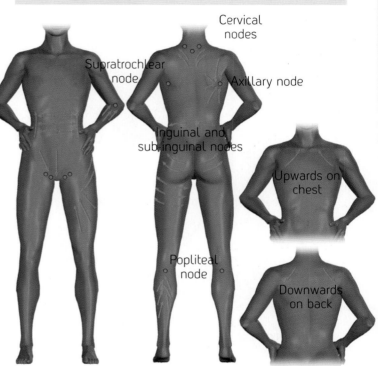

Vacuum suction movements work towards lymph nodes

Labels: Cervical nodes; Supratrochlear node; Axillary node; Inguinal and sub-inguinal nodes; Popliteal node; Upwards on chest; Downwards on back

Atomiser spray

Some machines have an atomiser spray for easy application of the body oil to the area. To operate:

▪ Unscrew the white top from the atomiser spray and fill the container with the product to be used.

▪ Screw on the white top and insert the metal prong into the spray tube.

▪ Set the main switch to the on position.

▪ Hold the atomiser bottle 20–25 centimetres from the area to be treated.

▪ To spray, place your finger over the air bleed hole on the top of the atomiser.

Body cups

There are two sizes of cups available for body work — small (40 mm) and large (52 mm). The size of cup selected will depend on the amount of fatty tissue present.

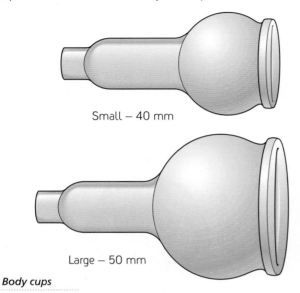

Small — 40 mm

Large — 50 mm

Body cups

Choose correct cup size to start treatment.

Cover the hole at the side of the ventouse to create the vacuum.

Place ventouse on client before turning up intensity.

Put on plenty of product to lubricate the gliding movements.

Work towards the lymph nodes in the area.

Remove ventouse by breaking the vacuum — release your finger from the hole.

Never flick or pull the ventouse from the skin.

Vacuum suction at a glance

Additional knowledge

High frequency

High-frequency treatment for the body is not covered in this unit — but it can be used in exactly the same way to the body as it is to the face and makes a really good treatment for either an indirect massage or directly on a congested back, for a drying germicidal effect.

Refresh your memory of the application of high frequency and its theory from Unit B14 Provide facial electrical treatments (page 279). The benefits and effects on the skin, safety precautions and contra-actions apply in the same way to the body as to the face.

Provide aftercare advice

After giving body electrical treatments to the client you should provide aftercare advice and recommendations for further treatments or suitable products, and give constructive advice for individual client needs.

Immediately after body treatments

- Remove any excess medium from the areas treated — the client should not leave the salon with galvanic gel or oil from vacuum treatment on the skin as it will get onto clothes and be uncomfortable. Always cleanse the area thoroughly with hot towels or flannels and/or apply a light tonic if desired.

- If the client has drifted off to sleep, allow them time to become fully aware of the surroundings, provide a drink of water to refresh and hydrate them and put their head up by raising the couch to a semi-reclining position, so they can gradually acclimatise to being upright. Never ask the client to jump straight off the couch — they may faint if there is a poor blood supply to the brain.

- Keep the client well wrapped up until they are fully awake and pass them their clothing.

- Spend a few minutes with them after they are dressed, talking the treatment through and updating the record card for likes and dislikes, any contra-actions and the client's preferred treatment moves.

- Talk to the client, recommending suitable and appropriate skincare products and the most suitable treatments to complement the one they have just had. It may be bath and shower products, exfoliators for the body, and/or moisturising products for dry skin. Clients often spend a great deal of time putting products on the face and forget that their bodies also need it.

Long-term aftercare

Talk to the client about their long-term goals: weight loss, firming and lifting or overall skin care. This will involve considerable personal commitment from the client with regard to changing lifestyle choices and eating healthily, drinking enough water and exercising regularly.

Discuss the possibility of a course of body treatments – most of the treatments in this unit have a much better cumulative effect than a single one-off treatment, but be sure the client understands the commitment in terms of cost (both in money and time).

You may want to discuss long-term goals for the client in terms of SMART planning – specific, measurable, achievable, realistic and timely. Putting a client on an egg-only diet for three months is just not realistic, neither is a five-hour daily exercise programme. However, small achievable goals, say of losing four pounds a month, if that is what the client wants to achieve, is realistic. Do remember it is the client's needs

and wants that count – do not assume it is weight loss she needs, if her desired outcome is to tone up.

Introduce the possibility of other complementary treatments to enhance the body treatments. If the client is stressed, then recommend a hot stone massage, or if when doing the legs you notice the feet need a pedicure, then recommend one! The fact that you have now passed your Level 2 qualifications does not exclude them from a client treatment plan – they should be offered a real treat or even an incentive. If the client achieves X as their goal, then offer a half-price treatment to keep them interested and motivated.

Think about it

When recommending products for home use that will benefit and protect the client, you should be careful to consider their individual needs, and never recommend a product you are not familiar with. Avoid encouraging expensive purchases with unknown benefits.

Salon life

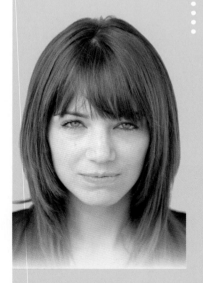

Marina's story

My name is Marina and I'm a third year student just finishing my studies. I was carrying out a faradic treatment on a client's thighs and buttocks and learned a valuable lesson about the importance of thoroughly checking my equipment after the treatment. The treatment had gone well and I'd given the client the necessary aftercare advice, but the next day she came to see me with something wrapped in some tissue paper. She wanted a confidential word so I took her into an empty treatment room. Inside the tissue was a black faradic pad and she explained that she was concerned about her 'insides' as she thought she'd 'passed it' while in the toilet. She was obviously worried and I felt so terrible because when I was removing the pads after treatment, I must have missed one. I'd told her that stimulating the muscles and digestive pathway may cause her to visit the toilet more and she obviously thought this was an extreme reaction. When she went to the toilet, the pad must have dropped off into the toilet bowl! I told her it was completely my fault and fully explained what had happened. She eventually saw the funny side, but I will be so much more careful in future.

Effects for the therapist:

- Don't assume clients understand everything you say – ask them questions about the after effects of treatments to ensure they are not taking them too literally
- Always check the equipment in and out after the treatment to ensure you are not missing anything and that nothing is still attached to the client

- Missing equipment is very expensive to replace and not all clients will return things

Effects for the client:

- Going home with a piece of equipment still attached to the body does not instil confidence in the therapist – especially if they think it is a side effect of treatment

Check your knowledge

1 What percentage of cup should be filled by the tissues?
   a) 10 per cent
   b) 20 per cent
   c) 30 per cent
   d) 40 per cent

2 Why is jewellery not recommended in electrical body treatments?
   a) It causes sparking.
   b) It causes a shock.
   c) The current is drawn to it.
   d) It gets hot.

3 What is the mono-phasic setting on a faradic machine for?
   a) Upward lift only
   b) Downward lift only
   c) Alternate lifting
   d) Sideways lifting

4 Galvanic treatment is used for:
   a) lymph drainage
   b) muscular toning
   c) circulation improvement
   d) anti-cellulite treatment.

5 The origin of a muscle is:
   a) the fixed part
   b) the moving part
   c) the end of the muscle
   d) the belly of the muscle.

6 The anti-cellulite gel effect on the body acts as:
   a) an irritant
   b) a diuretic
   c) a moisturiser
   d) an exfoliant.

7 Vacuum suction movements always go towards the:
   a) heart
   b) brain
   c) lymph nodes
   d) digestive tract.

8 Split padding is a type of faradic padding. It means:
   a) one pair of pads over the belly of the muscle
   b) two pairs of pads over a group of muscles
   c) one pair of pads over the same muscle on each side of the body
   d) three sets of pads on a muscle group.

9 Faradic exercise is classed as:
   a) passive
   b) aerobic
   c) anaerobic
   d) active.

10 An anti-cellulite treatment uses:
   a) desincrustation only
   b) iontophoresis only
   c) both desincrustation and iontophoresis together
   d) high frequency.

Getting ready for assessment

You are not allowed any simulation within this unit and you must practically demonstrate in your everyday work that you have met the Standards for providing body electrical treatments.

Your assessor will observe your performance on at least *five* separate performances, which must include at least *three* different clients.

From the ranges you must show that you have:

- used all types of equipment
- used all the body consultation techniques
- treated all the body types
- treated all body conditions
- carried out at least one of the three necessary actions listed
- met all criteria objectives
- provided all types of advice.

Unit B20

Provide body massage treatments

What you will learn:

- Maintain safe and effective methods of working when providing body massage treatments
- Consult, plan and prepare for treatments with clients
- Perform manual massage treatment
- Perform mechanical massage treatments
- Provide aftercare advice

Introduction

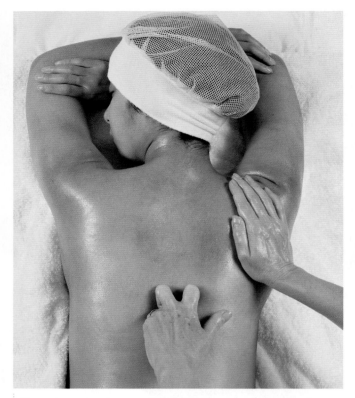

Manual massage is rewarding for both you and your client

Body massage is a satisfying treatment to give and receive. It is the stepping stone towards other qualifications within holistic treatments — aromatherapy, hot stones, sports massage and remedial massage all require a recognised Body Massage Certificate as a condition of entry. Indian head massage does not require body massage, but all forms of massage are enhanced and developed by gaining as much experience as you can. Successfully completing this unit could be the start of an exciting career path, using an ancient art form in manual massage techniques, leading into mechanical massage using equipment.

Swedish massage is the term most commonly associated with massage. It relates to the use of hands, rather than mechanical massage, and refers to the nationality of the man who developed the movements we still use today — Heinrich Ling. However, the Swedes were not the first people to recognise the benefits of massage. Centuries before, the Romans introduced massage to Europe. So massage has been with us for a long time — the term massage is thought to come from Greek meaning 'to knead'.

The Standards set out detailed performance criteria regarding:

- maintaining safe and effective methods of working when providing body massage treatments
- consulting, planning and preparing for treatments with clients.

The majority of these requirements apply to all beauty therapy treatments and are therefore covered in detail in Professional basics, Body treatments — theory and consultation, and G22 Monitor procedures to safely control work operations. You should also refer back to You and the skin, and to Related anatomy and physiology, as required.

Treatment-specific requirements for body massage are covered within this unit.

Maintain safe and effective methods of working when providing body massage treatments

In this section you will learn about:

- preparing your treatment area before the client arrives
- environmental conditions
- tools and equipment
- personal hygiene, protection and appearance
- preparing the client for massage treatment
- cost-effective treatments and commercial timing
- client record cards
- managing your working area.

Before beginning a body massage treatment, you will need to refer closely to the information in Professional basics and in Body treatments — theory and consultation.

Think about it

Throughout your massage course, you must uphold the professional image that all therapists involved in massage treatments have worked hard to maintain. Massage is a personal treatment and, unfortunately, has suffered from a sleazy reputation. However, a fully trained masseuse/masseur will have worked hard to achieve a recognised qualification.

Think about it

Massage should be given as a healing, soothing treatment, which requires calm and controlled movements. If you give massage in anything other than a composed way, the benefits of the treatment will be lost, and worse still, you may pass on your anger or irritability to the client. Your mood and the working atmosphere should be peaceful and welcoming.

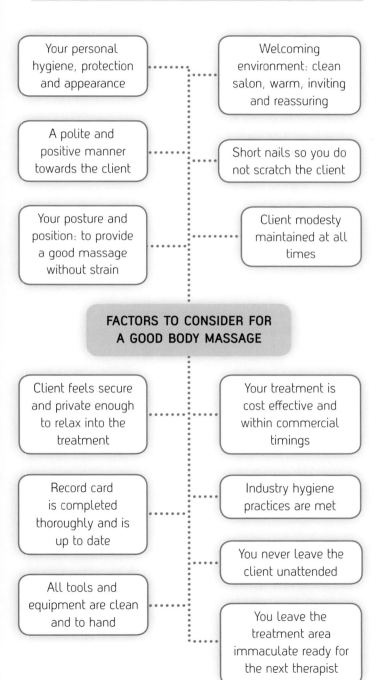

- Your personal hygiene, protection and appearance
- A polite and positive manner towards the client
- Your posture and position: to provide a good massage without strain
- Welcoming environment: clean salon, warm, inviting and reassuring
- Short nails so you do not scratch the client
- Client modesty maintained at all times

FACTORS TO CONSIDER FOR A GOOD BODY MASSAGE

- Client feels secure and private enough to relax into the treatment
- Record card is completed thoroughly and is up to date
- All tools and equipment are clean and to hand
- Your treatment is cost effective and within commercial timings
- Industry hygiene practices are met
- You never leave the client unattended
- You leave the treatment area immaculate ready for the next therapist

Things to consider when giving a professional body massage

Preparing your treatment area before the client arrives

The working environment should meet all legal, hygienic and treatment requirements — these are covered in Professional basics, 'You and your working environment', page 54. This unit also considers your professional appearance and personal responsibilities.

The working area — the treatment room, couch and trolley — and, of course, you yourself should be fully prepared shortly before the client arrives. This will allow you to give the client your total attention during the consultation.

Remember that a new client may be quite apprehensive about a body massage and will not know about the facilities of your salon: be polite and reassuring, spend a few minutes showing the new client around, explain the facilities, toilets and so on, where to put their outdoor clothing, and be generally welcoming and comforting in your approach.

Think about it

Both a full body massage and a back massage require clients to remove clothing, which may make them feel vulnerable, so along with equipment preparation, make sure you have either screens, a curtained area or a separate cubicle which will allow the client to undress in privacy and be certain of confidentiality.

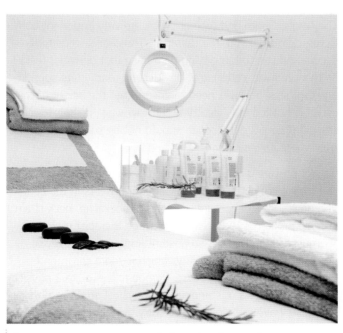

Prepare your treatment area before the client arrives

Environmental conditions

Room temperature

Consider the atmosphere of the area — too stuffy and the client may develop a headache and feel claustrophobic; too hot and the client may become overheated and faint, or end up with clammy skin, which is not comfortable to massage.

If the temperature drops too low, the client will automatically tense up, the muscles will be stiff and not easily massaged, and the relaxing benefits of the massage will be lost. So an even temperature should be maintained, with a good flow of air circulating, but without the draught from an open window.

Lighting

The most effective type of lighting is wall lighting, as it gives a soft glow of light, will not shine directly into the client's eyes and creates a warm feel, while providing enough light for you to work by. Too bright and the client is distracted — lighting which is too low will be a safety hazard.

Music

Soothing background music will create a calm ambience, but choice of music is personal — find out the client's preferences. Some clients dislike having the radio on during a massage as the chatter of the presenter may be disruptive. Always be guided by the client's wishes.

Tools and equipment

The couch – height, width and type

The height, width and type of couch are very important both to the client and you, the therapist. The client needs to feel secure and comfortable lying on a base that does not feel as though it will collapse at any second, and offers support and firmness. You will need to ensure that the height of the couch is not too low, ideally at hip/low waist height, to avoid stooping. Equally, the couch should not be so high that your movements are inhibited.

Correct posture is vital for the working therapist — after all, you may carry out several massage treatments in the course of a day, and poor posture will lead to backache, neck strain and hip problems. A full-time massage therapist may have six massages in a row — so posture and position is key to avoiding repetitive strain injury, which is more common in therapists than you may think. Our job role is quite a physical one, involving lots of standing and physical strain — most therapists have to be quite fit to carry out a busy week of appointments!

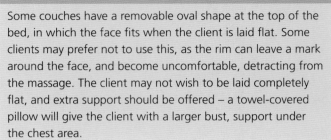

Think about it

Some couches have a removable oval shape at the top of the bed, in which the face fits when the client is laid flat. Some clients may prefer not to use this, as the rim can leave a mark around the face, and become uncomfortable, detracting from the massage. The client may not wish to be laid completely flat, and extra support should be offered — a towel-covered pillow will give the client with a larger bust, support under the chest area.

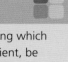

Think about it

Ensure you offer clients appropriately sized covering which maintains their dignity. If you have not met the client, be sure to have a choice of towel sizes, as you will not know the client's size or height! Not only will it protect the client's dignity, they will also feel secure and cocooned, which is going to make the treatment even more relaxing.

Working at the correct couch height will also ensure that the correct depth of pressure can be achieved to meet the client's requirements.

Preparing the couch

After wiping the vinyl cover of the unmade couch, fresh bed linen should be put on. This varies from salon to salon — the base of the couch is usually covered with a fitted sheet, but some salons use a quilt, with a cover, to create a feeling of getting into bed. However, it can be costly to keep washing the quilt covers and not always suitable in hot weather. Other salons favour open-weave blankets and towels, layering the towels over the blanket so that the blanket is protected and does not need to be changed after every client. Be guided by your training establishment.

Finally, place a layer of couch roll over the blanket and towels. The couch roll can be replaced after each treatment and will offer additional hygiene protection for clients. In some establishments, therapists put a split layer of couch roll along the length of the couch, ensuring all towels are protected. Others opt for just the head and foot areas to be covered. Care must be taken if the whole length of the bed is covered in couch roll as it is easily picked up within the massage movements, gets covered in oil and ends up sticking to the therapist's hands, again detracting from the massage movements.

The bedding set-up needs to be ready for the client to slip in to and for you to cover the client. Most establishments or training centres have their own uniform format for bed layout, so check this with your lecturer or trainer.

Massage stools or chairs

There are many adapted massage stools and chairs available from suppliers, if the treatment is not a full body massage. They provide support for head and shoulder massage, Indian head massage and foot massage.

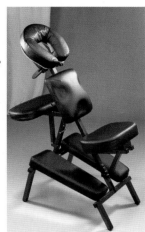
A massage stool

The floor area

Couch roll should be placed on the floor for the client to stand on once he or she has removed shoes and tights or socks. This prevents cross-contamination from the floor covering and can be disposed of after the treatment has finished.

Trolley layout

At this stage, you may not know the client's skin type, personal preferences or body type, which will affect the choice of massage medium, so ensure you have talc, oil and cream available, although the client may provide his or her own massage medium, particularly if the client has any known allergies or preferences.

Before setting out the trolley, wash the surfaces of each tier, and line each tier with a single sheet of couch roll if your training establishment recommends this.

> ### Think about it
>
> Before choosing equipment, try it out for your comfort and size, as well as the comfort of the client. Always buy from a reputable manufacturer and ask probing questions about the repair and maintenance service offered.

> ### Think about it
>
> All equipment must be to hand, so that you do not leave the client unattended, except to wash your hands, before and after treatment. Massage mediums should be put out within easy reach and you should not be stretching over the client to reach things.

First tier

- Talc, oil and cream, gel
- Medium-sized bowl to decant talc or cream into
- Large bowl for cotton wool squares
- Bowl or tub for tissues and spatulas
- Turban or headband (if not doing head massage)
- Client record card, if an existing client; blank one for a new client
- Pen
- Alcohol steriliser/hibitane and surgical spirit, or your preferred anti-bacterial wipe for the feet
- Eau de cologne, or similar, to remove any residue of oil after treatment
- Modesty towel. This is provided in health farms and spas, when the client has come from the sauna or steam room and has no clothing on. It is a long, small hand towel, covered in couch roll, which the client lies on, and then pulls up between the legs and over the pubic bone, allowing access to the upper thigh and gluteals, while maintaining client modesty. It can, however, be bulky to lie on. Most training colleges strongly recommend that

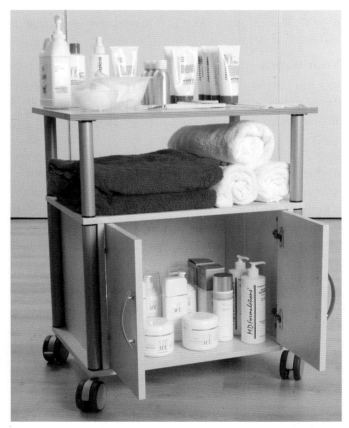
Another suggested trolley layout

female clients keep on their lower underwear or wear dry bikini bottoms and male clients wear boxer shorts or briefs. Be guided by your training establishment, but be prepared in industry for modesty towels or disposable pants to be provided.

Second tier

- 2 small hand towels
- Support props (these may be required to support the knees during leg massage, or to go under the ankles, taking the strain off the abdominal muscles)
- Bowl for the client's jewellery
- Space for the client's belongings, e.g. handbag
- Dressing gown or towelling robe

Third tier

Leave empty to store client's clothing, or store any spare products or equipment you may need

Personal hygiene, protection and appearance

Refer back to Professional basics, 'You – the therapist', page 4, for a full explanation of required personal hygiene and why it is so important to the treatment.

Your hands

Your tools of massage are your hands. Examine them, feel them, and rub your fingertips together. How do they feel? To give a good treatment your hands will need to be soft, supple and smooth. Long nails may scratch the client, so keep your nails short. A good rule to follow is: if you can see the free edge over the end of the fingertip, when your palm is facing you, your nails are too long. Start applying a hand cream at night to improve the texture, and a manicure will remove any jagged hangnails or rough cuticles which may catch on the client's skin.

Think about it

Remember that your tools and equipment should be cleaned and sterilised using the correct methods. Refer to Professional basics, 'You and your working environment', page 54, to find the most suitable cleaning products and how to use them.

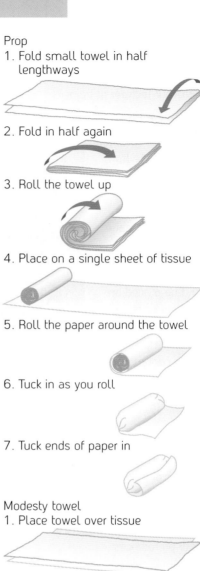

Prop
1. Fold small towel in half lengthways

2. Fold in half again

3. Roll the towel up

4. Place on a single sheet of tissue

5. Roll the paper around the towel

6. Tuck in as you roll

7. Tuck ends of paper in

Modesty towel
1. Place towel over tissue

2. Fold towel into centre, followed by tissue

3. Fold it in half again

Preparing a prop and modesty towel

Think about it

Your nails and hands should be clean, disinfected and germ free. Having dirty hands or nails is the quickest way to spread infection to the client and everyone else they may come in contact with.

Think about it

Students often say that initial use of the correct stance during massage treatments does not feel natural, but you must persevere, as this will prevent muscular damage and strain.

Your posture during treatment

Your lecturer will demonstrate the correct posture to use during massage. This will save your back and shoulders from aching, particularly as you will be doing more than one full body massage in the course of a busy salon day. It will also help you develop the right pressure, using your whole body, rather than all the pressure coming from your shoulders and upper back.

There are only two ways of standing for massage:

- walk standing
- stride standing.

Walk standing

Walk standing is usually used when working down the length of a muscle, with the feet, hands, hips and shoulders, all

facing in the same direction! The leg farthest away from the couch is placed in a walking position, slightly in front of the other one. Do not take a great big step, as if going hiking, just a gentle walking step in your natural pace is ideal.

This allows plenty of manoeuvring when massaging a long leg or back area. The body weight can be rocked from one foot to the other, without the need to shuffle or stretch. Do not be tempted to use the inner leg closest to the couch as you will then be working across your own body, which is awkward, and then if you have to come backwards, say from the top of the thigh, to the toes, there is a real risk of falling over!

Stride standing

Stride standing is used when working across the muscle bulk. The feet are evenly spaced apart, side by side, again in your normal comfortable stride, and the fingers, hips, toes and shoulders all face the same way.

Good massage posture	Poor massage posture
Upright spine	Bending at the waist
Shoulders gently back	Hunching over at the shoulders
Hips above knees and feet	Twisting at the hip
Soft knees	Poking a hip out and balancing all body weight on it
Body weight evenly spread	Locked knees

Massage posture – dos and don'ts

The client's position during treatment

There are two ways in which the client can lie on the couch:

- the supine position – face upwards
- the prone position – face downwards.

Think about it

A quick way to remember the meaning of the word supine is to think of the spine (cross out the 'u'!) touching the couch.

Preparing the client for massage treatment

Client comfort

You want the client to be physically comfortable but also mentally relaxed with the atmosphere and the expected procedure, too. Ensure you fully explain to the client what

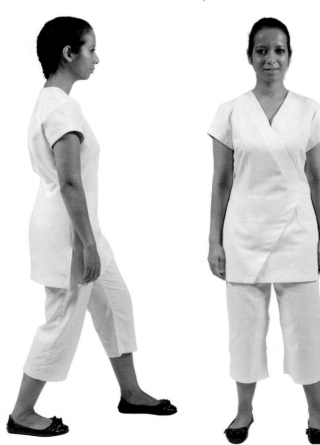

Walk standing   *Stride standing*

the whole routine involves — including removal of clothing except pants/boxer shorts — because if it's their first massage they will not know what to expect and this is quite daunting. Avoid keeping the bra on — it is uncomfortable to lie on and you may get oil on the straps, and if you take the straps halfway down the arm — off the shoulder — the client may be uncomfortable. Make sure the client understands they will be fully covered up and although they are topless, at no time will the breasts be exposed.

Ask the client to put on the robe provided, which you have already placed on the trolley. There may be a locker or hanger provided for clothing, and coats should be left at reception. If not, ask the client to place clothing on the third tier of the trolley along with handbag, briefcase, and so on. Assure the client of privacy while changing. You will be waiting outside the treatment room or cubicle and the client should call out when ready.

When you re-enter the cubicle, you may need to tidy away any remaining clothes or shoes. Ask the client to remove any jewellery, to prevent damage from the massage medium, and place it in the bowl provided.

Always use a turban towel or headband to protect your client's hair. If long, the client's hair should be restrained in a turban or headband, again to prevent oil or cream spilling on it, but also to stop your hands becoming entangled in it!

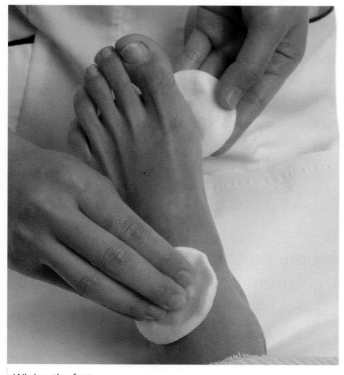

Wiping the feet

Think about it

If the client is booked in for facial massage, you will need to remove her make-up with suitable cleansers. If there is a cut or abrasion on the skin, it should be covered with a plaster, and the area avoided.

Some clients will have showered prior to coming to the salon, while other salons are able to offer the facility of a shower before the treatment.

Think about it

Head and scalp massage can be performed dry, with no medium and over a turban to avoid messing the hair.

Next, sit the client on the bed, with the robe closed, but not underneath the client. Hold a large towel in front of the client as he or she disrobes. Take the robe, fold it, put it away on the trolley, and then cover up the client.

Some establishments provide a modesty towel for the bust area, which the client holds in place with one hand while you help her with the robe. In this case, be guided by your training establishment.

At this point, you are ready to wipe the feet with a suitable cleanser, using one pad of cotton wool per foot, to avoid contamination, and then wash your hands. This should be the only time you leave the client unattended. Explain to them you are only going to the sink to wash your hands — then the assessor hears you say it as well!

Think about it

Always follow your Awarding Body's guidelines for hygiene and safety practice — refer back to Professional basics for all hygiene procedures and never put your client at risk through lack of knowledge or negligence.

Cost-effective treatments and commercial timings

As well as posture, hand movements and foot positions to consider, you also have to be cost-effective and time the massage treatment — both for assessment criteria and for commercial viability. You will need to ensure the massage does not feel rushed to the client, but that you are within your time limit and ready for the next appointment.

Massage area	Time allowed (minutes)
Arm	10 (5 per arm)
Leg	20 (10 per leg)
Neck and chest	5
Back*	20
Abdomen	5
Total time allowance	60

Suggested massage timings

*Gluteals optional — tops of gluteals are often included within the back massage time allowance.

Think about it

Standard salon practice is one hour for the massage routine.

If massaging the back of the legs and gluteals separately from the front of the legs, as in male massage, then split the leg time in half, that is 5 minutes only for the front, allowing 5 minutes for the back. As you will not be completing an abdominal massage, you can use those 5 minutes too.

Adapting massage for client needs

There will be times when client needs will require you to adapt the routine. For example, if the client is menstruating, she may not wish her abdominal area to be touched. Adjust the timing to allow for this, and perhaps spend more time on an area with lots of tension such as the upper or lower back, or the neck and chest.

Client record cards

You should also have your client's record card on your trolley, ready to record all the information pertinent to your client before and after the treatment, when your client can tell you which movements they preferred, which medium you used and any particular problems you encountered during the massage.

All of your questions, the client's replies and recording of client details should go on the record card. A completed example can be found on page 328 of Body consultation in the General Pathway unit, and general information in Professional basics.

A record card is the lynchpin to the whole treatment, as it contains all the information you will need to plan for the client's treatment and protection.

Managing your working area

After each treatment, remember to leave the treatment area as you would wish to find it — and remember, too, that it may not be your own working space or cubicle for the whole day — someone else may be working in it next.

So, if your client has dozed off and you have another client waiting, plus you need to prepare the area, this could be a problem. You should allow a little time within your appointment scheduling to gently wake up the client, allow them time to readjust and give them a glass of water, then wrap them up warmly in a cosy robe and take them to the rest area. Most health spas and saunas have rest lounges, with easy chairs and recliners where the client can relax, have a drink and perhaps continue dozing, which leaves your working cubicle free to prepare. The client does not then feel rushed.

If there is no rest area, then ensure your client is awake enough to safely get off the couch and get dressed, and then recommend they stay in reception with a drink, before driving or going back to work.

Think about it

As well as a full hour's body massage, you will need to allow time for:

- the consultation
- the client undressing and getting on the couch
- rousing the client after treatment
- the client re-dressing
- giving aftercare advice
- reviewing the consultation
- adding to your notes on how the treatment went, any adaption of treatment and further recommendations to benefit the client.

B20 Provide body massage treatments

Consult, plan and prepare for treatments with clients

In this section you will learn about:

- consultation techniques
- contra-indications and necessary actions
- treatment objectives
- the benefits of massage.

Consultation techniques

As with all other treatments, it is essential to carry out a full consultation. Clients' body massage requirements will vary, as will the necessary depth of pressure due to tissue density and differing body weight distribution. An athletic female client with lean tissue and little adipose tissue will require something different from a male client with poor muscle tone and quite a high proportion of fat. In fact, no two clients' needs are the same, so your massage techniques need to be adaptable, to suit each individual.

To refresh your memory on all aspects of the consultation process, look at the Professional basics unit. Also refer to Body treatments — theory and consultation.

Your consultation techniques should include the medical history, any physical characteristics and a lifestyle pattern analysis. You need to both observe the client and carry out a manual examination.

Observation

Your observation of the client should be subtle and tactful. For example, if the client is obese, make sure you have plenty of large towels to keep the client warm and comfortable.

The size of the client also directly relates to the amount of massage medium used — the larger the client, the more medium will be required. Massage depth and pressure will also need to be adjusted to penetrate into the muscular layer.

Manual examination

The observation should include a manual examination to assess the skin for texture, pigmentation, moles and other irregularities. This requires a keen eye and sensitive fingers.

Any condition that could be made worse through massage is contra-indicated. For example, a skin infection could spread not only to other areas of the client's body but also to yourself as the therapist and then from you to other clients. If the client had a condition such as infected varicose veins, stimulation of the blood flow in the area could make the condition worse, or be uncomfortable.

Often, the treatment can be modified and adapted, for example a pregnant client may prefer lying on her side during back massage, and the abdomen would be avoided. An ordinary varicose vein could simply be avoided and a protruding mole could be massaged around.

Think about it

It is always important to gain written consent from your client to confirm that they are happy for the treatment to go ahead, and that all aspects have been explained to them. This should be everything from what they will wear (just pants) to massage mediums, how long the treatment takes, and cost. Actively encourage your client to ask questions, and be patient with them — especially if it is their first treatment — and be sure to clarify any points they raise.

Contra-indications and necessary actions

Below is a checklist of all contra-indications to massage. An easy way to remember the contra-indications to massage is to visualise the body from the outside, going inwards. Start with the skin and problems you can actually see, and then work through the underlying anatomy of muscles, bones, blood and the organs.

Contra-indications to massage

More visible contra-indications:

- Skin which is thin or crêpey, or damaged
- Infectious skin diseases, for example scabies, where there is a risk of cross-infection
- Any fungal or viral disease, for example athlete's foot, warts, or verrucas
- Non-infectious skin disorders, for example eczema, dermatitis
- A bruise, sepsis, spots, boils — avoid the area as there is a risk of cross-infection, the treatment might spread or worsen the condition, and the client will experience discomfort
- Recent sunburn
- Varicose veins, phlebitis (inflammation of a vein) — avoid the area as massage worsens the condition, and the client will experience discomfort

- Tumours, unrecognisable lumps, bumps and swellings of either skin or the joints or painful areas
- Any damaged muscles or tissue swelling, for example sprains — avoid the area as massage worsens the condition, and the client will experience discomfort
- Any form of acute joint disease, or inflammation, for example rheumatoid arthritis
- Broken bones and recent fractures — treatment might cause client discomfort; if the area is in plaster, you will be unable to treat it
- Postural deformities, for example scoliosis or spastic conditions
- Avoid tapotement on extremely thin or elderly clients.

Less visible contra-indications (obtain a doctor's approval before treating):

- Clients with chronic diabetes tend to have thin, papery skin that bruises easily
- Clients with haemophilia may have no clotting capacity and could bleed
- Clients with epilepsy
- Clients with asthma or a lung condition — the treatment may require adaptation
- Clients with a cardiac condition, high or low blood pressure, including clients who have had a stroke or suffer from thrombosis; people with low blood pressure can feel faint when suddenly sitting up from a lying position
- High temperature
- During menstruation, avoid the abdomen — some clients may feel discomfort and the treatment could increase the flow
- Immediately before or after operations, for example hysterectomy
- In cases of stomach complaints, for example diarrhoea
- In pregnancy, ensure the client never lies on the stomach; after birth, always wait until the post-natal check-up
- Cuts/abrasions — cover with waterproof dressing and avoid area due to risk of cross-infection and client discomfort
- Allergies — select appropriate massage medium; carry out a patch test, if necessary
- Medication — if a client is on medication for a health condition that could be affected by massage treatment, a doctor's approval will be needed.

Additional knowledge

Pregnancy and position

The pregnant client should never lie on her stomach during treatment as this may cause pressure on the foetus, but recent advice also suggests that pregnant women should avoid lying on their back for any length of time. The increased weight of the uterus and foetus is thought to create pressure on the inferior vena cava. This vein returns blood from the lower body to the mother's heart. This may lead to lightheadedness and/or numbness, as well as being uncomfortable. Be guided by your client and allow her to choose the position she finds most comfortable. It would be advisable to check her comfort more often during the treatment and give her the opportunity to adjust her position if necessary.

Special considerations for certain conditions

You will need to give special consideration to clients with the following conditions:

- diabetes
- epilepsy
- heart disease
- high or low blood pressure
- pregnancy.

The elderly and clients who have recently had surgery will also require special attention.

Diabetes

Clients with diabetes have delicate skins, with a tendency to bruise easily. Their circulation may also may be impaired if it has been a long-term condition, with the consequence of poor healing if an infection has been present. Many people with diabetes have regular foot treatments from a qualified chiropodist, to avoid developing ingrown toenails or nail infections. Therefore, the lower legs and feet are delicate areas, and although foot massage helps improve the circulation, you should be on the lookout for infection in the area. Heavy massage movements can further damage the skin, so avoid these.

Check that the client has had enough to eat prior to the massage. Although a heavy meal would normally be a contra-indication, there is a risk that the blood sugar level will drop dangerously low if the client has not eaten recently. Then avoid the abdomen during the massage.

Epilepsy

Most epilepsy is controlled by regular medication, and although clients may not have had a seizure for many years, care must still be taken. Never leave the client unattended on the couch, and be careful that the client does not have a bright light shining into the eyes, as this is a known to be a trigger.

In some young people, the risk of a seizure is most likely as the person is waking up and brain activity is beginning. Since the client may fall asleep during a soothing massage, a doctor's approval for treatment is necessary.

High or low blood pressure, heart disease

Clients with high or low blood pressure and/or a heart condition should also be reviewed on an individual basis. The sufferer of low blood pressure may experience dizziness on getting up from a massage (as the blood flow is slower to the brain). The solution is to have the head raised slightly higher than normal, but be careful when turning the client over to massage the back, as it may be uncomfortable not to be lying flat out.

High blood pressure sufferers should also avoid being laid flat, and while massage has a calming, sedative effect, you are still stimulating the circulation, so again avoid any heavier movements. Keeping the head higher than the heart will ensure that palpitations are avoided and prevent the client hearing the blood pressure in the ears, which can be disruptive to the massage.

Pregnancy

Pregnant clients gain real value from massage, as long as the correct support is provided. Use a covered towel under the tummy, and ensure the client is not laid flat on her abdomen (see also Additional knowledge, 'Pregnancy and position', on page 393). When she is face up, use props to support the knees and head.

Some clients may not wish to reveal their body during pregnancy. If so, the neck and shoulder, face and scalp can be massaged with the client in a chair, but the real benefit is a massage to the lower back, where the muscles are put under strain to support the extra weight of the baby. Never massage a client who is pregnant directly over the abdomen. Be guided by your client – she knows what is best for her.

The elderly

The elderly also gain great benefit from massage. However, their skin may lack elasticity, have a tendency to bruise and be slightly drier in texture. Use plenty of oil, and avoid dragging the skin and heavy movements.

Recent surgery

Clients who have undergone surgery recently are unlikely to attend a massage appointment without a doctor's approval, but massage is recognised as very beneficial, as it improves the blood supply and so aids the healing process. Be careful to use light circular movements and avoid the area if the client prefers – you can show the client how to massage the area to promote the healing process.

Scar tissue and keloid tissue which has hardened can be visibly softened and minimised with massage.

The healing crisis

As well as talking through the contra-indications to treatment and the possible contra-actions, you should tell the client about other likely reactions to massage – often referred to as a 'healing crisis'. Massage has both a physiological and psychological effect on the client.

Physically, as the muscular tension is released, and the build-up of lactic acid in the muscle is dispersed, along with other toxins, the work of the lymphatic system is increased, filtering the lymphatic fluid through each of the nodes. This may result in a feeling of tiredness and aching in the groin, abdomen and underarms, where the nodes are situated. Instead of feeling uplifted, the client may experience flu-like symptoms. He or she might also suffer from a headache and slight nausea. Psychologically, the client may feel emotional, especially if he or she has been feeling very stressed.

All these symptoms are short-lived. They show that the massage has worked and is stimulating the body to heal itself.

Indentifying contra-indications

Do remember that, should you see any contra-indications present during the consultation stage, you are not a medical practitioner and are therefore unable to pass comment on any condition which you feel may require medical attention.

The necessary actions to take are to:

- suggest the client refers back to their own doctor for an appointment
- either avoid the area, or apologise and not carry out the treatment at all.

If there is any doubt, it is better not to treat a client rather than carry on regardless and possibly make a condition worse. Do not hazard a guess or offer an opinion regarding a possible medical condition, as you may frighten the client unnecessarily and cause upset.

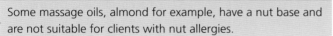

Think about it

Some massage oils, almond for example, have a nut base and are not suitable for clients with nut allergies.

Treatment objectives

At this stage of the consultation you should also give the client the full picture of the cost of the massage, the duration, what you would recommend as a treatment plan — i.e. how frequently they would benefit from a massage and the treatment itself, and what you and they hope to get out of it — this is called a treatment objective.

Treatment objectives could include:

- relaxation of the client
- giving a sense of wellbeing
- providing uplifting support
- anti-cellulite massage
- stimulating massage
- suitable massage movements to suit client needs.

You should choose your equipment and massage mediums to meet the treatment objectives and give maximum benefit to the client. Remember that not all treatment objectives will be carried out all at once — it may take time and patience to encourage a client to relax, or they may sometimes require quite a stimulating massage to help with muscular tension and on other occasions require uplifting support from you. So, not only will each client be slightly different, their needs may change and vary from week to week, depending upon what problems they bring to the salon and what stress they are under at any given time.

To understand how to achieve these objectives, you need to understand what the benefits of massage are.

The benefits of massage

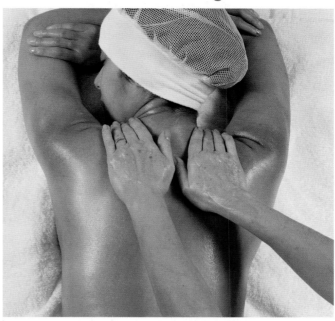

Massage has both physical and physiological benefits

The area	How the body benefits
Skin	• It gains moisture from the medium used, so becomes softer in texture • The sebaceous glands are stimulated by the pressure on the skin from the hands and so sebum is produced, helping keep skin lubricated • The pressure also helps the old dead cells come away easily (desquamation), allowing fresh cells to come to the surface. This gives the skin a clean, bright look • The blood supply to the skin is improved bringing food and oxygen to the cells, while taking away the waste products and carbon dioxide. This can be seen as a reddening in the area (erythema) • The stroking actions within the massage help soothe the sensory nerve endings • The motor nerve endings are stimulated and also receive a surge of blood to feed them, making them work effectively • Cellular functions are improved due to the stimulation • Small lesions or fibrous growths in the skin can be reduced • Dispersal of milia formation • Warming of the skin brings a small rise in body temperature, and the blood comes to the skin's surface (erythema)

Continued

The area	How the body benefits
Muscles	• Blood flow is increased to the muscles bringing oxygen and nutrients, while removing carbon dioxide and waste products such as lactic acid • The heat generated within the muscle fibres and the stretching action of massage allows the fibres to soften and relax, so eliminating bands of tension • Muscle tone is improved due to relaxation of fibres • Muscular performance is improved so that the muscle can perform to maximum potential • Muscular pain and tension is relieved • Tension headaches can be relieved through massage to the muscles at the top of the neck
Body systems	• As massage is always performed in the direction of the lymphatic flow, the lymph system is stimulated and therefore removal of waste and toxins is improved • The central nervous system is either relaxed or stimulated, depending upon the type of massage movements used. Slow stroking movements will help relaxation and sleep, vigorous movements will stimulate – both help the nerve endings and improve their functioning • General circulation is improved. The pressure on the superficial arteries helps aid the transportation of food and oxygen to all parts of the body, and veins are stimulated to bring back the deoxygenated blood to the heart faster. This promotes healing and regeneration of cells all over the body • Biochemical healing takes place not only by alleviating anxiety but also stimulating the production of antibodies, especially immunoglobulin, so enhancing the immune system • The systolic and diastolic blood pressure and heart rate are slowed down during massage and a cumulative effect of regular massage is beneficial to clients with blood pressure problems

What happens within the body, and what you see during massage

Think about it

Body massage not only benefits the client, it also has a relaxing effect on the therapist. Once the movements become automatic to you, the calming rhythm of your hands will bring down your blood pressure and you too will enjoy the stress-relieving benefits of the treatment.

Psychological effects – what happens to the mind

What happens in the mind and to emotions during massage?

- The stroking movements have a restful, relaxing effect.
- The client feels soothed and pampered, and the mind becomes still and calm.
- The rhythmic movements have a sedative effect on the brain and the client may feel drowsy or drift off to sleep.
- Accumulated emotional stress can be dispersed, put into perspective, or even forgotten for the length of the treatment.
- Stress and fatigue are diminished, and a general feeling of wellbeing takes over.
- A healthier outlook can be adopted, both mentally and physically, as the client is encouraged to look after themselves.
- The self-esteem of the client may be improved, through someone caring and nurturing the client.
- Sleep patterns improve, bringing a sense of calm, as sleep allows the brain to rest and process the day's information.
- The stress hormone, cortisol, has been shown to drop after a massage.

Basic massage movements are easily recognised and should be linked together in a continuous flowing rhythm. The actual routine followed is an individual choice, providing it meets client needs and makes sense. As you become more experienced (and qualified) and watch other professionals at work, you may adapt your massage routine; including particular movements used, say, in aromatherapy, and missing out the odd movement that you do not feel totally comfortable with. Most therapists would agree that they have not stuck rigidly with the routine they learned in training, but to start with it is a good idea to use the routine you have been taught until you develop enough skill and experience to change.

Perform manual massage treatment

In this section you will learn about:

- massage techniques and movements
- suggested massage routine
- massage procedures
- massage mediums
- contra-actions and prompt action.

Massage techniques and movements

When you are massaging your client always make sure that suitable support and/or cushioning for the specific areas requiring it are given – this may be a prop under the knees, to help take the strain off the tummy muscles, a prop under the knee during massage of the leg, or a cushion or pillow under the bust to help support the upper body, if the client is on her tummy.

Massage movements are divided into five main categories:

- effleurage
- petrissage
- tapotement
- vibrations
- frictions.

Think about it

Learning massage is like any other motor skill – you would not expect to play the piano in a day, nor drive a car. These are skills that require practice and supervision, so do not be despondent if you cannot do all the massage movements right away.

The table below lists the main massage movements and identifies the categories within each movement. All movements can be altered or varied by using differing pressure, direction, rate and rhythm.

Movement	Categories within the movement	Description	Reasons for use
Effleurage	Superficial and deep	A stroking movement The whole hand is in contact with the skin Slight pressure in the palm with deeper effleurage	• Introduces medium to the skin • Soothing first touch of the skin • Links movements together
Petrissage	Kneading – palmar, thumb, digital; ironing or reinforced stroking; wringing; skin rolling; picking up; pinchment; knuckling	Compression Deeper and firm kneading of the tissues	• Aids lymphatic and blood circulation • Helps release muscle fibres, so eases tension knots • Increases venous return to the heart
Tapotement	Clapping; cupping; beating; pounding	Often called percussion movements Heavy, stimulating movements	• Stimulates blood flow • Stimulates sensory nerve endings • Improves skin texture through erythema
Vibrations	Static and running vibrations	Literally, vibration of the fingertips or thumb, or the whole palmar surface can be used	• Relieve tension along the nerve path either side of the spine • When used along the path of the digestive tract, aid digestion
Frictions	Thumb or finger frictions	Regular, even pressure applied to areas of tension or fibrous build-up	• Aid relaxation • Relieve tight nodules in muscle fibres • Increase in lymphatic return and circulation to the area, creating heat

The five main massage movements

Effleurage

There are two types of effleurage:

- superficial
- deep.

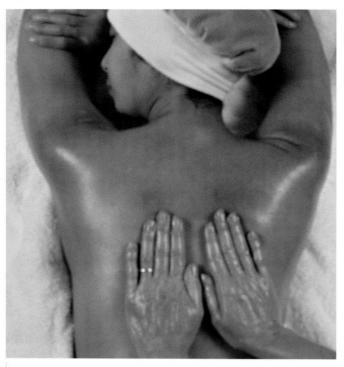

Effleurage

Superficial effleurage

This is a light flowing pressure used at the beginning and the end of most treatments. It introduces the therapist's hands on to the client and spreads the massage medium but is also a linking movement to help the massage flow. It heralds the start of the massage, so the rate and tempo of the massage are established from the beginning — if you start off in a rush, you will continue in that hurried fashion and possibly be under time for the treatment (therefore short-changing the client out of the full hour's body massage).

If you are applying the massage medium to the skin, use superficial effleurage. You can tell the client what you are doing, and that you may have to remove your hands to apply more oil, especially if the skin is dry and soaks up the medium. Once you are satisfied that both you and the client have sufficient medium to keep you going throughout the entire routine for that area, then make a definite statement of touch that you have started.

Try not to use a light, feathery touch, and never remove the hands — the client will not know whether you have started!

So how do I do it?

Glide the hand onto the skin, starting with the fingertips, so that the whole hand is in contact with skin. Try to keep the fingers relaxed. Your hands should feel as if they are moulded to the part of the body you are working on.

Use the entire palmar surface of the hands, keeping the fingers together, and still soft, with the thumb either close into the side of the hand, or open and out of the way. Depending upon the area being massaged, all or part of the palmar surface should cover it. Pressure should be light and even, with good contact with the skin, and the hands warm and relaxed.

Think about it

If in any doubt about which movement comes next in the massage routine, add in a little effleurage until it comes back to you. Don't take your hands off the client or tell him or her that you cannot remember the routine!

Superficial effleurage does not normally affect the circulation, as it is not a deep movement, and theoretically it can be used in any direction. However, massage should always be directed towards the heart (often referred to as centripetal) to aid the natural flow of blood back to the heart, from the limbs and trunk.

As effleurage can be used to link other movements, it will knit the routine together.

Think about it

Make sure you have enough massage medium on the skin, as too little and the hands become sticky and the movements will not flow; too much and it will run down the client's face or body! If at the first application the client's skin is dry and soaks up the cream or oil, then apply a little more at this point, rather than having to stop the massage to apply more.

Benefits of superficial effleurage

- Relaxes tense muscle fibres.
- Gives a general feeling of relaxation.
- Stimulates sensory nerve endings and gives a feeling of pleasure.
- Introduces the massage medium and cream on to the skin.
- Soothes and calms.

Deep effleurage

This is the same type of movement as superficial effleurage but with more pressure applied — not too much to make the sensation uncomfortable, but enough to encourage muscular relaxation and for you to feel the tension knots.

Maintaining contact with the skin helps avoid over-stimulation of the nerve endings. Otherwise, when contact is broken and then re-established, this sets up a reflex response in the nerve endings which prevents the muscles from relaxing. It can produce a very disjointed feel to the massage.

Benefits of deep effleurage

- Aids venous return and increases lymphatic flow within the area.
- Creates an erythema as the blood flow comes to the skin's surface.
- Stimulates glandular activity, helping a dry skin receive more sebum from the sebaceous glands.
- Aids arterial circulation by removal of congestion from veins.
- Aids desquamation.
- Has a relaxing effect.
- Can begin to generate heat in the muscle fibre and help disperse tension.

Petrissage

Petrissage is divided into the following categories:

- kneading
- ironing
- wringing — mostly used on body
- skin rolling — mostly used on body
- picking up
- pinchment
- knuckling.

Petrissage *always follows* effleurage.

Think about it

A petrissage movement requires the client to have a good covering of muscle and underlying tissue to be effective. It can be quite painful on an underweight, bony or elderly clients, so would be considered a contra-indication.

Too much pressure may result in damage to the skin – so adapt to suit the client's needs. Always use effleurage to link petrissage movements.

So how do I do it?

Petrissage involves compression movements, performed using intermittent pressure with either one or both hands using different parts. It requires practice and good hand mobility, to mould around the muscle for good manipulation. Most petrissage movements work on all or parts of a muscle and it is important that as a muscle is slowly released from application, pressure is reduced.

Petrissage movements must be applied rhythmically and in a repetitive pattern, not in a hurried way.

Petrissage movements

Kneading

Kneading uses small circular movements, with the whole hand in contact with the skin, but with the pressure coming from the heel of the palm — the fleshy part at the base of the thumb. The general pattern and direction should follow the direction of effleurage, but instead of big sweeping movements, these are smaller circles, going outwards and upwards.

It can be used with both hands in larger areas, such as the back, or single-handed on smaller areas like petite arms and legs, with the other hand offering support to the limb.

If when working the area, you find a tension knot, intersperse palmar kneading with some thumb or finger kneading to disperse the tension. Again, use small circular rotations, remembering not to press too hard.

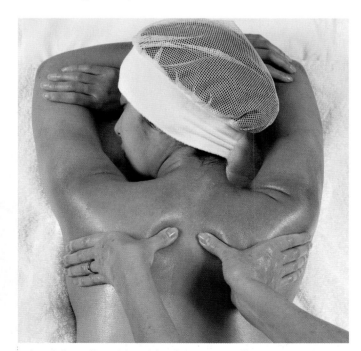

Thumb-kneading either side of the spine will remove tension

Ironing

Ironing, or reinforced stroking, is a deeper form of kneading. Place one hand on top of the other, and follow the direction of the kneading routine. It can be used along the length of the muscle, or across the muscle fibres, or in a figure of eight around the shoulder blades. This is a deep movement, so avoid using on a thin or bony client.

Wringing

Wringing is a very effective movement, but one which requires practice. The tissue is lifted away from the body and compressed between the hands — rather like wringing out a towel. The flow of tissue goes from the fingers of one hand to the thumb of the other, so that the movement forms an S-shape. This is continued along the perimeters of the back, and again, goes towards the heart. It is more difficult on the back, if there is little tissue to wring, so may be left out, but it is an excellent movement on limbs. Avoid pinching the tissue between the fingers and thumbs of the same hand, as this hurts!

Think about it

Try practising wringing on a rolled-up towel and create an S-shape with your hands.

Skin rolling

Skin rolling, as the name suggests, involves rolling the tissue by pulling it away from the skeleton, towards your body, using all the fingers, in a flat formation and then rolling the tissue back down with the thumbs. It works best on fleshy parts of the body, such as the perimeters of the back and the neck.

Keep a steady pace, work in the direction of your effleurage movements, and repeat as necessary. It is much easier to perform this movement on the opposite side of the client to you, as you are rolling the skin towards your body. When doing the side closer to you, take a small step back from the client, bend at the knee, and perform the roll in reverse, that is the tissue is rolled down and then pushed up by the thumbs.

Picking up

Picking up can be carried out with either or both hands, depending upon the area and the amount of tissue present. The tissue is grasped firmly between the index finger and thumb, with the hand forming a U shape. Using the whole hand, with fingers together, and flexion at the wrist, scoop up the tissue, squeeze and release. The index finger and thumb should be kept apart — if they come together, you will end up pinching the client's skin. Move along the length of the back and limbs towards the heart.

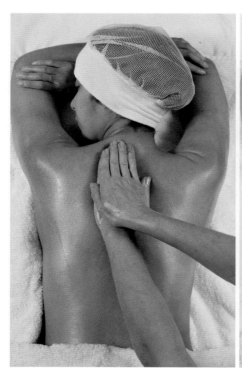

Ironing

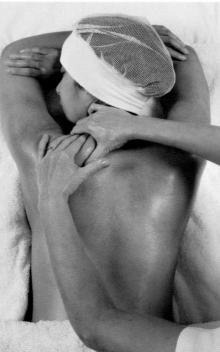

Wringing

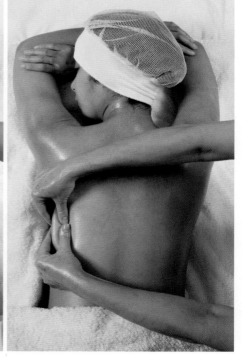

Skin rolling

Double-handed picking up is performed on larger muscle bulk, such as the upper thigh, and single-handed picking up on less muscular areas, such as the arms.

Pinchment

Pinchment tends to be used in facial massage only, and involves the skin and tissue being gently pinched between the index finger and thumb. A small compression is used and then the hands glide along towards the next pinchment. It is most effective along the length of the eyebrows and jaw line to remove tension and works very well on small muscles.

Knuckling

Knuckling is a form of circular kneading, but instead of using the ends of the fingers or thumbs, make the hand into a loose fist and use the knuckles. The circular movements can come from the wrist, so the whole hand is rotating over the area of tension, but also, with practice, the fingers can be rotated individually. This helps to break down tension nodules. Knuckling can be used on the face, in a light form, and on the body with more pressure.

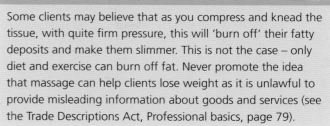

Think about it

Some clients may believe that as you compress and knead the tissue, with quite firm pressure, this will 'burn off' their fatty deposits and make them slimmer. This is not the case – only diet and exercise can burn off fat. Never promote the idea that massage can help clients lose weight as it is unlawful to provide misleading information about goods and services (see the Trade Descriptions Act, Professional basics, page 79).

Benefits of petrissage

- Relaxes aching, hard muscles, helping to prevent tension modules forming.
- Stimulates skin regeneration.
- Tones muscle tissue.
- Helps eliminate muscular fatigue by aiding the removal of lactic acid.
- Helps remove waste products and improves lymphatic flow.
- Increases circulation to the area.
- Helps to relax the client.

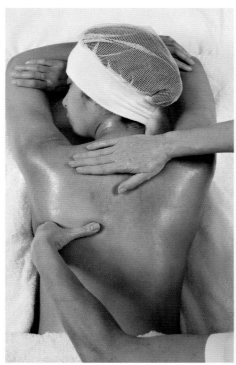

Picking up

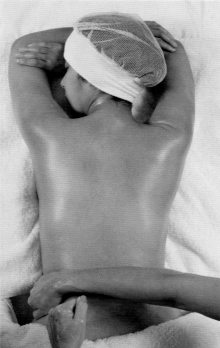

Tapotement

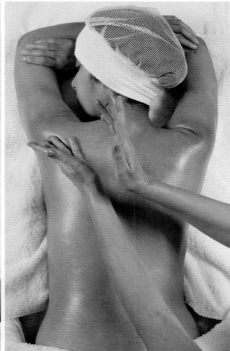

Hacking

Tapotement

Tapotement (drumming or tapping) comprises a stimulating set of movements which bring blood flow to the area very quickly. These include:

- hacking
- cupping
- pounding or beating.

Think about it

If the client wants a relaxing massage, you should use minimal tapotement, or leave it out altogether.

So how do I do it?

If done incorrectly, tapotement can leave the skin bruised and sore. The client also needs to have enough underlying tissue to absorb the movements – thin, bony clients would be contra-indicated.

Tapotement movements

Hacking

Hacking uses the outside edge of the middle, ring and little fingers of both hands. As the little finger makes contact with the skin, so the wrist is rotated and the outer ridge of the ring finger and then the middle finger make contact. The hand is loose and the palm slightly opens, so that the movement is firm, but does not produce a chopping movement – the key is keeping the wrists relaxed, which allows the hands to turn outwards as you complete the movement. Rigid, stiff hands will produce a chop using only the outer side of the little finger and hand, which will be painful for the client. The movement you are trying to achieve is a quick springy flick, not a dull heavy blow.

Think about it

Practise hacking on a hard surface such as a kitchen work surface or desk. Start slowly and keep the hands relaxed, rotate the wrists so that all fingers come in contact with the hard surface. Try to produce an even rhythm and do not go too quickly – speed will come later; you should be able to see your fingers touching the surface. If you hurt yourself, you are doing it too hard, or chopping when you should be rolling the wrist.

Hacking can be light or deep, depending upon where you are working and the amount of underlying tissue present. Light hacking uses only the ends of the fingers and has a tapping effect on the skin – deeper hacking, such as on the gluteals, can be performed using the whole hand and wrist, with a heavier force used. Light hacking on the face and neck are often referred to as point or digital hacking, as only the lightest of touches is suitable.

Cupping

Cupping uses the whole hand, held in a cup shape (hence the name!) with the thumb tucked over the forefinger joint. The fingers are closed and the wrists are soft and flexible. As the cup shape strikes the skin, a slight vacuum is created, and a hollow, cupping sound is heard. The hands cup alternately onto the area, and they should be light and springy. If the sound created is more like a slap, then the hand is not cupped enough, and the client will feel as though he or she has been slapped.

Think about it

Practise on a pillow or towel to get the cupping sound correct.

Pounding/beating

Pounding uses loosely clenched fists and performs the same rotation of the wrist that is used in hacking. The soft pounding as skin contact is made is followed by a flick of the wrist, so it almost becomes a flick of the skin.

Beating follows the same hand position, but the fists are dropped more heavily, and there is no flick of the wrist to remove the hand.

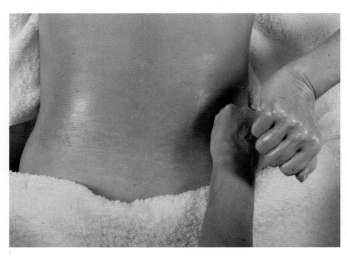

Beating

Benefits of tapotement

- Increases localised blood supply, bringing erythema to the skin's surface and causing a rise in local body temperature.
- Increases nervous response due to stimulation. If hacking is completed across the muscle fibres, it can cause them to have a momentary mini-contraction, as if responding to stimuli. Nerve paths can be cleared and therefore muscle performance and tone are improved.
- Stimulates the blood supply and produces a tingling and revived sensation in the skin.
- Light hacking aids digestion if it is done over the abdominal area – it should follow the direction of the digestive tract where stimulation will occur. It stimulates the wave of the gut as food passes through (peristalsis).

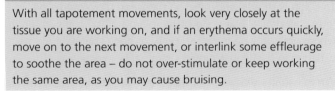

Think about it

With all tapotement movements, look very closely at the tissue you are working on, and if an erythema occurs quickly, move on to the next movement, or interlink some effleurage to soothe the area – do not over-stimulate or keep working the same area, as you may cause bruising.

Vibrations

Vibrations are fine trembling movements performed on or along a nerve path by the fingers. They can be static or running and you can use either the fingertips or the whole hand.

So how do I do it?

The muscles of the therapist's forearm are continually contracted and relaxed to produce a fine tremble or vibration, which runs to the fingertips. The tremor can run along the muscle length or side to side, depending on the size of the muscle bulk and the client's needs. The easiest way is to place one hand on top of the other, and tap the bottom hand with the top hand, using the fingertips, so that the vibration passes through to the other hand and then to the body below.

Benefits of vibrations

- Used at occipital region in facial massage.
- Can relieve pain and relax client due to its sedative effect.
- Soothes the nerve paths after stimulation.

Frictions

Frictions are often classified within the petrissage group, but their purpose differs. Friction movements will loosen adherent skin, loosen scars and aid in absorption of fluid around the joints.

So how do I do it?

These are stationary, concentrated pressure manipulations, exerting deep force on a small area at a time, with a gradual increase in pressure as you work along the muscle. This maximises the movements. Pressure is firm and the movement is usually applied in circular directions, with a regular pressure. On the face, fingertips or thumbs are mostly used. On large bulky muscle areas, one palm does the friction movement, reinforced by the other hand.

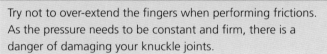

Think about it

Try not to over-extend the fingers when performing frictions. As the pressure needs to be constant and firm, there is a danger of damaging your knuckle joints.

Benefits of frictions

- Frees adhesions in the muscle.
- Creates warmth in the area, as blood is brought to the skin's surface.
- Stretches and loosens scar tissue.
- Aids relaxation.
- Helps break down the tight nodules found in stiff muscles (particularly useful on the trapezius).
- Stimulates lymphatic and blood flow in the area.
- Spinal frictions produce a tingling sensation – stimulates all nerves attached to the spine.
- Releases fluid trapped around the joints – make sure medical approval is sought first, and the swelling, or oedema, has no medical systemic origin, for example a kidney problem. If it is a swelling caused by poor circulation or tiredness, then relief can be given with frictions.

Think about it

Adjust the pressure and rhythm of the massage sequence to meet the client's individual needs. Not all massage movements will be appropriate for every client. Continue to monitor the effectiveness of the massage throughout the treatment – if the client falls asleep, you know it has been a success!

Think about it

Most Awarding Bodies do not dictate the order of these movements, so do not worry if you cannot remember the procedure without looking at your notes when you first start. As you become more practised and confident, so the routine will become second nature – your hands will automatically take over! Make each class of movements clear and recognisable – an assessment will depend upon your assessor being able to identify which movement is which.

Suggested massage routine

The massage procedure for a full body massage is as follows.

Client in a supine (face-up) position

- Front of right leg
- Right arm
- Left arm
- Front of left leg
- Abdomen
- Neck and chest

Client in a prone (face-down) position

- Back of right leg and gluteal
- Back of left leg and gluteal
- Back massage

This standard procedure ensures minimum discomfort for the client, as he or she only has to turn over once. The procedure will vary, depending upon your training establishment's preferences.

Variations on the theme

- Some therapists complete a leg massage from the front and do not treat the back of the leg separately.
- Gluteals are an option for massage. Some training establishments only do the top of the gluteal and include it within the back massage routine; others fully expose the gluteal for massage. (The latter option does not cater for the client's privacy, but some health spas would expect full gluteal massage to be part of the routine.) Commonly, one half of the gluteal is exposed at a time, both for client comfort and to stop the muscle from getting cold.

- If you are left-handed, you may wish to start on the left-hand side of the body – most students find they have a 'better' side, where they feel more comfortable, especially with posture corrections, and that is acceptable, too.
- Male massage will require adjustments within the routine – the upper thigh and abdomen areas are usually omitted, and more time given to the back and shoulder area, but most male clients would expect the back of legs to be part of the routine. If you progress to sports massage, the upper thigh would be included for pre-sport warm-up to maximise the muscle's performance.
- Facial massage is a range to be covered and depending upon client needs if the client is menstruating you can avoid the abdomen and include the face instead, which keeps the treatment time the same, or avoid treating the back of legs and include the face, or allow additional time to include the face.

To begin with, you will practise massage movements on fellow students. It is good to swap around the class, rotating whom you work upon, as a variety of body shapes and variation in tissue will provide invaluable experience.

When initially learning massage, it is best to begin on the back as it is a large area on which to practise, although you would not start the full treatment with the back massage. The client is prone so that eye contact is avoided, allowing you to concentrate on the massage.

Think about it

Each lecturer or therapist develops his or her own particular massage movements, through years of experience. Why not volunteer to be a model for another class being taught body massage? The fundamentals will be the same, but some of the massage techniques may be different. You will learn something new, and the students will be pleased to have a model on whom to perform an assessment. It's extremely useful to play the role of client in a different class, where you are not known, so you realise how vulnerable or nervous a client can feel.

Massage procedures

Arm massage – a step-by-step guide

Therapist in walk standing — outer leg in a comfortable forward position.

1. Effleurage to whole arm. Support at the wrist and supinate the arm for inner access so that the posterior and anterior aspects are covered. (×3)
2. Lock into the client's elbow with one hand for support and massage with the other.
3. Palmar kneading — single-handed to the deltoid, triceps and bicep muscles. (×3)
4. Picking up — single-handed to the deltoid, triceps and bicep muscles. (×3)
5. Thumb kneading to the deltoid muscle insertion on the humerus. (×1)
6. Light hacking to upper arm with one hand followed by effleurage. (×1)
7. Deep stroking to elbow joint. (×1)
8. Thumb kneading to elbow joint. (×1)
9. Deep stroking to the flexors and extensors of the forearm, supporting at the wrist, supinating for inner access. (×3)
10. Thumb kneading as above using one or both hands. (×3)
11. Thumb frictions to carpals. (×1)
12. Manipulations to carpals — flexion, extension and rotation at wrist. (×2)
13. Thumb kneading between metacarpals. (×2)
14. Thumb stroking to palms. (×3)
15. Effleurage to whole arm to finish arm massage. (×3)

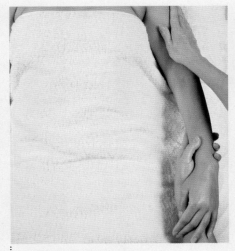

Effleurage to whole arm

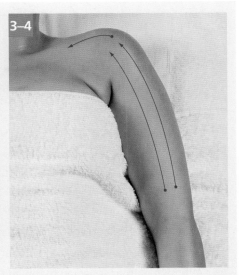

3–4

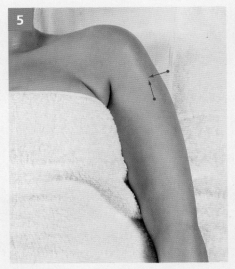

5

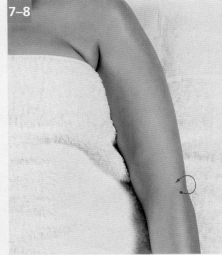

7–8

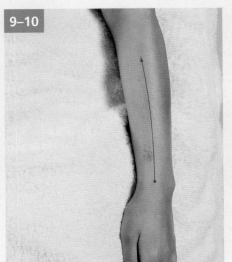

9–10

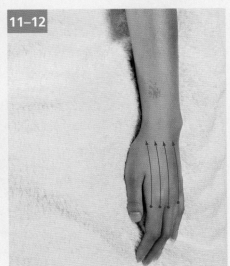

11–12

Front of leg massage – a step-by-step guide

Therapist in walk standing – outer leg in a comfortable forward position. Client fully covered, except the exposed leg. Prop at the ready. This massage covers the front and the back of the leg, all from the front.

1. Superficial effleurage to the whole leg from toes to thigh, with slight pressure in the groin to finish the movement. (×3)

Thigh only

2. Superficial effleurage to thigh only. (×3)

3. Palmar kneading – single-handed, to the outer, central and inner thigh (avoid going too high on the inner thigh). Support the limb with your free hand. (×3)

4. Picking up – to outer, central and inner thigh. (×3)

5. Wringing – to outer, central and inner thigh. (×3)

6. Alternate palmar kneading to outer and inner thigh. (×3)

7. Alternate palmar kneading to top and under the thigh (quadriceps and hamstring muscles). (×1)

8. Tapotement to all of thigh (depending upon client's needs). (×1)

Knee only (with support prop, if desired)

9. Effleurage around the knee joint. (×3)

10. Palmar kneading either side of the knee. (×3)

11. Thumb-kneading around the knee joint – fingers supporting around the back of the knee. (×3)

12. Effleurage around the knee joint to finish. (×3)

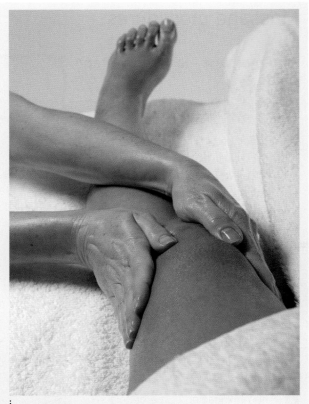

Client's leg positioned for massage

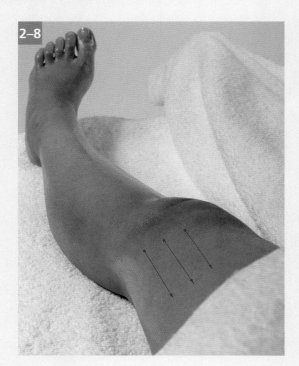

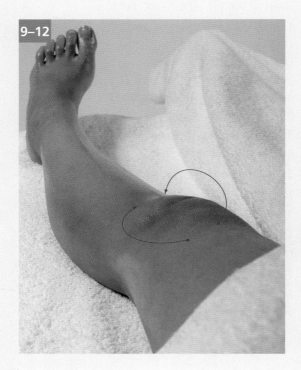

Front of leg massage – a step-by-step guide (*cont.*)

Lower limb – support under the knee and bend the leg so that the sole of the foot is flat to the bed, and hold up the leg in this position with one hand at the ankle

13 Superficial effleurage to the calf (gastrocnemius). (×3)

14 Deep palmar kneading to calf. (×3)

15 Picking up of calf. (×3)

16 Thumb-kneading along the length of the outer aspect from ankle bone upwards (tibialis anterior). (×1)

Place leg back down onto the couch (you may use your pedicure routine as massage to the foot, but be careful with timing)

17 Effleurage to whole foot. (×3)

18 Thumb-kneading to foot – top and sole. (×3)

19 Palmar stroking to sole of foot. (×3)

20 Scissor movements using thumbs, across sole. (×3)

21 Snatching/grabbing of toes. (×1)

22 Superficial effleurage to whole leg, as in the beginning of the leg massage. (×3)

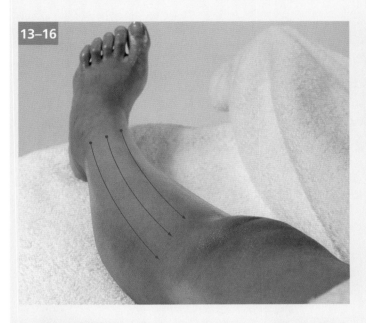

13–16

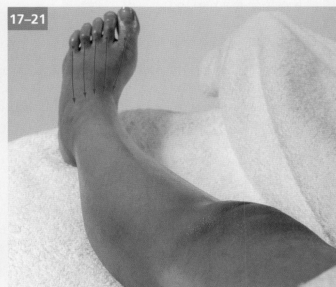

17–21

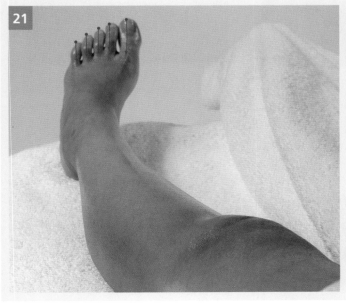

21

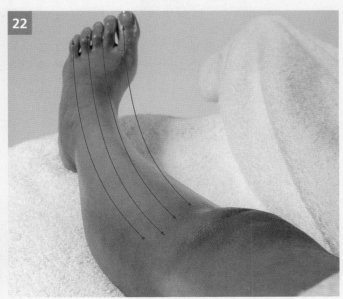

22

Back of leg massage – a step-by-step guide

Should the client prefer it, or your client is a male who is quite sporty and would like or needs a firm massage to the back of the leg, below is an alternative to the leg massage from the front. Adjust your time on the front of the leg massage, so that you have enough time to do the back of the leg and the top of the gluteal. Keep only the limb you are working on uncovered; the one resting should be covered and warm. Do the same movements in the sequence for the back, but avoid the back of the knee joint. The client will feel most comfortable with a prop under the ankle.

Therapist in walk standing, massaging the hamstring muscle.
(All movements ×3)

1. Superficial and deep effleurage with light effleurage back down.
   Deep kneading following same pattern.

2. Alternate palmar kneading.

3. Ironing.

4. Thumb rotations.

Therapist in stride standing, massaging the gastrocnemius muscle.
(All movements ×3)

5. Superficial and deep effleurage with light effleurage back down.
   Deep kneading.

6. Alternate palmar kneading.
   Thumb rotations.

7. Foot massage.
   Light stroking.
   Thumb kneading.

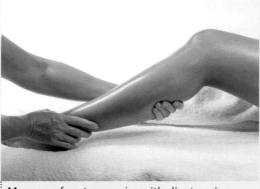

Massage of gastrocnemius with client supine

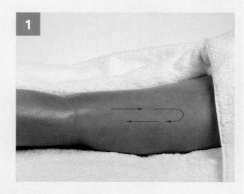

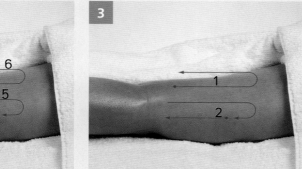

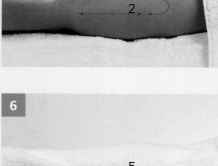

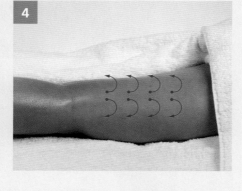

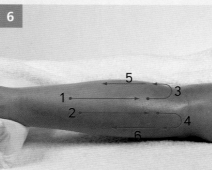

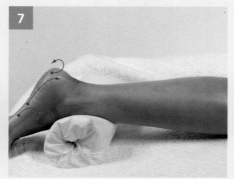

Chest and neck massage – a step-by-step guide

Therapist in stride standing, behind the head. (All movements ×3).

1 Superficial effleurage down the sides of the neck from chin, across chest, out to finish on shoulders.
Deep effleurage down the sides of the neck from chin, across chest, out to finish on shoulders.
Stroking down the sides of the neck from chin, across chest, out to finish on shoulders.

2 Deep kneading fingers following the same direction as previous movements encircling the deltoid, depressing slightly and continuing over the trapezius towards the spine, and with hands together, lift the occipital slightly to stretch the atlas and axis of spine.

3 Ironing over chest, going from shoulder to shoulder, using circular motions.

4 Knuckling, in circles, from chin, down neck, out to shoulders and return.

5 Picking up trapezius from shoulders towards spine.

6 Return to effleurage as No.1 to finish.

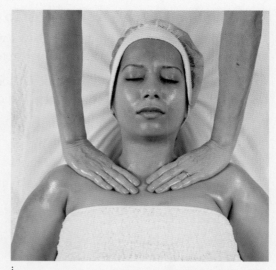

Client in position for a chest and neck massage

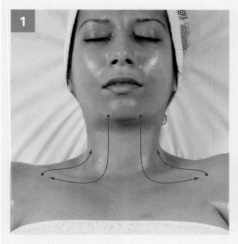
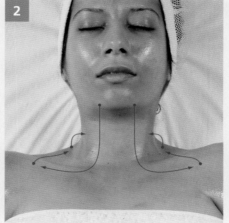
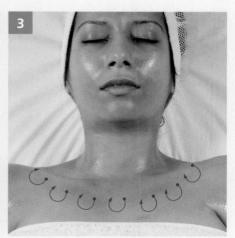
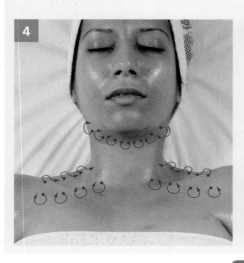
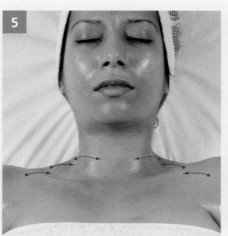
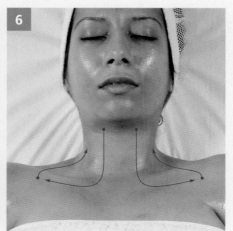

Abdominal massage – a step-by-step guide

The abdomen should only be included if the therapist is sure that it is appropriate. A specific contra-indication is early pregnancy.

Ask the client if she would like a prop placed under the knees to relax the abdominal muscles, and keep the pressure light at all times.

The client should have been given the opportunity to empty her bladder before starting the whole massage.

Therapist in walk standing, parallel to the client's hip.

1. Superficial effleurage from the pubis, up to the bottom of the sternum, out to the sides and then up over the iliac crest to the starting position.
2. Deep stroking following the same direction, pulling in slightly at the waist.
3. Circular kneading or ironing following the direction of the colon.
4. Wringing around the sides and front of the abdomen.
5. Picking up the perimeters – where possible.
6. Vibrations and light hacking – following the digestive tract.
7. Stroking/effleurage as for step 1 to finish.

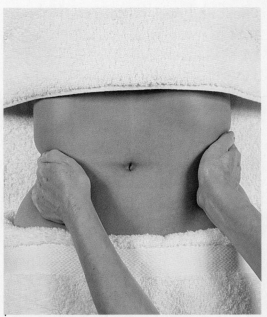

Client in position for a abdomen massage

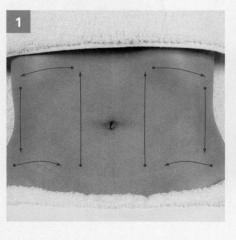

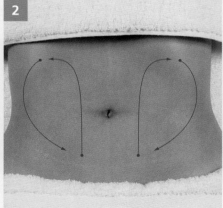

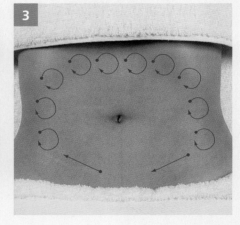

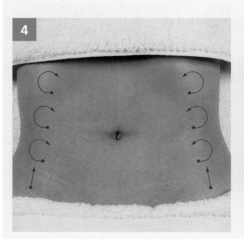

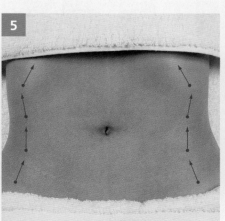

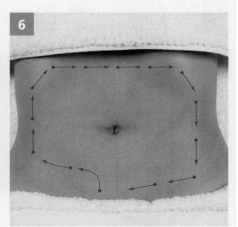

Back massage – a step-by-step guide

Therapist in walk standing.

Superficial effleurage – to cover the whole back. Three linked sequences are required.

1 Working from the sacrum to the trapezius, either side of the vertebral column, with light effleurage back down.

2 Work from sacrum to over the deltoid to cover the middle of the back.

3 Work from sacrum to under arms covering the perimeters of the back.
These three movements cover all of the back and the pattern is continued for the other back movements.

4 Palmar kneading following the same direction as steps 1–3.

5 Alternate palmar kneading following pattern of steps 1–3.

6 Circular kneading to scapula and thumb/digital kneading where necessary, following an upward flow towards the clavicle lymph nodes.

7 Reinforced ironing, starting at sacrum and covering all of the back.

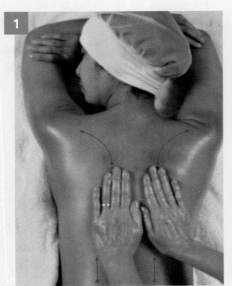

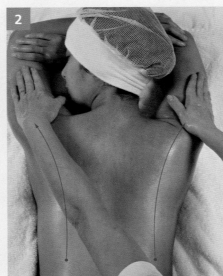

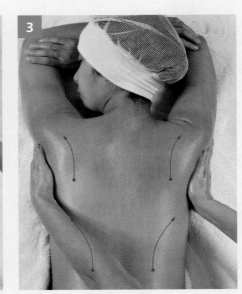

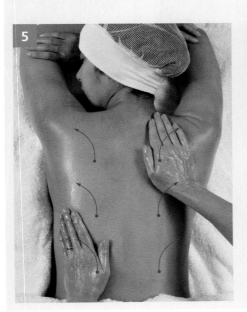

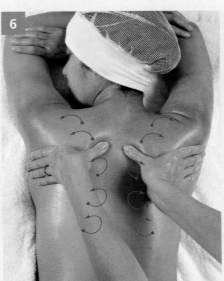

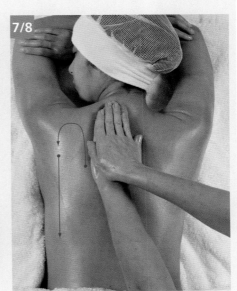

Back massage – a step-by-step guide (*cont.*)

8 Use a figure of eight over the scapulae.

9 Wringing following perimeters of body, where possible.

10 Picking up perimeters, where possible.

11 Skin rolling of perimeters, where possible.

Therapist in walk standing.

12 Thumb kneading or knuckling either side of spine from sacrum to occipital bone.

13 Spinal frictions following same pattern.
Therapist in stride standing.
Scissor movement up and down the back with light effleurage strokes.
Superficial effleurage to the top of the gluteals group.

14 Deep effleurage to the top of the gluteals group.

15 Reinforced ironing to the top of the gluteals group (figure of eight).

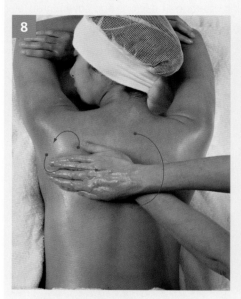

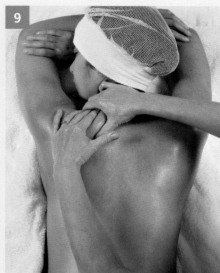

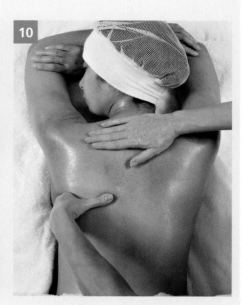

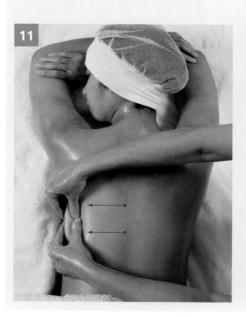

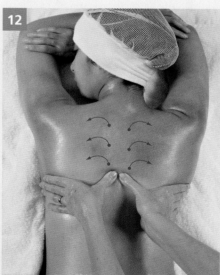

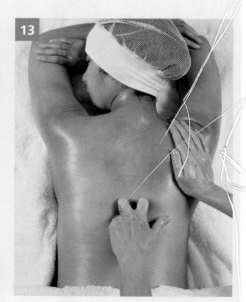

Back massage – a step-by-step guide (*cont.*)

16 Tapotement to the top of the gluteals group, depending on client size.

17 Hacking.

18 Beating.

19 Pounding.

20 Cupping.

21 Hacking to the whole back, or just trapezius area, depending on client size and amount of tissue present.

22 Light effleurage all over the back.

23 Reverse light stroking from head to sacrum to finish the massage.

24 Stretch the tissue out using the forearms.

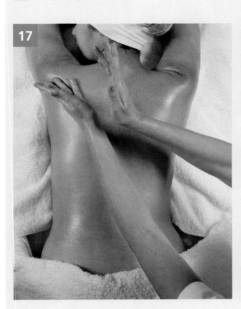

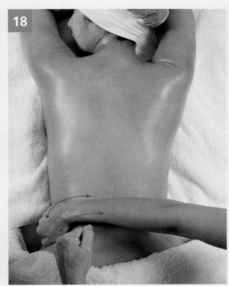

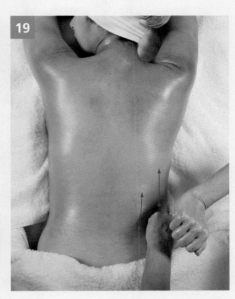

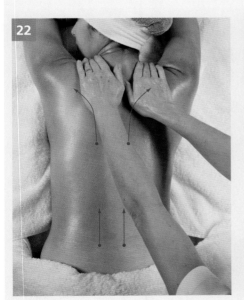

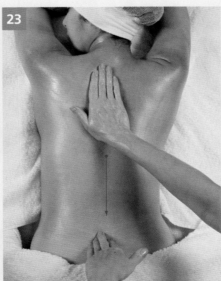

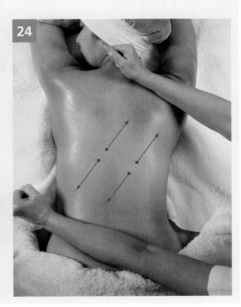

Head and scalp massage – A step-by-step guide

You can simply adapt your facial massage routine and add scalp massage movements. There are no set rules for scalp massage, but this is neither an Indian head massage routine (which is quite stimulating) nor an aromatherapy massage.

After a full consultation, prepare the client for a facial massage using your usual cleansing routine.

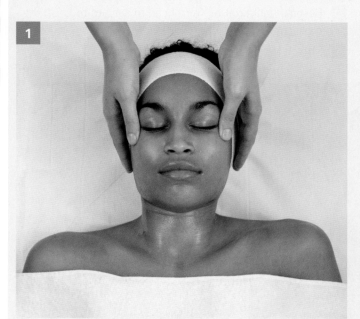

1 Cup the client's head with both hands, using light pressure, and breathe slowly with her three times to begin the massage.

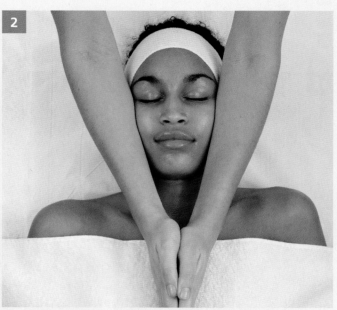

2 Put medium onto your hands and introduce your dry inner forearms to the cheek area.

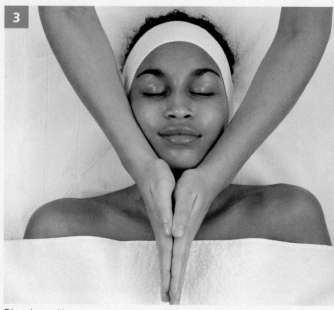

3 Slowly pull your arms upwards to introduce your palms and the massage medium to the face.

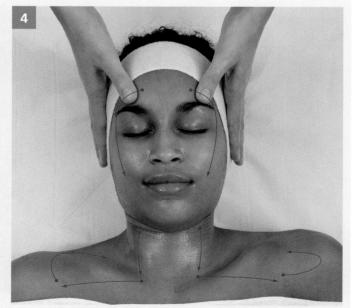

4 Carry out effleurage to the whole face, décolletage, along the shoulders and both under and over the trapezius to the occipitalis (×3).

Head and scalp massage – A step-by-step guide (*cont.*)

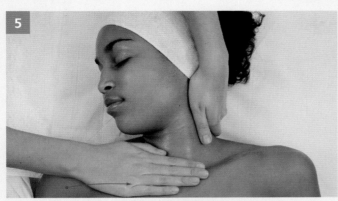

After the final effleurage strokes, hands are on the trapezius. Support the head with the palm of the hand, fingertips in occipital lift, and turn client's head to one side. Left hand reaches to elbow — with firm effleurage, come up the upper arm, over deltoid, over trapezius, back to occipital (×3). Lift client's head to centre, turn head to other side and repeat.

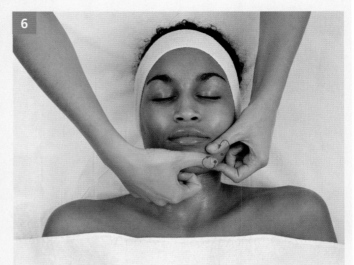

Come up to jawline and use small, thumb rotary movements.

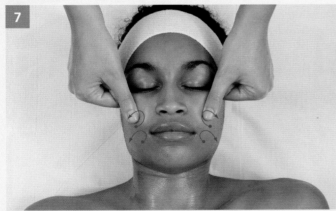

Work up to cheek area and continue thumb kneading outwards to preauricular lymph nodes.

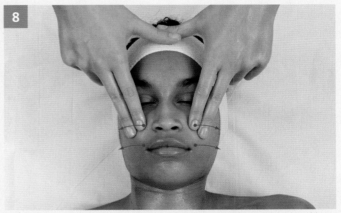

Pressure points — press fingers with pulsing pressure working outwards from nose to ear.

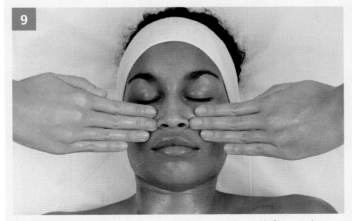

Follow same pattern from nose to ear using all fingers in a sweeping motion.

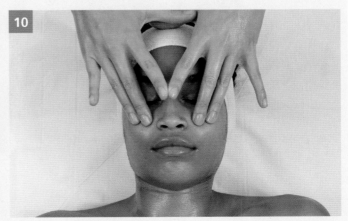

Light feather tapping (piano playing) movements around the eye socket.

Head and scalp massage – A step-by-step guide (*cont.*)

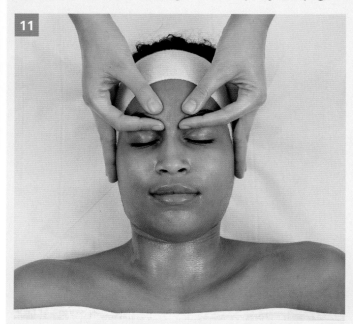

Stretch the eyebrow outwards between the thumb and fingers.

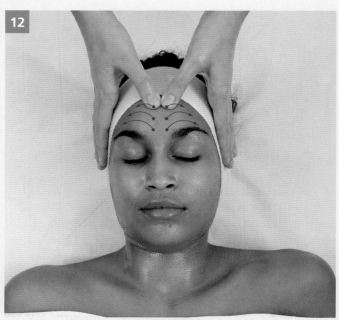

Thumb drainage across from middle to i) top of eyebrows, ii) middle of forehead, iii) along hair line.

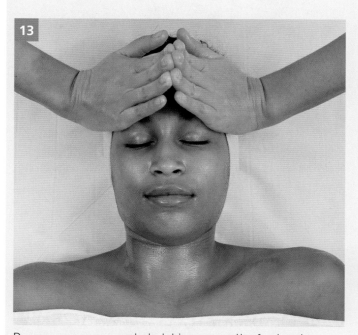

Deep prayer movement stretching across the forehead.

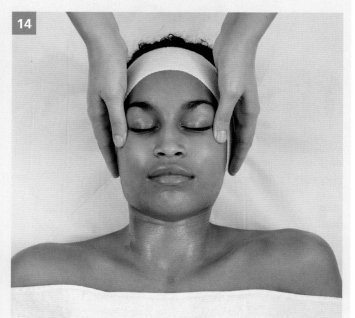

Cup face to signal end of treatment.

Massage mediums

Medium choice will largely depend upon the skin type. For a detailed description of skin types, see You and the skin, page 242.

If the skin is dry, oil is the best medium to choose, as it will help to nourish and moisturise the skin during treatment. A greasy/oily skin does not respond well to having more oil added to it, so cream or talc is more beneficial. When your massage techniques are perfected you may try a completely dry massage, with no lubrication on the skin, which is effective, especially if doing a pressure point massage; but clients would normally expect some products to be used.

Some skin conditions may not be contra-indicated to treatment, but need additional attention when choosing the massage medium. For example, mild eczema sufferers may be suitable for massage, but you should use a light aqueous (water-based) cream which will help the condition. Some clients will bring their own cream for you to use.

Decanting products

To avoid cross-infection, always decant products from salon-size containers into bowls and use a spatula for application. Never pour unused product back into the container as it will contaminate the remaining product. With experience, you will be able to judge the amount required, and not waste any. If you find you have product left over, decant it into a small jar and give it to the client to use at home.

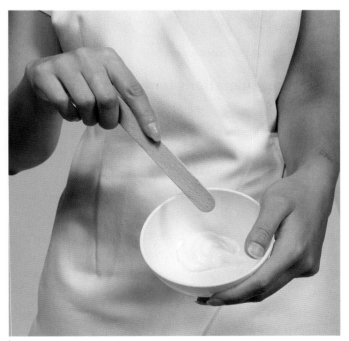

Decant products into a small bowl using a spatula

Think about it

The client's preference must always be considered. This needs to be discussed during the consultation, as some clients do not like the feel of oil on the skin, others prefer cream and some will bring their own products. Be cautious if using pre-blended aromatherapy oils should the client bring such a product. At this stage of your training, you are not trained or insured as an aromatherapist. Even diluted oils can be toxic, with potential to harm the client, especially if she is pregnant and does not yet know it. You may be better advised to pass the client to a more senior therapist if an aromatherapy massage is really what the client wants.

Allergies and contra-actions

Allergies can occur at any time, from any source, and the client may develop a reaction to a product he or she has been using for years. The most common visible skin reaction is itching, red irritation in the area, developing into swelling or heat. Lanolin is found in some massage creams, and can cause problems, as can perfume additives and some colourings. A client with a known nut allergy should always inform the therapist during consultation, as the reaction caused may be life-threatening (see You and the skin, page 234).

Actions for contra-actions

If the client develops an irritation caused by the medium during the massage, remove it immediately. Calm the area with a cool compress — a hand towel dampened in cool water should reduce the irritation immediately.

If the client has a history of reactions or irritability to products, do a small patch test. Place a small amount of product to be used in the inner elbow 24 hours before the treatment and ask the client to monitor the skin reaction.

Areas to be treated

Skin texture and conditions vary in different parts of the body. It is possible to use two mediums in the same massage. For example, the client may have an oily, slightly spotty back, requiring cream, but very dry legs, which require the richness of oil. This is perfectly acceptable and proves you are able to adapt to client requirements. (It also covers two ranges on the one assessment!)

During the consultation discuss the outcome of the treatment and the client's expectations, as these will also influence the choice of medium. If the client wants a soothing, relaxing massage to aid stress, then pick oil as it is designed to be smooth and flowing over the skin's surface, helping you achieve the right effect. Should the client want a heavier massage for muscular problems, when more vigorous movements are employed, use talc or cream. Many sports therapists prefer to massage with talc.

The client's schedule after the treatment should also be considered. Will the client be able to shower to remove any excess oil? Does the client need to return to work and therefore to be oil-free, or has the client come in loose clothing with the intention of leaving the oil on the skin to maximise the benefits?

Types of massage medium

Massage creams

Massage creams contain a mixture of wax, oil and water, and the consistency is determined by the ratio of ingredients. A cream that is too sloppy will drip off the skin and be irritating to the client, so most professional creams are of a whipped cream consistency, which is why they will not fall off the spatula as you decant the product.

The oil used is usually white soft paraffin, lanolin and mineral oil. The wax is white beeswax. These are mixed with water and an emulsifying agent is added to prevent the oil and water separating.

Oils and waxes condition and improve the skin's natural water barrier and some oils, like jojoba, can help prevent water loss.

Massage oils

Most types of oil make a suitable medium for massage. Vegetable oils such as olive oil, corn oil, sunflower or peanut oil can be used, although olive oil may be expensive in large quantities.

Mineral oil is a by-product of the oil-refining business and is inexpensive to purchase, so it is useful when you are first practising, although it is not used commercially.

> **Think about it**
>
> Vegetable oil goes off after a time, so do not buy in large quantities.

> **Think about it**
>
> Should you open a new jar of cream and find the ingredients have separated, return it to the supplier, as the product may be old stock and will have deteriorated.

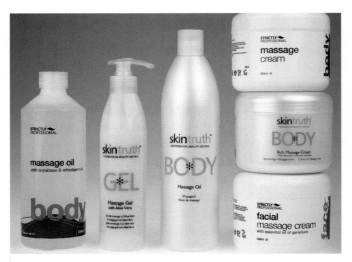
Massage creams

Talc

Talc is a dry powder which provides slip and smoothness if applied to a dry skin. Talc consists of magnesium silicate ground into a very fine dust. Corn starch is another common ingredient and iron oxides are added – quantities vary between products.

Talc	Ideal for combination or oily skins, skins with spots, and skins with a perspiration problem
Cream	Used for normal or dry skin. Suitable for clients who do not like the feel of oil on their skin
Oil	Can be used on most skins, ideally suited to a dry skin and lots must be used on a client with a hairy body

When to choose talc, cream or oil

COSHH considerations for each medium

 All ingredients are commonly used in cosmetic products.

- Non-hazardous.

- Non-inflammable.

- If ingested, drink milk or water.

- If in contact with eyes, wash well with water; if irritation occurs, seek medical advice.

- If spilled, use absorbent towels to clean the area, wash with detergent and water to avoid slippery floors.

- No special handling and storage precautions necessary.

- Avoid breathing talc deeply into the lungs; the fine particles if inhaled over a long period are known to cause lung damage.

- Store creams and oils in a cool, dark cupboard.

Think about it

The amount of product required will depend upon the client's size – the larger the client, the greater the skin surface, and if the client is hairy, you may need to use double the quantity of the medium. Skin texture also plays its part – a very dry skin will absorb a large amount of oil. Record details of the medium used on the client's record card and note if a reaction occurs.

For your portfolio

Investigate the products used in your salon or training establishment. Compare ingredients, prices and wholesale sizes from two local beauty therapy suppliers. How do they compare? Are more expensive products necessarily better than cheaper brands?

Which one to choose

Which medium you choose will depend on:

- the client's skin type
- the client's preference
- the client's allergies
- the client's contra-actions in previous treatments
- the area to be treated
- the desired effect
- other treatments combined with massage.

Think about it

Within your portfolio you will have very similar evidence for your body massage, however the depth, rhythm and pressure, medium, client needs and aftercare will be individual to your client, so each treatment will not be identical – and it shouldn't be, if your client care is in place.

Think about it

Remember to minimise waste, where possible.

- Decant only as much product as you need, it's easier to add more but you cannot pour oil, cream or talc back into the bottle once it is out.
- Save on laundry by covering your bedding with couch roll.
- Be conscious of the time and do not over-run.
- Only use as much cotton wool and tissues as you need.

Contra-actions and prompt action

A contra-action may occur randomly. For example, it might be caused by a product that the client has used for years with no ill effects, which suddenly causes a reaction. This is more likely if the client has changed regular medication or, in a woman's case, may be hormonal – because of the contraceptive pill, changes occurring in the menopause, or the early stages of pregnancy. The client should be advised that this may occur and what action she should take.

Think about it

A contra-action is different from a contra-indication. A contra-indication prevents the massage from being carried out, or means that the area should be avoided during massage. A contra-action is a reaction that occurs during the treatment.

Erythema

This may occur after a treatment and is a by-product of vigorous tapotement. It should subside after treatment.

Skin reactions

A skin reaction is not common in massage, but sometimes the client may suddenly develop an allergy (for allergic reactions, see You and the skin, page 234). The reaction should stop naturally, but ask the client to monitor the area for 24 hours and refer to the doctor if the reaction does not subside.

Identify the hazard	What is the risk?
Infection spreading	Low
Bruising to the skin	High
Spillage of products	Low
Scratching of skin through jewellery or long nails	High
Dragging of the skin	High
Falling getting on and off the couch	High
Slipping in the wet area	High
Postural problems for the therapist	High
Allergic/sensitive reaction to the massage medium	High

Continued

Provide body massage treatments **B20**

What should I do to prevent the hazard from becoming a risk?

- Follow full consultation and contra-indication checklist
- Carry out a patch test 24 hours before treatment. Ask clients to provide their own hypoallergenic creams if this is a known problem
- Adjust massage movements to suit depth of tissue and client preference
- Never carry out tapotement over bony areas
- Cut nails so that with the palm facing you, no free edge is visible over the fingertips
- Have sufficient product on the skin to keep it well lubricated
- Monitor for any developing contra-actions
- Provide suitable floor covering, e.g. woven matting or shower mats for wet area
- Never allow the client into the wet area with bare feet
- Decant products prior to use, and mop up any spillage immediately
- Remove all jewellery
- Provide a suitable step for the client to use when getting on the couch, not a chair
- Check posture and couch height to ensure good posture when massaging

Risk assessment for body massage

Updating treatment plan and record card

It is essential to review the massage treatment (both manual and mechanical) with the client to find out if the objectives of giving a relaxing massage and creating a sense of wellbeing were met. Before your client leaves, and whilst they are drinking a glass of water and beginning to come back into an alert state, just spend a few minutes checking client satisfaction and ask how the treatment was for them. Is there any aspect of the massage that the client would like to change? Was he or she comfortable at all times? Did he or she like the massage medium and all of the movements? Any adjustments can be noted on the record card, and you can move forward with the treatment plan, by agreeing that next time you will adapt the massage to suit what the client has said to you. It may mean leaving out a movement which they did not like, or putting more movements into a certain problem area, or they may ask advice about deeper mechanical massage.

Also check with the client (after all, they are paying for the service) that it meets the agreed treatment objectives that you started with and that the client is entirely happy, before they leave you.

Think about it

Do remember to allow post-treatment recovery time – the client is hopefully feeling relaxed and sleepy so will need to be allowed to wake up fully before going on to work or operate machinery such as driving. Relaxation is a good thing – but the client should be alert and with good reflexes before venturing out of the salon.

Perform mechanical massage treatments

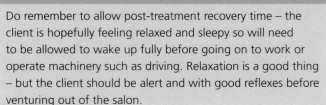

In this section you will look at infrared lamp, G5 and audio-sonic treatment. For each piece of equipment you will learn:

- how to choose mechanical or pre-warming equipment to enhance your body massage
- how to apply each piece of equipment
- the safety and risks of each piece of equipment
- treatment settings, intensity and duration of each treatment.

Pre-warming treatment for massage

Infrared lamp

Warming the muscles and tissue before starting the massage doubles the effectiveness of the massage movements and makes the tissue soft and more malleable to work with. If the client does not enjoy or does not have time for a spa or sauna, an infrared lamp is an invaluable form of pre-heating treatment. It is portable and gives out a warm deep heat. (See Unit B21 Provide UV tanning treatments, for a full explanation of infrared and its place in the electro-magnetic spectrum.) Any area of the body (and face) can be treated, although usually it is the back. It may also be used before electro-therapy (electro-muscular stimulation, galvanic, vacuum, etc.).

Salon life

Jonathan's story

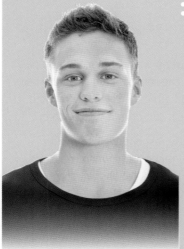

My name is Jonathan and I'm taking the massage route at Level 3. I know how effective massage is for tension, but I didn't realise what a dramatic effect it can have on a personality, too. One of my regular clients at college asked me if I would take her husband on as a client because he worked very long hours, was in the car for a lot of the day driving and suffered with back pain. She said it was making him irritable and depressed. We booked him in for a full body massage. The back pain was not severe enough to be a contra-indication so I was able to go ahead with the treatment. He was face down on the bed and absolutely rigid! It was like trying to massage an ironing board he was so stiff with tension. I worked and worked his muscular groups and did a really deep massage, but I felt I wasn't getting anywhere. I was worried that he wasn't happy with the treatment and wouldn't be back — he just didn't seem to relax, whatever I tried. But he did come back and next time he seemed more relaxed. We chatted about sport and his love of football. I felt the treatment was more beneficial this time — he just seemed more comfortable and less tense.

Eventually he became one of my regular clients. Over time, it became apparent that his back problem was a result of tension and bad posture in the car. He's now joined a gym to get fit and says he feels like a new man. I think some clients just forget how to unwind and their bodies hold on to all the tension.

Effects for the therapist:

- Don't give up on a client after just one treatment or prejudge them for being quiet or stand-offish — it could just be nerves

- What you consider to be normal and familiar — what happens during a treatment, what clothes to take off, where the toilets are, and so on — may be very daunting to a client and can have a detrimental effect on the relaxation of the treatment

- Realise that your treatment is not only about what happens in the salon — the client will take your lifestyle advice to heart and it can help to improve all aspects of their lives. A change in diet, taking more exercise and learning to take time out for themselves can improve their overall health

Effects for the client:

- Having someone take an interest in every aspect of their lifestyle problems can very often focus the mind and make them see clearly the changes they need to make

- Being given permission to take time out, to relax on the couch and be still, can be very therapeutic and restorative to both mind and body

- There are great physical side effects too: skin is nourished and moisturised, it feels softer, and even hands and feet get much needed attention

Provide body massage treatments **B20**

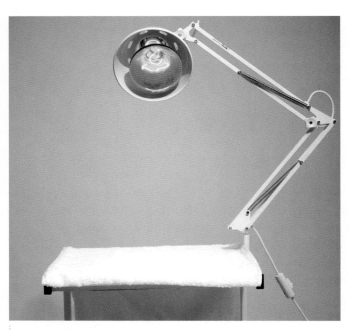

An infrared lamp

Contra-indications

- Circulatory problems, e.g. fluid retention, swelling, varicose veins (if treating the legs)
- Skin disorders – dermatitis, eczema
- Diabetes – because of less efficient circulation and lessened sensitivity to heat
- Respiratory problems and illnesses – congestion of the lungs, for example bronchitis
- Metal pins and plates
- Conditions requiring medical attention/approval prior to treatment
- Very low blood pressure
- Heart/artery problems
- Inflammation of any kind
- Remove contact lenses – these act rather like a magnifying glass and intensify the heat
- No oil or lubrication must be on the skin, as this intensifies the treatment
- Loss of skin sensation, or lack of response to the skin sensitivity test, which should always be carried out before starting the treatment
- Claustrophobia – especially when used on the face
- Hypersensitive skin
- Cuts, wounds or bruises in the area to be treated
- The nervous or highly strung client

When to use heat radiation treatment

Relief of pain

The mild heating will have a sedative effect and assist general aches and pains associated with muscular tension, poor posture, and so on.

Muscular relaxation

Muscles relax most readily when warm, so aches and pains can be relieved or avoided if the muscles are heated. Heat treatment is particularly good after exercise. Any muscle spasms or tension or tightness can often be alleviated.

Fibrous accumulations usually respond well to gentle heating and rapidly disperse, particularly when massage is applied afterwards. These accumulations are commonly found in the trapezius muscle of the back.

Regular heat radiation treatment should maintain beneficial preventative effects.

Physical and physiological effects of heat radiation treatments

- Circulation is stimulated – an erythema is produced. The improvement in circulation means that there is an increase of oxygen, nutrients are brought to the tissues under treatment and removal of waste is increased.
- There is a local rise in skin temperature, which is warming and relaxing. With a more prolonged or extensive treatment there may be a general rise in temperature. This should not exceed 0.5–1°C.
- As muscles become warmed and circulation is aided, the muscle tissue relaxes, enabling fibres to relax and contract more easily. The efficiency of muscle action is improved. Any tension should be relieved and stiff and aching muscles should ease.
- Mild heating has a sedative and calming effect on the sensory nerve endings. Intense heating, however, has an irritating effect.

Think about it

Therapists should only use infrared treatment for muscular aches or pains if given a doctor's consent. Heat does not help all pain, for example heating a sprained ankle will lead to vasodilation and cause bleeding. In this instance a cold compress, for example, would be more suitable.

- The higher temperature increases the rate of metabolism. Repairs to damaged tissues are speeded up and there will also be an increase in waste removal such as lactic acid and carbon dioxide.

- Sweating is induced as the blood in the treatment area is warmed and circulates. Temperature regulation centres in the brain are eventually affected and gentle perspiration occurs, which will have a cleansing action on the skin.

- The capacity of the skin to absorb oils and creams is greatly enhanced by the effects of warming, thereby increasing the effectiveness of subsequent treatments such as massage.

Use and storage of heating equipment

- Check plug and leads are intact.

- Check apparatus to ensure reflective surfaces are clean and free from dents, or 'hot spots' will result.

- Check the tightness of the angle-poise joints. They must hold the lamp in position and not allow it to fall on to the client. Tighten if necessary.

- Always ensure the client's and therapist's eyes are protected from the infrared rays. Wear goggles if necessary.

- If the lamp's outer casing becomes hot when in use, do not touch it. Use a towel if the lamp needs to be repositioned during treatment – this will reduce the risk of the therapist being burned.

- Do not move the lamp when it is turned on.

- Keep flammable material away from the lamp.

- Always ensure the client cannot touch the lamp or move closer to it during treatment.

- Never place the lamp directly over the client due to the risk of the lamp being accidentally knocked or the bulb shattering.

- Protect the working area – use a screen so others cannot accidentally walk into the lamp while it is on.

- Never leave the client or treatment area unattended.

- Never exceed treatment times – always gauge client responses carefully.

- When leaving the lamp to cool down, ensure it is left somewhere safe and protected with a sign to show that it is still warm. Similarly, if the lamp requires a warming-up period, ensure this is done in a safe and controlled manner. Never leave the lamp heating over a couch, for example, which might become hot and eventually burn.

- Store the lamp carefully – bulbs are delicate and are easily damaged!

Inverse square law

The law states that the intensity from the source – the lamp – varies with the square of the distance from the point of source. In other words:

- if the distance increases, the intensity decreases by the square of the distance

- if the distance decreases, the intensity increases by the square of the distance

- if the distance is doubled, the intensity is quartered

- if the distance is halved, the intensity will increase four times.

So if you double the distance, multiply the time by four. For example, if the original distance is 45 centimetres and treatment time is 5 minutes, after applying the inverse square law, if you double the distance to 90 centimetres you can multiply the treatment time by four to 20 minutes.

In this way the client will receive the same amount of radiation, but more slowly and gently.

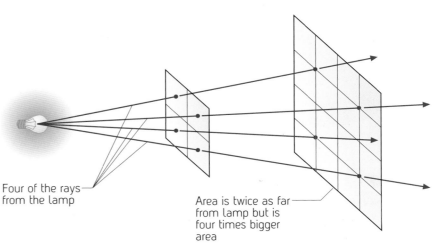

Four of the rays from the lamp

Area is twice as far from lamp but is four times bigger area

The inverse square law

Provide body massage treatments **B20**

Application of heat treatment – a step-by-step guide

1. Check the lamp for safe, correct working order.

2. Ensure the couch is prepared in readiness for the client's arrival.

3. Carry out a consultation, checking carefully for contra-indications.

4. Instruct the client to remove as much clothing as is necessary, depending on the treatment area, and make him or her comfortable on the couch.

5. To ensure the client is suitable for treatment, carry out a skin sensitivity test at the treatment site. If the client is unable to tell the difference between hot and cold and hard and soft, then the treatment is contra-indicated.

6. The area to be treated must be completely clean and free from any products, for example liniments. To avoid any possible reactions, such as burning, wash the area with warm, soapy water.

7. Ensure the client removes any jewellery that could get hot and burn at the treatment site.

8. Position the client so that he or she cannot move closer to the lamp or touch it. Heat radiation is commonly applied to the back so a good position is to have the client lying on the side supported by pillows.

9. Only expose the area to be treated and ensure the client is warmly covered.

10. Position a white reflective towel across the back of the client's neck and drape it in such a way that the eyes are shielded.

11. Explain the effects of the lamp and treatment to the client.

12. Position the lamp so that the rays strike the area at 90°, thus allowing maximum absorption. The lamp should never, at any time, be directly placed over the client. The treatment area should then be made into a 'safety zone' by placing a screen or something similar around it.

13. The lamp's distance from the client is usually 45–90 centimetres and the heat is applied for 5–20 minutes. However, it is essential to follow the manufacturer's instructions as lamps can vary considerably in their intensity and output. Guessing distances is dangerous, so always use a tape measure. The client should experience only a mild, gentle heating effect with the resultant therapeutic erythema.

If the client's tolerance of the heat is poor, the therapist must apply the inverse square law (ISL) which governs intensity of heat in relation to distance (see previous page).

14. During treatment, closely monitor the client's reaction by watching the area under treatment and also by obtaining feedback from the client.

15. If the lamp needs to be repositioned during treatment, handle the lamp carefully – use a towel.

16. When the treatment is complete, switch off the lamp and unplug it. The outer casing is likely to be very hot, so place a towel over the head of the lamp and then move it into a safe, screened area to cool down.

17. Reposition the client as necessary in readiness to perform subsequent treatment(s). If the client is not having another treatment, then assist the client into a sitting position before getting down from the couch. This is to avoid the dizzy feeling associated with the fall in blood pressure levels often accompanying a treatment of this type.

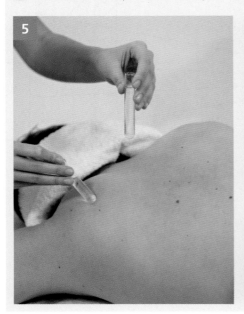

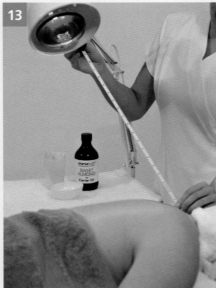

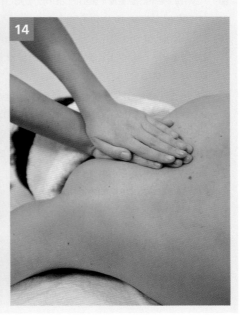

Identify the hazard	What is the risk?
Infection spreading	Low
Burning of the skin of client and therapist	High
Postural problems for the therapist	Low
Eye damage	High
Bulb falling onto the client's body	High
Allergic/sensitive reaction to the heat	High
Migraine	High
Fire	Low

What should I do to prevent the hazard from becoming a risk?

- Follow full consultation and contra-indication checklist
- Carry out thermal sensitivity testing
- Measure the distance of the lamp from the body
- Provide goggles
- Time the treatment
- Never leave the client unattended
- Monitor for any developing contra-actions
- Keep flammable substances away from the direct heat
- Remove jewellery which will get hot
- Position the lamp parallel to the body, never directly over the client
- Cover the client's neck with a towel
- Move the head of the lamp with a towel over the hand
- Check posture and couch height

Risk assessment for infrared treatment

Mechanical massage

Gyratory vibration

This is the most widely used mechanical massager in salons, health spas and cruise ships. The gyratory machine is often called a 'G5'. G stands for gyratory and 5 is the number of detachable heads which offer a variety of depth, pressure and sensation.

Why 'gyratory'?

A rotary electric motor inside the unit causes a circular massage movement similar to effect of ripples on a pond – superficial movements that radiate out from a central point.

Popularity of the G5

The G5 is popular because:

- it is labour-saving for the therapist
- it is ideal for large muscular areas, so is suitable for male clients

- it is economical to run
- it is collapsible, so ideal for the mobile therapist
- it offers a deeper massage and can therefore be extremely beneficial.

Vibratory treatments

There are three forms of vibratory treatment for the body:

- percussion
- vibration
- directional stroking.

These treatments may be applied by two types of machines – the more generally used large gyratory vibrators, or for localised effects, the smaller percussion or audio-sonic vibrators.

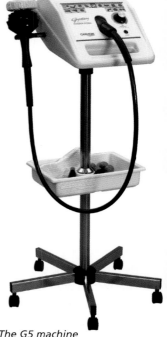

The G5 machine

Gyratory vibrators for general body work are normally floor-standing, with the weight of the motor supported by the main shaft or pedestal of the apparatus. This makes for greater safety as well as permitting long periods of use without undue fatigue.

Hand-held versions of these heavy-duty machines are also available. They produce similar effects for a lower cost but

Think about it

If vibratory treatments are used simply to complement and reinforce manual massage, rather than as treatments in their own right, a hand-held gyratory unit may well be adequate.

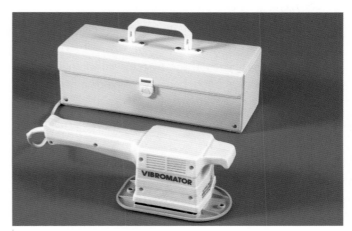

A double-handed gyratory vibrator

are more tiring to use. They look a little like an iron, and are quite heavy for the therapist. As they give quite a deep massage, they are really only suitable for dense muscle and clients with enough body tissue to take the pressure – a contra-indication would be a slight figure, or bony areas.

Whatever physical form the vibrator may take, it must be adequate for the task required and should have an air-cooled, heavy-duty motor capable of running for long periods without overheating.

The smaller vibrators normally used within facial therapy can be used on the body but are suitable only for localised areas.

Gyratory vibrators operate on a vertical and horizontal plane, creating a circular movement while vibrating up and down, thus achieving effects similar in action to manual massage. By altering both the applicator heads and the method of use, effects similar to effleurage, petrissage and tapotement can be achieved. This will help you to decide which applications are suitable and which contra-indicated.

Effects of gyrators

- Increases blood circulation.
- Aids desquamation.
- Increases metabolism.
- Promotes relaxation through warming of the tissues.
- Helps break down nodules of tension and relieves tightness in the muscles.
- Helps improve the texture of dehydrated and dry skins.
- Helps wellbeing if used alongside a diet and exercise programme.

Advantages of vibratory treatments

- They add variety to the treatment routines.
- They save time and prevent fatigue.
- They are less personal, so are useful in treating male clients.
- A deeply effective result can be achieved without the therapist using up a lot of energy, so helping her to conserve energy for other work.
- The time saving can help vibratory work to be more profitable.
- Clients enjoy vibratory massage and feel it is helping them in their fight against figure problems. They see value for money and have a sense that something is actually being achieved.

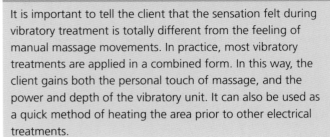

Think about it

It is important to tell the client that the sensation felt during vibratory treatment is totally different from the feeling of manual massage movements. In practice, most vibratory treatments are applied in a combined form. In this way, the client gains both the personal touch of massage, and the power and depth of the vibratory unit. It can also be used as a quick method of heating the area prior to other electrical treatments.

Contra-indications to gyratory massage

- Skin disorders/diseases
- Infected acne conditions
- Bruised areas
- Cuts and abrasions
- Recent scar tissue
- Sunburn
- Sensitive and fine skin
- Loose crêpey skin
- Oedema
- Glandular swellings
- Vascular conditions
- Bony areas
- Varicose veins, thrombosis or phlebitis
- Very hairy areas
- Over the abdomen during menstruation or pregnancy
- Clients with epilepsy or diabetes – a doctor's approval should be obtained
- Failure of the sensitivity testing on any area

Effects and benefits of vibratory treatments

- Vibratory treatments act as enormous encouragement to clients in their figure improvement plans, helping them to achieve results more swiftly and maintaining interest in their reduction programmes.
- As the effects of vibration are general stimulation of the circulatory system, the pattern of application can be varied to meet personal needs. The method of application follows body contours and works with the venous return towards the heart. It affects the subcutaneous tissues of the body, bringing about an increase in circulation, without any chemical or muscular contraction.

- The muscular system is improved by fresh interchange of blood through the tissue, but vibrations do not excite the muscle fibres to bring about a contraction.

- It produces a skin toning effect, both by improved nutrition to the skin's dermal layer and by increasing desquamation.

- Tense muscle fibres are relaxed and muscular pain relieved.

- Established fatty deposits are made more available to the general circulation and lymphatic systems, to be used up by the body when on a reduced food intake.

- Vibratory treatment can be extremely relaxing if combined with heat therapy and the more active stimulatory elements are excluded.

- Gyratory vibrators penetrate into the subcutaneous and cutaneous layers of the tissues, having their greatest effect on the skin's surface. Bony areas should be avoided to prevent resonance.

Method of use

The client is prepared for normal body treatments and may have had some form of pre-heating to aid relaxation of muscle tissues. Always explain the treatment to the client and test on yourself. Work as you would for a manual massage procedure, going towards the lymph nodes.

If the effect desired is relaxation only, then the application should concentrate on the soothing strokes and gentle vibratory effects of the treatment. If stimulation and figure reduction elements are needed, then a full range of applicators and a varied pattern of strokes should be used. The concentration then is local rather than general, working on areas of established adipose tissue and heavy muscle groups.

A smooth-surfaced applicator — sponge or soft rubber — starts the treatment. This is used with a light application of a talc medium, applied via the therapist's hands with effleurage strokes.

The treatment is applied with long sweeping strokes in an upward direction, towards the heart, as in a normal manual massage treatment. The strokes follow the natural contours of the body and can break contact gently or return with superficial strokes.

Different applicators may be used for variety — both simple round forms and those pre-shaped to mould around an area such as the leg.

Both legs may be treated superficially, one at a time, interlinking vibratory and manual strokes, and then using the ball-studded applicator deeply on the thighs. The deeper movements are performed in a kneading, compression

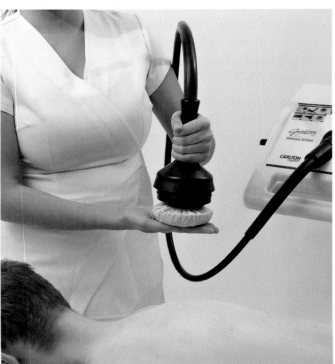

Always test G5 on yourself prior to treatment

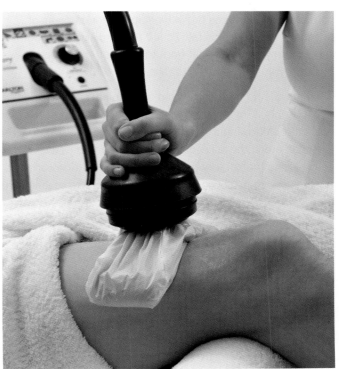

G5 application to the front of the legs using saddlehead with protective cover

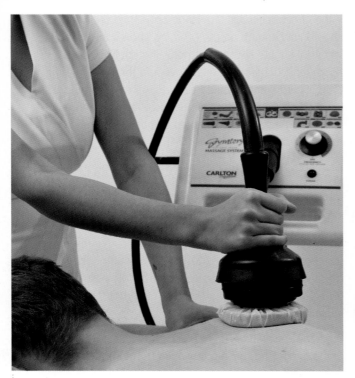

Place head onto skin prior to starting machine

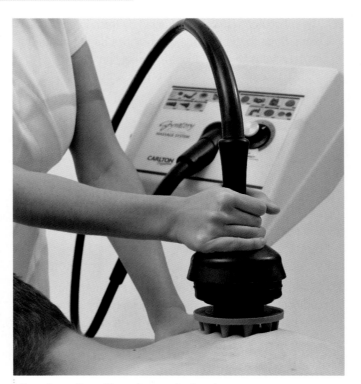

For a kneading effect, change the head

manner, with the therapist's hand providing support and resistance to the strokes, and interlinking them with effleurage. More superficial circular movements can then be performed using the brush type applicator on areas of adequate subcutaneous fat. Poorly textured skin and bad circulation will also benefit from the instant erythema produced by this method of treatment.

The legs should then be covered and the abdomen treated (if applicable). The application starts with the sponge applicator, following the body contours, and is followed by kneading along the ascending, transverse and descending colon, using the ball-shaped applicator. Manual movements interlink and re-establish relaxation, and then the routine can proceed to stimulating movements on the sides of the waist if indicated.

The studded or short-brush type rubber applicator is used to produce erythema and increase circulation in the area.

The abdominal area is then covered and the arms and chest are treated. It starts with stroking and progresses using the short spiky applicator on the upper arms. Softening of skin over the biceps and triceps muscles indicates the stimulating, abrasive effects of this application.

The arms only may be treated, or the strokes can be extended to include the chest on either side. Choice will depend on the amount of tissue covering the sternum area.

Turn the client over and treat the back of the leg and gluteals, remembering to keep the back and leg not being treated wrapped in towels to keep in the heat and keep the client comfortable.

The G5 is particularly effective on the back, and the ball-shaped applicator, the ball-studded applicator and the short brush can be used on top of the gluteals, just below the waist. When treating the top of the gluteals, be careful not to separate the gluteals fold, as this is very near the sciatic nerve and pressure should be avoided on the area, just as it should be on the vertebral column and borders of the scapula.

Think about it

Good technique depends on the smooth making and breaking of contact between the applicator head and the client's skin. Control of the heavy equipment comes only with practice and strength in the arms and wrists, and relies on working in the correct postural position.

Types of applicator

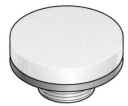

Sponge

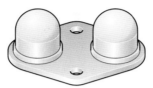

Blunt tipped firm rubber

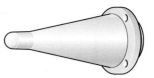

Pointed tip firm rubber

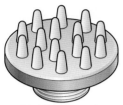

Multiple prong

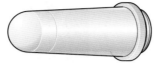

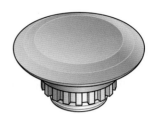

Hollow hot-cold use

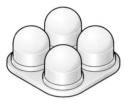

Four-ball firm rubber

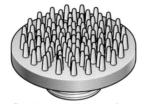

Two-ball firm rubber

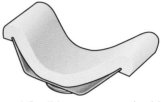

Curved flexible sponge and rubber

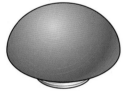

Half-ball firm rubber

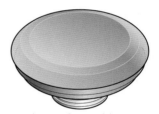

Scalp and skin surface

Large firm rubber

G5 applicator heads

Aftercare

Keep the client warm — to keep the heat in the muscles — while you prepare the equipment for the next part of the treatment.

If G5 is the finishing treatment, allow the client time to become aware of his or her surroundings, put the client into the semi-reclining position and offer a glass of water. Follow the aftercare and homecare advice detailed on page 431.

Mechanical treatments tend to have a superficial effect on the skin, rather like ripples in the water spreading outwards when a stone is thrown into a pond. Audio-sonic does not behave in this way on the tissue — it penetrates downwards rather than outwards.

Audio-sonic is not strictly a mechanical treatment, but as it is motor-driven (by electricity), it is included within this unit.

Think about it

The skin will be quite pink and hot in the area after the treatment if the full effects of vascular interchange and improved skin texture are to be effective.

Think about it

The size of the client will dictate the most suitable applicator head. Changing heads unnecessarily should be avoided as it breaks the continuity of the treatment and can be irritating to the client.

Audio-sonic treatment

The audio-sonic machine creates sound waves of 100–10,000 Hertz (in the range of human hearing) which cause all body tissue under treatment to vibrate simultaneously, resulting in nerve stimulation. Working like a tuning fork, the sound waves are transferred deep into the tissues up to around 6 centimetres. When applied to painful areas, for example tension in the shoulders, audio-sonic treatment speeds up the healing process through increased blood supply.

Hand-held audio-sonic has different applicator heads, ranging from a flat disc to a round knob and hedgehog type, depending on the machine you are using.

Contra-indications to audio-sonic

- Inflammation, sepsis, skin irritation
- Recent scar tissue
- Skin infections
- Extreme vascular skin conditions, dilated capillaries
- Sinus blockage – causes extreme discomfort
- Crêpey skin (percussion type only)
- Very bony areas – due to deeper penetration of audio-sonic. On less bony areas, audio-sonic may be used over the therapist's hands or fingers – the hands absorb some of the sound waves and this makes the treatment less penetrating and more comfortable for the client.

When to use audio-sonic treatment

- Any skin condition where stimulation is required but surface irritation needs to be avoided, for example sensitive skin, as little erythema is produced.
- To increase cellular function, improve sebaceous secretions in normal, dry or dehydrated skin.

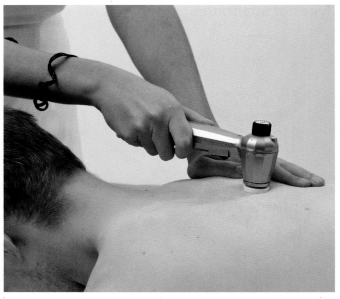

Audio-sonic treatment on the trapezium muscle

- If manual manipulations cause discomfort, audio-sonic can be used, for example to aid relaxation of tense muscle fibres.
- Mostly used on the body, rather than the face, for dealing with 'trapped fat' and is used with vacuum suction for reducing 'hard fat' in spot reduction.

Care of the machine

- As the equipment is motor driven, avoid lengthy, continuous use – about 15 minutes to avoid overheating.
- Keep applicator heads clean and sterilised with a suitable antiseptic anti-bacterial solution.
- Remove all traces of medium used from rubber applicator heads to avoid perishing.

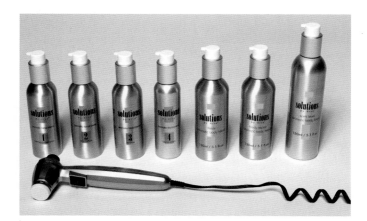

The audio-sonic machine

Think about it

Some areas of pain require a doctor's approval before being treated by a beauty therapist. If in doubt, ask the client to seek medical advice before treating.

Think about it

As an audio-sonic machine is small, it is most suited to treating specific areas of tension and is not cost-effective for a full body massage – it would take far too much time. It is a low-maintenance, portable piece of equipment particularly suitable for the mobile therapist.

Guidelines to method of treatment

- Normal application time: 5–15 minutes.
- Best to use with manual massage, as on its own the treatment may appear too mechanical for some clients.
- Can be used with either talc, cream or oil as a medium to cut down on friction and increase smoothness of application. Oil will benefit dehydrated skin.
- Adjust the speed in rhythm with the machine, if possible, or use the indirect method (over your hand/fingers) on bony areas.
- Alternate straight and circular patterns for client interest.
- Follow the natural contours of the muscle in a general upward direction.

Considerations to treatment

- Do remember to offer the most suitable support for all machines – props and pillows can be used to support the limbs.
- Always use the machines on the correct settings and always follow manufacturers' instructions.
- Always adjust to suit your client's physical characteristics and pick the most suitable equipment, for example an audio-sonic would be no use for a whole body massage as it would be too time-consuming, nor would you wish to give your client G5 on the face as it is far too heavy. So vary your equipment to meet the treatment objectives and to maximise the benefits of treatment to your client.
- Frequently check on your client's wellbeing throughout the treatment and ask if they are comfortable and relaxed – they should not feel that a mechanical massage is something to be endured!
- Do take remedial action if you can see the treatment is causing erythema or any other adverse reaction. Stop the treatment and take appropriate action – apply a cool compress or cool towel if the skin feels hot.
- Always allow sufficient post-treatment recovery time.
- After treatment, always confirm with your client that your mutually agreed treatment objectives from the beginning of the session have been met and that they are happy to pay for the treatment.

Think about it

There is no need for a risk assessment when using audio-sonic as the machine has little potential for harm.

- Write up any considerations or change of treatment on their record card for future reference.

Provide aftercare advice

In this section you will learn about:

- giving aftercare advice.

Aftercare

Procedure to follow immediately after the treatment:

- The client will be drowsy, or even asleep. Allow time to wake fully.
- Gently prop the client in a semi-reclining position on the couch.
- The client will not be sufficiently alert to take in details of aftercare – give the client a leaflet explaining long-term aftercare which he or she can read later.

Precautions after massage

- There is a risk that the client will become dizzy or light-headed if he or she gets off the couch too quickly. You may wish to help the client off the couch.
- Offer the client a glass of water to prevent dehydration.
- Allow time for the client to get dressed in a warm cubicle – rushing the client will undo the relaxation created by the massage. It is also important that the muscles stay warm, so suggest to clients that they wear loose, warm clothing, for example a tracksuit.
- You may find that the client's reflexes are very slow after massage, almost as if he or she has been sedated, so check to make sure the client is capable of driving.
- While not always possible, the client should avoid being thrown back immediately into the stresses of working – that is why an evening appointment is so beneficial. The client has time to rest and sleep, so will be more able to cope with everyday pressures at work.

Aftercare advice

- Recommend the client drink eight glasses of water a day for healthy functioning of cells, to improve the skin and aid digestion.
- Eat a light diet for 24–48 hours after the treatment. Avoid over-refined and processed foods, curries or other spicy foods.

- Avoid stimulants such as alcohol, tea and coffee. Try herbal tea, hot lemon juice or fruit juice.

- If the client smokes, recommend giving up.

- Take regular gentle exercise to help keep muscles flexible — encourage the client to join an exercise class, or take a gentle walk three times a week, or recommend a swim which keeps joints supple.

- Suggest the client sets aside time to relax.

- Try relaxation techniques and breathing exercises. The client may find that visualising a relaxing scene with eyes closed at times of stress will help keep the tension at bay, in between appointments with you.

- Any form of heat is very relaxing for tense, tired muscles, so a warm bath, a hot water bottle on the shoulders or a heat lamp will soothe aches and pains.

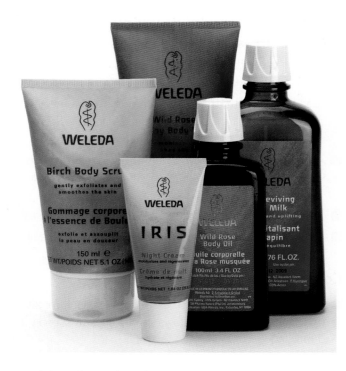

Homecare

As well as aftercare advice, you should recommend suitable products for the client to use at home.

Body scrub or exfoliation

This should be used weekly to prevent a build-up of dead skin cells so that the skin is kept smooth. Products contain finely ground olive stones, nuts, oatmeal or tiny synthetic micro-beads.

Body moisturiser lotion

Moisturisers are oil and water emulsions which help retain the moisture balance of the skin, keep the surface soft and smooth, prevent cracking and give some protection to the skin from the external environment. They should be applied morning and night for best results.

Loofah or body brushing

A variety of loofahs (body brushes) are available. They tend to be used in the shower when the skin is slightly damp, to remove dead skin cells and improve circulation and skin texture. Many cosmetic houses also produce abrasive gloves, which can be worn in the shower for really good exfoliation.

Your advice should be suitable and specific to the individual client's needs. If the client leaves feeling happy and pampered, with relaxed muscles, you will gain repeat business!

Check your knowledge

1 Manual massage is always carried out towards the:
   a) brain
   b) lymph nodes
   c) arms
   d) eyes.

2 Massage is very good for muscle tissue as it helps:
   a) remove hormones in the muscles
   b) improve balance
   c) tone the muscle
   d) increase blood flow and flexibility.

3 A client with a dry skin would most suit this medium.
   a) Oil
   b) Talc
   c) Cream
   d) Gel

4 Which of these movements is most relaxing on the body?
   a) Hacking
   b) Petrissage
   c) Effleurage
   d) Cupping

Check your knowledge (*cont.*)

5 Which of these movements would you avoid if the client had a varicose vein?
- **a)** Hacking
- **b)** Petrissage
- **c)** Effleurage
- **d)** Cupping

6 Hacking is done with:
- **a)** the whole hand
- **b)** the fingertips
- **c)** the knuckles
- **d)** the sides of the fingers.

7 The psychological effects of massage include:
- **a)** release of stress and anxiety
- **b)** release of tension in the muscles
- **c)** release of lymph into the lymph glands
- **d)** release of blood flow into the skin.

8 You should always use effleurage:
- **a)** to relieve tension in the muscles
- **b)** to link the massage movements together
- **c)** to manipulate the tissue firmly
- **d)** to bring blood to the skins surface.

9 A G5 machine is classed as:
- **a)** manual massage
- **b)** electrical massage
- **c)** mechanical massage
- **d)** Swedish massage.

10 An infrared lamp is used to:
- **a)** warm the tissue prior to massage
- **b)** warm the tissues after massage
- **c)** make the massage last longer
- **d)** make the client stay longer.

Getting ready for assessment

You are not allowed any simulation within this unit and you must practically demonstrate in your everyday work that you have met the Standards for providing body massage treatments.

You will be assessed on at least *four* separate occasions on four different clients and your assessments should include *two* full-body massages, including the face. One of the full-body massage treatments must include the use of mechanical massage and infrared treatment.

Treatment suggestions to cover all the ranges:

Back massage Male client	Infrared to warm the tissue Manual massage G5 on the trapezius muscle	Mediums: oil for manual massage talc for G5
Back massage Female client	Manual massage Audio-sonic to trapezius muscle	Medium: cream (if skin is oily)
Full body with face Male client	Manual massage to face and back G5 to legs, gluteals and arms (avoid abdomen)	Medium: cream and talc
Full body Female client	Manual massage to face and body	Medium of client's choice

Provide body massage treatments **B20**

Unit B23

Provide Indian head massage

What you will learn

- Maintain safe and effective methods of working when providing Indian head massage treatment
- Consult, plan and prepare for treatments, with clients
- Perform Indian head massage
- Provide aftercare advice

The Standards set out detailed performance criteria regarding:

- maintaining safe and effective methods of working when providing Indian head massage treatments
- consulting, planning and preparing for treatments with clients.

The majority of these requirements apply to all beauty therapy treatments and are therefore covered in detail in Professional basics unit, Body treatment – theory and consultation, and unit G22 Monitor procedures to safely control work operations. You should also refer back to You and the skin and Related anatomy and physiology, as required.

Treatment-specific requirements for Indian head massage are covered within this unit.

Introduction

Indian head massage is a massage delivered to the upper shoulders, face and scalp so is ideally delivered with the client in a seated position rather than lying down on a couch. This makes it a suitable treatment for the mobile therapist to perform and makes a lovely workplace massage. It is both relaxing and stimulating, and provides a sense of wellbeing and balance.

The physical effects and benefits to individual systems of the body are the same as any body massage treatment (for more information, see B20 Provide body massage treatments). On a purely physical level it relaxes muscle fibres, targets tension in the head, neck and shoulders and relieves stress, but on a more holistic level it is used to balance the chakras of the body and provides an alignment between all of the energy centres, making the client feel more grounded.

Indian head massage is an Eastern technique based on Ayurvedic philosophies, which date back 5000 years. Indian head massage is known as Champissage in India and is passed down in families as a ritual of massage and bonding and so is taught by example. Mothers perform massage on children; it is also performed by men in barber shops and even on the beach. These techniques have been adopted and have gained popularity in the West.

Ayurvedic medicine

'Ayurvedic' comes from the Sanskrit words 'ayus' and 'veda', meaning 'science of life'. Ayurvedic practices are a form of preventative medicine. They aim to balance flow of energy or 'prana' in the body in order to alleviate symptoms of 'disease' and prevent ill health.

Ayurveda is a holistic approach which treats the whole person, incorporating mind, body and spirit. Each person is treated as a unique individual rather than a set of symptoms. Ayurveda encourages people to achieve balance by living in harmony with themselves and their environment, and by taking control of every aspect of their life — thereby putting the body 'at ease'.

Chakras

An important element of Ayurvedic medicine is balancing the flow of energy in the body. The body is seen as having seven energy centres called 'chakras'. Chakras are termed as spinning vortexes of energy.

These are located in a vertical line running down the body and are classified as higher or lower, as shown in the table.

		Chakra	Location	Colour
HIGHER	1	Crown	Top of the head	Violet
	2	Third eye	Forehead in between the eyes	Indigo
	3	Throat	Base of the front of the neck	Blue
LOWER	4	The heart	In the chest cavity	Green
	5	The solar plexus	Sternum/stomach	Yellow
	6	Abdomen/sacral	Central abdomen by the navel	Orange
	7	Base chakra	Pelvis, coccyx	Red

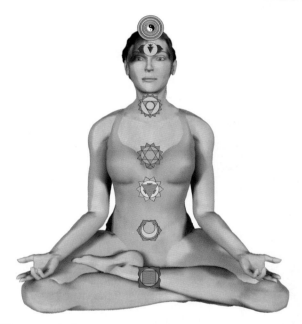

The seven chakras

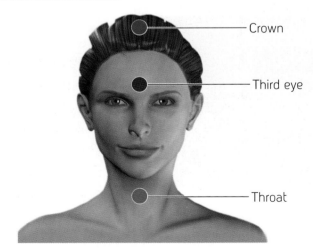

Position of the higher chakras

Crown

Third eye

Throat

Lower chakras

Base/pelvis/coccyx Element: earth Red Indian term: Muladhara Crystal/gem: Ruby	This relates to the pelvis and genital area. The Indian philosophy is that this energy is a serpent goddess lying coiled asleep around the base of the spine for protection. Its location means this chakra is concerned with the elimination of waste (both solid and fluid) and it also represents our foundations and connection to Mother Earth. If this chakra is not functioning properly a client is likely to feel as if they are on shaky foundations or ungrounded.
Abdomen/sacral/lumbar Element: water Orange Indian term: Swadhishthana Crystal/gem: Aquamarine or orange moonstone	This is connected to the bladder, the reproductive system and circulation. It is useful for the flow of creativity and is connected to the physical and emotional issues relating to sexuality. If this chakra is not functioning properly a client may feel they have lost their sexual drive or energy, and existence itself may seem pointless, with no creativity.
Stomach/solar plexus Element: fire Yellow Indian term: Manilura Crystal/gem: Topaz or citrine	This chakra relates to the energy we gain from food, and also our emotional energy, ego and personal power. When this is balanced and fine a client will find their vitality flows well and they enjoy a feeling of general wellbeing. As this is where the storage centre for life force is held, it is important that this chakra is nurtured otherwise a client may feel life draining away from them. We may say 'it felt like I was hit in the solar plexus' when we get upset about a major event in our lives. If this chakra is not functioning properly a client may become very low or feel despondent, making them hyper-sensitive to those around them and their reactions.
Chest/ heart Element: air Green Indian term: Anahata Crystal/gem: Emerald or rose quartz	This chakra mirrors its location: lungs and heart give oxygen and this chakra represents love and charity towards others. If this chakra is not functioning properly it is usually reflected in an unhappy social life. Clients may feel they have become fearful, bitter and even resentful.

Higher chakras

Throat Element: ether Blue Indian term: Vishuddha Crystal/gem: Sapphire or purple rainbow fluorite	This chakra of the throat, voice box and hearing represents communication and expression of ourselves to others. If this chakra is not functioning properly and clients are unable to communicate emotions, they may feel frustrated, misunderstood or tense.
Third eye/forehead Element: mind Indigo Indian term: Ajna Crystal/gem: Clear quartz	This is our inner vision and is the storehouse for imagination and memories. If this chakra is not functioning properly a client may experience nightmares, headaches, stress and sinus congestion. Irritability and tiredness may also occur.
Crown/top of head Element: spirit Violet Indian term: Sahasrara Crystal/gem: Diamond/amethyst	This is the master chakra – receiving and interpreting the information from the others. It is concerned with critical thinking, rational thought and decision-making. If this chakra is not functioning properly all the others may also suffer.

Indian head massage interacts with the three higher chakras: crown, third eye and throat. Each of these energy centres has an effect on the endocrine system and is allocated a particular colour (see table on pages 435–436).

With all the stresses of modern living and the fast pace of life, it is not surprising that the chakras become blocked, unbalanced or out of alignment with each other. We very rarely get the opportunity to be still and quiet and replenish our energy levels: there is always something to do!

Indian head massage will open up and balance the chakras and you will be giving a refreshing, caring treatment to your client who will feel restored, balanced and calmer afterwards.

Marma points

Marma in the ancient Indian language of Sanskrit means 'hidden or unseen' and Indian culture believes that this is where the physical meets the energy life force or *Qi*, in the body.

There are 107 marma points all over the body which represent where the vital energies flow – usually where muscle, veins and arteries meet or bone and tendons sit. There are also junctions where **Vata**, **Pitta** and **Kapha** gather. We work on the 37 marma points found in the head, neck and shoulders when delivering an Indian head massage. These points are similar to the pressure points used in acupuncture with either needle or manual manipulation and when stimulated they help release tension and help energy flow. Marma points can also be freed by the use of stimulating oils to help their function or soothing oils to calm and reduce inflammation.

Key terms

Qi *or* chi – life force.

Vata – a bio-energy formed from the elements metal/air and ether/wood.

Pitta – a bio-energy formed from the elements fire and water.

Kapha – a bio-energy formed from the elements water and earth.

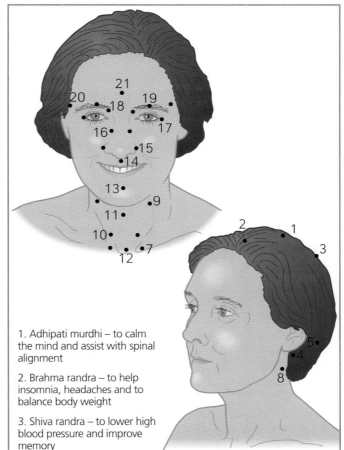

1. Adhipati murdhi – to calm the mind and assist with spinal alignment

2. Brahma randra – to help insomnia, headaches and to balance body weight

3. Shiva randra – to lower high blood pressure and improve memory

4. Vidhura – to help with congestion and to relieve tension and anxiety

5. Krikatika – to relieve spinal tension, relax the body and improve posture

6. Simanta – to help the body relax and to aid sleep

7. Arshak – to help digestion, anger management and to stabilise blood sugar

8. Manya – to improve facial circulation and ease sore throats or chest congestion

9. Sira matrika – to help improve circulation and the voice

10. Nila – to help improve the voice and ease a sore throat

11. Kantha – to help the thyroid and the expression of inner feelings

12. Kathanadi – to help with sore throats and upper respiratory congestion

13. Hanu – to help the heart connect with the heart feelings

14. Oshta – to prevent fainting, aid mental clarity and improve sexual desire

15. Phana – to balance brain function and aid ability to cope with stress

16. Gandu – to help clear the sinuses and brighten the eyes

17. Apanga – to relieve puffiness around the eye and clear the sinuses

18. Bhruh – to ease eyestrain and migraines

19. Avarta – to bring energy to the head and help with feeling centred

20. Shanka – to help calm and nourish the brain and mind

21. Sthapani – to relieve tension in the body and bring peace to the mind

Marma points on the face and neck

Consult, plan and prepare for treatments with clients

When consulting, planning and preparing for your Indian head massage treatment, you will need to refer closely to Professional basics, You and the skin, and Body treatments — theory and consultation.

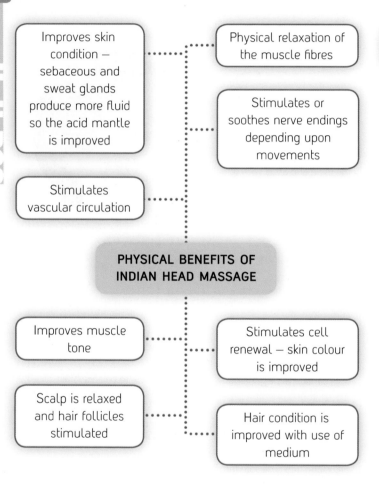

PHYSICAL BENEFITS OF INDIAN HEAD MASSAGE

- Improves skin condition — sebaceous and sweat glands produce more fluid so the acid mantle is improved
- Physical relaxation of the muscle fibres
- Stimulates or soothes nerve endings depending upon movements
- Stimulates vascular circulation
- Improves muscle tone
- Stimulates cell renewal — skin colour is improved
- Scalp is relaxed and hair follicles stimulated
- Hair condition is improved with use of medium

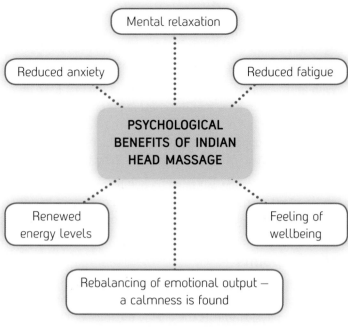

PSYCHOLOGICAL BENEFITS OF INDIAN HEAD MASSAGE

- Mental relaxation
- Reduced anxiety
- Reduced fatigue
- Renewed energy levels
- Feeling of wellbeing
- Rebalancing of emotional output — a calmness is found

Consultation techniques

You should always begin with the traditional consultation techniques of the massage consultation form, found in Body treatments — theory and consultation, page 328. However, if your client has the time, and you would like to incorporate a more holistic aspect, you can do the following consultation over a couple of visits and decide what dosha your client has and what characteristics they recognise in themselves. (See 'Doshas' below.)

This is not to be carried out in place of a more conventional full consultation, more as an enhancement. It allows the client to take an active part in the consultation — they are involved in their lifestyle choices and can often recognise the way forward to bring more balance into their lives. Sometimes it is difficult to tell a client that they need to make work/life balance changes — you must guide them, yet allow them to discover for themselves and recognise that wiser choices make for calmer, more balanced living!

Doshas

As well as energy centres, the body is seen to have three energies or forces known as doshas. These are:

- Vata dosha — the energy of movement and change
- Pitta dosha — the energy of transformation and metabolism
- Kapha dosha — the energy of structure and fluidity.

These three bio-energies determine an individual's physical, emotional and mental characteristics, since every person consists of a unique balance of these forces. The Ayurvedic practitioner offers advice and provides different treatments which aim to balance the three doshas, thereby promoting physical, emotional and mental harmony.

Characteristics of dosha types

Doshas are energies that influence body shape and size as well as physical and psychological characteristics. Each person contains a balance of the three doshas — Vata, Pitta

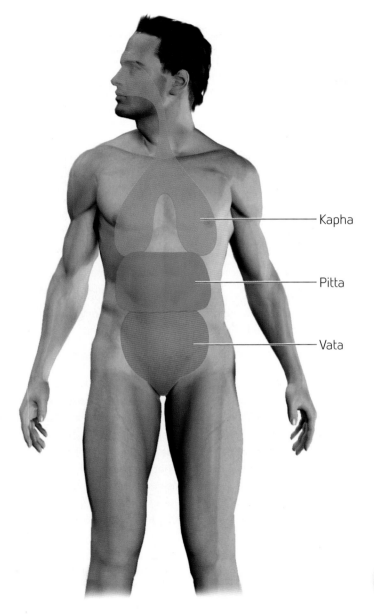

The three energy forces or doshas

Vata – physical characteristics	Vata – psychological characteristics
Thin and bony, and either very tall or very short.	Artistic and creative with a good imagination
Skin is generally thin, darkish and cool	Restless mind and poor memory
Hair is dark and coarse but thin and usually wavy	Fearful, anxious and prone to worrying
Moves quickly with short, fast steps	Spends money quickly
The face is usually long and angular	Often dissatisfied with and unable to sustain friendships.
Eyes tend to be small and dark brown/grey in colour	Active and sensitive nature
Small mouth with thin lips	Tends to avoid confrontation
Voice is low and speech is fast	Sexually, the most active

Factors thought to increase Vata

Exposure to cold	Suppressing natural urges
Lack of routine	Abdominal surgery
Eating too much dry, frozen or leftover food	Not oiling the skin
Travelling too much	

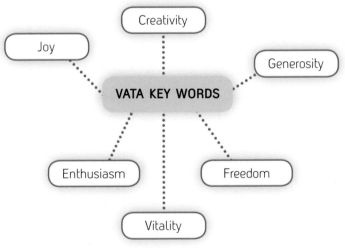

and Kapha — but one dosha is usually more dominant than the others.

A full description of the characteristics of each dosha type is provided below and overleaf. Each description includes a list of:

The physical characteristics	→	those factors believed to increase it
The mental characteristics	→	the key words associated with it

Pitta – physical characteristics	Pitta – psychological characteristics	Kapha – physical characteristics	Kapha – psychological characteristics
Moderately developed physique with muscular limbs	Articulate, intellectual, alert and focused	Well-developed, broad frame with large long limbs	Stable, steady, calm and patient
Strong, purposeful gait; moves at medium speed	Good organisational and decision-making skills	Large, rounded face with a wide, solid neck	Loyal, forgiving and honourable
Skin is fair, soft and sensitive to sun and allergies	Can be irritable, jealous and aggressive	Skin is thick, oily, pale and cold	Tends to be lethargic and sometimes lazy; is usually driven by others
Heart-shaped face	Argumentative and judgemental	Hair is thick, wavy and usually brown in colour	Analytic mind; takes time for consideration before reaching conclusions
Loud, strong voice	Good sense of humour		
Intense, light eyes of blue, grey or hazel	Excellent memory and fast learner	Big, attractive eyes which are blue or light brown	Too content to need fresh stimulation so can appear dull
Hair is fair or reddish, fine and soft	Money is usually spent on luxury items	Voice is deep and low, with slow rhythmic speech	Likely to spend money on food
Medium-sized mouth and lips; teeth which are yellowish	Moderately passionate in sexual pursuits and relationships	Mouth is large, lips are full, teeth are large and white	Strong, enduring sex drive and energy

Factors thought to increase Pitta		Factors thought to increase Kapha	
Over-exposure to heat Excessive red meat, salt or spicy food Indigestion and irregular meals Exercising at midday	Drugs and alcohol, especially antibiotics Too much intellectual work/thinking Fatigue Anger, fear and hatred	Over-exposure to cold Eating too much meat, dairy and fried foods Excessive water and salt intake Napping after meals	Doing nothing Sedatives and tranquilizers Doubt, greed and possessiveness Lack of compassion

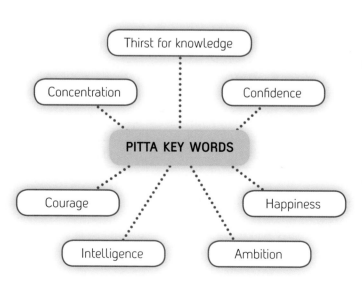

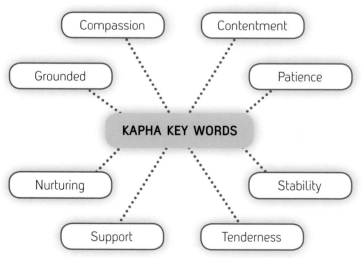

Dosha self-analysis test

This exercise will help to determine the dominant dosha, and can be used as a tool for consultation, treatment planning, and lifestyle and aftercare advice. Read through the different characteristics for each factor in the table below with the client, then tick the characteristics that apply. When you have finished, add up the scores in each column to find out which is their dominant dosha. You could try this yourself to enlighten your role as a holistic therapist.

FACTOR	VATA	✓	PITTA	✓	KAPHA	✓
Body frame	Thin and bony		Medium and balanced		Large and broad	
Weight	Underweight		Average		Overweight	
Skin type	Dry, dull and flaky		Soft, oily and rosy		Thick, moist and pale	
Hair	Dark, dry and wavy		Fair/red, soft, oily		Dark, thick, oily	
Teeth	Protruding, uneven		Medium, yellowish		Strong, white	
Nails	Dry, brittle, bitten		Soft, pink, strong		Large, white, soft	
Eyes	Small, dull, darting		Sharp, penetrating		Large with thick lashes	
Appetite	Variable		Healthy		Slow and steady	
Thirst	Variable		Excessive		Minimal	
Elimination	Dry, hard, constipated		Soft, oily, loose stools		Thick, heavy stools	
Urine	Frequent but sparse		Copious, very yellow		Infrequent, average amount	
Sweat	Minimal		Profuse, pungent		Slow to begin then heavy	
Pulse	Weak		Stable, strong		Slow, smooth	
Circulation	Sluggish		Good		Moderate	
Speech	High voice, fast		Loud, clear, strong		Slow, rhythmic	
Libido	Variable, based in fantasy		Passionate, excessive		Slow, strong, loyal	
Immunity	Low		Moderate		High	
Activity	Restless		Directed		Minimal	
Endurance	Minimal		Moderate		Very good	
Mind	Curious, restless		Clever, aggressive		Calm, slow	
Memory	Short-term good		Good, sharp		Long-term good	
Routine	Dislikes		Likes		Tolerates	
Faith	Changes		Fanatical		Devoted	
Dreams	Frequent, fearful		Fiery, vivid		Calm, romantic	
Opinions	Fluctuate		Firm, express forcefully		Change slowly	
Finances	Spends quickly, poor		Buys luxuries, moderate		Thrifty, rich	
Hobbies	Travel, philosophy, art		Luxuries, politics, sport		Leisurely, serene	
Food	Sparse, snacking		Regular meals		Gourmet, fatty foods	
Creativity	Original ideas		Technical, scientific		Entrepreneurial	
Sensitivities	Cold, dry		Heat, sun		Damp, cold, humid	
Temperament	Nervous, shy		Determined, motivated		Resilient, conservative	
Sleep	Minimal, disturbed, light		Moderate, sound		Excessive, heavy	
TOTAL	VATA SCORE		PITTA SCORE		KAPHA SCORE	

Provide Indian head massage Unit B23

Symptoms of dosha imbalance

Any imbalance in dosha is likely to have a negative effect on your client's physical and psychological wellbeing. They are also likely to display the negative aspects associated with dominant dosha. Negative emotions then aggravate the dosha associated with them, which in turn perpetuates the negativity.

The way to break this cycle is to pacify the aggravated dosha by restoring balance. The philosophy of 'like increase like' applies here — for example, if a client has a tendency to be impatient or over-critical (characteristics of excess Pitta) they should try to reduce those experiences which increase negative Pitta characteristics, such as eating spicy food or thinking too much.

Symptoms of Vata imbalance

Symptoms of excess	Nervousness and confusion Moodiness Impairment of sensory functions Loss of consciousness Fear and anxiety Sadness and grief Constipation	Tremors in limbs Insomnia Insecurity Dry, rough skin Lack of integrity Lack of creativity Poor communication
Symptoms of lack	Lethargy Nausea Depression Digestive disorders	

Symptoms of Pitta imbalance

Symptoms of excess	Ambition Anger Critical tendencies and scepticism Fear of failure Snappy speech Pride Burning sensations and fever	Excess thirst Loss of sleep Frustration Envy Craving for cold Hatred
Symptoms of lack	Irregular bowel movements Dull skin Indigestion Feeling cold	

Symptoms of Kapha imbalance

Symptoms of excess	Boredom and lack of interest Carelessness Lack of compassion for others Greed Excess sleep Obesity Obsessive or possessive behaviour Unkindness Disturbed digestion and nausea Feeling unsupported or unloved
Symptoms of lack	Thirst Muscular cramps Feeling giddy Aches and pains Dry mouth

Perform Indian head massage

In this section you will learn about:

- contra-indications to treatment
- treatment times
- client preparation
- massage mediums
- correct breathing techniques
- carrying out the massage, step by step.

Contra-indications to treatment

More visible contra-indications:

- Skin which is thin or papery, or damaged
- Infectious skin diseases, for example scabies, as there is a risk of cross-infection
- Any infestation of the head — for example head lice
- A recent head or neck injury/whiplash/operation to the head
- Non-infectious skin disorders, for example eczema, dermatitis
- A bruise, sepsis, spots, boils — avoid the area as there is a risk of cross-infection, the treatment might spread or worsen the condition, and the client will experience discomfort
- Recent sunburn, to the face or scalp (clients with very thin hair or bald patches can often have sunburn on the scalp)

- Tumours, unrecognisable lumps, bumps and swellings of either skin or the joints, or painful areas or unidentified lumps in the scalp
- Any damaged muscles or tissue swellings, for example sprains in the spine, upper back or shoulder joints – avoid the area, as massage worsens the condition and the client will experience discomfort
- Any form of acute joint disease or inflammation, for example rheumatoid arthritis in the treatment area
- Under the influence of alcohol or drugs
- Postural deformities, for example scoliosis or spastic conditions
- Avoid tapotement on extremely thin or elderly clients

Less visible contra-indications (obtain a doctor's approval before treating):

- Clients with chronic diabetes tend to have thin, papery skin that bruises easily
- Migraines or severe headaches
- Clients with haemophilia may have no clotting capacity and could bleed
- Clients with epilepsy
- Clients with asthma or a lung condition – the treatment may require adaptation
- Clients with a cardiac condition, high or low blood pressure, including clients who have had a stroke or suffer from thrombosis. People with low blood pressure can feel faint when suddenly sitting up
- High temperature
- Immediately before or after operations
- Stomach complaints, for example diarrhoea
- Cuts/abrasions – cover these with a waterproof dressing, and avoid the area due to risk of cross-infection and client discomfort
- Allergies – select appropriate massage medium and carry out a patch test, if necessary
- Medication – if a client is on medication for a health condition that could be affected by massage treatment, a doctor's approval will be needed
- Pregnancy – if a client is in the early stages and is suffering from sickness it is best to avoid the massage as it may induce nausea

Think about it

A contra-action is different from a contra-indication. A contra-indication prevents the massage from being carried out, or means that the area should be avoided during massage.

A contra-action is a reaction that occurs during the treatment. Should one occur during your treatment, always act promptly to remove the massage medium and apply a cool compress or soothing lotion to calm the skin.

Scalp and hair considerations

Alopecia is a degree of hair loss and it can be caused by a variety of reasons: hormonal influences such as pregnancy or the menopause, or stress can cause patchy hair loss and certain drugs such as chemotherapy cause the hair to fall out.

Indian head massage can help by stimulating the blood to go to the hair follicles (and it is generally stimulating to the whole skin/scalp), but if the client is still in the process of losing hair, they may wish to seek medical advice before having a treatment. Some of the movements include pulling on the hair shaft, and this may make the situation worse.

You may come across these terms used in discussion of alopecia:

Alopecia universalis or totalis	Total loss of hair
Alopecia areata	Circular areas or patches of hair loss
Alopecia androgenic senialis	Classic male pattern baldness: loss of hair from the top and crown of the head, with a circle left from ear to ear
Alopecia cicatrical	Hair loss caused by scarring burns or operations on the head
Alopecia traction	This is where the hair has been pulled too tight at the root in a constant pony tail – or from heavy hair extensions and the hair breaks off at the root, most common along the temples
Alopecia diffuse	General thinning that can occur in males or females especially with age and genetic inheritance

Treatment times

Your Indian head massage will last for 45 minutes in total, including consultation, massage and aftercare. You should follow all the advice and guidance about setting up for treatment in unit B20 Provide body massage treatments – the same principles of heating, lighting, warmth and inviting environmental conditions apply to all massage techniques.

> **Think about it**
>
> Remember to ask your client about their massage preferences, such as depth and pressure of movements. You may also need to adjust your movements to meet treatment objectives, such as light movements to aid relaxation or soothe the tender skin of a diabetic client, or to avoid contra-indicated areas. Check your client's comfort as the massage progresses and offer to vary the pressure if necessary.
>
> You will also need to adapt your massage and increase petrissage movements on clients with very short or no hair because some of the recommended movements will not apply.

Client preparation

- Ideally, if using oil, full removal of outdoor clothing is best, although in some cases a dry Indian head massage can be delivered over thin clothing such as a loosened shirt or blouse. For maximum benefit the client should be asked to remove all upper body clothing, and be wrapped in a large towel under the arms, to prevent oil dripping onto underwear. Trousers, skirts and socks/tights can be left on, and ensure the client feels warm and cosy in a towel.

- Advise the female client to keep her bra on, but remove the straps entirely – if they are draped over the shoulder you may get oil on them or rub against the skin which will be uncomfortable.

- Ask the client to remove shoes and plant both feet on the floor, slightly apart – this will ground them and provide a firm base for the client. (A Reiki practitioner wishing to use Reiki to enhance an Indian head massage may also remove her own shoes as it grounds the therapist, but do check with your Awarding Body about that – it may not be acceptable under assessment conditions.)

- Ideally, position the client on a suitable firm chair with a solid back rest and arms if possible. To allow the client to fully relax, the bottom needs to be firmly back in the base of the seat, spine supported and arms loosely at the side. Indian head massage can be performed on a massage stool or the client laying supine as for body massage but adaptation of the massage will be required. Breathing will be made easier if the client is upright. This massage is ideal for someone in a wheelchair as means the client can be treated in situ.

- Remove all jewellery, including earrings, and remove glasses. Check for hair pieces, extensions and wigs – the scalp massage is quite vigorous and may dislodge a hair piece or be uncomfortable if it is glued on.

- If the client has hair up, ask them to remove all the pins and grips and gently brush the hair out, so that oil does not mix in with hairspray – it can get very sticky and form clumps which, again, is uncomfortable and will detract from the massage.

- If the client has make-up on, perform a gentle cleanse routine to remove foundation and powder. Eye make-up can be left on, providing it has not smudged or run – and the eyes are not irritated.

- You are now ready to choose a suitable massage medium, based on client needs and preferences which you have discovered during your consultation.

Massage mediums

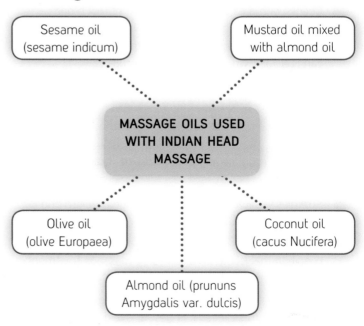

When choosing a medium remember the following:

- Client preference – they may just want a non-allergenic cream or a dry massage.

- Check your client is not allergic to nuts – most oils are nut-based, so a patch test is essential 24 hours prior to the treatment if there is any doubt.
- Pre-warm the oil to help spread the medium and prevent the client from jumping when you put it on the skin. Either use the infrared lamp for a few minutes or warm it between the hands. *Don't put it in a microwave to heat it as this constitutes a health and safety risk.*
- Oil will feed and nourish both the scalp and the hair shaft, rather like a deep conditioning treatment, but this may not be ideal if the client cannot wash their hair before going back to work.
- The best quality oils are unrefined and organic.

Type of medium	Characteristics and benefits
Sesame oil	The best quality sesame oil is warm-pressed from tiny seeds. It has a yellow colour and a nutty smell. However, there is a tendency towards bitterness with this oil. It is used for strengthening and nourishing the skin and scalp. Good for the relief of muscular aches and pains and used widely in India as it has hair colouring restorative properties – they believe it stops the hair losing its pigment and turning white. (Grey hair is really white, but mixed in with dark hair it looks grey.) Sesame oil is rich in vitamins and minerals and is a natural sun screen.
Mustard oil	This is usually mixed with almond oil. As this is a hot oil by nature it is good for increasing and warming the body temperature and tissues, so is good for pain relief and stiffness in the joints. It's good to use in a winter treatment, but can irritate sensitive skin because of its heat.
Olive oil	This oil is extracted from the olives when they are hard and unripened. It can be used to replace sesame oil as its properties are similar: it helps with muscular pain and stiffness, increases body heat and is ideal on a dehydrated, sore or inflamed skin.
Almond oil	This is from the sweet almond tree and is warm-pressed to release the oil from the nut. The oil is sweet, slightly thick and sticky in texture. Any irritated, itchy skin would benefit from almond oil treatment. It is widely used in facial massage and manicure treatments too. It warms the body and reduces pain, is soothing and moisturising.

Type of medium	Characteristics and benefits
Coconut oil	This oil is retrieved by solvent extraction from the dried flesh of a coconut, and is semi-solid until warmed. It retains the distinctive coconut smell, and often evokes memories of holidays as it is used in a lot of sun-screen preparations. It is moisturising and balancing, but can also be an irritant.
Cream	Cream may be preferred by a client who does not like the feel of oil on the skin, or who has an oily skin and does not want further oil applied. Use a non-allergenic, water-based cream, which is suitable to moisturise a dry or dehydrated skin – remember to decant the product with a spatula into a bowl before use.

For further information about oils, their properties, extraction methods, storage and safe use, see Unit B24 Carry out massage using pre-blended aromatherapy oils.

Positioning yourself

Remember it is important to position yourself comfortably with everything you need close at hand. Refer back to the detail in Unit B20 Provide body massage treatments for further information about your posture and how to avoid injury or strain.

Correct breathing techniques

Good breathing techniques should be incorporated into all massage techniques to help open up the body to receive more oxygen and get rid of carbon dioxide. In our modern, fast-paced society we are always rushing and many of us have got into the habit of short shallow breathing using only the upper part of the lungs, which is not only inefficient, it is counter- productive to relaxation.

As a therapist spend a few minutes really noticing your breathing and take time to breathe more deeply from almost your tummy, near the solar plexus at the bottom of your sternum, where the diagraph muscle will push up against the lungs to fully expand them. When doing your breathing exercises, clear your mind, visualise the healing colours of violet and white and calm yourself in for preparation for a good treatment.

Breathing with the client

When everything is fully prepared and you have your client in place, have washed your hands and are about to start — ask your client to breathe with you. Take five deep breaths in, through your nose and force it out through your mouth to the count of four — two seconds in and two seconds out. Ask the client to join you, and as they do so, place your hands over the throat chakra, but without contact, hovering just in front of it, then go over the face up to the third eye and then the crown chakra — all whilst you are both drawing life force breaths into your bodies, in harmony. You may wish to think a positive affirmation to the client such as 'I give this treatment with light and love and positivity' so that the energy transmitted in the treatment is for the good of the client and given without any negativity. The correct breathing techniques will also provide you with enough oxygen to encourage your full concentration and stamina throughout the massage.

You are now in sync with your client and can begin the treatment.

Indian head massage – a step-by-step guide

Repeat each massage movement three times before moving on to the next step, but remember to adapt the routine to suit your client's needs.

1 Hands placed on head, deep breathing for client and therapist. Add massage medium.

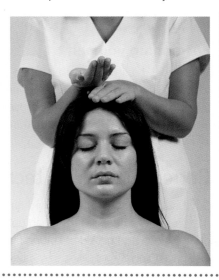

2 Honour the chakras of the throat by placing hands in front of it and deep breathing with your client.

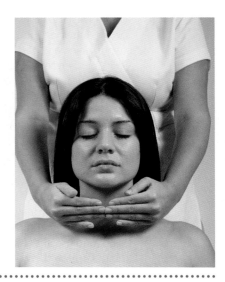

3 Carry out the same action for the third eye.

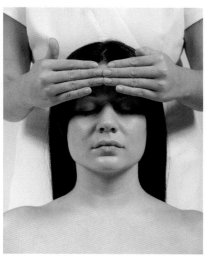

4 Carry out the same action for the crown chakra — they are now open to be balanced.

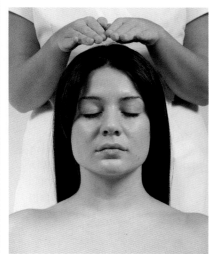

Indian head massage – a step-by-step guide (*cont.*)

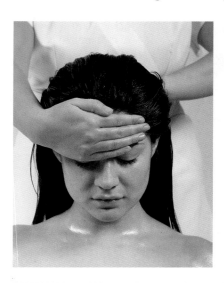

5 Move the head forwards ...

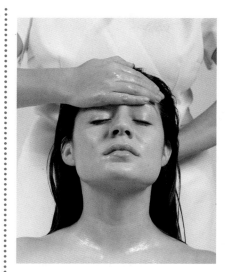

6 ... and backwards.

7 Then move the head from side to side.

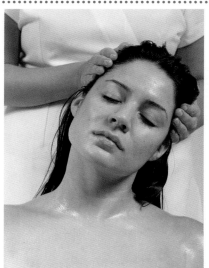

8 Smooth down, moulding around the head, neck, shoulders and arms. Perform thumb effleurage up the back with increasing pressure.

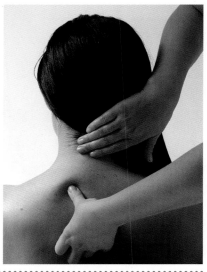

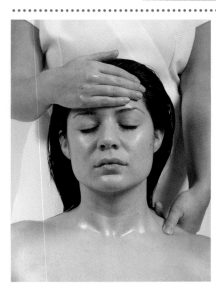

9 Carry out thumb circles across the shoulders and down the arms.

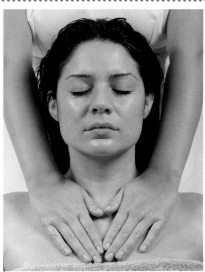

10 Perform effleurage to the neck and shoulders.

Indian head massage – a step-by-step guide (*cont.*)

11 Circle along the outline of the shoulder blade with the heel of the hand, starting at the base of the scapula. Repeat this movement, circling around each scapula with the fingers. Perform finger frictions from spine to scapula.

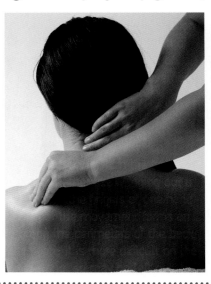

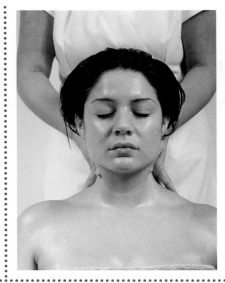

12 Perform skin rolls from thumb to fingers and vice versa across the shoulder.

13 Perform hacking movements to back and shoulders, followed by cupping to back and shoulders.

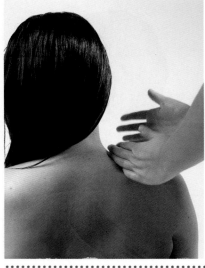

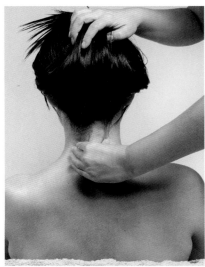

14 Perform neck squeezes at both sides of spine between thumb and finger.

15 Using heel of hand, create frictions along occipital bone.

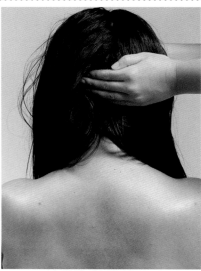

16 Using heel of hand, rub from front to back of head. Insert a neck support if required.

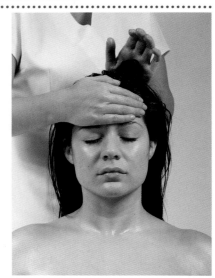

Indian head massage – a step-by-step guide (*cont.*)

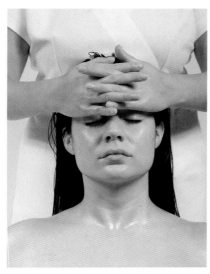

17 Link hands in front of client's face, moving upwards to connect with the higher chakras.

18 Perform effleurage to the face.

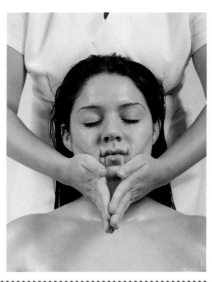

19 Continue with effleurage to the face.

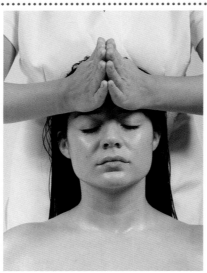

20 Circle at temples using palms of hands.

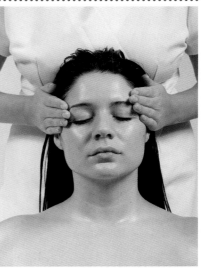

21 Perform finger frictions from front to back of head.

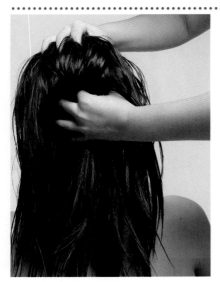

22 Pull hair upwards at the root, hold and release.

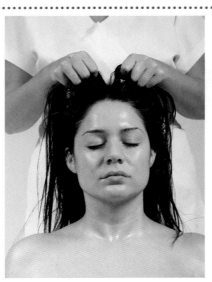

Indian head massage – a step-by-step guide (*cont.*)

23 Using the fingertips, create raindrop movements over the head.

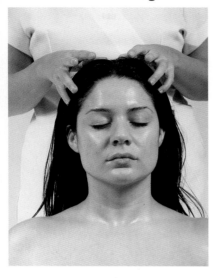

24 Using the fingertips, rake through the hair.

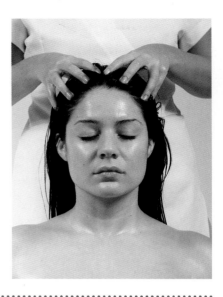

25 Gentle fingertip tapotement across the whole face, avoiding the eyes.

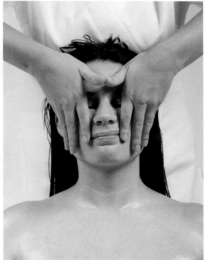

26 Perform finger circles in an arc from eyebrows to hairline.

27 Perform finger drainage from the midline of the face out towards the ears. Support the head by the jaw.

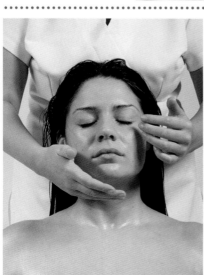

28 Knead the outer ears.

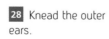

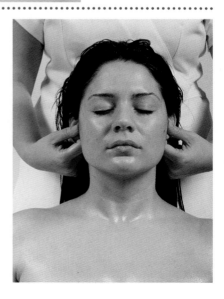

Indian head massage – a step-by-step guide (*cont.*)

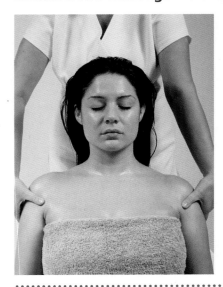

29 Effleurage from the outer edge of the shoulders up the neck to just under the ears, then down the arms.

30 Perform arm rolls using heel of hand from shoulder to elbow. Lift and squeeze between heel and fingers, working down arms.

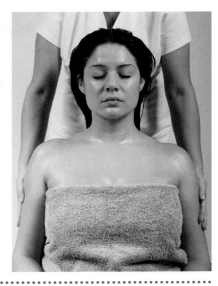

31 Lift shoulder joints, hold and release.

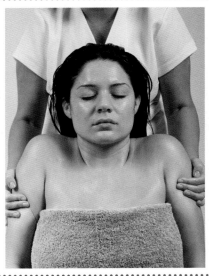

32 Shoulder hold to finish.

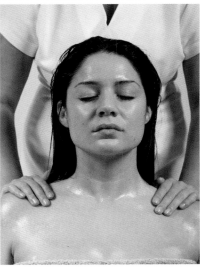

After treatment allow your client to wake up and become alert gradually – which may take some time!

Ideally, encourage your client to leave the oil on for the next 24 hours to nourish and replenish the scalp and skin.

Post-treatment advice is very important and you must spend time with your client to ensure they are fully functioning prior to leaving the salon. They should have a drink of water and not rush straight back to work or drive, as they may not be fully in charge of their faculties, which is dangerous.

Explain to the client that one Indian head massage is extremely beneficial, but a course of treatments is advisable as the cumulative effects of several treatments are even more noticeable. The client will develop a self-awareness of emotional and physical changes – especially if the client has been through a life-changing event such as bereavement, divorce or house/job changes.

Provide Indian head massage **Unit B23**

Salon life

Alice's story

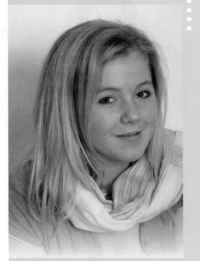

My name is Alice and I'm a second year student. I'm really enjoying my Indian head massage training and asked mum's friend, Carole, to be one of my case studies. She's a reflexologist so she understands meridians, chakras and health relationships. She has long dark hair, so sesame oil was an ideal choice for my medium. At our first treatment together, Carole had no contra-indications present. I sat her in the white beauty chair, with a backrest to support her spine. We began with deep breathing whilst I concentrated on opening her chakras. She began to see colours and the massage was going really well — I was under assessment so I was really working on getting my massage movements right and in sequence. Suddenly, I became aware that Carole was sliding sideways to my left and off the chair completely —

almost in slow motion — falling from her trunk with her feet still on the floor! I was massaging her scalp so I kind of caught her by her hair and kept her upright. She half-jumped and then looked at me really strangely so my assessor came over to find out what had happened. We think that Carole was so relaxed by the massage that she had fallen asleep and I woke her up by pulling her hair. She had completely zoned out of her surroundings and was not able to support herself in the chair. I gave her a drink of water and we moved to a firmer chair with arm and backrests to start the treatment again.

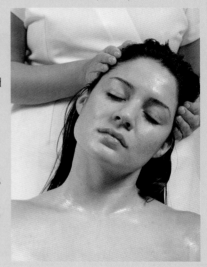

This has taught me that some clients are more reactive or susceptible to treatments than others. Carole was in need of more support than I or the chair was giving her. In her case, it may even have been best to give her a head massage laying on a couch, so she could really go to sleep in safety. I'm so glad I was able to catch her — if she had fallen right off, she could have been hurt. Health and safety is always so important for every treatment.

Effects for the therapist:

- Realise that clients can take holistic treatments very deeply and that people's reactions may vary
- Understand that health and safety is important, no matter what the treatment is
- All aspects of the treatment should be taken into account — client care is more important than getting the massage sequence right. The client is not aware of the order of treatment, only the effect it has on them

Effects for the client:

- The client may feel insecure and not fully 'let go' during the treatment if they are worried or inhibited about falling off the chair, snoring or falling asleep
- Muscles may become stiff if the client is holding a posture which is not comfortable or relaxing — the exact opposite of what the treatment is supposed to achieve
- The client may be aware that they fall asleep easily and 'zone out' of their surrounding — it is worth asking so that the therapist is forewarned and can take appropriate precautions

Provide aftercare advice

- contra-actions to Indian head massage
- aftercare
- homecare advice
- lifestyle changes.

Contra-actions to Indian head massage

Contra-actions are really reactions to the treatment, and they occur within 24 hours of the treatment. They can be physical symptoms, as the body clears itself, or mental, due to emotional cleansing of the mind or general lethargy and tiredness. They are collectively referred to as the healing crisis.

Do explain to the client that they may experience all, or none, of these contra-actions — or mild versions of them, depending upon their personal situation. There is a fine line between informing the client of possibilities and implanting the notion that all of these will occur. A simple aftercare leaflet is a good way of helping the client — they can take it away with them and look up any symptoms and feel reassured that it is normal. Obviously if symptoms last a lot longer than 24 hours then it could be a serious illness so a doctor's advice should be sought.

Worsening of current ailments	To promote healing, the body must first acknowledge the problem and expel it, in order to rebalance and heal. Suppressing symptoms means the body is in denial and Indian head massage will bring on dormant symptoms in order to flush them out. If a client has been struggling on with a cold and has not given in to it, massage will bring it right out so the body can get rid of it, and move on. It is important the client understands this — and doesn't blame poor hygiene or the therapist for giving them the cold! Whatever the symptom, stifling it will not work. It must come out and may get worse before it gets better.
Cleansing reactions	This is the body physically cleansing itself — through extra perspiration, producing more urine, more frequent bowel movements — often diarrhoea and/or an upset tummy, rashes, or cold and flu-like symptoms. Mucous production may increase so that nasal congestion occurs, sore throats and nausea may appear. These are normal cleansing reactions to your body rebalancing.
Tiredness	Tiredness is the body's way of telling you that sleep is required for healing, growth and repair of tissues. Give in and go to sleep early, or advise your client to cat-nap or have a siesta for twenty minutes during the day, where possible. The toxins released from the muscular massaging combined with emotional rebalancing can make a client really tired — this is a good thing and necessary. Tiredness may be combined with aching limbs and a headache. Overriding the tiredness mechanism can lead to accidents and poor performance.
Emotional disturbance	It's not unusual for a client to feel very wobbly, tearful or slightly depressed and low after Indian head massage. Again, this is a cleansing act for the emotions — especially if the client has been holding on to too many issues or has not yet dealt with big resentments which have been dormant in the subconscious. Tears are the body's way of washing and healing and, again, should not be denied.

Aftercare and homecare advice

- Possible healing crisis and contra-actions — ranging from a headache or cold to flu-like symptoms and lots of tears
- Reduce all stimulants to allow healing to happen — less tea and coffee, no alcohol and more herbal teas and fresh juice
- Eat a light diet with protein and vitamins to promote cellular renewal and healing
- Reduce or give up (if possible) smoking
- Relaxation promotion — relaxation tapes, visualisation, meditation or yoga, or just taking ten minutes to breathe and empty the mind

- Take gentle regular exercise such as walking in the fresh air and touching earth through gardening to help ground and reconnect them

- Reading prior to sleep will help still the mind

- Avoid over-stimulation — violent films or loud music and aggression will over-stimulate the brain and is not conducive to sleep and relaxation

- Remember to stress the importance of regular treatments and the cumulative effect

- Drink plenty of still fresh water to flush out toxins and rehydrate the body

- Advise the client on correct procedure for removal of the massage medium — when removing oil, apply neat shampoo before the hair is wet (it doesn't lather but the action of the shampoo will dissolve the oil molecules) and wash off as normal

- Regular warm baths and the use of a hot water bottle or heated wheat pillow will help alleviate sore or tense muscles, especially in the upper back

- Hair care is essential for maintaining the benefits of the massage stimulation — encourage the client to have regular trims and to use the correct skin and scalp products

Lifestyle changes

This is a delicate subject to broach with clients and it has to be dictated by them. Take their lead if they ask you for advice, but clients will take offence if you give them a long list of what is 'right and wrong' and you may end up losing your client altogether. Do not set them up to fail with extreme diet or lifestyle restrictions. Nor is it about judgement and implying you are morally superior with clients. It is about helping your client achieve what they can to feel better about themselves.

It is better to talk through one positive, achievable aim rather than being unrealistic on client lifestyle changes. It could be suggested that the client cut down cigarette use per day, or have a couple of alcohol-free days per week — or swap fizzy drinks for water. Small achievable goals will make the client feel empowered and in control — rather than hopeless and a failure!

Clients are usually very aware of how to enjoy a healthier lifestyle and will often not need to be told — but it isn't easy for a busy person to get more sleep/relaxation/time off and so on. Especially if the client is a carer with dependents, or works really hard to support a family and has financial restrictions — so be realistic, supportive and make the time the client is with you as enjoyable and relaxing as can be.

Check your knowledge

1 The chakras are:
   a) pressure points of the body
   b) energy channels in the body
   c) meridians of the body
   d) lymph points of the body.

2 Green is the colour associated with:
   a) the crown chakra
   b) the third eye
   c) the heart/chest
   d) the base chakra.

3 Sesame oil is thought to:
   a) help keep the hair colour
   b) keep in body heat
   c) help cool the tissues
   d) make the nails grow strong.

4 Almond oil comes from:
   a) seeds
   b) olives
   c) nuts
   d) leaves.

5 A contra-action to treatment may be:
   a) dry skin
   b) crying
   c) alopecia
   d) dandruff.

6 Which of the following is *not* a contra-indication?
   a) Baldness
   b) Alcohol consumption
   c) Skin infection
   d) Heart conditions

7 Where does Ayurvedic treatment originate?
   a) Turkey
   b) India
   c) Japan
   d) China

8 How many marma points are there on the head and neck?
   a) 28
   b) 37
   c) 56
   d) 107

9 The benefits of an Indian head massage include:
   a) clearing of chakras and rebalancing
   b) body lifting and toning
   c) deep-cleansing the skin
   d) removing the hair.

10 Homecare advice should include:
   a) eating spicy food
   b) doing strenuous exercise
   c) drinking coffee
   d) drinking water.

Getting ready for assessment

You are not allowed any simulation within this unit and you must practically demonstrate in your everyday work that you have met the Standards for providing Indian head massage treatments.

Your assessor will observe your performance on at least *three* separate occasions, each time on different clients. *One* massage must include massage oil and *one* must exclude massage oil.

From the ranges you must show that you have:

• used all consultation techniques
• dealt with all the client characteristics
• dealt with at least one of the necessary actions
• used all massage techniques
• covered all treatment areas
• given all types of advice.

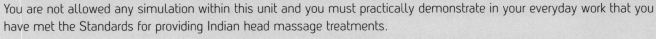

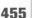

Provide Indian head massage **Unit B23**

Carry out massage using pre-blended aromatherapy oils

What you will learn

- Maintain safe and effective methods of working when providing massage using pre-blended aromatherapy oils
- Consult, plan and prepare for treatments with clients
- Massage the body using pre-blended aromatherapy oils
- Provide aftercare advice

The Standards set out detailed performance criteria regarding:

- maintaining safe and effective methods of working when providing massage
- consulting, planning and preparing for treatments with clients.

The majority of these requirements apply to all beauty therapy treatments and are therefore covered in detail in Professional basics, Body treatments – theory and consultation, and unit G22 Monitor procedures to safely control work operations. You should also refer back to You and the skin and Related anatomy and physiology, as required. Unit B13 Provide body electrical treatments explains the physical characteristics of a client and the postural problems you may encounter, such as lordosis, kyphosis and scoliosis.

Treatment-specific requirements for pre-blended aromatherapy massage are covered within this unit.

Introduction

Aromatherapy involves the use of **essential oils** to promote physical, mental and emotional balance. It is the use of fragrance, combined with the properties of the oils, which enhances a person's frame of mind to promote relaxation, to stimulate, to give a sense of wellbeing, to uplift and to help with detoxification and cellulite.

However, there is more to aromatherapy than just the action of essential oils. Aromatherapy consists of a combination of the essential oils and their actions, the benefits of massage, the personal input of the therapist, the relaxing ambience of the treatment room, the active participation of the person seeking help and the subtle power of healing.

In aromatherapy massage, essential oils are blended with a carrier oil to provide the massage medium to enhance the treatment, but there are also other methods by which the client can enjoy oils, such as inhaling oils, burning them, aromatherapy candles and adding oils to a bath.

For your Level 3 qualification you will be using pre-blended oils, already made up by the manufacturer for use, and you will not need, nor will you be qualified, to blend your own. However, you still need to understand the properties, characteristics and the origins of the oils. As you will not be blending, some information is not required, such as chemical composition, ratios and synergistic blending and this is therefore not included within this unit.

Key terms

Aromatherapy – the use of fragrance and smell to alter or affect a person's mood or behaviour.

Carrier oil – a base oil used to dilute essential oils before they are applied to the skin in massage and aromatherapy treatments.

Essential oil – natural essence, in the form of oil, that is extracted from plants, herbs, flowers, leaves, berries, fruit, bark, resin, seeds, wood, roots or grasses.

Fragrance – one or a blend of fragrant or volatile plant oils. Fragrance is added to products to give them a pleasant aroma.

Perfume – a mixture of essential oils, aroma compounds (chemical fragrances), stabilising and preserving agents, and solvent to create a pleasant-smelling liquid.

The following table outlines the key terms used in the description of odours.

Term	Explanation	Example
Animalic	Odours associated with animals	Underlying heavy notes in jasmine, orange flower absolutes
Balsamic	Sweet and vanilla-like	Benzoin, resinoid
Citrus	Odours of citrus fruits	Lemon and orange oil
Coniferous	Fresh green and resinous notes of cut green pine cones	Rosemary oil, pine and fir oils
Earthy	The smell of rain-moistened earth	Patchouli oil
Floral	Odours of fragrant flowers	1% rose or 1% jasmine absolute in a carrier oil
Fruity	Odours of edible fruits	Any of the citrus oils, roman camomile oil
Green	Odours of crushed, green leaves	Violet leaf absolute
Herbaceous or herbal	Odours of culinary herbs	Thyme and sage oils
Medicated	Odours suggesting medication	Wintergreen and ylang-ylang oils
Minty	Notes given by spearmint or peppermint leaves, when stroked	Spearmint and peppermint oils
Resinous	Odours of fragrant resins	Myrrh and frankincense
Spicy	Odours of culinary spices	Clove, cinnamon and coriander
Woody	Odours of exotic woods	Sandalwood and cedarwood oils

A brief history of aromatherapy

Throughout the centuries, plants have been used for their healing properties. Ancient cultures such as the Egyptians used temple incense, perfumes and fragrant oils. In their quest for a comfortable afterlife, wealthy Egyptians would have many expensive oils in their burial tombs and

B24 Carry out massage using pre-blended aromatherapy oils

pyramids. When King Tutankhamen's tomb was opened 3000 years after his death there were calcite pots which he was buried with, still giving off a faint smell of the spices, such as frankincense. The embalming process, especially for royalty, involved wrapping the corpse in bandages soaked in frankincense, myrrh, clove, cedarwood, cypress and other oils for fragrant and antiseptic properties.

The ancient Greeks had the word *aromata* to describe the various spices, medicines and incense they used. The Romans introduced the concept of communal bathing to Great Britain, and this involved pouring oils into the waters and also oils being massaged on the body, to keep the body smelling nice and to keep the skin supple, in our colder climate.

The Normans liked to put aromatic leaves on the floor as it was believed (quite rightly) that the antibacterial properties would ward off disease and deter fleas and lice. It also helped to reduce the smell in houses which were un-plumbed and had poor sanitation.

A French chemist, Renée Maurice Gattefosse, is often referred to as 'the father of modern aromatherapy' and is credited with introducing the phrase *aroma* — meaning fragrant or sweet-smelling — and *therapy*, which means healing treatment. So, the word itself was not introduced until the twentieth century. Gattefosse wrote a book about aromatherapy in 1937 and in France aromatherapy is still regarded as a science. Marguerite Maury developed his theory in the 1950s and it has evolved into the therapeutic practice we still use today.

Now aromatherapy is a big business, worth millions of pounds. It is used widely in salons for treatments, and in retail it is included in everything from pillows to aid sleep (lavender) to bath products, pot pourri and even neat oils sold over the counter. Health professionals use it — but both its healing properties and its toxicity are not to be under-estimated.

Think about it

This unit is about pre-blended oils, and is not the same as having a full practitioner qualification to blend oils and dispense them. This unit is perfectly acceptable for employment in health spas, salons and cruise ships, but you need a full Diploma to become a clinical aromatherapist. If you begin to blend undiluted oils it will null and void your insurance and you will be unprotected, should anything go wrong.

What you must know

To enable you to complete this unit, it is important that you firstly understand and can perform a body massage, as aromatherapy techniques build upon your basic massage skills and develop those skills further, as advanced movements. Therefore, before teaching this unit, your tutor will need to guide you through B20 Provide body massage treatments. Otherwise this unit will not make sense to you, and you will not have the skills in place to build upon.

You will also need to know about:

- pre-blended aromatherapy oils
  - what essential oils are
  - what carrier oils are and how to choose them
  - which essential oils are used for different effects
  - how essential oils get into the body
  - the effects of using pre-blended aromatherapy oils on the individual systems of the body
  - the physical and psychological effects of massage using pre-blended aromatherapy oils
- organisational and legal requirements
- how to work safely and effectively when carrying out massage using pre-blended aromatherapy oils
- how to carry out the client consultation
- preparation for treatment
- contra-indications to treatment and possible contra-actions
- treatment-specific knowledge
- aftercare advice for clients.

Maintain safe and effective methods of working when providing massage using pre-blended aromatherapy oils

All the topics required for this performance criteria are covered in Professional basics, Body treatments — theory and consultation, and G22 Monitor procedures to safely control work operations. The following topics relate to aromatherapy only.

You must set up your working area to meet organisational requirements and following manufacturers' instructions, exactly as it would be for a body massage. In aromatherapy massage it is particularly important for the client to feel warm, relaxed and pampered for the treatment to be effective.

The environmental conditions should also be as for body massage: the client needs to feel at ease in their surroundings and confident in your abilities to enable them to gain maximum benefit from the treatment. For a full explanation of environmental conditions please refer to the Professional basics unit, page 58.

Timings

Stand-alone treatment times:

Massage	Time
Full body treatment	1 hour 15 minutes
Back massage only	30 minutes
Face and scalp massage only	20 minutes

Treatment breakdown for a whole body treatment:

Massage	Time
Consultation	10 minutes
Back	20 minutes
Back of legs	5 minutes each = 10 minutes
Front of legs	5 minutes each = 10 minutes
Abdomen	5 minutes
Arms	5 minutes each = 10 minutes
Face and scalp	10 minutes
Completed treatment	**1 hour 15 minutes**

Think about it

Remember that when aromatherapy oils are used, the room should be adequately ventilated (see Professional basics, 'You and your working environment', page 60, for more detail on ventilation). It is possible to get a build-up of the essences and you or your client may overdose on the heady mixtures, causing headache and lethargy. The room should ideally be for your treatment alone, but if you are sharing a teaching/assessing room with others, using differing oils, you may get a conflict of smells which will negate the good works the oils are suppose to achieve!

Think about it

As you are using pre-blended oils it is easiest to select and bring the bottle to your working area, and then decant it into a bowl ready for use. If you pour the oils into a bowl at a central working station and then walk with it, you are more likely to spill it and create an unsafe, slippery floor for others.

Decant oil into a small bowl to avoid cross-contamination

Only use enough oil and carrier oils to cover the area used, so there is minimum waste

HOW TO BE COST-EFFECTIVE WITH PRE-BLENDED AROMATHERAPY OILS

If you have oil left over, give it to the client for the bath

Always stick to the treatment times

Always do a patch test 24 hours prior to treatment, so you do not waste the oils or put the client in danger of an allergic reaction

Client record cards

Always ensure the client record card is up to date, accurate, complete legible and signed by both the client and the therapist – this is most important. You need to have written consent to perform the treatment. An example record card, completed for a body massage treatment, can be found in the Body treatments – theory and consultation, page 328. You must ensure you also record the essential and carrier oils you have chosen for the treatment with an explanation of why.

Think about it

Always remember to leave your treatment area and equipment in a suitable condition for future treatments – there may be someone else working in your room. Imagine it is you coming in after you – ask yourself, is this working area suitable to begin a treatment?

Consult, plan and prepare for treatments with clients

Your consultation techniques should be polite, sensitive and in a friendly manner — you need to gain the client's trust to enable a full consultation to take place and to determine the most suitable type of treatment for your client's needs. Refer to the Professional basics unit, from page 29, for questioning techniques and all aspects of consultation requirements, as they all apply to aromatherapy.

Using the consultation card as a guide, you should ensure that all areas of the treatment are covered and remember to obtain a written confirmation that the client is happy for the treatment to go ahead — you will also need signed, parental consent for a minor and make sure that the parent or guardian is present throughout the treatment.

You need to fully explain the treatment in a way the client can understand, including what you hope the particular blend of oils will achieve and enhance for them. Avoid jargon — it really is not helpful and the client may not wish to appear silly by asking questions. Be prepared to repeat yourself, if necessary, and ask them about their hopes for the treatment.

Contra-indications, contra-actions and allergies

Remember to ask specific questions about the client's contra-indications — it may be that a small contra-indication, e.g. a bruise on the leg, will require the treatment to be modified — i.e. you avoid the area. It may be that the treatment has to be halted and you need to explain to the client the reasons why and gently suggest they go to a doctor for an appointment. Remember that you are not a trained physician and not able to make a diagnosis on the client's symptoms. It is not your place and you may alarm them. However, it has been useful for therapists to suggest the client see a GP for all sorts of reasons, especially if a client cannot see an angry mole on their back, and so on.

If the client has any allergies, then you need to be very careful to avoid the source. It may be an allergy to nuts, or cotton wool or lanolin: so be careful to avoid any irritants. The topic of allergies is fully explained in You and the skin, page 234. Allergies can be life-threatening and under no circumstances should you underestimate them.

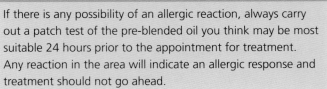

Think about it

If there is any possibility of an allergic reaction, always carry out a patch test of the pre-blended oil you think may be most suitable 24 hours prior to the appointment for treatment. Any reaction in the area will indicate an allergic response and treatment should not go ahead.

You must also be cautious if the client has any of the following conditions:

- High blood pressure — don't use blends containing rosemary, thyme, black pepper or basil.
- Epilepsy — don't use blends containing rosemary or fennel.
- Breast or ovarian cancer — don't use blends containing clary sage or fennel (oestrogen-imitating oils).
- Pregnancy — avoid blends containing clary sage or jasmine, as these may induce labour.

Contra-indications to pre-blended aromatherapy massage include:

- substantial cuts and abrasions
- contagious skin diseases and disorders
- any infections
- fever
- varicose veins
- if alcohol has been consumed
- after heat treatments such as sauna, steam bath
- any inflammation or swelling
- diabetes
- high/low blood pressure
- pregnancy without GP approval for treatment
- cancer patients who are undergoing chemo- or radiotherapies
- deep vein thrombosis.

Also remember that contra-indications to body massage also apply to aromatherapy massage too.

You are now ready to select the pre-blended aromatherapy oils that marry up to the treatment objectives in your client consultation.

Think about it

Some medications interact with complementary preparations, so take that into account when choosing your blends. Carrier oils, essential oils, sprays and other topical aromatherapy prescriptions may interfere with the absorption and action of topical creams from the doctor. Massage may also disperse topical medication over areas where it is not desirable and get onto the therapist's hands. Avoid massaging and applying preparations to all areas being treated by topical medication.

This is another reason to ensure your consultation is full and thorough – the client must inform you of any and all medications.

How essential oils get into the body

The essential oils can enter the body in a variety of ways:

- *The skin*: During massage – the method you will use for your client – essential oils penetrate the dermis and are absorbed into the bloodstream and then become transported all round the body. This is also how a small portion of the oils from a bath enter the skin, and you may also inhale the steam. Carrier oils are not absorbed, as their molecular structure is too big, so they stay on the skin's surface and allow the massage to flow, by providing slip and lubrication.
- *Lungs*: They are inhaled through the lungs and pass into the bloodstream through the lining of the lung tissue, again to be transported to the rest of the body.
- *The nose*: Via the olfactory system (see below and Related anatomy and physiology, page 217, which will explain the mechanics of olfaction).
- *The digestive system*: But only a clinical aromatherapist would give dilutions of oil in an ingestible form (a drink, for example); we would not advise this for clients.
- *Through the vagina or anus in pessary form*: Again, only a clinical aromatherapist or medical practitioner would recommend this.

Elimination of oils

The body will get rid of the oil by either exhaling it through the lungs, passing it through urine, or through the breath, and (in the case of garlic) skin will also release oil during perspiration.

Olfaction

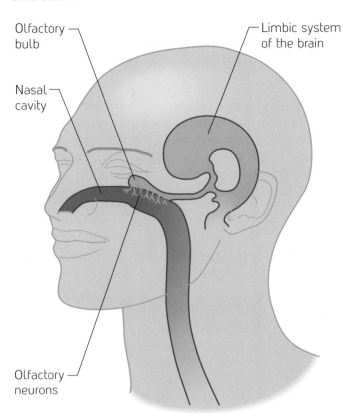

The olfactory system

Olfaction is the sense of smell. When you breathe in an essential oil two quite separate things happen:

- the sense of smell is stimulated
- substances are taken in by the lungs, and respiration in general.

In the first, the message contained in the oil molecules are passed on to the brain and begin their therapeutic effect. In the second, the molecules themselves are inhaled with the incoming air and carried into the lungs. Here they take part in a process called the 'exchange of gases', which enables them to be absorbed by the body tissues and continue their beneficial effect as the massage progresses.

A nose can detect the difference between thousands and thousands of different smells – far more individual smells than the number of individual sounds that can be detected by the ear.

Because the hairs in your nose (cilia) are in direct contact with the source of smell, and then connect directly with the brain, the sense of smell has a powerful and immediate effect on the body, which is a crucial part of the aromatherapy massage. It does so because the area of the brain associated with smell is very closely connected with that part of the brain known as the limbic system (the 'primitive' part of our brain). In simple terms it is the seat of our primeval instincts and is concerned with the emotions, memory, sexual drive, intuition, etc.

Virtually every function of the body is controlled by the brain, via the central nervous system, so any process which can send messages directly to the brain can be used to influence both the physical body and the emotions, and the implications of this effect of the sense of smell and its immediacy are very important to the practice of aromatherapy.

Think about it

We respond to smell emotionally rather than intellectually, so smells can bring back powerful memories: happy memories of childhood, holidays by the seaside or even people, if they had a distinctive smell – for example a granddad smelling of pipe tobacco! Coconut smells may be linked to holidays and freshly mown grass may be linked to spring. Certain smells can also bring back fear; if the smell is linked to an unpleasant memory, such as a fear of water, then the smell of the sea may link that emotion to the smell. List your own top three happy smells – your linked memories and why you remember them. Do you have any particular smell that fills you with dread, fear or loathing? School cabbage may be an example!

The following table lists the beneficial effects on the various body systems when massage and essential oils are combined.

System of the body	Effects of oils	Relevant oils
Skeletal	Oil and massage help maintain a full range of movement in the joints because the circulation is stimulated, so joints and bone receive oxygen and nutrients from the blood cells to help maintain growth and repair.	Arthritis – choose caraway, lemon or cypress oils Rheumatism – choose cajeput, coriander, sage or camomile oils Sprains – choose marjoram or rosemary oils
Muscular	Massage helps muscles in two ways: they function on full capacity because of stimulation of the bloodstream, so feeding muscle fibres oxygen and nutrients; they also benefit from the muscular stimulation from the massage movements. Fibres are relaxed and fibrocystic nodules are removed, the blood flow improves, muscular tension is relieved and so aches and pains are alleviated. Muscles are then able to function better.	Cramp – choose basil, cypress or marjoram oils Lack of tone – choose lemongrass, black pepper or lavender oils Aches and pains – choose caraway, eucalyptus, lavender, clary sage, rosemary, ginger or black pepper oils
Circulation	When the circulation is stimulated every cell in the body benefits, as more nutrients and oxygen are given to them, and waste and carbon dioxide removal is speeded up. This in turn benefits all areas of the body. During massage this is seen as erythema on the skin: cellular regeneration for growth and repair is improved and this creates more healthy cells.	High blood pressure – choose lavender, geranium, marjoram, ylang ylang or clary sage oils Low blood pressure – choose black pepper, rosemary or peppermint oils Varicose veins – choose lemon, cypress or geranium oils
Lymph	The function of the lymphatic system is increased, both through massage and oil use. Massage will help relieve swelling and mild oedema and some oils are diuretic so elimination is also stimulated. (Remember that excessive swelling or oedema is a contra-indication as it indicates a systemic illness.)	Poor circulation – choose fennel, geranium or juniper oils Infection – choose lemon, eucalyptus or tea tree oils

System of the body	Effects of oils	Relevant oils
Nervous	The nervous system can be stimulated by oils and encouraged to work at maximum efficiency, so parts of the body affected by nerves – muscles, the senses and so on – will also work well. Conversely, the nervous system can also be calmed and slowed, so nerve endings are relaxed by massage and oils – nerve endings can be soothed and stretched out, so relieving pain and tension.	Tension – choose basil, bergamot or camomile oils Insomnia – choose marjoram or neroli oils Depression – choose sandalwood, lavender or clary sage oils
Endocrine	The endocrine system (concerned with hormone production and transportation) has a big influence on the body, so it follows that massage and oils can have a big effect, too. The problems associated with hormonal changes such as puberty, pregnancy, labour and menopause can all be helped with massage and the right oils. The immune system can be balanced and regulated, hormone production stimulated in all the endocrine glands, and endorphins and serotonin production increased, giving a 'feel-good' high to the body in much the same way that exercise does. Emotional balance can be restored and the body strengthened.	Painful periods – choose cajuput, clary sage, melissa or camomile oils Pre-menstrual syndrome – choose clary sage, rose, neroli or geranium oils Menopause – choose clary sage, cypress, fennel, rose or geranium oils
Digestive	Digestion is stimulated both with oils and massage. Peristalsis is accelerated, aiding digestion. Tension in the abdomen area is also calmed and excretion stimulated – there may be an increase in bowel movements. Clients with irritable bowel syndrome and other digestive disturbances find massage soothing and restorative.	Laxatives – choose black pepper, peppermint or ginger oils Indigestion – choose fennel, basil or peppermint oils Diarrhoea – choose eucalyptus, sage, camomile or sandalwood oils, or neroli if due to nerves Constipation – choose marjoram, rosemary or ginger oils
Metabolism	Cell metabolism can be stimulated, so all the body's systems benefit as growth, repair and cellular activity is increased and improved.	Poor growth and repair – choose lavender, tea tree or camomile oils Sluggishness – choose eucalyptus, lavender, sandalwood, rosemary, juniper or lemon oils
Respiratory	The intercostal muscles in the ribs are the muscles of respiration along with the diaphragm, and they can be soothed and relaxed with aromatherapy. This helps the lungs expand and inhale more oxygen; this in turn means more oxygen gets into the bloodstream and all the cells of the body benefit with an extra hit of oxygen. Respiratory conditions such as asthma can be reduced and the lungs cleared of mucus. The general functioning of all the body is improved when respiration works properly.	Mucus – choose eucalyptus, lemon, myrrh, benzoin, frankincense or eucalyptus oils Asthma – choose basil, lemon, marjoram, frankincense or clove oils Flu – choose lavender, pine, tea tree, eucalyptus or benzoin oils

Continued

B24

Carry out massage using pre-blended aromatherapy oils

System of the body	Effects of oils	Relevant oils
Olfactory	The smells of the oils have a huge effect on the limbic system in the brain, as smell is very emotional: moods are affected, memory stimulated, and smells of oils can calm or stimulate, depending upon which oils are chosen.	Hay fever – choose hyssop, camomile or melissa oils Congestion – choose rosemary, lemon or myrrh oils
Reproductive	See endocrine system. Associated problems with the reproduction system can be helped: pre-menstrual syndrome, irregular periods, infertility, and menopausal problems can all be improved with oils.	Irregular periods – choose clary sage, camomile, rose or lavender oils Lack of periods – choose fennel, cypress, rose or myrrh oils Aphrodisiac – choose ylang ylang, rose or patchouli oils
Skin	Massage of the skin can be exfoliating and improve the skin's texture and suppleness. Sebaceous secretions are regulated and the glands stimulated for more production, thereby helping a dry skin. Massage in combination with the oil used helps to make the skin smooth and soft. The pressure exerted on the nerve endings in the skin is very calming and soothing to body, mind and spirit.	Acne – choose lavender, bergamot or tea tree oils Eczema – choose camomile, lavender or rose oils Psoriasis – choose bergamot, camomile or lavender oils

About pre-blended aromatherapy oils

What are essential oils?

Essential oils are highly concentrated and very complex substances, which are extracted from a plant. They contain all the special properties of the plant and carry its distinctive aroma.

An essential oil is never exactly identical to the essence of the plant from which it is extracted, because the essence is changed by the process of distillation.

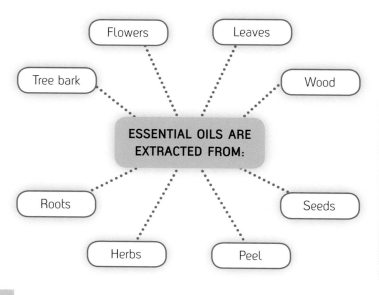

Flowers · Leaves · Tree bark · Wood · **ESSENTIAL OILS ARE EXTRACTED FROM:** · Roots · Seeds · Herbs · Peel

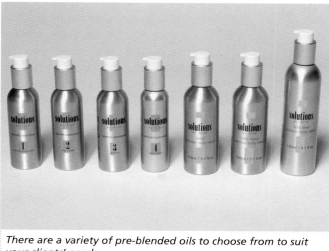

There are a variety of pre-blended oils to choose from to suit your clients' needs

Think about it

When they are distilled from a plant, the oils become a hundred times more concentrated and their effects on the body are increased, so proportion, dilution and ratio to carrier oil is the key to safe aromatherapy practice. The untrained general public do not realise how toxic or strong essential oils can be, or the physical, physiological and **pharmaceutical** effects on the body.

Key terms

Pharmaceutical – relating to drugs. A pharmacist is qualified to prepare and dispense drugs.

Herbs	Rosemary or thyme
Flowers	Jasmine, geranium, rose or lavender
Leaves	Petitgrain, marjoram, basil, sage or clary sage
Fruits	Mandarin, tangerine, lemon or grapefruit
Berries	Juniper and cypress
Bark	Cinnamon
Resin	Made into incense, e.g. myrrh and benzoin
Wood	Sandalwood, rosewood
Seeds	Caraway or fennel
Roots	Vetivert, ginger, angelica or caraway
Nuts	Nutmeg
Grasses	Lemongrass

Some plants produce slightly different essences in different parts of the same plant. For example, the orange tree gives us neroli from the petals, petitgrain from the leaves and orange from the fruit (rinds). The three oils all have similar properties but each one has unique therapeutic qualities.

Examples of essential oil origin

Additional knowledge

Extraction

There are several methods of extraction used by commercial companies to obtain essential oils but you do not require this knowledge for pre-blended oils. If you would like to research them yourself, there are some very good websites which give detailed explanations. Try www.aworldofaromatherapy.com or carry out an internet search for 'essential oil extraction'.

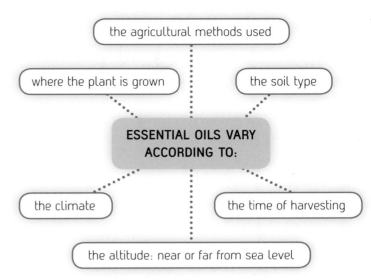

the agricultural methods used

where the plant is grown

the soil type

ESSENTIAL OILS VARY ACCORDING TO:

the climate

the time of harvesting

the altitude: near or far from sea level

Additional knowledge

Plant knowledge

It is important for the therapist to know which part of the plant the oil is obtained from, as there may be differences of quality or therapeutic effect. For example, juniper berry oil is superior both in smell and in therapeutic effect to the cheaper oil which is obtained from the juniper needles. Cinnamon bark yields oil which is a violent skin irritant, even in tiny amounts, while the oil from the cinnamon leaf can be used on the skin, with discretion.

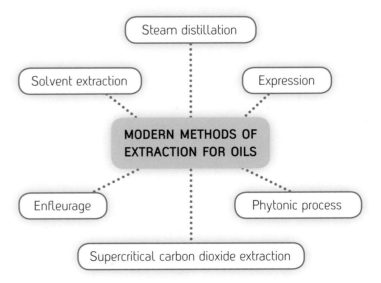

Steam distillation

Solvent extraction

Expression

MODERN METHODS OF EXTRACTION FOR OILS

Enfleurage

Phytonic process

Supercritical carbon dioxide extraction

The physical characteristics of essential oils

Essential oils differ from more commonly known oils, for example vegetable oil used in cooking. They are not fatty like vegetable oils, and are much lighter. In some respects they are more like alcohols.

- Essential oils are non-greasy or oily.
- They do not dissolve in water.
- They are sensitive to sunlight.
- They are sensitive to heat.
- They dissolve easily in fatty oils.
- They dissolve fairly easily in alcohol.
- They are aromatic and fragrant.
- They are volatile (turn into vapour very easily).
- The colour of essential oils can vary from a pale straw colour to deep brown. A very small number of essential oils are brightly coloured.
- They mix well with alcohol, mineral and vegetable oils.

Additional knowledge

The classification of oils

Essential oils are divided into top, middle or base notes, depending upon how quickly they evaporate. They also vary in other properties of absorption, how long they last in the body and where they originate from.

Classification	Properties and examples
Top notes	Evaporates really quickly Sharp aroma Absorbed quickly by skin Lasts approximately 10 hours in the body Thinnest of the oils but stimulating, e.g. sage, bergamot, lemon
Middle notes	Evaporates fairly quickly Floral aroma Absorbed fairly quickly by skin Lasts for approximately 24 hours in the body Balancing oils Slightly sedative, e.g. lavender, geranium, black pepper
Base notes	Evaporates slowly Woody and spicy aroma Absorbed slowly by skin Can last up to 5 days in the body Fixes the top and middle oils Relaxing and sedative, e.g. cedar wood, jasmine, marigold

Carrier oils

Essential oils should *never* be applied directly onto the skin. You will be using oils diluted in carrier oil. The best quality of vegetable oils should be used: they are found in the seeds of plants from around the world.

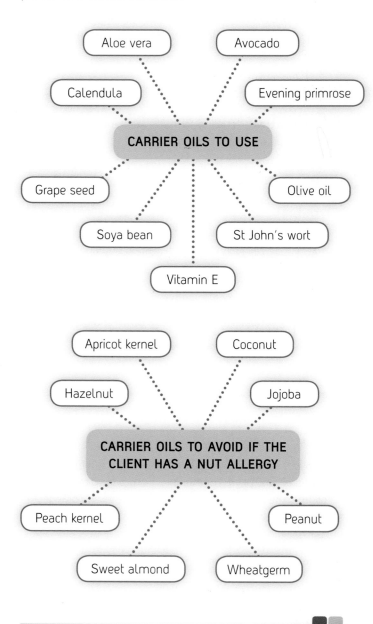

Think about it

Wheatgerm oil should be avoided as a carrier oil if the client is a coeliac – that is, they cannot tolerate gluten, the protein constituent of wheat and other grains. Coeliacs may also have a problem absorbing some fats and can become very poorly with vomiting and diarrhoea – this condition is thought to be hereditary and the client will certainly know if they have it.

Carrier oil	Botanical name	From where	Colour / Shelf life	What it contains	Properties	Suitable for
Apricot kernel (quite expensive if used on its own, more commonly mixed with grape seed)	*Prunus armeniaca*	Seed kernel from the apricot fruit	Pale yellow Shelf life: 2 years	Vitamin A and minerals	Easily absorbed, soothing and nourishing	All skin types, especially dry skins. Thought to help hyperactivity in babies and young children
Avocado (cloudy appearance with residue)	*Persea americana*	Flesh of the avocado	Dark green Shelf life: 1 year	Protein, lecithin, essential fatty acids, vitamins A, D and E	Highly penetrative, soothing and relieves itching	All skin types
Calendula (pot marigold)	*Calendula officinalis*	Macerated from the marigold flowers	Orange-yellow Shelf life: 1 year	N/A	Anti-inflammatory, astringent and soothing	Oily or combination skins
Evening primrose (very expensive)	*Oenothera biennis*	Extracted from the seeds	Pale yellow Shelf life: 6–9 months	Polyunsaturated fatty acids and linoleic acid	Soothing and nourishing – thought to help the healing process	Oily, combination, acne-prone and inflamed skin
Grapeseed (very light)	*Vitis vinifera*	Heat extracted from the grape pips	Pale green Shelf life: 1 year	Linoleic acid, protein and vitamin E	Emollient	Dry and ageing skins
Hazelnut (expensive)	*Corylus avellana*	Extracted from the nuts	Yellow Shelf life: 1 year	Oleic acid, linoleic acid and vitamin E	Slightly astringent, and stimulating to circulation	Oily or combination skins
Jojoba (expensive)	*Simmondsia chinensis*	From the bean of the plant	Yellow Shelf life: 2 years	A waxy substance which mimics collagen, vitamin E, minerals and protein	Anti-inflammatory and highly penetrative	Oily, combination, acne-prone and inflamed skin
Macadamia nut	*Macadamia integrifolia*	Pressed from the plant	Peach Shelf life: 1 year	Fatty acids	Rich and nutritive	Dry and ageing skins

Continued

Carry out massage using pre-blended aromatherapy oils **B24**

Carrier oil	Botanical name	From where	Colour / Shelf life	What it contains	Properties	Suitable for
Olive oil (very heavy oil)	Olea europaea	Unripe olives	Yellow-green Shelf life: 1 year	Vitamin E	Rich and nutritive	Dehydrated and inflamed skin
Peach kernel (regenerative and toning)	Prunus persica	Extracted from the kernel	Pale green Shelf life: 2 years	Vitamins A and E, essential fatty acids	Emollient	All skin types, especially dry and mature
Rosehip (rich texture)	Rosa canina	Seed of the rose bush	Rose Shelf life: 6–9 months	Polyunsaturated fats	Regenerating and healing	Scar tissue, stretch marks and dehydrated skins
Safflower (inexpensive and light)	Carthamus tinctorius	Pressed from the seeds	Yellow Shelf life: less than 3 months	Essential fatty acids and vitamin E	Nutritive	All skin types
St John's wort (soothing and healing)	Hypericum perforatum	Macerated from flowers and leaves	Mauve, red-brown Shelf life: 2 years		Heals and soothes, anti-inflammatory and astringent	All skin types, especially dry and sensitive
Sunflower (fine and light)	Helianthus annus	Pressed from sunflower seeds	Golden yellow Shelf life: 8 months	Fatty acids and high levels of vitamin E	Nutritive	All skin types, especially dry
Sweet almond (very popular)	Prunus amygdalus	Kernel of the sweet almond tree	Pale yellow Shelf life: 4–6 months	Vitamins A, B^1 B^2, B^6 and E and protein	Therapeutic and nutritive	Dry, ageing and inflamed skins
Wheatgerm (quite sticky)	Triticum sativum	Warm-pressed from the germ of wheat kernel	Orange-brown Shelf life: 6–8 months	Vitamin E and protein	Soothing, nourishing and healing	Inflamed and ageing skins

Which carrier oils to choose

As there are no essential oils or carrier oils named specifically within the Standards for this unit, we need to look at the treatment objectives and recommend a carrier oil and pre-blended oil, or oils which will best achieve your objectives.

Client complaint or need	Recommended carrier oil
Muscular tension, pain and stiffness	Sweet almond oil, olive oil Sesame oil (but can irritate sensitive skins) Wheatgerm (for tired muscles)
Moisturising	Avocado oil (recommended) Jojoba (recommended) Sweet almond oil, apricot kernel oil, coconut oil, grapeseed oil, olive oil, peach kernel oil, wheatgerm oil Sesame oil (but can irritate sensitive skins)
Inflammation	Sweet almond oil, avocado oil, jojoba oil, wheatgerm oil Coconut oil (but may irritate sensitive skin)
Itching associated with conditions such as eczema and psoriasis	Sweet almond oil, calendula, evening primrose oil, jojoba oil, peach kernel oil
Itching associated with dry skin	Apricot kernel oil, evening primrose oil
Sensitive, dry and ageing skin	Macadamia oil (recommended) Apricot kernel oil, peach kernel oil Wheatgerm oil (recommended for ageing skins)
Healing skin, scars and stretch marks	Avocado oil, calendula oil, evening primrose oil, rosehip oil, wheatgerm oil Sunflower oil (especially for bruises)
Premature ageing	Avocado oil, macadamia oil
Dandruff	Evening primrose oil
Help with the control the release of sebum	Jojoba oil
Help with leg ulcers	Sunflower oil
Help with acne and skin disorders where there is dryness and inflammation	Sunflower oil
Symptoms of dermatitis	Wheatgerm oil
Stimulation to local circulation of the skin	Hazelnut oil
Oily skin	Hazelnut oil
Dehydrated skin	Avocado oil, olive oil
Cell regeneration to improve the skin's condition	Wheatgerm oil

Carrier oils and their properties

The following table gives examples of pre-blended oils within a carrier oil and their effects on the body.

Treatment outcome/ranges to be covered	Where to use and skin type	Carrier oil	Essential oils
Refreshing and stimulating	Facial blend for normal/combination skin	Sweet almond oil	Lavender, peppermint and bergamot
Soothing and moisturising	Facial blend for a dry skin	Grapeseed oil	Lemon, sandalwood and geranium
Calming and soothing	Facial blend for sensitive skin	Sweet almond oil	Camomile, lavender and sandalwood
Healing and antiseptic	Facial blend for a congested and dull skin	Sweet almond oil	Grapefruit and tea tree
Pre- and post-exercise	Body repair mix for muscles and joints	Grapeseed oil	Black pepper, lemon and lavender
Stress relief and sense of wellbeing	Body blend for deep relaxation and indulgence	Grapeseed oil	Jasmine, lavender and camomile
Detoxification to treat cellulite	Body blend to reduce fluid retention and improve the appearance of the skin	Grapeseed oil	Juniper, bergamot and lavender
Uplifting and invigorating	Body blend to uplift and invigorating and awaken the senses	Grapeseed oil	Mandarin, bergamot and peppermint

(Source: table courtesy of Hive of Beauty Ltd)

The oils you are using are pre-blended by the manufacturer. However, there is no reason why you should not be able to explain to your client during consultation the origin of the oil, the way it has been extracted, its benefits and effects on the body and why you have chosen it, as well as how it is diluted.

Dilution

Essential oils are measured in drops because they are very concentrated, so generally the rule of dilution is: *half* the number of drops to the number of *millilitres* in volume of the carrier oils. So:

- 25 drops of essential oil to 50 millilitres of carrier oil
- 5 drops of essential oil to 10 millilitres of carrier oil.

For a full body massage you will require approximately 20 millilitres of carrier oil – so there should be 10 drops of essential oil in your pre-blended bottle.

If you are recommending the client puts oil in the bath, they will need about 6–8 drops and it *must* be dissolved into carrier oils first, as essential oils are not soluble in water. This will prevent irritation to the skin. For maximum effect they should be added just before the client gets into the bath, rather than first – although adding under running hot water also creates a fragrant steam, which makes the bathroom smell lovely! This is a great way to use up any leftover oil from a massage, and the client continues to gain the benefits at home.

Most oils contain a top note, middle note and base note as they work well together, and generally the botanical families that the oils come from blend well too. This is called a **synergistic blend**.

You can mix:

- floral + citrus + herbs
- citrus + herbs + trees
- herbs + trees + spices
- trees + spices + resins
- spices + resins + floral
- resins + floral + citrus.

Key terms

Synergistic blend – the interaction of two or more agents or ingredients or oils so that their combined effect is greater than the sum of their individual effects.

Here are some examples of these categories. For a full list, refer to individual oils.

Trees	Bay, birch, pine, sandalwood
Herbs	Basil, coriander, rosemary, thyme
Spices	Cinnamon, cloves, black pepper, tea tree
Resins	Myrrh, frankincense
Citrus	Lemongrass, lime, neroli, orange
Floral	Geranium, rose, violet, lavender

The following table provides terms of medical reference for the effects of oils.

Term	Effect	Term	Effect
Anti-	A prefix denoting against: effective against, to counter the effect of or opposed to something	Antiseptic	Stops bacterial growth
Anti-allergic	Effective against allergies, or allergens which cause a reaction in the body, e.g. food, drugs, animal fur etc.	Anti-toxic	Neutralises poison
Anti-catarrhal	Effective against catarrh, which is inflammation of a mucus membrane in the nasal passages	Astringent	Dries the tissue
Anti-convulsive	Effective against convulsions – involuntary contractions of muscles in groups, as in fits or spasms	Bactericidal	Any agent which destroys bacteria
Antihistaminic	Effective against the development of histamine – a chemical in the body which causes a violent reaction in the tissue and blood capillaries, and can bring on an allergic reaction or anaphylactic shock	Balsamic	Balsam is a healing pharmaceutical preparation containing resinous substances used for healing and soothing
Anti-rheumatic	Effective against rheumatism	Calmative	Reduces wind or flatulence in the digestive tract
Anti-spasmodic	Effective against spasms	Cellular regenerator	A stimulus to the cells for growth and repair
Anti-viral	Effective against viruses	Cholagogic	A stimulus to aid increase in bile flow into the intestine
Anaphrodisiac	Lessening of sexual desire	Carminative	Helps coughing
Aphrodisiac	Increasing sexual desire	Cephalic	Stimulates the brain
Aperitif	Stimulation of the appetite	Cicatrisant	Helps form scar tissue
Analgesic	Pain relief	Cordial	An invigorating preparation for stimulating the heart and circulation
Antibacterial	Destroys or inhibits the growth of bacteria	Cytophilactic	Encouraging cell regeneration
Anti-depressive	Stops depression	Depurative	Detoxifying and clearing of impurities
Anti-inflammatory	Reduces inflammation	Decongestant	Relives catarrh

Continued

Term	Effect
Diuretic	Stimulates water balance and urine formation
Diaphoretic	Induces perspiration
Euphoric	Induces bodily calm
Emmanagogue	Regulates menstruation
Expectorant	The elimination of mucus from the body
Febrifuge	Reduces fever
Fungicide	An agent which is lethal to fungi
Hepatic	Liver tonic
Hypertensive	Raises blood pressure
Hypotensive	Lowers blood pressure
Haemostatic	An agent which stops bleeding
Hypnotic	A drug or treatment which induces sleep
Insecticide	An agent which kills insects
Laxative	Aids digestive excretion
Nervine	To strengthen the nervous system

Term	Effect
Neurotonic	Support or help with the nervous system or emotional stability
Parasiticide	An agent which destroys parasites
Phlebotonic	Support or help with the veins
Photosensitising	Sensitivity to light
Rubefacient	Producing redness in the skin
Sedative	Helps sleep
Splenetic	Pertaining to the spleen
Stimulant	Increases something
Stomachic	Relating to the stomach – increasing appetite and digestion
Sudorific	The promotion of sweat
Tonic	An energiser or boost
Uterine	Pertaining to the uterus
Vasodilator	Dilation of the blood vessels
Vermifuge	An agent which causes an intestinal worm or parasite to be expelled
Vulnerary	Healing of cuts

Essential oils

There are approximately 39 essential oils and their properties and benefits could fill a book of their own. The following table gives a brief summary of each oil and its properties. For a fuller breakdown of each oil, including the areas of mind and body that can be helped through the oil's use in massage, please visit the Pearson website: www.pearsonfe.co.uk/BeautyTherapyLevel3units

As an holistic therapist you need to be aware of the holistic effects essential oils can have. Aroma is an essential part of Eastern practices and principles such as yin and yang. Refresh your knowledge of them by referring to the section on 'Becoming an holistic therapist', in Professional basics, page 25, and to unit B23 Provide Indian head massage, page 434.

Essential oil	Properties
Basil	Analgesic, antibacterial, anti-depressive, antiseptic, anti-spasmodic, digestive, hormone balancer, neurotonic
Benzoin	Anti-inflammatory, antiseptic, carminative, deodorant, diuretic, expectorant, sedative, vulnerary
Bergamot	Analgesic, anti-depressive, antiseptic, anti-spasmodic, aperitif, deodorant, disinfectant, expectorant, healing, insecticide, photosensitising, sedative
Black pepper	Analgesic, antiseptic, anti-spasmodic, diuretic, febrifuge, rubefacient, splenetic, stimulant, stomachic, tonic
Cajeput	Antiseptic, antibacterial, anti-catarrhal, insecticide, tissue stimulant

Essential oil	Properties
Camomile	Analgesic, anti-allergic, anti-convulsive, anti-depressive, anti-inflammatory, antiseptic, anti-spasmodic, diuretic, sedative
Cedarwood	Antiseptic, astringent, expectorant, fungicide, insect repellent, tonic
Clary sage	Anti-convulsive, anti-depressive, antiseptic, anti-spasmodic, aphrodisiac, astringent, deodorant, diuretic, sedative, tonic
Cypress	Antiseptic, astringent, a vasoconstrictor for blood vessels
Eucalyptus	Analgesic, antiseptic, anti-viral, bactericidal, decongestant, deodorant, depurative, diuretic, kidney tonic, stimulant
Fennel	Antiseptic, anti-spasmodic, anti-toxic, aperitif, diuretic, expectorant, laxative, splenetic, tonic for urinary tract
Frankincense	Antiseptic, astringent, cicatrisant, cytophilactic, digestive, diuretic, expectorant, sedative, tonic, uterine, vulnerary
Geranium	Analgesic, anti-depressive, anti-inflammatory, antiseptic, astringent, deodorant, diuretic, healing, tonic
Ginger	Analgesic, antiseptic, decongestant, laxative, stimulant, tonic
Grapefruit	Aerial antiseptic, digestive stimulant, lymphatic decongestant, stomachic
Jasmine	Anti-depressive, anti-inflammatory, antiseptic, anti-spasmodic, aphrodisiac, expectorant, sedative
Juniper berry	Anti-rheumatic, antiseptic, anti-spasmodic, astringent, diuretic, parasiticide, sedative, tonic
Lavender	Analgesic, anti-depressive, anti-fungal, antiseptic, anti-spasmodic, anti-viral, astringent, bactericidal, cardiac tonic, decongestant, disinfectant, deodorising, fungicidal, insect repellent, parasiticide, sedative, tonic
Lemon	Anti-rheumatic, antiseptic, anti-spasmodic, astringent, insecticide, laxative

Essential oil	Properties
Lemongrass	Analgesic, anti-depressive, antiseptic, astringent, bactericidal, carminative, deodorant, digestive, diuretic, febrifuge, nervine, tonic
Marjoram	Analgesic, anaphrodisiac, antiseptic, anti-spasmodic, carminative, diaphoretic, emmenagogue, expectorant, hypotensive, nervine, sedative, stomachic, tonic, vasodilator
Mandarin	Antiseptic, anti-spasmodic, carminative, digestive stimulant, hepatic, light hypnotic, lymphatic stimulant, mild diuretic, sedative, tonic
Melissa	Anti-depressive, anti-histaminic, cordial, digestive, febrifuge, hypotensive, insect repellent, nervine, sedative, stomachic, sudorific, tonic, uterine, vermifuge
Myrtle	Anti-catarrhal, antiseptic, astringent, bactericidal, expectorant, mild sedative
Neroli	Anti-depressive, antiseptic, anti-spasmodic, deodorant, sedative, tonic
Orange	Anti-depressive, antiseptic, carminative, digestive, hypotensive, sedative (nervous), stimulant (digestive and lymphatic), stomachic, tonic
Palmarosa	Antibacterial, anti-depressive, anti-fungal, anti-inflammatory, anti-viral, astringent (mild), calmative, cellular regenerator, minimises infections
Patchouli	Antibacterial, anti-inflammatory, anti-fungal, cicatrisant, decongestant, digestive stimulant, febrifuge, immune tonic, insect repellent, minimises infection, phlebotonic, stomachic, tissue regenerator
Petitgrain	Anti-depressive, antiseptic, anti-spasmodic, deodorant, digestive, nervine, stomachic, tonic
Pine	Adrenal cortex stimulant, analgesic, antiseptic, bactericidal, balsamic, expectorant, insecticidal, rubefacient, tonic, vermifuge
Rose	Anti-depressive, antiseptic, anti-spasmodic, antiviral, astringent, laxative, sedative

Continued

Essential oil	Properties
Rosemary	Adrenal cortex stimulant, analgesic, antiseptic, anti-spasmodic, astringent, bactericidal, cardiac tonic, cephalic, cholagogic, diuretic, emmenagogue, hair and scalp tonic, hepatic, hypertensive, nervine, parasiticide, stimulant, stomachic, sudorific
Sandalwood	Anti-depressive, antiseptic (urinary and pulmonary), anti-spasmodic, aphrodisiac, astringent, carminative, diuretic, expectorant, sedative, tonic
Spikenard	Antibacterial, anti-fungal, anti-inflammatory, deodorant, laxative, sedative, tonic
Tea tree	Antibiotic, antiseptic, anti-viral, bactericidal, cardiac tonic, expectorant, fungicidal, immune stimulant, sudorific
Thyme	Anti-infectious, antiseptic, anti-spasmodic, aphrodisiac, diuretic, emmenagogue, expectorant, hypertensive, hypnotic, stimulant, stomachic, sudorific, tonic
Vetivert	Anti-depressive, anti-infectious, anti-rheumatic, anti-spasmodic, calmative, digestive stimulant, emmenagogue, general tonic, hepatic stimulant, immune tonic, pancreatic stimulant, phlebotonic
Yarrow	Anti-inflammatory, anti-rheumatic, antiseptic, anti-spasmodic, carminative, cicatrisant, diaphoretic, digestive, expectorant, haemostatic, hypotensive, stomachic, tonic
Ylang ylang	Anti-depressive, antiseptic, euphoric, hypotensive, regulator of sebum and hormones, stimulant of circulation, tonic

Additional knowledge

Oils to avoid

The following oils are not recommended and are not suitable for use:

- Bitter almond
- Bolda leaf
- Calamus
- Camphor
- Horseradish
- Jaborandi leaf
- Mugwort
- Mustard
- Pennyroyal
- Rue
- Sassafras
- Savin
- Southernwood
- Tansy
- Thuja
- Wintergreen
- Wormseed
- Wormwood

For your portfolio

These oils do take some revision. To help you remember them, buy a flip-type photo album, where you can see the photos staggered down the album. Each of the plastic wallets takes a postcard size insert, which any stationery shop will sell. You can write out the key points to all the oils and insert them into the photo album. This gives you an at-a-glance guide to the oils and their uses. This is a very good revision tool. Keep it with you for referral all the time!

Safety and storage of oils

Oils react to sunlight and require the correct storage to keep them at maximum strength for the duration of their shelf life, which is six months to two years depending upon the oil.

They should be:

- in dark glass bottles
- only used with a dropper for actual measuring
- kept in an airtight container
- out of sunlight
- kept in a dry, cool area
- locked away so no one untrained can get them – especially children
- fully labelled so you know what they are
- never used in a high dilution with a carrier oil
- never applied directly to the skin neat
- not used for too long on any one client
- not used too frequently
- usage must stop immediately if irritation occurs
- always used with a patch test prior to use
- never used with homeopathy treatments – they may counteract the effects
- never used in the first five months of pregnancy
- used only after a full consultation.

Massage the body using pre-blended aromatherapy oils

Now you have all the information to be able to pick your pre-blended oil and your working area is all set up and ready. Make sure you have enough towels and props for your client – they need to be supported and cushioned so that they can completely relax and 'give in' to the treatment, both physically and mentally. Refer to the section on 'Becoming an holistic therapist', in Professional basics, page 25, for detail on creating a relaxed and inviting environment.

For a full breakdown on the client's physical characteristics and various postural problems see Body treatments – theory and consultation, pages 331–335. Your client may need extra support or adjustment.

Massage procedures

Your Swedish body massage movements are very acceptable for use with aromatherapy pre-blended oils, and you can add some more advanced techniques to further increase the benefits of the treatment.

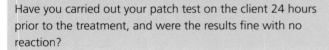

Think about it

Have you carried out your patch test on the client 24 hours prior to the treatment, and were the results fine with no reaction?

Neuromuscular massage is much firmer to feel and apply, and the direction is aimed at the sensory and motor nerve pathways rather than towards the heart and lymphatic glands. This is why you will sometimes work away from the heart, as in reverse effleurage down the back, from the head to the coccyx. The pressure is very firm and if it causes the client any discomfort it is because the nerve pathways are blocked and/or there may be tension nodules present that need dispersing. So the client will get a lot of benefit from this type of movement.

Static pressures can also be applied to areas of the body that correspond to shiatsu massage – these are called tsubo points, and during aromatherapy massage these points are pressed firmly with the fingertips, using the whole weight of the therapist's body. This will unblock the energy flow and restore harmony and balance. See the section 'Becoming an holistic therapist' in Professional basics, page 25. This gives a full explanation of energy flow, yin and yang and meridians of the body. All can be relaxed, freed and unblocked with a combination of massage, pressure point manipulation and the benefits of the correct oils.

Massage movement	Application	Effects on the body
Effleurage	Deep or superficial – as in Swedish body massage. Using the palms, hands relaxed	Introduces medium to the body Relaxes and helps spread the medium Warms and increases blood flow to the area Establishes rate and rhythm of the massage
Petrissage	Kneading moments using the palms, fingers and thumbs with more pressure	Promotes deeper movements within the muscles, so starts to warm and relax the muscle fibres Stimulates blood and lymph flow and releases tension or fibrocystic nodules in the muscles – felt as knots in the tissue
Pressure points	Finger, thumbs or heel of the palm	Eases congestion within the nervous system and opens up nerve pathways Eases pressure, releasing tension
Neuromuscular frictions	Along the nerve pathways with the finger pads	Can be both stimulating to the nerves and calming for the client
Vibrations	A tremor or shake using the pressure of the hand	Increases blood flow and lymphatic drainage, cellular activity is increased Softens scar tissue and tension Relieves tension and warms
Tapotement	Hacking, cupping, pounding, beating	A stimulating set of movements which brings bloodflow to the area quickly Caution required as it can leave the client bruised or sore if done incorrectly. The client also needs to have enough underlying tissue to absorb the movements

Massage movements

Salon life

Ulrika's story

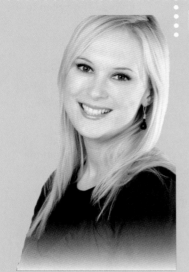

I have learned a valuable lesson about aromatherapy oils being strong and highly **flammable**. When I was doing my Level 2 qualification we all took it in turns to assist the Level 3 therapists set up the spa, sauna and wet areas — it was part of the course. My senior therapist asked me to get some eucalyptus oil for the sauna, as it was a cold winter morning and she said that it would warm the sauna, make it smell nice and help the clients with their breathing, if any of them had a cold coming. I thought this was a really nice touch and good client care. I asked the receptionist for the oil, which she took out of storage, and went back to the sauna. I already had it warming up so the coals were hot and the sauna was lovely and warm. The senior therapist was just outside and I heard her say add three drops — so I put three drops onto the hot coals. There was an almighty flash and then flames appeared — the sauna coals were on fire! I stepped backwards in panic, and fortunately she came into the sauna and poured water onto the flames from the bucket. Her quick thinking saved the day. We switched the sauna off at the mains and got out of the area quickly. I was in tears and shaking like a leaf. The senior staff all came running in to see if we were all right, and smoke was everywhere.

Our senior tutor decided it wasn't bad enough to call out the fire brigade and we opened all the windows to ventilate the room — and of course the sauna was no use, so we had to let the clients know.

I was made a cup of tea and I had to explain what happened. I heard my senior therapist say 'add three drops…' but I hadn't heard her adding '…to the water bucket'. I put the oils straight onto the coal, undiluted and as oils are highly flammable, the fire was almost instant.

I was in the wrong, but they were very understanding, and no one was hurt, thank goodness. I had to write out an accident/incident report form and we claimed on the insurance for the repair to the sauna coals. If the pine wood cabin had caught fire, then we would have been in trouble, but as I say, the senior therapist's quick thinking saved the day.

I will never underestimate the power of essential oils again. It took a long time before my confidence returned enough to use them.

Effects for the therapist:

- Concern for health and safety for all — compromised through fire
- Broken confidence concerning the wet area
- Realisation of how flammable oils are
- Learning curve on listening properly and the consequences of not doing so
- Risk assessment required for the use of oils in the sauna
- Poster required for the safe use of oils
- Loss of business through lack of confidence and repairs required

Effects for the client:

- Danger of fire from oils on the coals
- Danger from fumes in the confined space of the sauna
- Lack of confidence in the therapist — feeling unsafe
- May wish to move elsewhere

Key terms

Flammable – easily set on fire, easily ignited and capable of burning rapidly.

skin diagnosis – this is very popular). There is a strong relationship between the fascia in the muscles of the back and the nerve supply running from the vertebrae. This will show up as bodily weakness in other areas, like the face. Patchy, blotchy skin, rather than full erythema can be seen, indicating specific facial sensitivity. When the client turns over, there may be corresponding redness on the facial skin.

- Massage of the back is the most relaxing part of the treatment, so by starting with the back the client gets instant relaxation.

- It stops eye contact with the client, and there is less temptation to make conversation – the object is total relaxation and if the client is lying supine, face down, they feel less obliged to talk.

The order is:

- back
- back of legs
- front of legs
- abdomen
- arms
- chest
- face and scalp.

Think about it

You must always adapt your massage movements to suit a client's needs; if they require complete relaxation and intend going to sleep during the massage it would be best to avoid tapotement movements and anything too stimulating. If they have lots of muscular tension your massage needs to be firm and work on pressure points. Never continue if the client experiences sharp or sudden pain and adapt your movements to the amount of tissue present – deep tissue movements may not be possible on a very thin client.

Massage routine

The massage routine for aromatherapy massage is slightly different to a Swedish body massage – in aromatherapy we start on the back first, rather than last.

The reasons for this are:

- It is a wider surface area so the oil penetrates easily and therefore starts being effective straight away.

- It is a good diagnostic tool (many commercial companies offer a facial but do a back massage first as part of the

Back massage – a step-by-step guide

Caution: Never massage directly onto the spine.

1. With the towel still covering your client, place one hand at the top of their spine and the other at the base. Both take three deep breaths and relax.
2. When exposing the back for massage don't short-change your client: expose the whole of the black to the top of the gluteals, you should be massaging it all, not just half-way up! The room will be warm enough for you to do this.
3. Place oil on your hands and apply to the back in long, slow, sweeping movements.
4. Place one hand on your client's shoulder and the other on the opposite hip, get them to take a deep breath in and when they breathe out stretch the tissue so it stretches up with the shoulders and down with the hips. Swap sides and repeat.
5. Do some effleurage movements up the back (ironing, reinforced effleurage).
6. Move back to one side of the client and run your thumbs up the erector spinae muscles either side of the spine. (x3)

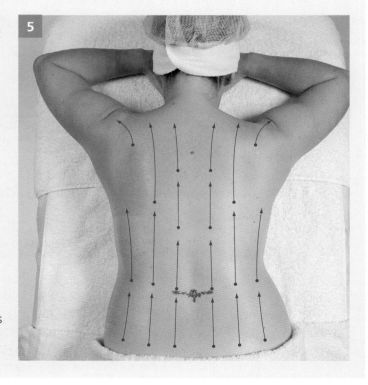

Back massage – a step-by-step guide (*cont.*)

7 Using circular movements with the thumbs or index fingers, massage the erector spinae muscles moving from the base of the spine to the top. (×3)

8 With the thumbs either side of the spine, press in between each and every vertebrae. (×3)

9 To clear any blocks along the energy pathway use the thumbs alternately each side of the channel pushing upwards towards the head. Swap sides and repeat.

10 Finally, run the thumbs up either side of the spine. (×3)

11 Stand to the side of the client and with a kneading movement massage the large muscles of the back starting at the base and finishing at the shoulders.

12 Do the raking vibration stroke down the side of the spine opposite to where you are standing, starting at the base of the spine and gradually moving upwards. Swap sides and repeat.

13 Stroke firmly up the whole back. (×3)

14 Apply circular pressures with your thumbs around the sacral area of the lower back.

15 Work the whole sacral area and sacral rock.

16 Place one hand over the lower part of the spine above the sacrum and the other hand over the lumber thoracic part of the spine and gently pull apart giving a lumbar stretch. Do the same on the other side. (×3)

17 Cover the lower back; use effleurage movements to move up to upper back.

18 Stand on one side of the client and use a kneading motion with both hands over the opposite shoulder. Swap sides and repeat.

19 When you have massaged each shoulder individually do both at the same time, this will allow you to see if the muscles in both shoulders are equally relaxed.

20 With a kneading motion massage the back of the neck.

21 Press into the occipital area with your index fingers.

22 Stand at the head of the client and use a circular movement with your forefingers around each shoulder blade at the same time. (×3)

23 Use effleurage movements around the shoulder blades.

24 To finish, stroke from top to bottom of back until the muscles feel completely warm and relaxed.

25 Place one hand on the client's shoulder and one on the opposite hip, stretch the muscles in the opposite direction. Swap sides and repeat.

26 Use cat strokes down the spine – the middle finger one side of the spine, the index on the other. Use alternate strokes, the first time quite firm, the second a little lighter, the last like a feather.

27 Place the forearms together in the middle of the back and firmly pull them apart with one arm sliding down towards the base of the spine and the other sliding towards the top of the spine.

28 Cover the client with a towel and hold at the top and bottom of the spine for a few moments.

29 With the top hand still in position, move your bottom hand from the base chakra and onto the heart chakra, hold for a few moments, then gently take your hands away.

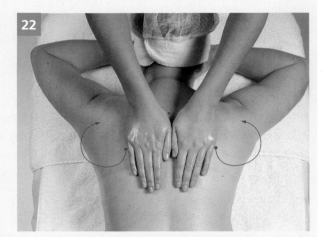

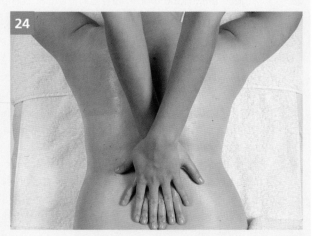

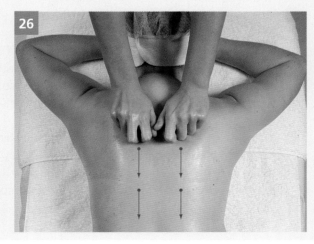

Leg massage – a step-by-step guide

Back of leg

1 Before you start the massage make sure that both legs are covered with a towel (the towel should be long enough to cover the feet as well).

2 Hold both feet firmly in your hands and pause for a few moments.

3 Uncover the leg you are about to massage.

4 Put oil on your fingers and with both hands pointing towards one another on the leg (and one placed above the other) slowly and gently sweep up from the foot to the top of the leg.

5 Lift and support the client's ankle with one hand and then with the heel of the other hand stroke up towards the popliteal nodes to assist lymphatic drainage.

6 With both hands either side of the leg run both thumbs up the centre of the leg (side by side) with firm pressure on the muscle. Go lightly over the back of the knee, then more deeply into the back of the thigh. (×3)

7 Face towards the client's feet and use a cat stroke with the pads of your fingers from ankle to knee and then back of knee to thigh.

8 Turn back to face the client's thigh and then with your palms facing down and your thumbs linked, press the palms down and slightly vibrate as you move towards the inside of the thigh, then the outside of the thigh and finally up the middle of the thigh.

9 Knead the thighs to work the muscles, starting from the back of the knee and moving to the top of the leg; make sure you work the whole area.

10 Once again lift and support the client's ankle with one hand and with the heel of the other hand stroke up towards the popliteal nodes.

11 Stroke the leg with both hands from bottom to top. (×3)

12 Cover both legs with a towel.

13 Hold the foot for a few moments.

14 Repeat massage sequence for the other leg.

Front of leg

1 Repeat the first three movements for back of leg massage.

2 Put oil on your fingers and with both hands pointing towards one another on the leg (and one placed above the other) sweep slowly and gently up from the feet to the top of the leg. Avoid going straight over the kneecap. (×3)

3 Repeat this movement a little more firmly. (×3)

4 Move to the thighs and carry out a tunnelling movement, one hand above the other, to help lymphatic drainage.

5 Use a kneading stroke to the upper thighs.

6 Put your hands together as if in prayer and run them up either side of the upper thigh with the tips of the fingers meeting as you move up.

7 Face the client's thigh and then with your palms facing down and your thumbs linked, press the palms down and slightly vibrate as you move towards the inside of the thigh, then the outside of the thigh and finally up the middle of the thigh.

8 Hold the knee with both hands (fingers either side of the knee for support) and run your thumbs around the outside of the kneecap. (×3)

9 On the inside of the knee, with reinforced fingers use circular movements around this area.

10 Press around the knee with your thumbs.

11 On the lower leg use a kneading movement with just the web of your hands. (×3)

12 Stroke the leg from the ankles to the top. (×3)

13 Cover both legs with the towel.

14 Hold the foot for a few moments.

15 Repeat massage sequence for the other leg.

Abdominal massage – a step-by-step guide

1 Place both hands, one above the other, over the solar plexus.

2 Dip your hands into the oil and spread it over the abdomen using a clockwise, circular movement.

3 Use the 'diamond effleurage' movement starting over the pubis, over the iliac crest, round to the back of the waist, up to the solar plexus and then back again.

4 With one hand over the other, from the belly button to the solar plexus, use the ironing movement across this area.

5 Still with one hand reinforcing the other, gently go around the solar plexus in a clockwise direction.

6 Lift across the sides of the abdominal wall.

7 With the fingers of both hands in a clockwise direction, trace gently but firmly around the abdomen, remembering to go lightly over the bladder.

8 Using the thumbs, trace up the ascending colon, along the transverse and down the descending colon to help with digestion.

9 Finish with a gentle circular movement around the abdomen.

B24 Carry out body massage using pre-blended aromatherapy oils

Hand and arm massage – a step-by-step guide

1. Uncover one arm and start to spread the oil over the entire arm and hand.
2. With one hand reinforcing the other, stroke firmly around the cup of the shoulder, covering the upper trapezius and front of arm.
3. Using alternate hands make circles around this shoulder area.
4. Take the arm out at an angle to the body and hold onto one hand, with the other using the web of the hand to work into the muscles of the upper arm. Swap your hands so that you can work on both sides.
5. Rest your client's hand on your shoulder and with a tunnelling movement use both your hands to push any lymph released towards the axillary nodes.
6. Place the elbow on the bed, support the lower arm in your hand and using the web of your other hand push any lymph etc. towards the supratrochlear nodes. Swap hands in order to do both sides.
7. Still holding the hand, use your thumb in a creeping, pressing movement to move up the membrane between the radius and ulna.
8. Then use the thumbs alternately to drain in between that membrane. Repeat technique on inside.
9. Rotate your fist into the palm of the hand.
10. Turn your client's hand over and rub each finger thoroughly between your thumb and forefinger.
11. Gently pull each finger upwards (as if you were pulling it out of its socket) and slide your thumb and forefinger up the entire length of their fingers.
12. Place each of your hands either side of your client's hand and massage the back, rubbing gently between each of the bones.
13. Push and release with your thumbs between the metacarpal spaces.
14. With the client's elbow resting on the couch, tunnel down using the webs of both hands towards the elbows.
15. Finish with some effleurage strokes.
16. Repeat massage sequence for the other arm.

Neck, chest and shoulder massage – a step-by-step guide

1. Begin by using sweeping strokes across the upper chest over the upper arms, round the shoulders and up the back of the neck. (x6)
2. Stretch out the shoulders by cupping your hands round both shoulders and pressing down using the pressure of your body weight, then extend it gradually down the arms.
3. Roll the head to one side and use smooth stroking movements around the shoulder up to the top of the neck to stretch out the area.
4. Using small friction movements massage up the same area with your thumbs or forefingers.
5. Place one hand at the back of the neck with fingers resting just below the occipital area (hollow at base of skull) with the other hand cupping the shoulder, ask your client to take in a deep breath. When they exhale, gently stretch this area by pulling your hands apart. (x2)
6. Repeat the last three steps on the other side, then place the head back to its original position.
7. Lift the head, support it at the base of the occipital and cradle it. Steer the head gently in circles creating a figure of eight from side to side. Take the full weight in your hands, then place it back down.
8. Using the tips of your second, third and fourth fingers, press up either side of the top vertebrae into the occipital region.
9. With one hand at the base of the skull and the other hand on the forehead, pull the head back to create a space use a kneading action to the neck.
10. Swap the hands and work on the other side.
11. Place one hand on the base of the skull and the other on the top of the shoulder: ask your client to breathe in. As they exhale press the shoulder down with one hand and pull up at the base of the skull with the other.
12. Swap sides and repeat the movement.
13. Using circular movements with your fingertips, massage over the whole upper chest area.
14. Place your thumbs just beneath the clavicle in the middle and press each thumb out towards the lymph nodes under the arms, then use the heel of your hands over the same area. (x3)
15. Finish by using sweeping strokes across the upper chest over the upper arms round the shoulders and up the back of the neck. (x6)

Face massage – a step-by-step guide

1. Start by applying the oil with your fingertips from the clavicle up the side of the face to the forehead and then return.
2. Press into the pressure points on the forehead with your thumbs. (x3)
3. Start with your thumbs together just above eyebrows and pull them apart stretching out the frontalis muscle. When you reach the sides of the forehead make gentle circles with your thumbs over the temples. Move up towards the hairline and do the same movement, finishing just under the hairline. (x3)
4. Using the index finger press all the points along the brow line working towards the hairline. Then with your index finger and thumb 'pinch' along the brows. Repeat both movements three times.
5. Press under the eye sockets with the index fingers.
6. Press in all the pressure points either side of the nose, being careful not to block the nostrils.
7. Finally, with your index fingers press under the cheekbones working towards the drainage points in front of the ears, then sweep out towards the ears; repeat several times.
7. Place your hands either side of the nose, palms down, and push out towards the outside of the face.
9. Squeeze the points along the jaw line working towards the ears.
10. Using the pads of the fingers make circular movements all over the face.
11. Placing your fingers together underneath the jaw, pull up either side of the face and meet your fingers above the forehead.
12. Squeeze around the outside of the ears and then gently block the ears.
13. With palms flat on the forehead stroke up towards the hairline, alternating hands.
14. Place both hands on the forehead.

Think about it

You must take immediate remedial action and stop the treatment if your client develops any contra-actions during any part of the treatment: when using preblended essential oils these would commonly be a rash, headache, nausea, light-headedness or irritation of the skin. Pain of any kind should also be reacted to quickly. Remove all oil on the area and apply a cooling compress – a cool, damp towel would soothe the area. Notes should be added to the record card so that it doesn't happen again.

Provide aftercare advice

The healing crisis

The client may have unexpectedly strong physical and emotional responses to their aromatherapy massage because they have had a rebalance and blockages have been cleared.

Think about it

Pre-blended oils come directly from the manufacturer and therefore you will have a limited range of mixtures and dilutions. You may feel that your client could benefit from more advanced treatment from a clinical aromatherapist and you can refer them on, perhaps to one of your colleagues taking a full diploma in aromatherapy, as this includes customised blending.

Aftercare advice

The client will certainly be sleepy and, probably, very relaxed! Do warn your client that they have had a strongly sedative treatment and they should not drive or do anything too strenuous until their mental functioning returns to normal. Give the client a drink of water and allow them to gradually sit upright and awaken — just as if they have had a deep and replenishing sleep. There may be some adverse effects as the body heals and clears any blockages; light-headedness, headaches and nausea are common if the client had lots of pent-up tension or emotional issues they had been holding on to. This is part of the healing crisis, mentioned above. Ginger biscuits are good for nausea and a quiet lie-down will help with a headache. If the client expects it, they will cope in the knowledge that it will pass and it is part of the body healing itself.

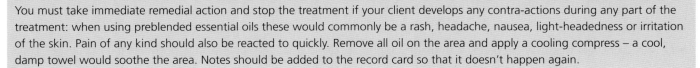

The following aftercare should be advised:

- Do not bathe for at least six hours after treatment as the oils should penetrate the skin fully and get into the system — bathing will wash them off.

- Keep the feeling of relaxation going by avoiding over-stimulating the brain: driving, television and loud noises should be avoided where possible — even conversation is hard when you have just woken up.

- A light diet of fruit and vegetables will help throughout the day — avoid stimulants such as tea, coffee and alcohol.

- Keep drinking lots of water or herbal teas.

- Keep the skin moisturised by applying body lotions throughout the week, to reinforce the effects of the massage.

Talk the client through the findings from the massage regarding muscular tension, preferred movements, blends of oils used and any problems and add the information onto their record card. Offer some tips about getting more sleep, taking gentle exercise two or three times a week and trying to relax more.

Allow the client enough time to be comfortable standing up. They can then get dressed and you can talk them through the aftercare.

Check with your client that they are happy with the resulting treatment and make any notes on the record card of movement to be avoided or included if the client especially disliked/liked it. Also note the oil and carrier oil used and the client satisfaction with the treatment.

For your portfolio

Create an aftercare leaflet that explains everything to the client. Cover both immediate aftercare, and then longer-term aftercare and lifestyle changes which may help the client: diet, relaxation, exercise, sleeping and healing, both mind and body.

Avoidance of activities which may cause contra-actions

As well as discussing your client's future treatments, modifications to their lifestyle to help with the treatments and a healthy eating and exercise plan, you should ask the client to avoid any activities which may cause a contra-action, later in the day. Remind your client that the oils are active within the body for a long time, depending upon the blends.

The following advice should ideally be given on an aftercare leaflet, which they can take away with them.

Advise the client:

- not to apply any other oils to the skin, in case of over-stimulation of both the area and the brain

- to avoid other treatments such as waxing, heat treatments or sunbathing

- to avoid the application of perfumed products for 24 hours

- to avoid alcohol and smoking, as most oils are detoxifying and the client could cause an over-reaction.

Check your knowledge

1   When performing a patch test for suitability of essential oils, how long should you leave it?
   a) 2–4 hours
   b) 4–6 hours
   c) 10–12 hours
   d) 24–48 hours

2   Which part of the plant does benzoin come from?
   a) The twigs
   b) The bark
   c) The flower
   d) The leaves

3   An analgesic is used to:
   a) help with growth and repair
   b) stop sickness
   c) relieve pain
   d) stop water loss.

4   To describe a smell as citrus means it is:
   a) zesty
   b) floral
   c) spicy
   d) herby.

5   An aromatherapy full body treatment should take:
   a) 1 hour 15 minutes
   b) 1 hour
   c) half an hour
   d) 1 hour 30 minutes.

6   Sandalwood is a good oil for:
   a) acne
   b) depression
   c) nail growth
   d) muscles.

7   A good oil for treating cellulite is:
   a) spikenard
   b) tea tree
   c) ylang ylang
   d) thyme.

8   An oil you should never use is:
   a) rosemary
   b) calamus
   c) lavender
   d) fennel.

9   Tea tree is said to have what property?
   a) Analgesic
   b) Anti-inflammatory
   c) Antibacterial
   d) Anti-fungal

10 Sage is a:
   a) middle note
   b) top note
   c) base note
   d) lower base note.

Getting ready for assessment

You are not allowed any simulation within this unit and you must practically demonstrate in your everyday work that you have met the Standards for providing massage using pre-blended aromatherapy oils.

Your assessor will observe your performance on at least *four* separate occasions, each time on different clients. At least *two* must be full body treatments including the face.

From the ranges you must show that you have:

- used all consultation techniques
- dealt with all the client characteristics
- dealt with at least one of the necessary actions
- used all massage techniques
- covered all treatment areas
- given all types of advice.

To show a good understanding of the oils and the treatment outcomes, it would be a good idea to have at least one male client and to try to incorporate more than one range in your assessment, for example:

- Client A — male, with treatment objectives of uplifting and wellbeing required
- Client B — female with treatment objectives of relaxing and anti-cellulite required.

Carry out massage using pre-blended aromatherapy oils B24

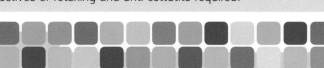

Unit B28

Provide stone therapy treatments

What you will learn

- Maintain safe and effective methods of working when providing stone therapy treatments
- Consult, plan and prepare for treatments with clients
- Perform stone therapy treatments
- Provide aftercare advice

The Standards set out detailed performance criteria regarding:

- maintaining safe and effective methods of working when providing stone therapy treatments
- consulting, planning and preparing for treatments with clients.

The majority of these requirements apply to all beauty therapy treatments and are therefore covered in detail in Professional basics, G22 Monitor procedures to safely control work operations, and Body treatments – theory and consultation. You should also refer back to You and the skin, Related anatomy and physiology and B20 Provide body massage treatments, as required.

Treatment-specific requirements for stone therapy are covered within this unit.

Introduction

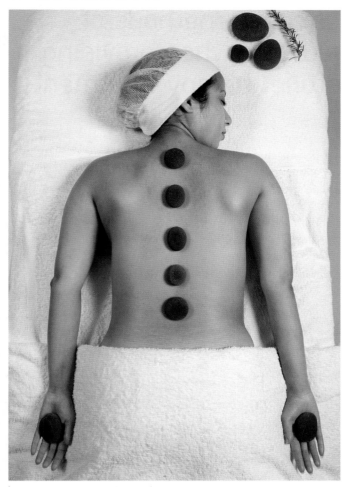

Spinal placement of hot stones is done for publicity only – the stones are not placed over the vertebrae in treatment and would be too hot for direct contact with the skin

The use of stones for healing has been used for centuries, and stones have been around since the earth was formed. The correct term for stone use is geothermotherapy – *geo* referring to the rocks of the earth; *thermo* relating to the use of heating and cooling effects to stimulate the body's natural functions; and *therapy* for healing.

Indigenous people from countries with volcanic landscapes have always used both hot and cold stones for healing, and therapists have harnessed this as an extension of their massage techniques. Native Americans, the Incas and Egyptians were known to hold ceremonies, treatments or healing sessions with precious stones and rocks and the Inuit people use hot rocks worn in papooses close to their bodies for muscular ailments. In Russia, hot stone therapy is used with bathing, with the client lying on the stones so that the main **marma pressure points** throughout the body are

stimulated, promoting healing and a feeling of wellbeing. In Japan hot stones are placed on the abdomen after eating to aid digestion. So, many cultures use hot and cold stones to restore balance and health and to promote wellness and relaxation in the body.

How does it work?

The hot stones are heated in a big electrical heater base with an inner water reservoir (a bit like a slow cooker used in domestic cooking). The stones are placed in the order that they are going to be used, on a towel to eliminate noise, and then water is poured over them and heated up. The use of a waterproof thermometer indicates when the working temperature has been reached and, when the client is fully prepared for massage, you remove the stones, drain and dry them and work them over the body, both as massage instruments and as placements.

The cool stones are chilled and kept in a small refrigerator or cool box, ready for use with alternate hot stones, or can be used on their own.

On a superficial level, hot stones within massage are a labour-saving device for the therapist. The stones aid penetration of movements by the heat emitted, warming the underlying tissue, and the stones are a smooth extension of the hands, making contact with the skin in place of the therapist – so reducing the repetitive strain that hands and wrists endure.

Additional knowledge

Stone therapy in Western culture

Mary Nelson from Arizona is widely credited for introducing stone therapy back into Western focus with the introduction of La Stone Therapy™. She used stones from a sauna to help her with her Swedish massage clients, as she was suffering from repetitive strain injury to her shoulders and was told by her **spirit guide** to pick up the stones and use them.

Key terms

Marma pressure points – there are 107 marma points all over the body which represent where the vital energies flow.

Spirit guide – according to some people's beliefs, a spirit guide (also known as a spirit teacher or a guardian angel) is a wise pure soul who has lived many times before and who acts as a guide and teacher to each human being, helping them to gain insight and learn life lessons during their time on earth.

On a deeper holistic level, the stones have their own high vibrational energy, connecting us to Mother Earth, Father Sky and the five elements: water, ether/wood, earth, metal/ air and fire. These elements are provided by the earth and are the building blocks of every living thing in the universe, including the human body. Holistic therapists believe that we should honour the five elements as they are gifts from the universe and relate deeply to our bodies on all levels — physically, emotionally and spiritually. The stones can be used to open up the **chakras** of the body and chilled stones can be used on areas of inflammation and injury — just as a sports massage therapist would use ice. In fact hot and cold stone therapy is often advertised as a 'fire and ice massage'.

More detail on chakras and ayurvedic principles can be found in B23 Provide Indian head massage, page 435.

Think about it

Stone massage therapists believe in 'the power of ten': that one stroke with a stone is worth ten of the hands and that treatment is ten times more effective and deeper than manual massage, with ten times less effort involved.

Think about it

Stones are used in two ways:

1. as *tools* held in the hand for deeper movements and more penetration into the tissues
2. as *placements* onto the body for deep penetration of heat, rather like a stone hot water bottle.

Key terms

Chakra – spinning vortexes of energy. The Sanskrit word for chakra means 'wheel of light'.

Thermotherapy – the application of heat and cold to alleviate pain and stiffness in muscles and joints and increase blood flow to the area.

Cryotherapy – cooling the body using extreme cold, either locally in the form of ice packs or generally, where the whole body is artificially cooled.

Maintain safe and effective methods of working when providing stone therapy treatments

In this section you will learn about:

- manufacturer's instructions
- environmental conditions
- personal hygiene
- stones
- tools and equipment
- caring for your stones
- protection of the skin
- client modesty
- treatment time.

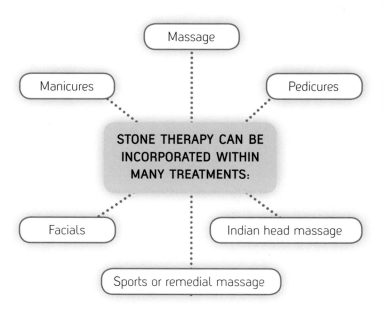

STONE THERAPY CAN BE INCORPORATED WITHIN MANY TREATMENTS: Massage, Manicures, Pedicures, Facials, Indian head massage, Sports or remedial massage

Manufacturer's instructions

- Hot stone heaters do vary with each manufacturer and you must not assume that all heaters operate in the same way.

- Some may take longer to heat up in relation to the water capacity (the larger the heater capacity in litres, the longer it take to heat) depending upon the size bought, which varies between a 6- and 18-stone heater.

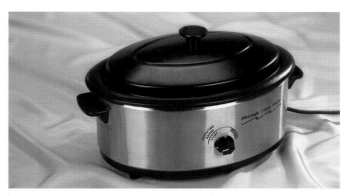

A hot stone heater

- The way you lift out the stones may vary; some manufacturers supply gloves, others supply tongs or a slotted spoon.
- Some manufacturers name their stones, for example Grandfather stone, Grandmother stone, Father stone and so on.
- Some will recommend you turn on the heater prior to use for the first time and set it to preheat and run for an hour to burn off any odour or smoke from the heating element. (This will not occur again during normal use.)

The more familiar you become with the instructions and the more you work with the stones, the more you will understand how to use them to maximum effect. Do not use any other heater than the one supplied with your stones. A domestic slow cooker is *not* a substitute heater for the stones and, by not providing enough room for the stones to heat evenly, you risk burning the client if the stones develop hot spots. You will need more than one heater if you build up a regular clientele and you should allow for more than one set of stones, as they will need cleaning and reheating between clients. They will also need re-energising and you should never use dirty stones on a client, both for hygiene reasons and possible cross-infection, but also because the negative energy will build up and the stones will stop working effectively and will not hold the heat for very long. You risk transferring negative energies between clients and the idea is that they leave refreshed with open chakras, not weighed down with the accumulation of every client's troubles!

Environmental conditions

The environmental conditions for stone therapy should be exactly the same as for massage – the heating of the room, the lighting and ambience of the treatment areas should be one of relaxation and calm. The only real difference for the

client with a stone massage is that it can be noisy as you get the stones out, and when you first start, you may find you drop a stone or bang them together unintentionally, which can make the client jump! With practice and the placement of a towel in the heater and a towel lining a bowl or trolley to place the stones on after use, the noise can be cut down – and you will develop confidence the more you use them.

The massage techniques also vary with stones, because you do break contact with the client when you add stones or put stones down after use. However, as you develop your routine, the contact of the placement stones on the body keeps the continuity going and the client is not really aware you have taken off your hands to get more – they will just be enjoying the heat generated and relaxing.

Personal hygiene

Personal hygiene should be identical to your massage routine and it is important that you still recognise your hands as important massage tools, so keep nails short and unpolished and hands flexible.

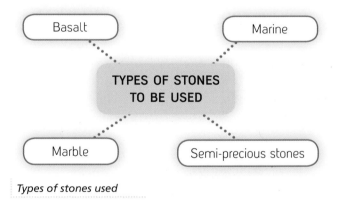

Types of stones used

Stones

Basalt stones

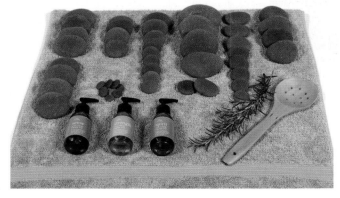

Basalt stones are dense, heavy volcanic rocks which have been naturally shaped and polished by the sea or riverbed over thousands of years. They are various shades of grey/green to black and will change in colour once they are oiled and used regularly. For use in stone therapy they should be smooth and regular with no chips in them. The stones are sourced from Arizona, Greece and Mexico — areas of previous volcanic activity. The basalt stones are formed under immense pressure and heat, creating their unique qualities. This molten rock contains pyroxene (a mineral), plagioclase (crystallised from magma activity from volcanoes), very high levels of iron and magnesium and other minerals which compress under weight and produce these compact basalt stones.

The stones are able to hold their heat for up to four times longer than any other natural stone. Once heated, the stones retain heat for a long time and release it slowly, thus making them the ideal massage tool.

During treatment the stones are skilfully applied to the skin using the medium of aromatic essences and specific massage techniques. The stones are self-adjusting to the body's own temperature requirements and will transfer heat according to the areas of greatest need, promoting thermal balance.

Marine stones

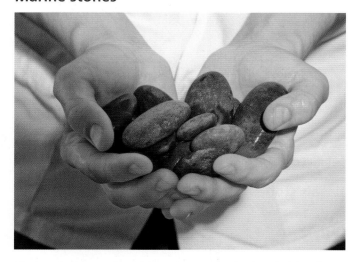

Marine stones are found in waters around volcanic islands such as Hawaii and come from the sediment on the ocean floor. They are formed from the coral reef and shaped by plant life in the sea. They are used within cool massage as they contain lots of minerals. This makes them ideal for detoxifying and they also have anti-inflammatory properties. They are often green in colour, very smooth and some have distinct patterns, looking like two eyes.

They can be used:

- for broken capillaries on the face
- over the eyes for instant relaxation and cooling of the area
- to reduce puffiness and dark circles around the eye area
- to reduce headaches and tension.

Marble stones

The cool marble stones are organic rocks, mostly made from calcite and limestone. Marble stays cool due to its calcium content and it is really metamorphosed limestone (calcium carbonate re-crystallises under heat and pressure to form marble). The benefits of using marble stones are that they are able to retain cold for long periods and they are less messy and cooler than ice. They need to be handcrafted so they are more expensive than basalt stone, but because of being polished by hand the shapes can be made to fit particular contours of the body, with half wedges, rounds, corner stones and crescent shapes for use on the contours of the face and body. Marble creates heavy stones, yet they are more delicate than basalt stones and vulnerable to scratching. Marble is often the choice of building materials in hot climates; it remains cold to the touch and draws heat from its surroundings, so cooling the atmosphere. Marble stones in massage regulate temperature and cool over-heated areas of the body. This can often appear in cases of inflammation. They are also of great value to tone and firm the skin, especially the facial tissue.

Semi-precious stones

Most stones and rock have some degree of crystal within them, so all rock could be called crystal — but what we think of as beautifully coloured crystal, with distinctive, easy recognition, are really gem stones. Massage that incorporates semi-precious stones is frequently a specialised treatment delivered by holistic therapists. The stones are often polished and used as part of a placement massage for spiritual healing and altering the mood in treatment rooms. Semi-precious stones have been used within ceremonies and traditions of ancient cultures and often symbolised wealth and importance. This is continued in modern day: do you know what your birthstone is?

There is a basic set of twenty crystals ranging from amber to quartz, and its most popular method for use is to open the chakras. Crystals can also be used with reflexology, aroma therapy and Indian head massage. See the detail on chakras and their relevant crystals/gems in B23 Provide Indian head massage, page 435.

The most common of the stones used are basalt stones, with a stone heater, and marble stones in a cool box for alternate use on the body. Crystal use is a separate therapy on its own and therapists spend many years honing their skills. Be careful of using the term 'crystal healing', because of its medical overtones. The crystals do have some powerful cleansing effects on the chakras and can open the emotions to free blockages, but this should in no way imply a cure from any ailment or medical condition. You are not medically trained and cannot claim to treat any conditions that require medical attention.

Size of stones

Get used to the feel and weight of the stones and choose stones which fit easily into your hands for massage – if you are too clumsy with a bigger stone than your hands can comfortably hold and use, the awkwardness will transfer to the massage movements, which will not flow nor be enjoyable for the client. So, take some time to practise with those stones that feel best, and stick with them – obviously a male masseur with larger hands will use a bigger stone and be able to handle it with ease. A petite therapist may only use several of the smaller stones. This doesn't matter to the client. They will be unaware and not at all critical, and the larger stones make lovely placements on the lumber/sacral area, under the knees and under the couch for energy balancing.

Sensation of the stones

Stones come in all sorts of shapes, sizes and weights – in fact no two stones are identical, because of the way they are formed. You use similar ones in size on the body for symmetry, so facial stones will be the same size to keep the sensation of the massage even. Marble stones do have more uniformity of shape because they are hand-crafted and can be made to fit the purpose (for example, crescent-shaped to fit over the limbs).

Stone therapy uses a variety of shapes for differing purposes:

- round, small and large – which suits most massage strokes of effleurage and should fit nicely into the palm of the therapist's hands
- oblong – for deep tissue use, as the outer rim is ideally suitable as a finger-kneading and thumb-kneading substitute (saving wear and tear on the therapist's own joints)
- large half-crescent shaped stones with a flat side for placement either on the sacrum, under the neck or under the feet or knees
- C-shaped stones in marble, shaped for use on the limbs.

Whichever shape they are, the stones need to be smooth so they glide over an oiled skin and are workable. They should feel like an extension of your hand and be level, even and almost soft – that is the illusion because, of course, the stone is very hard, which is why the heat stays in the stone for up to ten minutes. The rougher stones can be used as placement stones only, and under either a towel or sheet so the client just feels the warmth and not the texture of the stones. For the client the stones feel warm, induce a comforting pleasant heat in the muscles and keep the continuity of the massage going, even when the therapist has broken contact to get more stones.

Removing and handling of stones

- When they are brand new, unpack and wash all the stones and oil them thoroughly, using this time to familiarise yourself with the stones and their feel and weight. Pick the most suitable ones for your hand size. Don't oil the marble ones as they absorb it and this softens them and may cause cracking. The oil doesn't stay on the stones – this is just when they are new and you need to become familiar with them. Oil will also darken new stones slightly.
- The stones take up to 45 minutes to heat up to their full temperature, which should never exceed 66°C. The normal reading on your thermometer should be in the region of 120°F or 50°C but always refer to manufacturers' recommendations.
- Never place the stones on to a client without testing them on yourself first.
- Use the tongs or insulated rubber (waterproof) gloves or slotted spoon to remove the stones on to a towel by the client, ready for use.
- Always have a bowl of water on the trolley to immerse a hot stone in to cool it – if it is too hot for your hand it is too hot to place on the client.

Tools and equipment

Always clean the unit thoroughly after each day's session and leave all equipment as you would wish to find it in the morning.

After removing the stones, the water reservoir can be emptied and removed, washed in warm soapy water and dried with a towel. The bottom heating part of your unit must never be fully immersed in water – it just needs wiping over with a damp cloth. Do ensure it is cool enough.

Rinse the removed stones in warm water with a small amount of mild detergent, then rinse in clean, warm water and allow to dry thoroughly before storing them.

Never move the heater when it is full of water and plugged into the mains — you risk tripping over trailing wires or spilling hot water.

Never add the stones to the hot water; always place them in the heater and then add water.

Use a towel to line the water reservoir as it muffles the sound, aiding relaxation. If the room lighting is quite dim, a white towel will enable you to see the stones' layout better, making it easier to pick them up quietly.

Never pour boiling water on top of the stones for a quick heating effect — you risk splashing and scalding yourself.

Only fill the water reservoir to just cover the stones and no more than 1 inch below the top rim — the heater will heat more efficiently with the lid on.

Caring for your stones

Sterilising

You should have a system of sterilising your stones between clients — and ideally have two sets and two heaters to prevent clients from being kept waiting, or spread out the treatments to allow cleaning and heating time. As the stones will have oily residue from the treatment on them, and any skin particles they may have picked up, they should be sprayed with surgical spirit, alcohol solution or a manufacturer's recommended bacterial cleaner.

Even if they have only been used once during the day, they will still need cleaning and sterilising.

Recharging

On a monthly cycle the stones will also need recharging to restore their energy levels, to discharge all the negative energy they have absorbed throughout the treatments and to reconnect to their roots in nature. You can tell when the stones need recharging as they do not hold the heat for very long and are not hot to the touch, even if the water is at the correct temperature.

The stones can be charged by being:

- immersed in sea water — if you practise your therapies near the coast then washing the stones in natural salt water is ideal and they should then be left out in the sun and wind to dry

- cleansed and left in the sunlight for a day to absorb the rays (this is not suitable for crystals as they fade in sunlight)

- cleansed and left out overnight in the moonlight (cold stones and crystals are better cleansed in moonlight)

- allowed, if possible when the stones are not in use, to have 24 hours out in both sunshine and moonlight to rebalance, so allowing the perfect balance of **yin and yang** to be restored

- allowed any contact with the elements — left out in a thunderstorm, or in the rain, held under natural running spring water or soaked overnight in bottled natural spring water

- cleansed with crystals — labradorite or moonstone for cold stones

- cleansed with Reiki therapy, if you are a practitioner

- stored with wild sage sprigs

- placed on a bed of natural salt or you could sprinkle salt onto heated stones for a quick recharge. Never do this with marble stones as the salt will be absorbed and soften them, making them more likely to crack or split.

Protection of the skin

- Use a towel or a sheet between the skin and the placement stone, if required, to cushion and avoid burning the skin.

- Some manufacturers suggest and provide bags, socks or small pillow cases to put small stones in for placement around the joints — even a facial flannel would be suitable as a barrier (but remember the thicker the insulation the more heat it will block).

- Remember that it is possible to burn a client with cold stones, too. If you remove the stone from the cold box and place it straight onto the skin it can give a cold burn. If this were to happen, apply a warm (not hot) moist cloth to ease the stone away.

Key terms

Yin and yang – in East Asian thought, the two opposite but complementary forces or principles that make up all aspects and phenomena of life.

Consult, plan and prepare for treatments with clients

In this section you will learn about:

- consultation for stone therapy
- physical characteristics linked with treatment objectives
- using stones within other treatments
- how to do a test patch
- contra-indications to treatment.

Consultation for stone therapy

As with all your treatments a full consultation should take place to ascertain the client's needs, treatment objectives, whether any contra-indications are present or the treatment requires adaptation in any way. You can use the body massage consultation form in Body treatments – theory and consultation, page 328, as many of the contra-indications are the same. Full consultation techniques are covered within Professional basics and all you need to do is adapt your consultation to the treatment you are currently doing. As always, the fundamental principle of any consultation applies: the client is the most important person and deserves your full and professional attention!

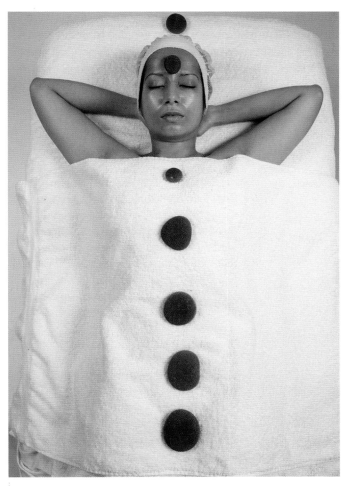

Protection of the skin

Physical characteristics linked with treatment objectives

When using hot and cold stone therapy not only should you adapt the treatment to suit the physical characteristics of the client in terms of height/weight ratio and muscle/fat ratio (see Body treatments – theory and consultation, page 341) but also noting whether the client is a hot or cold person and their preferences. If a client is quite thin and feels the cold, does not have good circulation or suffers muscular tension, then they are an ideal candidate for a hot stone treatment. They need warming and soothing heat massage to raise body

Client modesty

Client modesty is exactly the same as for any massage and sufficient towels and blankets are required to keep a client's body fully covered and the heat in the muscles once the treatment areas have been worked upon. Please refer to B20 Provide massage treatments for a full towel and couch layout.

Treatment time

Treatment time for stone therapy will vary – depending upon whether you are doing hot and cold stones, rebalancing of chakras and using crystals. The general rule of thumb is that treatments generally last slightly longer than Swedish manual body massage and are similar to an aromatherapy treatment in both time and cost involved. Approximately 90 minutes for a full stone treatment is standard – but you should compare with differing salons to ensure you are providing a fair and comparable service for your clients.

Think about it

Remember you will need written consent to enter into a treatment plan with all clients and especially those who require parental permission for a treatment. Refer to Professional basics, page 23, for more detail on treating minors.

temperature and create relaxation in muscles that may be tense due to the cold. However, if a client has a hot body, muscular and sporty with a tendency to sprains — then cold marble massage is going to suit them far better. You may want to start with hot stones to open up the muscles, but the majority of your work will be with cold stones.

Whichever treatment plan you mutually decide upon with your client, do ensure that they fully understand what the treatment involves: that they will be massaged with stones and have stones placed upon the body, and or be lying upon them, be undressed and in a prone position on the couch, as for manual massage.

Encourage the client to ask lots of questions — and perhaps show them the stones, the heater, how it works and let them hold a hot or cold stone or crystal during your consultation period. Just holding a smooth stone in the hand and stroking it will relax the client and fill them with enthusiasm for their treatment. Explain the physical, physiological and emotional effects of massage and what you hope to achieve. If you are also doing chakra work and placement to open and balance them, then explain to the client about a possible healing crisis and how the body develops contra-actions to rid itself of negativity and restore calm. Possibly, with a new client and as an introduction with a first treatment, it is better to focus on the physical effects and allow them just to relax and enjoy the release of tension in the muscles and even to induce sleep. As you build up your relationship and the client trusts you, you can then introduce the concept of chakras and the emotional balancing and cleansing of them.

Using stones within other treatments

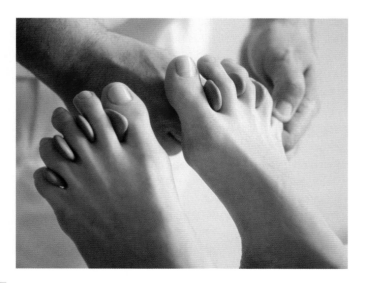

Another way to introduce the use of stones is to use them for other treatments such as pedicures and manicures, so that the client can literally see the stones being used and feel their benefits — and you can talk them through the treatments.

Manicures	• Use a large stone which has been heated instead of a pad on your manicure work station. The client rests a hand on the stone whilst you work on the nails and can enjoy the heat in the palm releasing tension • Use the smaller stones in the bowl when soaking the hands — and encourage the client to play with them, stroke them and twist them around the fingers. Do explain that they are there, though, as if you use hand soak that bubbles up, they may not be visible. The bowl should be deep enough so there is no splashing of water to cause a spillage • Do your normal manicure massage routine but use the hot stones and pick a suitably sized one for the client to hold in the hand that is not being massaged • You can use hot stones to work in the exfoliant hand scrub • The cosy toe stones can also be placed between the fingers when you are painting the nails
Pedicures	• Ideal for clients who suffer with cold feet and poor circulation • Use a large hot stone or several small ones to put under the feet on a towel at the beginning of the treatment • Use the smaller stones in the bowl when soaking the feet • Work in foot scrub exfoliants with the stones • Use hot stones for the massage • Put the cosy toe stones between the toes when nail painting • Give the client hot stones to hold and play with in their hands whilst you are working on their feet. This give you the opportunity to discuss body treatments using the stones and how beneficial it is

Indian head massage	• The stone can be used along with the fingers for parts of the massage involving palmar movements and kneading • The client can be holding stones in the hands during treatment • You can use stones as placements under the feet (as shoes are removed) • If massaging through the clothing the stones will need to be hot enough to penetrate through
Sports or remedial massage	• Deeper movements can be used with hot stones to aid penetration into muscular tension • Hot stone massage will aid lymphatic drainage • Placement stone can be used in the hands and under the neck, or either side of the spine as well as used within the massage movements • Cool stones can be used in conjunction with hot to help vasoconstriction and reduction of fluid retention
Facials	• Use placements under the knees, in the hands of the client and under the neck and, if the client requires it, over the abdomen over the towel or blanket (just as a hot water bottle would be placed for period pains) • The client can hold the stones in their hands • Small stones can be used for manual massage • Cool marine stones can be used over the eyelids during the mask or used as a massage tool to reduce puffiness around the eyes and aid congestion of the sinuses • Exfoliant products can be applied with the stones

How to do a patch test

Whichever use of the stones you choose, you should always carry out a thermal sensitivity patch test using hot and cold test tubes, in the areas to be worked, to determine the client responses to hot and cold (just as you would with electrical equipment – see B13 Provide body electrical treatments, and B14 Provide facial electrical treatments). Not only will this reveal if there is any nerve impairment in the area, which would be a contra-indication, but it will also show the skin's reaction to hot and cold and help you form a treatment plan based on the skin response and the client's personal preferences.

Contra-indications to treatment

- Skin or scalp infections, ulcers, open cuts and abrasions, bruises
- Recent injury, operations or recent scar tissue
- Any infectious conditions because of the risk of cross-infection
- Clients undergoing treatments which require chemo- or radiotherapies
- Pregnancy or clients who are breastfeeding
- Diabetics and epileptics – GP approval should be gained and the letter attached to the record card
- Medication taken which would make the client sensitive to heat, or which thin the skin – Roactane or steroids either applied topically or taken orally
- Osteoporosis
- High or low blood pressure or clients who are very heat-sensitive
- Acute inflammation in an area or over joints
- Loss of sensation and failure to distinguish hot and cold thermal testing
- The very elderly or the very young
- Clinical obesity
- Any other contra-indications from a general massage treatment (see unit B20 Provide body massage treatments, page 392)

During your treatment consultation remember to keep the client informed about the cost, duration, frequency and the type of treatment you are agreeing with them, and your recommendations for further treatments.

Stone massage will be more expensive than a normal body massage and last about 90 minutes as opposed to a manual massage lasting an hour, and you may like to charge a small addition to your normal manicure and pedicure prices as you are offering a deluxe version of a standard treatment.

> **Think about it**
>
> Always check for the suitability of the oil you wish to use, both to meet client needs and prevent an allergic reaction. Suppliers of stones also sell a lovely range of products to be used with them, some including essential oils. You can also choose from your usual body massage medium range.

Salon life

Jaina's story

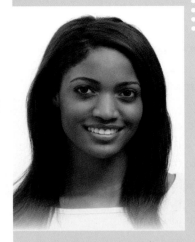

My name is Jaina and I have been in my salon for about a year. I love hot stone massage treatments but something happened to me recently which reminded me just how different my clients are and what a mistake it is to treat everyone in the same way.

I had a young male client who wanted a full body massage. During our consultation, he explained that he was into sport, had lots of muscular tension and wanted a deeper massage. I explained the beneficial effects of hot stone massage on the muscles and told him he would get much better results with the weight and strength of the stones.

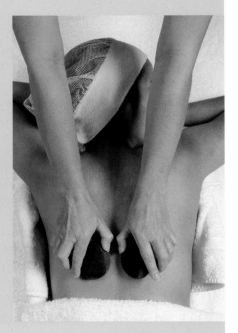

He told me that he was interested in a hot stone massage but had never had one because he was quite sensitive to heat. I told him that, although the treatment is called 'hot stone', they aren't really *hot* but warm and that we would do a sensitivity test so he could feel the heat of them before the massage, so he signed up for a course of six treatments.

At his first massage, I performed the sensitivity test by placing a warm stone on his forearm — one of the least sensitive areas. He flinched and said it was far too hot. So I let the stone cool in cold water and placed it on a higher part of his arm. He said it was still too hot. After I had done this three or four times, he said the stone was at a temperature he could tolerate. They were practically cold! I explained that he wouldn't get as many benefits without the heat but he said he didn't mind — he liked the feel of the stones and felt he was getting a deeper massage.

He really enjoyed his course and now comes in twice a month but I have to remember to turn the heater off! Some clients can take a really hot massage and others just can't. Everyone is different and I needed to adapt the treatment to suit him.

Effects for the therapist:

- Taking time to explain treatments in detail can lead to big sales
- Realise that no two clients like the same thing — it is very important to learn to adapt your treatments to suit the individual
- There is no set way to carry out a treatment, and you shouldn't make the client uncomfortable — the client is always right, and meeting their needs will determine how successful your treatment is

Effects for the client:

- Care and attention to detail really enhances the treatment
- Having their personal preferences taken into account means the client will trust their therapist
- If the client can discuss adaptation of the treatment they will have a treatment that is tailor-made for them — it will be more effective and more enjoyable

Check out your own local salons and spas for prices for both hot and cold stone massage therapy. Have a look at which other treatments the business incorporates the use of stones with and how much additional fee they charge. A stone heater and kit price list can be found on any beauty supplier website and they will vary depending upon the size bought. How many treatments would you need to do to recoup the price of your equipment and what profit margin is there in stone treatments?

Perform stone therapy treatments

In this section you will learn about:

- the effects of hot and cold stones
- the benefits of using hot and cold stones
- stone therapy techniques and massage movements
- what you need for treatment
- client preparation
- the treatment procedure
- contra-actions.

The effects of hot and cold stones

Thermotherapy is the application of hot and cold temperature to restore balance to the mind and body.

The practice of thermotherapy can be traced as far back as the hot and cold bathing methods introduced by Hippocrates in 430 BC as a means of promoting positive circulation, boosting the immune system and relaxing the mind. More recently Sebastian Kneipp, a German monk and doctor in the nineteenth century, achieved optimum health in his practice with the use of alternating hot and cold baths and showers. So, his principles are used in beauty therapy to restore health and balance with hot pools, cold dips, saunas, steam rooms and plunge pools. The same principles apply with hot and cold stones.

Vasodilation occurs – blood vessels open and blood flow is increased

Metabolism increases so cellular functioning is improved

EFFECTS OF HOT STONES ON THE BODY

The warmth has a sedative effect on the nerve endings

Deep relaxation occurs within the muscle fibres

Pulse rate quickens with the heat

Effects of hot stones on the body

Reduction in erythema

Vasoconstriction occurs – blood vessels narrow reducing blood flow

Cools inflammation – ideal after waxing treatment

EFFECTS OF COLD STONES ON THE BODY

Balances the hot stone effect on the body's temperature

Decongesting as the cold constricts blood vessels

The cold causes nerves to constrict and this numbs the area (analgesic effect)

Effects of cold stones on the body

The benefits of using hot and cold stones

Stone therapy application of hot and cool temperatures stimulates the body's own natural functions, especially the circulatory and lymphatic systems, along with the nervous system. The nerve endings in the skin pick up the changes in temperature, move along the nerve fibres to the spinal cord and to the related organs and the brain. Generally the skin over a main organ is where its relative reflex point is — so any stimulation of the skin over an organ improves its function. When all these systems are working normally, all the body's organs and tissue and cell functions improve, promoting optimum health and giving more energy.

Benefits to the client

- Boosts circulation — increased blood flow serves to bring more oxygen and nutrients to the area whilst speeding up the removal of carbon dioxide

- Speeds up cellular metabolism — increased in the area by 10–15% due to the local rise in body temperature of between 1–2°C

- Increases immune function — increased lymphatic circulation speeds up the body's own natural elimination process, boosting energy levels and ensuring full removal of waste

- Improves muscle and skin tone — positive circulation of blood and lymph serve to nourish and stimulate the skin's reproduction of healthy cells and the muscle fibres, leaving them healthy and toned

- Improves joint flexibility — increased circulation and lymph flow aids flexibility in supporting joint muscle by relaxing the connective tissue, as well as removing excess waste that can often lead to aches, pains and joint stiffness

- Alleviates deep muscle aches and pains — the hot stones heat the muscles and additional movement of the stones provides deeper penetration into the muscle structure than traditional massage; often the massage is able to reduce muscle spasms and chronic muscle tension and stiffness, especially sports-related tension

- Deeply relaxes the nervous system — positive circulation and lymph flow, especially to the spinal nerves and muscles, help to stimulate a poor nervous system inducing feelings of wellbeing, positivity and vitality

- Calms the mind — as all of the body's natural process are boosted the body feels less challenged, allowing the mind to be quiet and relaxed; at the same time the application of different temperatures unlocks deep emotional tension

The treatment aims to gain complete homeostasis — a perfect peak of balance for the body.

Benefits to the therapist

- One stroke of the stone is equal to ten strokes of manual massage, so it is labour-saving for the therapist

- Prevents over-use in the joints of the thumbs and wrists and upper body — avoiding repetitive strain injury and hypo- and hyper-extension of the joints; the stones are perfectly shaped tools for giving the same effects of thumb and finger kneading

- The stones keep the therapist in contact with the client, even when the physical contact is broken

- The heat of the stones benefits the therapist — it will soothe the therapist and make the treatment relaxing for them too

- The stones act as a barrier against the client's negative energies, absorbing them so the therapist does not have to

- Offers the therapist a chance to give a deeper, more holistic treatment by clearing the chakras

Stone therapy techniques and massage movements

Providing you use your techniques wisely, have the best interests of the client in mind, and the treatment is suitable for their physical characteristics, there is no set method of working. As you gain more experience, the movements you feel most comfortable with will become the ones you use most often. You will continually adapt your depth of pressure, your rhythm and techniques to meet clients' needs and preferences. Remember, all considerations when choosing massage strokes still apply with the stones.

Here is a guide to changing your Swedish massage techniques to incorporate stone use.

Effleurage	All of the normal benefits of effleurage, such as spreading the oil, warming the tissue and so on, are gained using stones. The stone should be held flat in the hand. You may wish to begin with the back of your hand and stroke with superficial effleurage along the area to be massaged first, then gradually turn the hand over to introduce the texture of the stone to the skin. This gliding of the back of the hand gives the therapist time to judge the heat of the stones; it also warms the therapist's hand and allows the client to get used to the sensation. Remember to take care over bony areas and that you can do more transverse effleurage – i.e. down the body, working along the length of the muscle fibres.
Stroking	A superficial gliding stroke is often performed with the outer edge of the stone, which reduces the amount of pressure applied, and it is really useful for finishing the movement at a lymph node to aid drainage.
Combing/ stripping	This is a deep, intense stroke using the stone on its edge, working the muscle along its entire length from its origin to its insertion. This helps pull the muscle fibres outward and removes tension, and is best performed when the stone has lost some of its heat, so use this after the first round of effleurage and stroking. It can be incorporated with the piezoelectric effect (see below) to create a deep release and stretch of soft tissue.
Petrissage	All the effects of kneading, squeezing, pressing and releasing of the tissue that you would achieve with the hands can be achieved with the stones – either flat or, for deep concentrated work, using the edges. Do remember, though, that you do not have as much contact with the body as you do with manual massage, and cannot judge the extra depth which the stones give. These kneading movements can be very deep – always check with your client that they are comfortable. It is not supposed to hurt! You do not want to cause bruising – clients may think that pain is part of the treatment and that they must put up with it, but whilst it's true that there is a certain painful pleasure in having tension knots removed, it should not be continuously sore. The client should not feel tender afterwards – if they do, this is a sign you are going too deeply into the tissue.

Frictions	Frictions can be simulated with stones by using the edge of the stone, to give mild pressure for a soothing feeling, or more concentrated pressure, to stimulate the nerve endings. This will entirely depend upon the client – whether they just need tension released or deep tissue manipulation. Alternatively, you may miss this movement out altogether if the client wants to fall asleep!
Piezoelectric effects/ vibrations	Swedish-massage tremors from the hands (vibrations) can be achieved with the stones very successfully. Vibrations can also be achieved by rhythmical tapping of two stones together creating sound – one stays in contact with skin while the other taps it at the top. This causes a transfer of energy – mechanical energy to electrical vibration that penetrates deeply into the soft tissue. You should gently remind the client of the noise. It may be momentarily uncomfortable, but this method is highly effective at removing tension knots.
Stone placing	The stones are placed on or underneath the body, covered by a towel or sheet to prevent burning. Never place stones directly onto the spinous processes of the vertebrae or over bony areas such as the scapula. Using placements before the massage softens and prepares the tissue; placement after massage continues the good relaxing work of the stones and keeps heat in the muscles.
Holding	The heated stones can be held in the hands or used as a prop during treatment for any specific problems in any region. Just choose a suitably sized stone to fit the area, and keep referring back to the client to check that they are comfortable.

Think about it

As with Swedish body massage, provide suitable cushioning and support if required.

Trigger points

Trigger points are knots of tension which form from adhesions within the muscle fibres; they can be deeply imbedded and be present for years. They are most commonly formed in the shoulder, in the trapezius muscle, but can occur in any muscle. These can be dispersed by using the edge of the stones and maintaining pressure for between 30–90 seconds in the one area, when you feel the knot ease away; it melts underneath the stone. Use warm (not hot) or cold stones for this work and apply deep but firm pressure. There is a certain amount of discomfort whilst these are being manipulated, but they do diffuse quite easily with the use of stones and save the therapist using lots of finger and thumb kneading, cutting down the risk of repetitive strain injury on the joints. You can complete trigger work though clothes but if this is required make sure the stone is warm enough to penetrate through the clothing. If the stone used is very cold then use a child's cotton sock to hold it, so that you do not have a chilled hand.

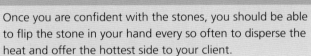

Think about it

Once you are confident with the stones, you should be able to flip the stone in your hand every so often to disperse the heat and offer the hottest side to your client.

Tucking

This refers literally to tucking stones under the client for additional heat – if you have some spare. This is a nice touch and feels very cosy. It can be done under the shoulders, under the knees, in the small of the back and even under the arms – in fact, in any nook or cranny! The key is to ask the client, and to continually check if it is comfortable, and do not place stones directly onto the skin if they are hot. Tucking of either hot or cold stones allows the stones to do the work for you and often by the time you get to the area where you tucked a stone, the area is lovely and soft ready for massage.

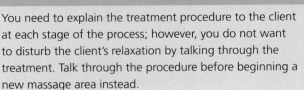

Think about it

You need to explain the treatment procedure to the client at each stage of the process; however, you do not want to disturb the client's relaxation by talking through the treatment. Talk through the procedure before beginning a new massage area instead.

What you need for treatment

The stones

Kits vary in size and price and range from anywhere between 6-stone sets to 54 pieces. The number of stones you require will also depend upon the size of your client, what type of treatment you are doing and if you are using both hot and cold and/or precious stones to finish. There are many variations and the treatment must be tailored to suit your client's needs: you may do a full body with face, placement stones and toe stones, or just a back massage with a stone on the sacral area, under the knees and under the head as a support, or just the limbs or just the face. This will depend upon your client and what you decide upon after consultation, the time available and how many treatments the client has already had. (You may wish to start with just a back massage to introduce the concept of the stones to your client, working up to a full treatment with positioning of stones a little later in their plan, when they are fully comfortable with the procedures.)

There are no set rules about how many stones to use, or how to use them.

An average facial set will contain 38 stones made up of:

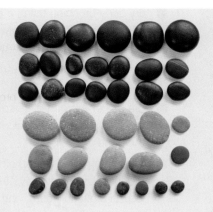

6 medium basalt stones
14 small
8 toe
4 medium cold stones
4 small cold stones
2 eye stones

An average body set will contain 47 stones made up of:

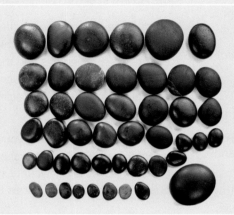

1 extra large basalt stone
6 large
20 medium
12 small
8 toe

An average semi-precious stones set will contain 7 crystals made up of:

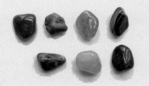

amethyst
blood stone
turquoise
tiger's eye
rose quartz
jasper
sodalite

An average manicure and pedicure set will contain 28 stones made up of:

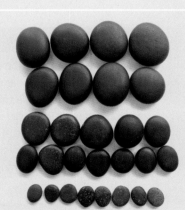

8 medium basalt stones
12 small
8 toe

You can also buy stones individually and in packs of two and four, or specialised half moon cold marble eye stones specifically shaped for the eyes.

You will also need:

- your heater on a flat surface with a towel underneath it
- a towel to dry and tuck the hot stones in when they come out of the water
- your tongs, gloves or slotted spoon for removal
- a water-resistant thermometer probe to test when the water is up to optimum temperature
- a bowl of cool water to cool the stones in (if required) or to warm up a very cold stone
- a cool box with ice or freezer packs for cold stones
- massage oil
- all towels and blanket as for normal body massage to maintain client modesty, and to keep them warm and cosy
- a bowl or a tray nearby (on the second tier of a trolley or shelf) with a towel in the bottom to place the used stones, ready to be cleaned and reheated.

Client preparation

When you have your treatment area set up, the stones fully heated and the temperature checked, you are ready to greet your client. For the consultation, many salons have a pedicure bowl filled with warm water and small stones in the bottom that you can use for the client. Ask your client to sit comfortably and soak their feet, getting them to rub the stones with their soles. Also give them a glass of water, in case they need some hydration. Using the pedicure bowl ensures the client's feet are cleansed and it grounds the client: they also get a few minutes to relax into their treatment and leave their problems behind, outside the salon. It starts the benefits of the treatment right away and they get to leave their negativity in the pedicure bowl. If you cannot offer this service, do make sure you wipe the client's feet prior to treatment, just as you would with Swedish massage – it does help the client to become centred on the treatment.

Other client preparation could include:

- the use of hot towels on the feet or on the area to be massaged

- dry body brushing using a bristle brush or disposable mitt all over to stimulate the skin
- exfoliation with a suitable product and removal with hot towels – just as you would prepare the skin before a self-tanning application
- the use of a pronged scalp brush and/or kneading brush for use on the head, feet, shoulders, thighs and palms of the hand.
- If the treatment is being offered in a salon with spa facilities, the client may already have been in the sauna, jacuzzi or steam room, and showered – so no further cleansing of the skin or heat application will be necessary.

All of these suggestions for client preparation will depend upon the facilities available, the time restriction of the client, the treatment objectives and the client's personal preferences – but however limited your working space and facilities, you can still offer a thereputic beginning to the treatment and set the tone for the client.

If working on the face, and your client is female and wearing make-up, then this should be removed. Glasses, hair accessories and jewellery should also be removed and placed on the trolley – just as for massage.

When the environmental conditions of heat, soft lighting, warmth and relaxing music are set, the client is fully prepared and there are no contra-indications present, you are able to begin treatment.

Remember to carry out your thermal sensitivity testing on the client to check that there are full nerve responses prior to treatment.

Think about it

Stone massage is exactly the same as Swedish massage in that if you are relaxed and confident, the treatment will be peaceful and enjoyable for the client. This is why it is important to practise with the stones a lot when you first start – and that the stones fit snugly into your hands. They should be an extension of your hands and become part of you. Relax and enjoy it as much as the client.

Think about it

The stones hold their heat for about 20 minutes, so don't worry about them going cold once they are out of the heater – if you have the facility to wrap them in a hot towel then do so, as most salons have a towel heater.

Think about it

If you are doing cold stones after hot then you will need your marble stone in a cool box by the stone heater, and these can be used in exactly the same way as hot stones, either as placement stones or massage tools over muscles that need decongesting or are injured.

The treatment procedure

Working on the back of the body

You will need the large sacral stone, four stones for the sides of the body and four for the legs. Four slightly bigger stones are needed for the back. You also need cloths, towels or sheets for protection of the skin, and your bowl to place the used stones in.

1 Go to the head of the bed and prepare yourself and the client to receive the treatment. Connect with the client and ground yourself with deep breathing.

- Go to the crown chakra, and with your feet firmly planted and connected to Mother Earth, close your eyes and breathe deeply. (A Reiki practitioner wishing to use Reiki may also remove her own shoes, as it grounds the therapist, but do check with your Awarding Body about that – it may not be acceptable under assessment conditions.)

- Rub your hands together to generate heat and imagine a bright white light beaming into your body to cleanse you. You can silently offer a small chant or wish to say that you give this treatment with care and love for the client, with goodness and purity.

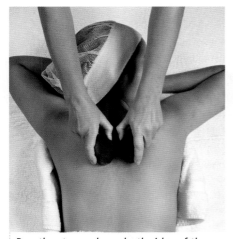

Run the stones down both sides of the spine avoiding the edges of the spinous processes.

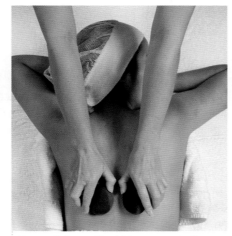

Be careful over the kidneys – ease the pressure slightly.

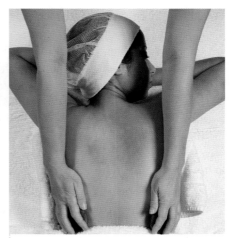

Move along the perimeters of the body and come back up to the lymph glands under the arms.

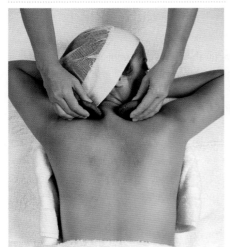

The edges of the stones can be used as finger kneading to release muscular tension.

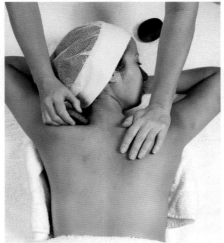

Really knead into the top of the trapezius muscle to release the tension.

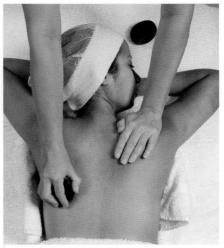

One or both hands can be used in the massage – if using one hand, hold a stone in the other like a hot water bottle.

- Stop rubbing your hands and hold them over the crown chakra, either hovering over the client's aura or making physical contact with the head.

- Ask the client to close their eyes and breathe deeply with you; co-ordinate so you are breathing rhythmically together. Ask them to visualise a bright white cleansing light and to blot out all external thoughts. If the client's mind starts wandering and thinking about other things, just encourage them back to the light visualisation and breathing easily.

- To protect yourself against any negativity from the client, visualise yourself cocooned in a white or violet egg shell, which nothing can penetrate.

2 The client is in the prone position with just the back exposed – keep legs covered at this stage with a large towel. Remove the sacral stone from the water, with gloves, tongs or a slotted spoon (never your bare hands – you risk burning yourself), and place it on the towel in front of the heater. Test it with your finger and, if it is too hot, dip it into your cold water bowl for a few seconds; it should be at a suitable temperature for holding in your hand. Dry it off and place it on top of a towel on the client's sacrum, not directly onto the skin. Immediately the heat will start to transfer into the client's base chakra.

3 Take out four stones and place them in front of the heater on the towel to dry off. Stand at the side of the client in stride standing position and place one hand on the sacral stone and the other between the client's shoulder blades. Gently rock the client back and forth for a few seconds and keep your breathing at a steady, slow, deliberate pace. Then place one hand on the client's hips and the other on the opposite shoulder and rock again, then repeat on the opposite shoulder and hip.

4 There are two ways to work on the posterior of the body. Either massage the back only, as you would for Swedish body massage, and then do the back of each leg, or all of one side of the body together – so you need to expose one leg and keep the other covered. It is a matter of personal preference. Either way, take two medium stones and put them beside the client ready for use. Apply your chosen massage medium to the area to be worked and pick up a stone in each hand. In stride standing, introduce the stones to the client by gliding the back of your hand either up the ankle or, if working just the back, start at the base of the back near the sacral stone – but at either side of the spine, never over it. Glide and turn the hands over, to make contact with the client's skin. Follow your

normal manual massage routine, using superficial and deep effleurage movements, but using the stones. You can use the edges of the stones for: kneading around the scapula; deep kneading for the subscapularis muscle, with the client's hand placed in the small of the back to open the scapula up; or a combing and stripping action down the erector spinae muscle. You can also tap either side of the spine to release nervous tension along the pathways (see 'Piezoelectric effects/vibrations' in the table on page 497, for more explanation). When you have covered the whole area twice, turn the stones over in your hand and repeat. Continual movement of the stones ensures there is no overheating of the skin. Once the stone starts to lose heat on the side that is being used, turn it over and keep it moving. Intersperse your massage with lighter effleurage linking movements, just as you would with manual massage.

5 Before you begin the back massage, you may wish to put placement stones in the palms of the client for them to hold whilst you massage the back. Remember to test them prior to placement.

6 Some manufacturer's instructions work the back from the head, using transverse effleurage movements down the back, rather than towards the heart. The therapist stands in the stride standing position above the head, and works the stones down the length of the muscles. Either method of working is acceptable and may depend upon the size of the client – you may not be able to reach the length of the back, to cover all areas from the head on a larger/male client and may need to work up the back, as you would with Swedish massage. Be flexible and try both ways – see which one suits you and your client.

7 If working the entire length of one side of the body, start at the ankle and work up towards the knee. When you get to the back of the knee, turn to face the feet so that you are pulling the stones over the hamstrings to the top of the leg.

8 Break contact from the leg and go to the hand. (Remember your sacral placement stone is still keeping contact with the client.) Slide one of your stones over the palm of the client's hand. Keep your stone and one hand statically in their hand and, with the other hand and stone, work up the arm to the top of the shoulder.

9 Gently slide the stone all down the client's back and back of leg and return to the ankle.

10 Repeat twice and turn the stones over and repeat twice again.

11 Finish with effleurage all over. If there is still heat in the stones, continue to use them; if not, use manual massage to end this part of the massage. When the stones are finished with, place them in your collecting bowl and cover the side of the body you have massaged.

12 Repeat on the other side of the body.

Legs

1 Take out four stones, and follow the drying, testing and cooling procedure of the stones from step 2 as necessary. Place them by the legs ready for use. Either uncover one leg at a time and apply massage oil, or uncover both legs and treat them together with a hand and stone each. Either method is acceptable. Start with some manual effleurage to spread the oil and then pick up two stones and introduce them by gliding the back of the hand and then turning them over to work the stones into the gastrocnemius and hamstring muscles. Perform slow pressure circles over the muscles with the stone flat and then turn them on their edge for some combing and stripping work, finishing with light pressure on the lymph nodes at the back of the knee, to promote draining.

2 Finish with effleurage all over. If there is still heat in the stones, continue to use them; if not, use manual massage to end this part of the massage. Remove the sacral stone.

Working on the front of the body

Hold the towels and ask the client to turn away from you, so that their modesty is protected.

1 Remove eight medium flat stones from the heater and follow the drying, testing and cooling procedure of the stones (from step 2) as necessary. Help the client sit up. Place the eight stones in two rows on the couch so the stones are at either side of the client's spine, between the hips and the scapula, when the client lies down again. There must be space for the spine to sit in between the stones (these stones should not be too small as it will feel uncomfortable for the client). Make sure there is either a sheet or towel covering them, to protect the client's skin from the heat. Lay the client back down, so they are resting comfortably — this feels like lots of hot water bottles either side of the spine and holds the heat into the nicely relaxed muscles that you have just massaged.

2 Take out the seven chakra (basalt or semi-precious/gem) stones and follow the drying, testing and cooling procedure, as necessary. Place them on the client

starting at the crown, then the third eye (check the temperature as it will go directly onto the skin) and then, over a towel, place the throat chakra, heart, solar plexus, sacral and then the root stone just above the pubic bone.

3 Remove another four stones and follow the drying, testing and cooling procedure. Place two stones under the hands and then two under the knees. Remember to check these are not too hot as they are going directly onto the skin. To disperse heat, immerse them in the water.

4 Remove the cosy toe set from the heater and follow the drying, testing and cooling procedure. Place them between the toes. The client is now fully heated and ready for your facial massage.

Think about it

Never put basalt stones in an autoclave to sterilise them. If the inner core is still wet and the stone is heated to a high temperature, the stone may explode with great force.

Scalp, face and décolleté massage

Refer back to Related anatomy and physiology, page 190, to refresh your memory of the different facial muscles. Remove two stones from the heater and follow the drying, testing and cooling procedure. Place them by your client's head.

1 Position yourself behind the client as in a normal facial. Remove the crown and third-eye chakra stones and use these stones (provided they are still warm) to perform a scalp massage, with deep circular kneading all over the head, then place them either side of the couch.

2 Apply the massage medium all over the face, chest (décolleté) and tops of arms over the deltoid muscle. You may need to move your placement stone for the throat down a little to gain access to the chest.

3 Using the stones flat in the hand, hold a position at the temples to start, then work up to the middle of the forehead and perform slow, light drainage massage movements along the hairline, finishing at the lymph nodes in front of the ear (sub-auricular nodes). Go back to either side of your starting position and repeat until all of the forehead is covered. Work slowly over the entire face and then turn the client's head to one side and perform light combing and stripping movements with the edge of the stones to the sternocleidomastoid muscle and trapezius muscle to relieve tension. Be careful not to put any pressure on the clavicle bone — this will cause discomfort.

4 Use the stone flat and get right under the shoulders to the trapezius muscle. Leave the stones tucked in under the shoulders. Replace the crown and third-eye chakra stones back in position and allow the client to doze off.

5 You can also place the cold marine eye stones over the eyes to aid any decongestion and to cool the area.

Abdomen

The use of stones on the abdomen is optional. It can be really nice to place a hot stone on the abdomen if the client suffers with period pains or IBS (over a towel or flannel, or encased in a sleeve), but it can be omitted if the client is contra-indicated and would prefer more work on the back. Follow Swedish massage procedures: always work in the direction of the digestive tract and avoid bony prominences of the iliac crest of the pelvis and sternum in a client with little body tissue.

Arms and hands

1 Take two stones from the heater and follow the drying, testing and cooling procedure.

2 Wrap one stone in the hot towel and use the other stone as a tool for massage, following your normal massage routine for the arms. Use your free hand to support at the wrist and use your stone for circular movements in the palm of the hand, then supinate the arms and work all the muscle groups – flexors and extensors of the forearm, biceps, triceps and deltoid in the upper arm. Avoid the bony prominence of the elbow, but work around it with the edge of the stones.

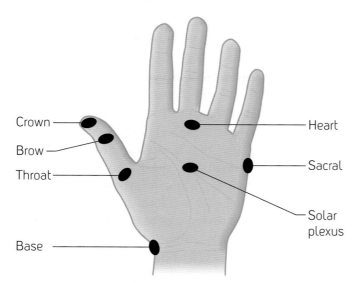

Chakra meridians of the hand

3 You can close down the chakras by working the matching reflex points along the edges of the thumb, top of the middle finger and top and base of the little finger. Repeat on the other arm and hand using the other stone.

Front of legs and feet

1 Remove the last four stones from the heater and follow the drying, testing and cooling procedure.

2 Uncover one leg at a time, remove the cosy toe stones and place in the used stone bowl. Apply massage medium and replace a warm stone under the knee as a prop, if not too hot. Follow a normal massage routine for the legs, repeating the same movements as for the back of the legs and taking care on the tibia bone.

3 You can perform light effleurage movements on the front of the foot and deeper movements with the stones to the soles. Combing and stripping can be done in between the metatarsals and up the tibialis anterior muscle if there is tension present. Close down the chakra points on the foot, starting with the big toe, but reverse the direction of the movements if the client is a male.

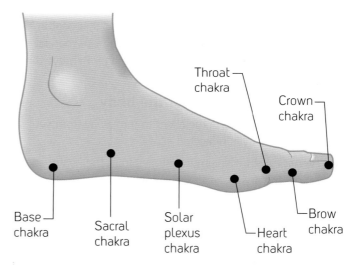

Chakra meridians of the foot

Think about it

When thinking about the direction in which you move the stones and the effect on the chakra you wish to have, remember a female spin is anti-clockwise, a male spin is clockwise.

Closing down the treatment

- To complete the treatment and clear the chakras, begin at the head of the bed, standing at one side of the couch.

- Take the crown chakra stone in one hand, the third-eye chakra stone in the other, and lifting them above the client, tap the crown stone on the third-eye stone three times and place the crown stone on the couch.

- Then take the third-eye chakra stone and use this to tap the throat chakra stone, then place the third-eye stone on the couch.

- Work down the body's chakras, until all the stones have been tapped and set down. Place them in the bowl ready for cleaning and gently wake up the client.

- Gently sit the client up into a semi-reclining position and offer a drink of water.

- Allow them to get up in their own time and offer the client the option of keeping on the massage oil, or removing it with extra towels or rosewater on a cotton pad.

- Whilst they are waking up and reviving their consciousness, you must wash your hands thoroughly to get rid of the negative energy you may have absorbed from the stones. Do not begin tidying up and cleaning the stones yet – it is too noisy for the client. Wait until they have left the treatment room.

- Allow the client to rest and check that they are happy with the treatment they have received, and note anything they would prefer for next time on their record card.

- Talk through the aftercare and long-term health benefits of regular treatments, and your further treatment plans or combinations of treatment specifically for their needs.

Think about it

- Always follow the drying, testing and cooling procedure.
- Always make sure the skin is protected from the direct heat of the stones by using face cloths, towels or sheets as a barrier.
- Always ensure that the skin is sufficiently lubricated – check that the client has no allergies to the chosen oil.
- Minimise excessive noise and therefore disturbance to the client by using towels to line both the used stone bowl and the heater.
- Always allow sufficient post-treatment recovery time – the body needs to readjust. Allow the client sufficient time to become fully aware of their surroundings, especially if they are going to be driving and/or going back to work.

Contra-actions

Never underestimate both the effect of the heat from the stones on the body and the effects of clearing the chakras. There may be mixed contra-actions and reactions to treatment, ranging from excessive erythema under a placement stone – to a slight dizziness when becoming upright.

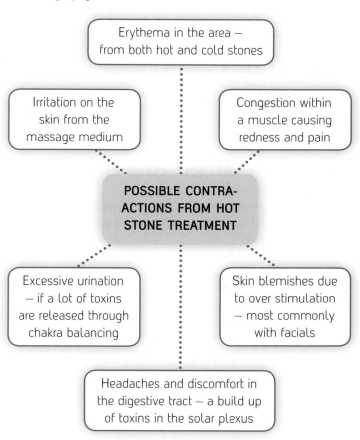

Possible contra-actions from treatment

These contra-actions should not last long and are an indication that the treatment has been successful but stimulating. Make sure the client is aware of the possibility of these contra-actions and allow time for the body to balance itself out and heal – obviously if the client has a strong reaction to the oil, you should act immediately and remove it, apply a cool compress or the cold stones to the area and stop the treatment.

A healing crisis (see Professional basics, 'You the therapist', page 27) may also occur if the client has bottled-up emotions and been over-doing things, has high stress levels, suffered a bereavement or stored up lots of negative energy. The treatment often relaxes the client so much that the blockages are removed. Tears are not uncommon and the client may feel completely drained and very tired. This is the body's way of asking for rest and recuperation time. On the client's next visit ask them about their reactions and make some notes on the record card about how the treatment affected them. The removal of toxins and emotional balancing may also show as disturbed sleep, disturbed digestion, upset tummy, irregular bowel movements and bloatedness. All of these are signs of rebalancing and the body ridding itself of the toxic build-up.

Once the client is prepared for this to happen and gives in to it with rest, and you explain that with regular treatments the balancing gets easier, the client feels more centred and balanced and this gives their whole outlook a lighter more positive feel.

Provide aftercare advice

In this section you will learn about:

- aftercare advice.

Aftercare advice

Immediate aftercare advice

- Ensure the skin is left grease-free and all the massage medium has been removed (unless the client wants it left on the skin, if it is excessively dry).

- Make sure the client gradually becomes vertical after lying down for so long, as this allows the blood flow to the brain to increase and so prevent any dizziness or faintness occurring.

- The client should be rehydrated with a glass of water and encouraged to drink lots of water within 24–48 hours.

- Avoid electrical or heat treatments for 12–24 hours.

- Avoid loud or aggressive people if possible to maintain the calming effect of the treatments.

- Avoid heavy mental stimulation where possible – ideally recommend that the client doesn't go back to work straight away after treatment.

- Avoid alcohol and spicy foods for the remainder of the day.

- Avoid or minimise any stimulation such as loud or aggressive films, loud music or games.

- Rest if possible and sleep – even if it is a siesta for half an hour in the middle of the day. It allows the body to restore balance.

Additional knowledge

Fainting

Fainting is the body's way of making sure that the brain is on the same level as the heart and therefore receives enough vital blood flow and oxygen – the body's quickest way is to make the body limp and horizontal.

Long-term aftercare advice

- Be constructive and kind to your client and give specific advice relating to their individual needs. Everyone has differing stress levels and trigger points so what is stressful for one person is not the same as for another. Stress is not necessarily a bad thing and keeps us focused and in peak condition for important events or performances – but too much stress will have a negative effect, and how we cope with it differs greatly between individuals.

- Look at the client's work/life balance or any other lifestyle patterns that may be causing stress and pressure on the body and find ways to minimise and reduce it. Sometimes it needs an outside observer (the therapist) to be able to see where improvements can be made. The client often doesn't see that their high stress levels or own internal pressure can become the norm to them – but is not good for the body, long term. This is often the case with the perfectionist who cannot possibly maintain a perfect everything, but cannot stop striving for it, so causing immense pressure, resulting in tension, eating disorders and an irritable bowel, or other symptoms.

- Encourage the client to take up yoga, meditation, learn a musical instrument or join a choir – anything that allows them to enjoy an activity to the extent that they are living 'in the moment' and are completely absorbed, so cannot worry about anything else. Children have that ability and adults need to copy it – rather than worrying about what is next to do, or worrying about tomorrow.

- Promote good health in the client by encouraging a balanced diet, gentle exercise and less salt and alcohol. Smoking, alcohol and drugs are toxins to the body and clients who rely on them for relaxation are only over-stimulating an already over-loaded body. By cutting down, it reduces the stimulation and promotes relaxation.

Give the client permission to take time out and enjoy simpler pleasures. Activities which connect back to Mother Earth, such as gardening, are excellent for grounding, as are unselfish deeds or help given to others

Encourage positive thoughts with the client so that they feel better about themselves, rather than getting caught in a cycle of negativity, which is often very difficult to break. Ask the client to name one thing they enjoy and are good at — it could be handwriting, cooking skills, organisation, playing an instrument, card making or home making. Whatever it is, the client should give a positive affirmation of it, rather than focusing on what they cannot do, or have not got.

Home treatments between the salon treatments should include moisturising and caring for the skin's condition, the use of heat such as a hot water bottle on muscular areas of tension, relaxing baths and relaxation periods for enjoyment — hobbies are essential for mental well-being. Spending time with family and sharing laughter

and food with good friends is as therapeutic as some salon treatments. Discourage clients from buying oils for aromatherapy over the counter and adding them to the bath; recommend pre-blended ones from the salon — then at least you know the composition and strength of the products.

Discuss further options and treatments with the client that may also promote good health and mental well-being. Stone therapy complements aromatherapy — oils can be added to massage oil or added to the water which is heating the stones. Indian head massage, if the client wants a shorter treatment which is not full body or Swedish massage, is another option. Other treatments which will make the client feel better about their appearance can be good morale boosters — so introduce your Level 2 treatments too. Even a simple eyebrow shape, skin improvement or a manicure for someone who bites their nails will encourage self awareness and confidence.

Check your knowledge

1 What are the five elements to stone therapy?
   a) Water, ether/wood, earth, metal/air and fire
   b) Earth, wind, fire, rain and wood
   c) Ice, hail, wind, rain and snow
   d) Earth, moon, stars, sky and sea

2 Which of these is *not* a contra-indication to treatment?
   a) Contagious skin diseases
   b) Loss of skin sensitivity
   c) Varicose veins
   d) Radiotherapy

3 Which of these is *not* a type of stone used?
   a) Basalt   c) Marble
   b) Marine   d) Purbeck

4 The test for thermal sensitivity will show if:
   a) the client has good skin
   b) the client has any loss of sensation
   c) the client goes red with heat
   d) the client likes hot treatments.

5 The chakras can be described as:
   a) spinning circles of cells
   b) spinning vortexes of energy
   c) the control panel for the body
   d) the central core of the body.

6 The Piezoelectric effects are achieved by using which movements?
   a) Effleurage
   b) Tapotement
   c) Vibrations
   d) Tapotement

7 The average time it takes for heaters to heat up the stones is:
   a) 20 minutes   c) 45 minutes
   b) 30 minutes   d) 60 minutes.

8 The heater/water temperature should never exceed:
   a) 45°C   c) 60°C
   b) 50°C   d) 66°C.

9 Vasoconstriction is when:
   a) blood vessels narrow, reducing blood flow
   b) blood vessels open, encouraging blood flow
   c) blood and lymph flow work together
   d) muscles and nerve paths are soothed.

10 Hot stones hold their heat for approximately:
   a) 10 minutes   c) 20 minutes
   b) 15 minutes   d) 30 minutes.

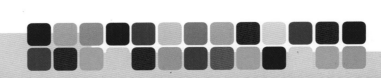

Getting ready for assessment

All the practical assessments for this unit must be carried out with clients in the salon, in a realistic working environment setting, including the client paying for the treatment and it being carried out in a commercial time.

Your assessor will observe your performance on at least *four* separate occasions, each time on different clients. This should include *two* full body stone therapy treatments. Within the practical element of this unit you must also show that you have met the ranges expected for the types of stones in your assessment book and the use of *three* out of the *four* types.

Tip – when choosing your ranges think carefully about the types of stone you wish to use. Crystal therapy is regarded as a specialised in-depth subject in its own right, and you may feel you want to be a more experienced therapist before using crystals in your stone treatments.

You should be able to use all the equipment and adapt your treatment to suit the client's physical characteristics and meet all the treatment objectives listed in your ranges. However, the actual massage movements for the stones are not assessable and you can adapt your massage to suit the client and how comfortable you feel with both hot and cold stones. As with Swedish body massage, as long as the movements are recognisable and the assessors can see you have adapted the movements to suit the client, you will be considered competent. It would be good practice for you to have at least one male client and you could try to incorporate stones into treatments such as manicures and pedicures, or facials.

Never feel that if the assessor asks you a question it is a criticism or that you are doing something wrong – it is for clarification and they may not have been watching a particular movement or procedure.

The more you use the stones the more confident you will become under assessment conditions.

Section

6

Other practical units

Unit B29

Provide electrical epilation treatments

What you will learn:

- Maintain safe and effective methods of working when providing electrical epilation treatments
- Consult, plan and prepare for treatments with clients
- Carry out electrical epilation
- Provide aftercare advice

Introduction

Unwanted hair is a common problem affecting most women to varying degrees throughout their lives and prompting the use of various temporary methods of hair reduction or hair management systems. However, electrolysis is still the only proven permanent method of **epilation** and many women and men have benefited from this tried and trusted treatment. Electrolysis, when performed correctly, is a safe, effective, progressive and permanent method of removing unwanted hair. It is the only permanent method of hair removal and is therefore a treatment in great demand.

From its humble beginnings as a medical treatment for ingrowing eyelashes in 1875, electrolysis has become a sophisticated, effective, comfortable and affordable modern treatment. A fine probe (about the size of an eyelash) is introduced down the hair follicle where a tiny burst of electrical energy is targeted at the root of the hair. This burst of energy gradually prevents nutrients feeding the hair and the hair becomes progressively weaker and finer. After repeated treatments the hair is no longer able to grow and hair-free results are eventually obtained.

Each hair requires repeated treatment because every individual hair has its own growing cycle and blood supply. Electrolysis works by weakening the hair and eventually destroying it. Results take a little time but, just like dieting, it is not the crash diet that works but a long-term healthy eating plan.

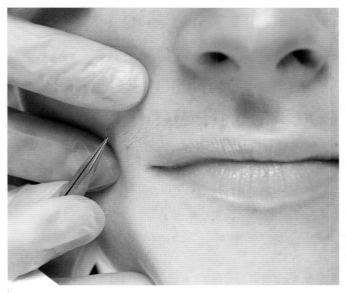

Permanent hair removal will often result in a happier, more confident client

As you work through this unit, you will need to refer closely to the Professional basics and Related anatomy and physiology units. References are provided throughout.

Think about it

Electrolysis was first developed and documented in the USA by Dr Charles E. Michel in 1875 to treat ingrowing eyelashes. He used a direct (**galvanic**) current to achieve this.

In 1924 Henri Bordier invented the **short wave diathermy** method, which utilises an alternating current and is often referred to simply as diathermy or thermolysis.

Key terms

Epilation – removal of unwanted hair, including the hair root, by means of electrical device, tweezer, or wax.

Galvanic – permanent hair removal, first documented in 1875. It uses a direct (or galvanic) current which flows down the needle into the follicle and mixes with the natural tissue fluids in the follicle to form a chemical known as sodium hydroxide or lye. This natural chemical is highly caustic and destroys the hair bulb and cuts off the blood supply to the hair.

Short wave diathermy – a method of epilation consisting of an alternating current and known by many names, for example high frequency, radio frequency, electro-coagulation amongst others. It produces intense heat in the base of the follicle created by the release of high oscillations of current and coagulates or cauterises the blood supply feeding the follicle.

Additional knowledge

Dr Plym S. Hayes

Dr Plym S. Hayes, a professor of chemistry and toxicology at Chicago College of Pharmacy wrote his book *Electricity in facial blemishes*, published in 1910. This featured many other facial blemishes suitable for treatment using electrolysis. Qualified electrologists can go on to study Advanced Electrolysis (NVQ Level 4) or the more complex Advanced Cosmetic Procedures courses run by Sterex Electrolysis International Limited. Courses are also run by other establishments including the British Institute and Association of Electrolysists (BIAE).

Maintain safe and effective methods of working when providing electrical epilation treatments

In this section you will learn about:

- the treatment area, equipment and materials
- minimising personal risk and injury
- health and safety
- cost-effectiveness and commercial viability.

The treatment area, equipment and materials

It is important to set up and monitor the treatment area before, during and after a treatment. Ensure guidelines and procedures set out by your salon or college are followed, and that you adhere to manufacturers' instructions for equipment and materials.

Suggested trolley layout

On a clean and sterile trolley, lay out the items suggested below. The tiers of the trolley may be lined with couch roll for hygiene purposes. However, always read manufacturers' instructions, as some epilation units, designed for continuous use, require clear surfaces as they have built-in cooling fans which may get blocked by the use of couch roll.

First tier:

- Epilation unit and accessories
- Bowl with cotton wool pads
- Client record card/treatment plan
- Alcohol steriliser (for example Steritane)
- Aftercare creams/gels (small selection)
- Kidney bowl with a sterilised pair of tweezers
- Timer
- Sharps box

Think about it

Ensure the trolley, couch, stool and working area are freshly cleaned with a suitable disinfectant and that there are no hazards. Refer to Professional basics, 'You and your working environment', page 54, for detailed advice on maintaining a hygienic working area.

Second tier:

- Box of tissues
- Boxes of needles — a good selection
- Aftercare leaflets
- After creams/gels (further selection)
- Skin and hair visual aids

Third tier:

- Bowl for the client's jewellery
- Box of disposable gloves
- Box of disposable masks
- Mirror
- Sterilising fluid container (if room)
- Covered container with sterilised chuck cap and tweezers
- Covered container for used chuck caps and tweezers

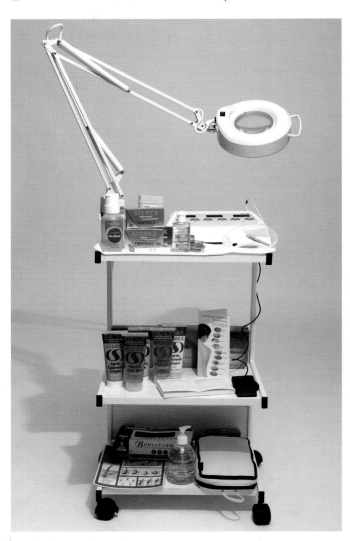

Trolley layout for epilation

The working area

The trolley and magnification lamp should be within easy reach of the couch.

Ensure the treatment room is not too hot, otherwise the client may perspire, which will make epilation more difficult as the skin will become moist. This can cause the electrologist to 'slip' and be unable to stretch the skin properly. Remember that an electrical current can be intensified when the skin is moist, and that perspiration forming on the skin will make the hair difficult to grip. The skin will have to be blotted with tissue frequently if this occurs.

Lighting is of major importance with epilation. Good basic lighting is required as well as additional lighting from a magnification unit, which also serves as a protection screen between the electrologist and the client.

Magnification lamps

There are many different types of magnification lamp available including fixed or free standing, with attachments for the wall or attachments for trolleys. Some offer individually operated lights on both sides of a square-shaped glass (these allow shadows to be cast to assist removal of very fine blonde hair). Others offer natural light or a high level of flexibility and are lightweight. If you opt for a flexible, lightweight round lamp, without the individually controlled lights that the square lamps offer, then a tip is to have a flexible wall light near to the your work area. This will enable you to use this to cast shadow. An additional flexible wall light can be used to illuminate blonde hairs (which can be particularly difficult to see) by casting a shadow when angled across the skin.

Keys to good practice

Use of magnification lamps is strongly recommended. For good clear vision, safety, hygiene and sometimes discretion, they are essential. The positioning of the lamp is vital in order not to distort vision or limit probing. Look through the centre of the magnification lamp and not the edges as this can distort the image and result in a sensation of dizziness. Position the lamp so that it is equidistant between the client and the electrologist.

It will also protect your eyes and your back from strain, because you will not have to crouch so close to the client to see. When working on intimate areas such as the bikini line, a lamp will offer the client some discretion.

Think about it

Always release each section of a magnification lamp by turning the nut to slacken and then move the section into position. Once positioned, tighten nut. This will ensure the magnification lamp remains stable. Failure to do this will result in a 'floppy' or unusable lamp.

Minimising personal risk and injury

Repetitive Strain Injury (RSI)

RSI is a collective term for a number of conditions affecting the neck, shoulders, arms, wrists, hands, legs and feet. RSI can present itself when repetitive movements are performed on a regular basis, for example needle-holder and tweezer use in electrolysis treatments, or foot-pedal use of an epilator. There are two forms of RSI:

- Distinct RSI — which includes a number of different conditions such as carpal tunnel syndrome (CTS), tennis elbow (epicondylitis) and tendonitis
- Diffuse RSI — where multiple areas of diffuse pain in the muscles and other soft tissues are experienced due to nerve compression etc. When a healthcare professional refers to a condition as just 'RSI', this is the condition they mean.

Both types of RSI can be suffered simultaneously, with multiple occurrences being experienced at the same time. Many electrologists who carry out repetitive treatments over long hours of work may be susceptible to RSI, so regular rest breaks, a break in routine movement, and treatments being varied as much as possible are advisable. You should also take great care with your posture and positioning to help protect against RSI.

Think about it

RSI can result from incorrect tweezer technique. There are a number of different tweezer methods — experiment to find out the one that suits you referring to the techniques shown on page 533.

The correct working position

Keep your back as straight as possible

Do not cross your legs

Have both feet firmly planted on the ground

Ensure your neck and shoulders feel relaxed

SOME TIPS FOR GOOD POSTURE

Take regular short breaks, vary treatments and avoid repetitive movements as much as possible

Change positions when working on different areas of the body

Ensure your stool is the correct height

Ensure the couch is in a central position in the room so you can move around it.

Occasionally, you may need to lean on the client – use body weight lightly and regularly check the client's modesty, privacy and comfort levels.

Do not be afraid to move the client into a position that is comfortable and effective for you but regularly check the client's wellbeing so you are assured it is equally comfortable for them.

To assist with accurate insertions, position yourself so that the wrist and elbow are aligned with the direction of hair (when possible).

Correct positioning of the magnification lamp helps ensure the back and neck are kept straight, and a correct height for the stool also helps to prevent leaning over the client, which can cause back and neck strain or possible injury.

Think about it

Using a disposable mask and disposable plastic apron is a matter of personal preference, but they are useful as they offer a degree of privacy and minor protection. If you or the client has a cold, or if you feel it appropriate for the client or area you are working on, they can be used. Some clients may prefer the use of masks, particularly clients of different cultural or religious backgrounds or transgender clients. Others just feel it more professional and are comforted by the outward appearance of professionalism and hygiene levels.

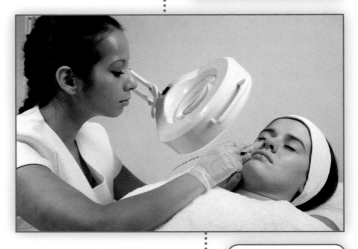

Ensure correct positioning of the magnification lamp – the lens should be parallel to the treatment area, with enough space left to move the hands freely without touching the lens and with similar distance from the lens to the therapist's face.

Ensure equipment is easily accessible.

Ensure a clear view of the epilation unit at all times for adjustment of the dials.

If right-handed, the therapist should sit on the right side of the client as he or she is lying down and vice-versa for left-handed therapists.

Tips for positioning during epilation

Risk assessment

You should always be aware of the hazards and risks involved in a treatment, and they can be particularly serious when involving electricity. Further detail can be found in Unit G22 Monitor procedures to safely control work operations, page 92, and Professional basics: 'You and your client', page 48, and 'You and your working environment', page 54.

Hygiene	
Hazard (What can go wrong)?	• Cross-infection, contamination of equipment
Who could be harmed?	• You, the client, other therapists and colleagues and visitors to the salon
Prevention (How can I prevent this?)	• Use the most up-to-date effective methods of sterilisation • Use sterilisation equipment and products in accordance with the manufacturers' recommendations • Ensure your immunisation certification is valid • Ensure regular maintenance of autoclave and other methods of sterilisation • Ensure scrupulous personal and salon hygiene • Work to HASWA recommendations
Monitoring (How can I check this?)	• Regularly test equipment • Maintain immunisation records correctly • Ensure regular inspection visits from professional bodies for insurance validation • Ensure regular inspection by self and colleagues of all surfaces, floors and equipment working to a standard of hygiene excellence
Corrective action (What do I do if things are not right?)	• Replace and regularly update equipment • Follow the correct procedures for reporting infectious diseases and disorders (RIDDOR) (see Professional basics, 'You, your client and the law', page 77) • Follow the correct procedures for dealing with any hazards of accidental exposure to clinical waste and organise rosters and procedures to ensure there will be no repeat of any occurrence

Equipment	
Hazard (What can go wrong?)	• Ineffective treatment • Damage associated with faulty equipment, possible burns, and skin blemishes. See contra-actions on page 551.
Who could be harmed?	• The client; the salon owner and/or electrologist because of possible litigation
Prevention (How can I prevent this?)	• Ensure regular testing and maintenance of equipment • Hold a valid certificate of insurance • Ensure regular training and updating of skills
Monitoring (How can I check this?)	• Maintain equipment correctly • Machinery should have a visible sticker noting last PAT test date
Corrective action (What do I do if things are not right?)	• Ensure manufacturers' recommendations are followed • Ensure spare accessories are available

B29 Provide electrical epilation treatments

Magnification lamp

Hazard (What can go wrong?)	• If a lamp is left uncovered by a window on a sunny day, it will generate enough heat to burn or set fire to fabrics close by • Injury to the client due to a loose-fitting joint connecting the lamp and its support
Who could be harmed?	• If a fire starts, everyone is at risk
Prevention (How can I prevent this?)	• Cover the lamp – follow manufacturer's instructions • Avoid keeping lamp near a window • Use correctly following manufacturer's instructions • Loosen nuts to move and tighten when positioned
Monitoring (How can I check this?)	• Be aware of possible dangers • Ensure regular maintenance of equipment
Corrective action (What do I do if things are not right?)	• Maintain fire extinguishers and hold fire drills – all staff should be aware of evacuation procedures (see Professional basics, 'You and your working environment, page 63) • Immediately withdraw from service if faulty

Needles/tweezers

Hazard (What can go wrong?)	• Needle stick injuries
Who could be harmed?	• Client/electrologist
Prevention (How can I prevent this?)	• Follow manufacturer's instructions when loading and unloading needles • Ensure correct treatment procedure is followed
Monitoring (How can I check this?)	• Follow manufacturer's instructions
Corrective action (What do I do if things are not right?)	• Injury to electrologist – stop treatment immediately and follow first aid procedures • Injury to client – immediately apply pressure to assist clotting and help prevent bruising

Allergies (see You and the skin, page 234)

Hazard (What can go wrong?)	• Skin reaction or contact dermatitis caused by allergy to nickel/cotton wool fibres/product ingredients/latex and powder used in gloves
Who could be harmed?	• Client/electrologist
Prevention (How can I prevent this?)	• Hold a full consultation with client • Use alternative products and specialised needles designed for allergies • Use latex-free gloves without powder
Monitoring (How can I check this?)	• Monitor client reaction during treatment • Hold a consultation update each visit/specifically check for delayed reactions • Follow manufacturers' instructions for products and gloves (see Professional basics, 'You and your client', page 43, for detail on choosing gloves)
Corrective action (What do I do if things are not right?)	• For client – immediately stop treatment, remove product if necessary and apply cool compress • For electrologist – wash hands and change gloves

Risk assessment for epilation

Health and safety

Your legal responsibilities

As an electrologist treating hair follicles using diathermy, galvanic and **blend** epilation techniques, you have responsibilities as laid down by:

- Health and Safety at Work Act
- The Control of Substances Hazardous to Health Regulations
- Electricity at Work Act
- local by-laws relating to electrical epilation registration and approval from the local environmental health office.

It is your responsibility to contact the local environmental health office to register with them and obtain a license to practise epilation. An environmental health officer will visit the premises and check on a number of criteria including sterilisation and disinfection methods used. In order for them to grant a license they will want to satisfy themselves that you are aware of and will abide by their high standards. This includes safe and correct disposal of single-use items, hazardous waste and waste materials, the rules and regulations of which vary throughout the UK, depending upon the individual county or borough.

For more information on hygiene and safety legislation, see Professional basics, 'You, your client and the law', page 68.

> ### Key terms
>
> **Blend** – epilation technique using both galvanic and diathermy currents; this method is said to be kinder to the skin and less uncomfortable.

> ### Think about it
>
> Each treatment requires a new needle, a fresh sterile chuck cap, a fresh sterile pair of tweezers and new gloves (washed in antibacterial hand wash).

Keeping equipment clean and sterile

Throughout the treatment, safety and hygiene are of vital importance for both the client and electrologist's health and safety. For example, any waste products such as cotton pads or tissues used for wiping the skin must be disposed of immediately in a covered waste bin. Under no circumstances should they be placed on the trolley or machine as this may cause accidental exposure to contaminated waste.

At the end of each treatment (or day at the salon) the treatment area(s) and equipment used must be left as found – in a pristine condition for immediate use or use the following day. Always be mindful of the electrologist who may 'take over' your working area and leave absolutely everything as pristine and sterile as you would wish to find it. This will also encourage efficiency and allow treatments to be performed in a cost-effective manner and carried out within a commercially viable time. Used chuck caps and tweezers should be gently scrubbed in hot water using a mild antiseptic wash and a special brush (for example a baby's toothbrush) kept specifically for the purpose. This will ensure that any contaminated material present will be removed, and should be performed by the electrologist with gloved hands for protection. The items should then be rinsed, dried and put in either an autoclave or liquid sterilant. This will ensure that any contaminated waste is not baked onto instruments used and that the sterilant is not contaminated or diluted, thereby allowing it to work effectively. (For information on the autoclave, see Professional basics, 'You and your client', page 53).

Personal hygiene and safety

When ready to begin the treatment, wash your hands with an antibacterial hand wash, then dry with tissue, hot air or a clean towel. It is imperative that gloves are worn for the treatment. There are a variety of types available to choose from, and these are covered in detail in Professional basics, 'You and your client', page 43. Have everything ready and prepared prior to treatment as it is pointless once gloved to perform other tasks such as placing the client's belongings on the trolley, positioning the bin nearer you, blowing your nose or coughing, as the gloves will have picked up bacteria prior to treatment.

> ### Think about it
>
> Always protect your hands with gloves when dealing with blood, chemicals or body fluids. But remember, disposable gloves are not sterile. Therefore it is recommended that you 'dry wash' your gloved hands in a good quality antibacterial product especially designed for the purpose.

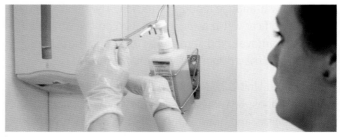

Dry-wash your gloved hands using a product such as Stericleanse

Needle stick injury

In the event of a needle stick injury to the electrologist the following steps should be followed.

- Immediately encourage bleeding to occur at the point of injury by applying pressure.
- Immerse under warm running water as soon as possible and wash thoroughly with antibacterial soap.
- Dress the area to cover and protect wound.
- If continuing treatment, apply a fresh pair of disposable gloves before proceeding with treatment.
- Any blood waste should be disposed of in yellow clinical waste bin.
- All injuries should be recorded in accident book within the salon.
- The electrologist may wish to visit their doctor for further advice.

You will also need to take preventative measures against cross-infection – see the risk assessment table on page 515. Viruses such as HIV and hepatitis B and C are transmitted by blood and blood-stained body fluids. Prevention of cross-infection can be achieved through:

- strict attention to personal hygiene
- thorough cleaning, including washing and disinfecting of treatment rooms and all surfaces
- correct and thorough washing followed by sterilisation of all equipment, tweezers and chuck caps
- using pre-sterilised disposable needles and following correct disposal procedures
- keeping cuts and abrasions covered
- hand washing before and after all client contact
- gloves worn at all times – a fresh pair for each client and for different areas worked
- 'washing' gloved hands with antibacterial hand cleanser
- correct disposal of clinical waste – an approved refuse collector must remove sharps boxes and contaminated waste. Contact your local council refuse department, which will arrange regular collection. The health and safety officer will provide information on contaminated waste removal, and sometimes local pharmacists or hospitals may dispose of your sharps boxes.

Refer also to Unit G22 Monitor procedures to safely control work operations, to ensure you are familiar with potential workplace risks and hazards, and what to do when you discover one.

Cost-effectiveness and commercial viability

It is important to perform treatments in a cost-effective manner and within a commercially viable time. Efficiency and organisation in all aspects of working practice are required to achieve this, including equipment maintenance, setup and preparation of the treatment area, prepared sterilisation, ensuring adequate supplies to hand, timed consultation and efficiently carried out verbal and written aftercare etc. Some electrologists have a small timer which, once the client is prepared and ready for treatment, they set for the required and paid time. Once this timer 'beeps', the treatment finishes, the aftercare product is applied and advice is given.

Think about it

You should always consult the client's record card before you begin any treatment, and update it once the treatment is complete. Client records need to be up to date, accurate, complete and legible to ensure whoever treats the client is fully informed of any problems, contra-indications or personal requirements.

It is also important that both you and the client sign the record card to agree treatment before it begins and to accept treatment once it is complete. This gives you legal protection should any problem arise in the future, and it may also be a condition of your insurance.

More detail on client records can be found in the next section: 'Consult, plan and prepare for treatments with clients'.

Consult, plan and prepare for treatments with clients

In this section you will learn about:

- explaining the treatment
- establishing and recording client information through consultation
- the epilation record card
- planning the treatment
- contra-indications to treatment.

1 As part of a thorough consultation, a detailed skin analysis should be carried out to assess the area requiring treatment.

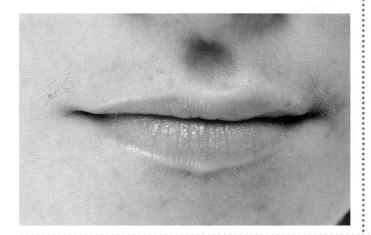

2 Carry out a thorough skin cleansing procedure using an antiseptic lotion designed for electrolysis.

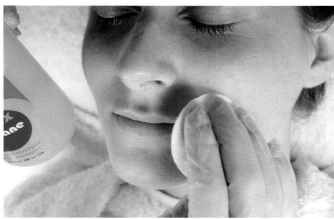

3 The probe is inserted, charged with a tiny amount of electrical current. The client will experience either a build-up of warmth concentrated in the locality or a sensation similar to a slight sting depending on the method used.

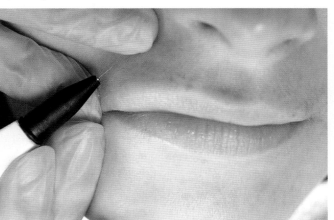

4 The hair is gently released from the follicle with tweezers. If the hair has been adequately treated, no traction or 'plucking' should be required and the hair should be easily lifted from the follicle.

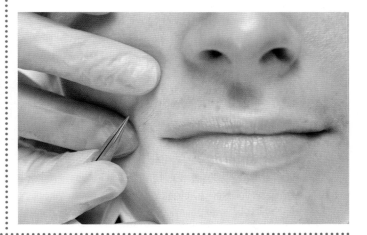

5 Following the application of aftercare product and the delivery of verbal and written aftercare and home care advice, the next appointmment is made. This ensures regular treatments are maintained and the client continues to be pleased with her progress.

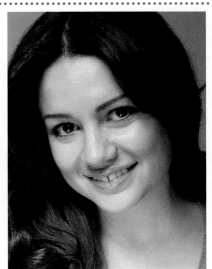

6 Showing the client the collection point at the end of the treatment and allowing her to see the amount of hair that has been removed can encourage, enthuse, inspire and motivate the client.

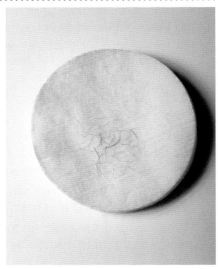

With any new client, you will need to discuss their medical history, any potential contra-indications, hair type, causes of hair growth, skin type and condition and, within reason, to ascertain the client's emotional condition before beginning treatment.

It should be explained to the client from the outset in a clear, concise manner that although the results of epilation are permanent, it is a progressive treatment. Each hair has to be treated separately and a number of times. The hairs will become finer, lighter in colour, less dense and eventually disappear, but this may take a considerable length of time. Clients may ask for an estimation as to the expected number of treatments, but this is difficult. It is not advisable to guess, as every client is different and any number of factors can affect progress.

Explaining the treatment

You will need to explain the treatment fully to the client. If possible, show step-by-step visual graphics or photographs with a 'summary' under the pictures.

Ensure that you cover the following points.

- A tiny probe (some clients have a fear of needles), the same diameter as the hair, is inserted into the follicle opening — an opening that is already present in the skin, so no discomfort should be felt as the skin is not pierced.

- The probe is charged with a small amount of electrical current and the client will feel a sensation very similar to a slight sting. This sensation will feel more noticeable in some areas than others, where there are more nerve endings in the skin. (It is important to have experienced the treatment yourself to clearly explain the sensation the client is likely to experience in a way that they can understand.) The hair is then gently lifted from the skin with tweezers. There will be no plucking or pulling of the hair as the electrical current has released the hair from the follicle. Each hair must be treated individually with enough current and correct insertion to provide a solution that is eventually permanent.

- Explain to the client the stages of hair growth — anagen, catagen and telogen.

- The client will need to tell the electrologist the areas that he or she would like treated. This should be clearly noted on the consultation card.

- All elements of the treatment should be recorded in great detail before and after treatment.

- Realistic outcomes of treatment must be explained to the client, who should be made aware of the commitment required.

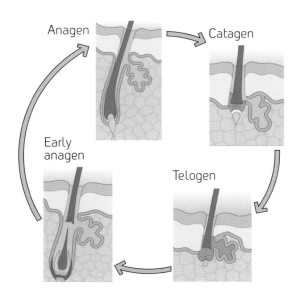

The hair growth cycle

Visual aids

During the consultation, illustrations, pictures or graphs can be used to assist your presentation to the client. You can draw your own or obtain them from manufacturers, who supply skin and hair charts and even three-dimensional models of the skin. A good electrologist understands that it is his or her job to give the client as much relevant information regarding the treatment as possible. Certainly, visual aids can help clients to 'see' rather than 'hear' explanations and will greatly assist in demonstrating that the skin is not pierced in epilation but rather the needle or probe travels down an already existing cavity (the hair follicle).

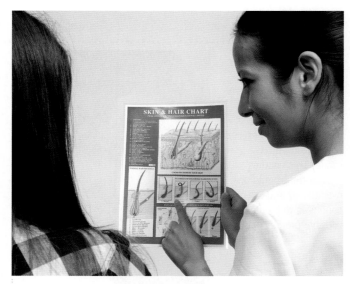

A graphic can be used to explain to the client exactly what is involved

To support your work on advising clients, you should refer to the following sections in Related anatomy and physiology: the structure and function of skin, page 166; the endocrine system, page 207; and the circulatory and lymphatic systems, pages 194 and 201.

Treatment options

A treatment plan should be completed with the client. If the unwanted hair problem is severe, it may be necessary to 'clear' one area at a time, which means the client will need to continue to use his or her own personal 'hair management' system.

Different **modalities** could be used on one client, for example blend and/or diathermy. Diathermy on the majority of the area will ensure that the client leaves the salon hair-free, as a greater number of hairs can be removed at any given time, but blend concentrated in a small area will ensure the quickest results. Once this chosen blend treatment area is permanently cleared, an additional blend area could be started.

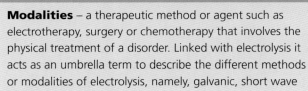

Key terms

Modalities – a therapeutic method or agent such as electrotherapy, surgery or chemotherapy that involves the physical treatment of a disorder. Linked with electrolysis it acts as an umbrella term to describe the different methods or modalities of electrolysis, namely, galvanic, short wave diathermy and blend.

Think about it

Demonstrating to the client the quicker results achieved with blend is a tried and tested way of successfully changing diathermy clients onto blend.

Think about it

Actively encourage clients to ask questions and clarify any points of which they are unsure, especially during the consultation and at any time during and after the treatment. This must all be recorded accurately by the electrologist. The more informed a client is, the more effective the treatment is likely to be, so directly ask the clients if they have any questions and offer to explain anything again if they are uncertain.

Additional knowledge

Client diversity

Every client will require different care and treatment. Areas requiring epilation may include the face and neck, underarm, bikini-line, chest (male and female), and for experienced electrologists, the most intimate areas — pre-operative transgender clients' genitalia. (See You and the skin, page 245, for male skin behaviour, structure and product use; also the section on ingrowing hair, page 536.)

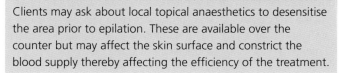

Think about it

Clients may ask about local topical anaesthetics to desensitise the area prior to epilation. These are available over the counter but may affect the skin surface and constrict the blood supply thereby affecting the efficiency of the treatment.

Here are some common unrealistic aims that clients may hold or express, and which you should politely clarify with a more realistic aim or explanation.

Unrealistic aims	Realistic aims
Hair will never grow back again after one treatment	Each individual hair will need to be treated a number of times
It's quick and easy	It is a slow but permanent treatment requiring great skill from the electrologist
No skin reaction after treatment will occur	Mild erythema and oedema is normal and expected. This very quickly subsides and any redness can be camouflaged with a specialised mildly medicated foundation
It doesn't hurt at all	A level of discomfort is involved – it must be remembered that the treatment sensation will vary depending on the area worked. Some areas are far more sensitive than others, e.g. just underneath the nose is particularly sensitive with a high number of nerve endings. The high frequency current is usually reported as a short sting which will last just a second or two. With blend, a more gentle build-up of warmth is often experienced for 3–5 seconds. Galvanic feels similar, with a build-up of warmth, and can feel relatively painless for a number of clients

Continued

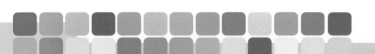

Unrealistic aims	Realistic aims
It works well on large areas	Large areas can be treated, but electrolysis works best on small areas because each hair has to be treated individually
It won't matter if I don't keep appointments	Regular appointments and a good deal of commitment are required from the client in order to achieve satisfactory outcomes
The hairs grow back with a sharp, spiky feel	The hair is removed from the root, therefore the hair grows back with its natural tapered end, feeling smooth to the touch
All the hairs grow back at the same time	Hairs grow back spasmodically, as the hair growth cycle varies for each follicle and area

Realistic and unrealistic aims of electrolysis

Epilation clients

Epilation clients are very varied, and may include both men and women and clients who may be minors — i.e. legally under age for the treatment. (See Professional basics, 'You the therapist', page 23, for further detail on treating minors.)

Prior to any electrical epilation treatment it is imperative that informed and signed parent or guardian consent is obtained (as well as the GP's written agreement) and that the parent or guardian is present throughout the treatment. This is not only for the client's emotional support but for their and your legal protection.

With the law constantly tightening up legislation, it may be necessary in the future for electrologists to have police checks to treat minors and the current legal situation should also be ascertained by the electrologist prior to treatment. A referral from the GP is also strongly recommended and may be a legal or insurance requirement prior to treatment.

In the interest of moral and ethical fairness and behaviour, it is imperative that no discrimination against clients with illnesses and disabilities takes place. The Disability Discrimination Act requires that everyone is treated equally. It is also important to 'pitch' the consultation at the correct level for effective communication and understanding, irrespective of whether that client differs from you in cultural and religious background, age, or gender, or has a disability.

Present and past hair management techniques

Epilation currently offers the only permanent method of hair removal. However, there are many different ways to remove unwanted hair temporarily and the client may well have used some of these, including waxing, plucking, depilatory creams, shaving and laser. The use of any other method will have a bearing on future epilation treatments and can affect the client both psychologically and physiologically. It is important for the electrologist to establish how the client has been managing the hair problem and to suggest the best way forward.

Think about it

If you suspect that the client might have an underlying medical condition which is exacerbating the hair growth problem, refer the client to his or her doctor for advice. Be sensitive and careful in the language you use to avoid causing undue alarm or concern. It is not your place to suggest what may be wrong, merely to suggest the client seeks further advice.

If the client has been using temporary methods of hair removal, you will need to establish whether he or she was under the false impression that these methods were permanent. Then, with this knowledge, you will need to carefully consider the treatment programme and decide whether it should be revised as the hair growth, skin, and the client's sensitivity may well have been altered in some way.

Another factor that might affect treatment will be the client's own need to 'manage' hair growth between treatments to make it acceptable to him or her. Only cutting is recommended, although occasional shaving is acceptable. Cutting does not damage the hair follicle in any way. It may also be necessary to recommend alternative treatments or products which are suitable for the client if contra-indicated for electrical epilation treatment.

Hair removal methods and how they may affect epilation

Method	Effect
Facial discs/ abrasives	Gently abrasive, rather like an ultra-fine sandpaper. Only really suitable for very fine hair. Not suitable prior to epilation as it makes it difficult to follow the line of the hair into the follicle and weakens the body of the hair resulting in possible breakage when removing from the follicle following epilation
Hair removal creams	Establish how long these have been used for and if any allergies or soreness resulted. Was there any indication of skin sensitivity or infection? When was the last treatment? If very recent, it may be necessary to wait for the skin to desensitise before electrolysis. Depilation creams can also result in brittle hair, making hair difficult to release from the follicle without breakage during electrolysis
Bleaching	Clients may bleach their hair to disguise it, using a number of specialised colourants. While this minimises the appearance of unwanted hair, it can result in the hair becoming brittle and liable to break, as well as sensitising the skin, both factors causing difficulties for the electrologist
Plucking/ threading	Plucking can sensitise the skin. Has the client caused skin damage from over-enthusiastic plucking? If so, this must be brought to the client's notice, recorded on the record card and if new scarring (less than one year old) is apparent, this would be a contra-indication to treatment and the immediate area would have to be avoided. Has incorrect plucking been carried out, e.g. causing breakage of the hair or performed in the opposite direction to the hair growth? When the hair is plucked out in the opposite direction to the natural fall of the hair growth, the follicle is likely to have been distorted. Therefore, blend or galvanic epilation should be the preferred choice of treatment. It is widely believed that plucking may cause topical stimulation to the area and encourage the growth of more hair, although the evidence does not always support this theory

Method	Effect
Electrical appliances/ shaving	Shaving can sensitise the area and products used, e.g. aftershave, may contain alcohol that can further sensitise the skin. Therefore, special consideration must be given to the condition of the skin. Also, any nicks or cuts that may have resulted from shaving would be a contra-indication to treatment. Shaving cuts the hair, leaving it feeling blunt to touch and thicker and can also result in ingrowing hairs. As with plucking, it is claimed that shaving results in topical stimulation (massage of the area stimulates the blood supply that 'feeds' the hair), so exacerbating the problem. However, some experts claim that encouraging the client to shave a few days prior to treatment can show the electrologist exactly which hairs are in anagen by the longer appearance of those hairs. This then ensures that the hairs treated are the active growing ones, thereby resulting in the most effective treatment.
Electrical plucking	Electrical plucking rips the hair out from the root. However, this is not always successful and hairs often break. Electrical plucking can result in distorted follicles and sensitised skin as well as ingrowing hairs and hairs which have been dislodged from the dermal papilla, sometimes resulting in infected follicles and affecting an electrolysis treatment
Waxing/ sugaring	Waxing is also said to cause topical stimulation, although the evidence does not always support this. Waxing rips out hairs in the opposite direction to growth, which in turn causes distortion of the hair follicle, and this will have a bearing on the method of epilation used. Blend or galvanic methods, which both allow the treatment of distorted follicles, should be chosen
Laser/intense pulsed light (IPL)	Laser is the most recent newcomer to hair removal. Legally, laser manufacturers can claim permanent hair reduction but not (to date) removal, and it is said to be an effective method of hair management. Currently, laser cannot successfully treat light blonde or white hair and indeed can strip the colour from some hairs, often leaving white hair remaining which can only then be removed permanently with electrolysis

Hair growth definitions

Your hair performs three functions — it protects you, regulates your temperature and acts as adornment.

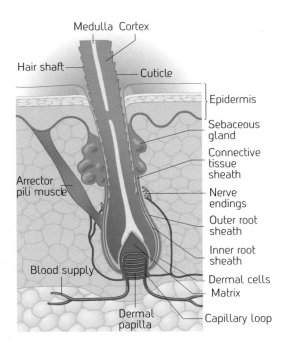

The structure of the hair and its follicle

Superfluous hair growth

Superfluous (excess) hair growth is a general term. Females with low levels of female hormones (oestrogen and progesterone) and higher levels of the male hormones (androgens) can develop superfluous hair growth. Superfluous hair is, however, a matter of opinion and cultural preferences, and only the client can judge what is excessive for him or her.

Key terms

Hirsutism – term usually reserved for females. It refers to the growth of hair on the face and body, which is usually characteristic of masculinity. Caused by an over-abundance of the hormone androgen in the blood. The dormant follicles are stimulated to grow hair, and existing vellus (fine) and terminal (coarse) hairs grow larger in diameter.

Hypertrichosis – term used for both men and women. It describes a general overgrowth of terminal (coarse) hair affecting the entire body surface. It is not hormone-dependent, and results from ethnic or genetic predisposition.

Hirsutism and hypertrichosis

Hirsutism and hypertrichosis describe excessive hair growth. Some men may have excessive hair growth on the bridge of the nose, ears, cheekbone area, neck, back, chest, arms and hands, and may also have unusual amounts of hair on the legs.

Establishing and recording client information through consultation

The electrolysis consultation provides an opportunity:

- to build a rapport between the client and the electrologist
- to discuss client expectations and agree on the treatment
- to advise the client on the achievable outcomes of the treatment
- to aid client understanding of the treatment
- to discuss suitability of the client for treatment
- to allow the client to ask questions about the treatment
- to explain all possible reactions to the treatment
- to discuss the probable causes of hair growth
- to examine the client's skin and hair type
- to discuss any previous methods of hair removal
- to plan the course of treatments
- to discuss costs
- for the client to experience the treatment
- to record in detail client hair growth and, where appropriate and whenever possible, take before and after photographs of the treatment area as visual evidence
- to obtain signed, written, informed consent from the client prior to carrying out the treatment
- to ensure the client has no contra-indications to epilation treatment and that they are of the legal age of consent for treatment.

With electrolysis, the consultation and record-keeping are of utmost importance and new levels of empathy and consultative skills will need to be developed. A balance must be found so that the client feels confident about the electrologist's professionalism and skills but also relaxed and able to communicate on the subject of unwanted personal hair growth.

You should use a polite, sensitive and supportive manner to determine the client's treatment needs. This is a firm foundation for the start of a developing bond and good professional working relationship between the client and electrologist.

It is one of the most difficult and awkward subject matters for some clients to talk about. Clients will often feel apprehensive, emotional and intimidated. A good electrologist is one who can make the client feel relaxed and special, but most importantly feel like a normal human being and not unusual or abnormal. A polite and reassuring manner should be shown to the client at all times, throughout the preparation process, the treatment itself, through aftercare and homecare advice to the end of the treatment.

No two clients are the same, even when the underlying cause of the problem may be the same. All clients vary in their response and commitment to treatment. Each treatment and each course of treatments must be tailored to suit the needs of each individual client.

This is where careful and accurate record keeping is important. Every client is different, so you cannot expect to remember every detail about their individual treatments. Write down your client's responses to questioning on their client record and consultation cards, and update their treatment plans as their course progresses and any further information comes to light.

Timing

The first electrolysis consultation should last at least 30 minutes, with 20 minutes allocated to the consultation and 10 minutes for a patch test treatment. A patch test area should be carefully chosen. This is of prime importance, especially if working on the face. A small area should be chosen, as unnoticeable as possible but with similar skin and hair type as the desired treatment area. This small area and how it reacts gives invaluable feedback to the electrologist as to the treatment effects on any individual client. This includes:

- the ability to identify any allergies to needle type or products used
- establishing any pigmentation issues
- the degree of skin reaction
- the healing response
- which method is most suitable
- the pain threshold of the given area at time of treatment
- skin characteristics and skin type of client and ethnic group
- any idiosyncrasies pertaining to that particular client.

Think about it

Verbal and written aftercare should be given after the initial patch test treatment and with every subsequent visit.

As with any epilation treatment, aftercare product advice and written aftercare procedures must be explained in detail and given to the client. It is advisable to encourage clients to start the course of treatments straight away if possible; otherwise they may get 'cold feet'.

Pain sensitivity

Most individuals describe electrolysis as uncomfortable — a warm, burning or stinging sensation — rather than painful.

Think about it

Pain thresholds and sensitivity vary from client to client, area to area and appointment to appointment.

Factors which increase discomfort

- Poorly motivated clients
- Age — young clients are less motivated
- Sensitive body areas, for example upper lip
- Too long a treatment, too soon
- Too high a current, for too long
- Poor insertions
- Defective needles
- Defective equipment
- Inflamed skin (reworking over the same area)
- Failure to adjust settings
- Too small a needle
- Individual sensitivity changes, for example tiredness, headache, nervousness, menstruation
- Hairs requiring high current
- Dry, sensitive skin type
- Mature, sensitive skin type

Factors which relieve discomfort

- Motivated client
- Relaxed and comfortable atmosphere
- Using the minimum effective current
- Varying intensity/duration and techniques with blend
- Medicinal pain relief (a personal option clients may occasionally take)

- Acclimatising the client — start with less sensitive areas
- Concentrated treatments rather than jumping to other areas
- Ice packs to cool and help numb the area
- Aftercare products to reduce oedema and erythema
- Electrologist acting in a confident and professional manner
- Ensuring an efficient and effective treatment
- Upgrading and improving skills with further training
- Finger pressure as a distraction
- Distraction for the client, for example music and/or aromatherapy scent
- Choice of modality to suit client
- Treatment planning to avoid times of heightened sensitivity, for example menstruation

Demonstrating progress

It is recommended, where possible and with the client's agreement, to take clear, high-quality photographs of

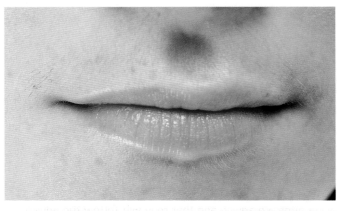

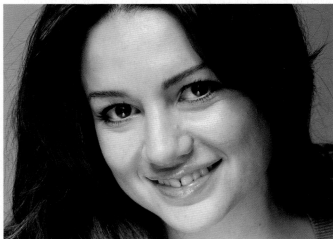

Your client will be encouraged through the use of 'before and after' photos

the treatment area, prior to and following a course of treatment. With a slow process such as epilation, this visually demonstrates to the client the progress made, as it is sometimes difficult for the client to 'remember' how significant the original problem may have been. It is also encouraging for the electrologist to see ongoing results and alerts them if progress is not as expected, thereby allowing in-depth analysis for the client's benefit of the potential causes for any discrepancy. These pictures are ideally used only for a specific area, rather than a whole headshot where the client can be easily identified. Either way, the pictures must remain private and confidential, securely stored and never be shown to anyone without the written permission of the client.

The epilation record card

In addition to the standard information, the epilation record card should include:

- detailed information on previous hair removal treatments
- hair type
- skin type
- method of epilation
- intensity of current
- needle size and type
- date and timing of sessions
- treatment remarks and details, length etc.
- machine settings
- reaction to treatment
- aftercare advice
- products purchased.

During consultation and throughout a course of treatments, the condition of the client's skin is vital to the success, effectiveness and comfort of the treatment. A full skin diagnosis should be carried out and details noted on the client's record card. Any previous record cards must be referred to and taken into consideration where appropriate. As well as general skin type, great care must be taken to record, in great detail, the condition of the skin in the direct working area. Any changes in the skin (good or bad) throughout the treatment should be recorded.

After a full consultation, the content of the record card should be clarified with the client to ensure that the correct information is recorded and that no misunderstandings have arisen.

ELECTROLYSIS HAIR REMOVAL CONSULTATION CARD

STEREX ELECTROLYSIS INTERNATIONAL LIMITED

Client Name: _____

Date of Consultation: _____ Recommended By: _____

Address:

Occupation:

Postcode:

Home Tel No:

Work/Mobile No: Date of Birth:

Medical Information

Doctor's Name: Medical History:

Address & Tel:

Are you currently under medical care? Yes No

Do you take medication, if so why? Yes No

Do you or have you ever smoked? Yes No Do you currently smoke? Yes No How many? _____

What is your weekly alcohol consumption?

Contra-indications Definitive - * in area (recommendations only - please check your insurance specifications)

A.I.D.S. / H.I.V	Haemophilia	Metal plates/pins	Recent scar tissue *
Cancer	Heart conditions	Moles/pigmented naevi	Rosacea (active) *
Circulatory disorders	Hepatitis	Pacemaker	Skin diseases/disorders *
Dermabrasion (recent)*	Keloid scarring	Phlebitis/Thrombosis *	Sunburn *
Diabetes (Type 1)	Laser/IPL (recent) *	Pregnancy (1st trimester)	Varicose veins
Drugs (eg blood thinners)			

Plus any other conditions you may not be insured to treat:

Contra-indications Restrictive - * in area (recommendations only - please check your insurance specifications)

Asthma/respiratory disorders	Diabetes (Type 2)	Loss tactile sensation *	Pregnancy
Cancer (history of)	Drugs (e.g. steroids)	Lupus	Skin diseases/disorders *
Cuts & abrasions *	Endocrine disorder	Minor	Swelling/oedema *
Dermabrasion (ongoing) *	Epilepsy	Nervous client	Other:
Dermagraphia	High blood pressure		

Plus any other conditions you may not be insured to treat:

Evidence Gathering

Before photos taken:	Yes ☐	No ☐	Date (s) taken:	
Photo taken mid course:	Yes ☐	No ☐		
Photo taken on completion of course:	Yes ☐	No ☐		

Needle Choice

Needle Type:	Gold ☐		Stainless Steel ☐		Insulated ☐
Needle Size:	F2 ☐ F3 ☐ F4 ☐	F5 ☐ F6 ☐ F10 ☐	1 Piece ☐	2 Piece ☐	
Needle Length:	Short ☐		Regular ☐		

Skin Analysis

Previous treatment? Yes No Date:

Laser/IPL ☐ Waxing ☐ Plucking ☐ Depilatory Creams ☐ Cutting ☐ Other:

Any tissue damage present? Skin healing rate:

Skin Type: Coarse ☐ Combination ☐ Dehydrated ☐ Dry ☐ Mature ☐ Normal ☐ Oily ☐ Sensitive ☐

Pigmentation: Prone to pigmentation Yes No Existing pigmentation Yes No (if Yes, record detail)

Known Allergies: Topical/local anaesthetics ☐ Cosmetics ☐ Latex ☐ Metal ☐ Products ☐ Vinyl ☐

(if Yes, record details)

Hair Analysis

Area to be treated:	Top Lip ☐	Chin ☐	Neck ☐	Breast ☐	Abdomen ☐
	Underarms ☐	Legs ☐	Bikini ☐	Other ☐	

Hair type: Terminal ☐ Vellus ☐ Coarse ☐ Fine ☐ Curly ☐

First noticed Growth: .... Hair density: ....

Cause of Growth: Congenital ☐ Topical ☐ Systemic ☐

Treatment plan

Client's pain threshold:	Good ☐	Normal ☐	Poor ☐
Healing rate:	Good ☐	Normal ☐	Poor ☐

Frequency of treatments:

Result & reaction of electrolysis patch test: ....

Current choice:	Short Wave Diathermy ☐	Blend ☐	Galvanic ☐

Current settings:

Treatment strategy:

Comments:

Aftercare

Advice given for management of hair growth:

Recommendations: ....

Written aftercare advice given: Yes ☐ No ☐

Client signature: .... Date:

Declaration

I confirm I have received a thorough consultation and understand the nature of the treatment. I declare I have disclosed all necessary information in order that my treatment may be carried out safely. A treatment plan has been discussed as well as the importance of regular treatments in order to achieve success. I understand there is a healing process following treatment and I must adhere to the aftercare advice. I have received, read and understood the written aftercare advice given to me. I understand I must follow the advice given for hair growth management between treatments.

Client signature: Therapist signature:

Client name in print: Therapist name in print:

Date:

An epilation record card (Source: Sterex Electrolysis International Ltd)

Think about it

A skin in good condition ensures for the client:

- more comfortable treatments
- more effective treatments
- quicker healing time
- less erythema.

A good skin condition ensures for the electrologist:

- easier treatments
- satisfied clients.

Obtaining signed, written, informed consent

Ensure your client carefully checks, signs and dates the record card at the end of the consultation, stating that all the information is true to the best of their knowledge. It is imperative that the electrologist also dates and signs/initials the consultation/record card on every client visit, as generally this is also a legal requirement. It is also advisable to ask clients to sign and date a statement that they have been given aftercare advice and that they will follow the advice, for example 'I agree to follow the written and verbal aftercare advice which has been given'.

The information on the client's record card should be checked every time the client visits the salon to ensure that there are no changes; for example, has the client started HRT and not informed you? This could affect her hormonal balance and therefore her hair growth, skin and general wellbeing.

Think about it

Failure to keep up-to-date, accurate, complete, legible and signed records could result in unsafe treatment and possibly to legal action being taken against you and/or the salon.

Planning the treatment

The treatment plan should include:

- area to be cleared and a consistent, organised visual aid showing how to attain the final desired result
- date
- time and timing of treatment
- area worked
- size and type of needle
- hair removed (clients should be told how many hairs are removed and with the 'treat and leave' technique, it is easy to count them).

All hair management techniques should be discussed as part of the treatment plan to manage the client's hair growth between treatments and whilst the course of epilation is continuing (see the section on hair management techniques, page 522).

Working cost-effectively

It is important to complete services in the given time so that you are cost-effective. It is not advisable to over-treat or go over time and you must ensure the client pays for work carried out and is not overcharged.

The costs of individual epilation treatment and courses of treatment vary considerably around the UK and depend not only on region but location, standard of premises, experience of electrologists and client base. In addition, single treatments vary in time to suit a variety of clients and their own personal hair-growth problems. Appointments can range from 5 minutes to 2 hours or longer. Prices usually get less expensive the longer the session and a course usually offers a reduction of some type. Alternatively, many electrologists offer a free aftercare product if a course is booked. This way you can ensure the client receives an excellent product, which will ensure good aftercare.

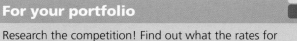

For your portfolio

Research the competition! Find out what the rates for epilation treatments are in your area.

Regular treatments

Regular treatments are essential to achieve permanent hair removal. The following factors will affect the regularity of treatments and the speed of results:

- the scale of the hair growth problem
- the financial considerations
- the area to be treated

- regrowth time
- the size of the area to be treated
- the type and strength of hair
- the type of skin
- any underlying medical problems
- the healing rate of the client
- the client's pain threshold.

Causes of hair growth

Causes of abnormal hair growth range from illness to hormonal reasons. What is considered excessive hair growth in one country can be considered normal in another, and what is considered unattractive by some can be appealing to others. Some clients may feel they are abnormal and all clients must be taken seriously. If a client feels that he or she does not fit into the 'norm' in a society, it can seriously affect his or her general wellbeing.

The human body is covered with hair follicles that can be dormant or active and can grow no hair, fine **vellus** hair or thick **terminal** hair. All hair growth – normal or abnormal – is controlled by hormones and it is the over-secretion of male hormones that causes excessive hair growth. Hormones are chemical messengers that are circulated by the bloodstream. Research has shown that most excess hair is due to a combination of over-abundant androgen (the male hormone) secretion and an enzyme in the follicle that is sensitive to androgen increase.

Key terms

Lanugo – downy fine hair which grows on a foetus.

Vellus – short, fine, non-pigmented hair which replaces lanugo after birth.

Terminal – longer, coarser, pigmented hair which replaces vellus during puberty.

Classification of hair growth

Causes of hair growth are classified as:

- congenital
- topical
- systemic.

Congenital

This is hair growth that is present from birth. Some people are born with greater amounts of facial and body hair that is both normal and hereditary, for example eyebrows, eyelashes, nostrils, scalp and body hair. People vary considerably in their skin sensitivity to androgens and females who have low levels of the female hormones (oestrogen and progesterone) and higher levels of androgens can develop superfluous hair.

Topical

Friction or stimulation to an area of skin can cause excess hair growth. Topical causes include plaster casts, plucking and waxing. This hair, formed as a protective mechanism of the body, grows deeper and coarser because of stimulation of the blood supply to the skin in that area. Moles and birthmarks often have excessive hair growth because of the multiple and unusual development of capillaries near the surface of the skin.

Systemic

These are normal and abnormal hormonal changes that can stimulate hair growth — see the table below.

Normal systemic causes of hair growth

At puberty, hormone levels start to rise. The process starts when the hypothalamus stimulates the anterior pituitary gland to secrete gonadotrophic hormones which activate the sex glands. Hormones secreted by the anterior pituitary gland at this time are:

- adrenocorticotrophic hormone (ACTH) — this stimulates the adrenal cortex to produce oestrogen and progesterone in the female, testosterone and a little oestrogen in the male, and androgens in both sexes
- follicle-stimulating hormone (FSH) — stimulates the development and ripening of ovarian follicles and produces oestrogen
- luteinising hormone (LH) — stimulates the formation and secretion of the corpus luteum, which in turn secretes progesterone.

Normal	Abnormal
Puberty	Cushing's syndrome
Pregnancy	Adrenogenital syndrome
Menopause	Archard-Thiers syndrome
Medication	Polycystic ovary syndrome
Stress	Anorexia nervosa
	Acromegaly

Systemic causes of hair growth

During pregnancy, women can have increased hair growth which may be temporary and will disappear without treatment after the birth. However, often the fine vellus hair appearing throughout pregnancy can develop into terminal hair and electrolysis is required. The many hormonal changes and often temporary imbalances result in the androgen level being raised, resulting in superfluous hair growth.

During menopause, the ovaries begin to degenerate as their reproductive function is no longer required and a reduction in the levels of oestrogen, progesterone and androgens occurs. However, the adrenal cortex continues to produce androgens and this can lead to the production of superfluous hair in the male growth pattern. A premature menopause can be brought about by surgical removal of the ovaries and womb (total hysterectomy).

Long-term stress causes secretion of hormones from the adrenal cortex and these androgens will stimulate superfluous hair growth in the male pattern.

Many types of medication can encourage superfluous hair growth, including anabolic steroids and some makes of the contraceptive pill. It is estimated that there are over 500 different drugs that can affect hair growth.

Anorexia nervosa is a psychological disorder, mostly affecting adolescent girls, and involves the nervous, endocrine and digestive systems. A strong conviction that the sufferer is overweight and a general lack of self-esteem cause the sufferer to become malnourished and severely underweight, and can even be fatal. Lanugo hair (baby hair) develops all over the body, and there is a thinning of the hair on the head.

Endocrine disorders affecting hair growth

To learn more about the endocrine system, see Related anatomy and physiology, page 207.

Endocrine disorders include the following:

- Cushing's syndrome — increased levels of ACTH lead to an excess of androgens, which possibly lead to hirsutism. Symptoms include osteoporosis, muscular weakness and wasting of the limbs, thinning skin, rounding of the face, high blood pressure, oedema, and obesity of the trunk.
- Adrenogenital syndrome — a very rare condition, it is present from birth and is a genetic defect causing overproduction of androgens by the adrenal cortex. Symptoms include enlargement of the genitals, dehydration, weight loss, low blood pressure and hypoglycaemia.

- Archard-Thiers syndrome — another rare condition, its symptoms are similar to Cushing's syndrome. Women with diabetes can suffer from this where the adrenal glands and ovaries produce too much androgen.

- Polycystic ovary syndrome — this produces symptoms including enlarged ovaries with numerous follicular cysts, irregular or absent menstrual cycle, and weight gain. Polycystic ovaries are capable of secreting large quantities of androgens, causing the development of excess hair.

- Acromegaly — this is caused by the hypersecretion of growth hormone. Symptoms can include large hands and feet, coarse facial features and the secretion of excess androgens that stimulate excessive hair growth in the male pattern.

Contra-indications to treatment

Electrolysis guidelines about restricting treatments or requiring medical referral are given below. This is not necessarily a comprehensive list. For any condition you are uncertain of, a doctor's permission must be sought.

The following contra-indications will either prevent or restrict treatments and are in place for the health and safety of the client and the protection of the electrologist. Carrying out an epilation treatment on a contra-indicated client could result in a number of different reactions, ranging from skin irritation, discomfort or infection to potential cross-contamination of infectious disorders and diseases. At its most serious, treatment could cause serious health issues such as cardiac arrest.

- Bacterial infections, for example impetigo
- Circulatory discorders
- Contagious or infectious disease or disorder
- Cuts and abrasions (treatment area)
- Dermagraphia
- Drugs, e.g. blood thinners or steroids
- Electronic implants, for example pacemakers
- Fungal infections, for example ringworm
- Haemophilia
- Heart valve disorders
- Hepatitis
- High blood pressure
- HIV or AIDS
- Hyperpigmentation and hypopigmentation
- Infestations, for example scabies

- **Keloid** scarring
- Loss of tactile sensation
- Metal plates or pins (treatment area) — this is especially important with blend or galvanic currents
- Moles
- Phlebitis/thrombosis/varicose veins
- Pregnancy — first three months
- Pregnancy — avoid breasts or abdomen particularly during the last three months
- Pregnancy — below neck area with blend or galvanic currents
- Pre-malignant/malignant lesions
- Recent scar tissue (treatment area — advisable to wait 12 months)
- Rosacea
- Severe active psoriasis/eczema/acne/dermatitis (treatment area)
- Severe stress or anxiety
- Skin cancer (treatment area)
- Sunburn
- Swelling/oedema
- Viral infections, for example herpes simplex.

Seek medical advice if your client has:

- auditory devices
- history of cancer
- emphysema
- endocrine disorders/hormone imbalance
- epilepsy
- hairs from moles, moles and pigmented naevi
- heart problems
- hiatus hernia (affects positioning of client)
- insulin-controlled diabetes
- lupus
- pregnancy
- psoriasis
- severe asthma requiring medication.

Key terms

Keloid – elevated fibrous enlargement of the skin, most commonly found at the site of a scar. A skin reaction to injury, keloids are usually raised, smooth and firm. They are most frequently found on black skin and the person will usually have a congenital disposition to keloid scarring.

Minors will also need a doctor's permission before treatment can be carried out.

In addition to these contra-indications, skin sensitivity can be affected by other skincare treatments that may inhibit or prevent epilation, for example glycolic peels, microdermabrasion and laser.

If epilation is contra-indicated for a client, refer to page 523 and the alternative methods of hair removal which they can be informed about.

Carry out electrical epilation

In this section you will learn about:

- carrying out a treatment
- hair growth rates
- electrologist positioning for treatments
- skin and hair types
- sizes and types of needles
- loading and unloading the needle holder
- working safely to avoid contra-actions
- methods of epilation
- possible faults
- contra-actions.

Carrying out a treatment

During consultation, a treatment plan to cover the course of their treatment will be discussed with the client. This will ensure the client is fully aware of the necessary commitment required and that regular appointments, often for long periods of time over months, if not years, may be necessary for desired results.

Good skincare and product advice, to ensure the skin is in the best possible condition, will make the treatment more comfortable and effective for the client and easier to perform for the electrologist. Facials, particularly light exfoliation, can assist epilation treatment, ensuring ease of operation. When aftercare is discussed, products to calm, soothe and assist with healing should be recommended and sold to the client. It is imperative that clients follow the electrologist's advice, as the use of incorrect products could be detrimental to their skin and health.

It is important to organise treatment time carefully — clients will want value for money and not to be rushed. Always start each treatment with the darkest, most noticeable hairs first. Ask clients which hairs bother them the most (never presume as the answer may not necessarily match your opinion).

With a dense growth it is advisable to treat every other hair to prevent over-treatment of the area and cause either the build-up of heat (diathermy) or **lye** (blend or galvanic) as this can cause tissue damage, oedema and/or erythema and sensitisation of the skin. Treat all hairs of the same type, texture and diameter. When these have been treated, it may be necessary to reduce the needle size to complete the treatment. It is important to work in a systematic manner so that you are not jumping from area to area, for client comfort, to prevent touching areas that have been treated and for healing and regrowth purposes.

Key terms

Lye – or sodium hydroxide (NaOH), is a strong, caustic alkali produced as a result of a direct current and salt water solution (as found in a hair follicle). It provides the destructive force for blend and galvanic.

Think about it

A skin in good condition will yield the hair on removal, preventing breakage and will ensure smoother insertion, making the treatment more comfortable.

Hair growth rates

The growth pattern of the hair will influence present and future treatments. All hair goes though a life cycle that is timed by genes. This cycle can vary from a few months for an eyebrow hair to up to six years or even longer for a scalp hair — see the table below.

Type of hair	F = Female M = Male	Regrowth time
Upper lip (vellus hair)	F	8–9 weeks
Upper lip (terminal)	F/M	4–6 weeks
Chin (vellus)	F	6–7 weeks
Chin (terminal)	F/M	5–6 weeks
Bikini line (terminal)	F	5–6 weeks
Eyebrows	F/M	5–6 weeks
Underarms (terminal)	F/M	7–8 weeks
Neck/nape (terminal)	F/M	5–6 weeks
Breast (terminal)	F	7–8 weeks
Chest (terminal)	M	6–7 weeks
Abdomen (terminal)	F	8–9 weeks
Fingers, toes (terminal)	F/M	6–8 weeks

Guideline estimates for regrowth of hair

It is advisable to be aware of the estimated rate at which hair grows on different parts of the body so that you can prepare an effective treatment plan and to understand that hairs that grow in treated areas before the normal regrowth time are hairs growing from untreated follicles. The client must understand that latent early anagen hairs account for the largest percentage of the 'regrowth problem'. If you feel at any time that progress is not being made or that the hair growth problem is getting worse, then it is advisable to refer the client to their GP for investigation into any possible underlying medical problem.

Each area of the body has a set number of hair follicles from birth. Most hair follicles are dormant or grow hair invisible to the human eye. New hair grows only if a dormant follicle becomes active. There can be approximately 5000–10,000 hair follicles per square inch depending on the part of the body.

Electrologist positioning for treatments

The images below are intended for right-handed electrologists; it is vice versa for left handed electrologists.

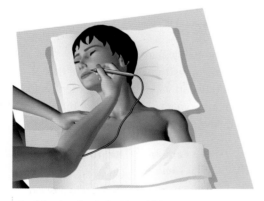

Positioning for left side of face

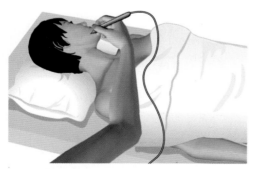

Positioning for right side of face

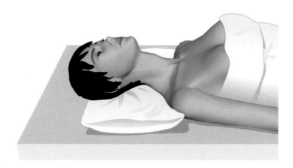

When working on chin and throat, position the neck so it is supported by a pillow, raising up the client's chin and exposing the area

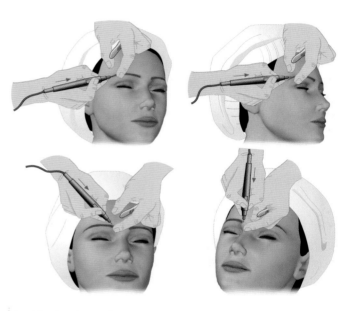

Positioning for eyebrows

Think about it

The images on pages 532–534 are intended for right-handed electrologists; it is vice-versa for left-handed electrologists.

If right-handed, position yourself on the right side of the client as he or she is lying down; vice-versa for left-handed electrologists. The electrologist can also position herself behind the client for eyebrows or other areas when the direction of hair growth demands it.

Refer also to Unit G22 Monitor procedures to safely control work operations, page 99, for information on needle health and safety.

Tweezer methods – a step-by-step guide

Technique 1

1 Hold needle holder in your right hand and tweezers in your left hand. Rest the tip of the tweezers between your thumb and the palm of your hand

2 Slide the needle holder between your first and second or second and third fingers, using your thumb. Take the tweezers from your left hand, with the thumb and forefinger of your right hand

3 Grasp the epilated hair and gently release from the skin

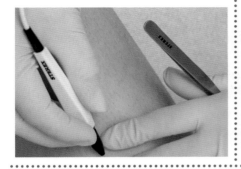
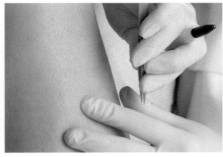
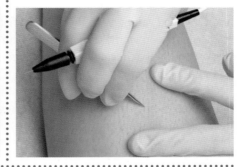

Technique 2

1 Hold the needle holder in your right hand and tweezers in your left, with the tip facing away from your client

2 Slide the needle holder between your first and second or second and third fingers, using your thumb. Take the tweezers from your left hand, with the thumb and forefinger of your right hand

3 Grasp the epilated hair and gently release from the skin

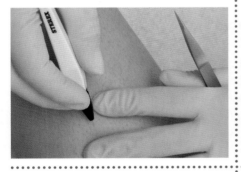
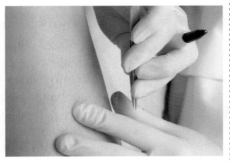
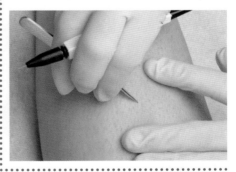

Technique 3

1 Hold the tweezers and needle holder in the right hand and approach the hair for epilating as in techniques 1 and 2

2 After treating, slide the needle holder between your first and second or second and third fingers, using your thumb to push it into place

3 Manoeuvre the tweezers into position between your thumb and forefinger, and gently release the epilated hair

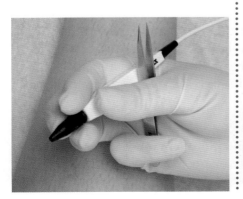
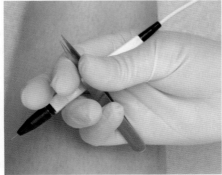
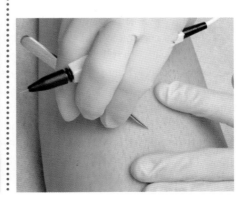

Skin and hair types

The outer appearance of the skin and hair both act as a guide for different strategies when giving an effective electrolysis treatment.

The thickness of the epidermis affects the treatment. For example, a thin epidermis will react with almost immediate erythema because the epidermis is nearly transparent and the blood can be seen through it, whereas a thicker epidermal region with a deeper hair follicle may not react so quickly and may require deeper than normal insertions with a regular needle rather than a short one. The length of the needle depends on the average depth of the hair follicles in the area to be treated. In general, dark terminal hairs lie deeper than fine dark and vellus hairs.

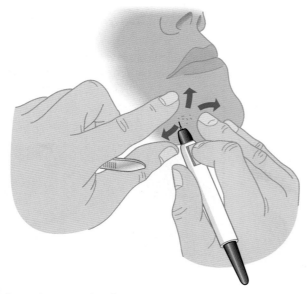

A steady, supportive three-way stretch helps ensure accurate insertion

Always aim for a steady, supportive three-way stretch positioning to help ensure the needle holder and needle are used at the correct angle, direction and depth for the hair follicle and the area to be treated. It will also make the treatment as comfortable as possible for the client. A three-way stretch with a firm but light touch opens up the follicle, allowing easy clear entry. Down pressure is not required but, rather, a gentle pulling open pressure. To secure an effective stretch, the fingers should be close together and the index and second finger (or thumb and index) are used. The needle holder hand utilises the second, third or even the fourth finger to attain the stretch, thus creating an effective three-way stretch.

A firm or soft skin can also affect an epilation treatment because of the ease or otherwise of needle insertion.

- The chin is an example of a firm area.

- The breast is an example of a soft area where a greater stretch will be required with difficult insertions because of the skin's resilience in this area.

- The abdomen is surprisingly sensitive with the hair often proving very strong, therefore a firm stretch is required due to the resilient nature of the skin and lack of underlying bone support. The skin of the abdomen area behaves very similarly to the breast area.

- Fingers and toes are sensitive and hair can be difficult to remove. The depth of insertion generally is superficial, so a low intensity for a longer time is recommended.

Type of hair growth

The type of hair growth — vellus, terminal, fine, curly, straight or **compound** — will affect the choice of method of epilation, intensity and timing. Fine hair is often accelerated lanugo or vellus hair and although the hair is fine, it will be anchored into the follicle very firmly and will require more time on a lower intensity. Fine vellus hair may have no papilla and may be located in and feed off the sebaceous gland. Darker and thicker hairs require higher intensity than finer, less dense hairs. Curly hairs may have distorted hair follicles and probing accuracy can prove difficult with no obvious or clear insertion, with the blend method offering most success.

Insertions too close to each other result in over-treatment of the area (often performed on dark, deep terminal hairs with a close proximity to each other) and can cause hyperpigmentation and possible pitting. If the hairs are too long to treat, cut them, allowing the angle of growth to be seen more easily. The darkest and heaviest growth should be removed first so that the client can see immediate progress. Red and non-pigmented hair types often prove exceedingly difficult to treat. Red hair and non-pigmented white hair is often coarse, strong and firmly rooted, proving difficult to treat, and frequently requires a substantial current level. This poses a dilemma for the electrologist as the skin is often extremely sensitive and therefore can react quite fiercely. Both hair types appear to respond well to diathermy treatment. Spacing out insertions, short treatment sessions, varying areas when possible and using a gold needle for sensitive skin are all options which can be utilised.

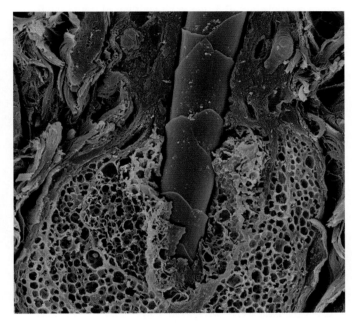

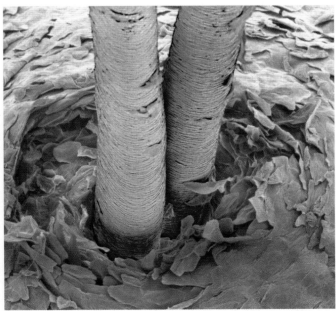

Different types of follicle – single and compound

Curvy follicle growth

- The hair replacement cycle of curly hair is just the same as straight hair.
- Curved follicles can be found on white as well as black skin, but are predominantly found in black skin.
- The amount of follicle curvature is related to the flatness of the hair shaft.
- In most curved superfluous hair, the lower quarter of the follicle turns at an obtuse angle from the follicle proper and this angle causes the flattening of the hair structure. It is the flattened shape which gives rise to the curling of the hair shaft.
- The curl of the hair above skin level is greater than the follicle curvature in the skin. This is because the part of the root encased in the root sheaths is still in a newly formed, moist condition — the hair does not begin to curl until it has left the sheaths and it begins to dry.
- Treatment for curved follicle growth must be given special consideration. Insert the needle on the underside of the hair. It may be necessary to push past a tissue obstruction and continue down about half as far again and release the current. When the hair releases, check the depth and use this depth as your guide.

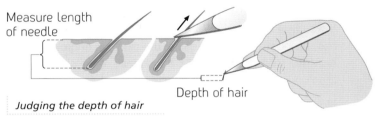

Measure length of needle

Depth of hair

Judging the depth of hair

Corkscrew hair

This is a distorted hair follicle and is produced by the remains of an almost destroyed pilosebaceous unit, which has become disorientated and has not re-formed properly. To treat, see curly follicle growth above.

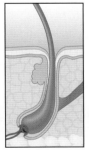 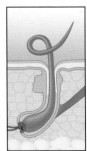 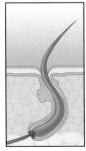 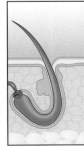

| J - shaped | Corkscrew | S - shaped | U - shaped |

Distorted hair follicles

Single hair

A single hair grows from a single follicle and is treated by lining up the needle with the hair and inserting gently into the follicle. Adequate current is used and the needle is removed. The hair is then gently released from the follicle by the use of tweezers.

Compound hairs

These are also known as **pili multigemini**. The follicle has two or more dermal papillae, which results in two or more hairs growing from the same follicle. Treat the larger hair with the current. This may well affect both hairs. Gently release the treated hair and then try to remove the second hair; if it has been successful, the hair will epilate easily. If using the blend method, wait to see if the hair releases after some time has passed. If not, the hair can be treated as a single hair when deemed appropriate and not over-treated. If the hairs are 'blasted' separately, then too much current may be unnecessarily used and could cause skin damage.

Ingrowing hair

An ingrowing hair is one that grows abnormally under the skin, having been covered by an overgrowth of skin. There are several reasons for this: some people are genetically disposed towards them; waxing or tweezing hairs often cause them, when the hair breaks at the weakest point just below the surface of the skin. Waxing, in particular, can distort the hair, especially if pulled against the direction of growth. The hair then tends to grow under the surface of the skin rather than up and out of the hair follicle.

Men with heavy hair growth can have this problem. When they shave closely, the hair pulls back into the hair follicle and sometimes its direction of growth is altered, causing ingrowing hairs. The hairs can continue to grow just beneath the skin's surface and may become infected. If not infected, the trapped end should be freed from the skin to release it, either using a one-piece needle, a microlance or a professional sterilised pair of sharp-tipped tweezers. Once released, if not infected, the hair can be treated with epilation or allowed to heal as required. If infected, antiseptic cream should be applied and if necessary antibiotics prescribed by a GP. Ingrowing hairs often resolve soon after electrolysis is started.

Embedded hair

These can be recognised by the appearance of bumps on the skin, irritation, erythema and hair being seen under the skin. There are many causes including friction, irritation and dry skin. To treat this condition, see 'Ingrowing hair' above.

Unshed telogen hair

Telogen hair that fails to shed appears in the form of a shaved or clipped stump and can become infected. It is usually colourless and occurs when a telogen hair that is quite wide reaches the skin's surface. Telogen hair is difficult to see and does not usually grow in length. It lacks pigmentation because the hair has lost contact with the source of pigmentation after separating from the dermal papilla. Treat these hairs as normal in telogen stage.

Tombstone hair

This is a small hair that has been epilated in the anagen stage of hair growth, but remains in the skin. The electrologist will probably have removed a hair from a follicle in the telogen stage, without realising a new anagen hair was forming underneath. Such hair is thick, very dark, brittle and looks like a 'foreign body' or 'rotting stump' at the surface of the skin. It does not usually need to be epilated — cleansing and exfoliating the skin or tweezing it out is usually sufficient.

Lanugo comedones

These are a tiny bundle of lanugo hairs protruding from a follicle or follicles. They may appear as a short, thick brown hair, resembling a comedone. When examined closely, this is made up of a number of very fine lanugo hairs held together by sebum, as they can arise from the sebaceous gland. There is a tendency for them to be found on oily, seborrhoeic skin. These comedones can be tweezed out without traction.

Skin types

Refresh your memory about skin types and the skin's structure and functions by referring to You and the skin and Related anatomy and physiology (see pages 242 and 166).

The following skin-type information applies mainly to white skin, although it is possible to have several aspects relating to other skin types. Clients must be treated as individuals based on the information obtained at consultation, especially clients who may have a combination of the differing skin categories.

Oily/combination skin

Sebum is found in abundance in this skin type. It is the insulating properties of sebum that are of benefit during a short wave diathermy treatment. Provided there is correct probing technique and intensity of current, as it reaches the surface of the skin the sebum will protect the epidermis from the effects of the current. However, any surface oil should be completely removed. The moisture content of this skin type is usually good, which plays an important part in conduction of the current. Insertion of the needle will usually be relatively easy because of dilated pores common in this skin type. Care must be taken when working near any papules or pustules as the pH balance of the skin may also be affected, which could cause infection in the area. The skin texture is often thicker than that of normal or dry skin.

Dry or dehydrated skin

Dry skin is usually lacking in sebum and moisture content and will take longer to heal, so additional space should be left between probes as well as a longer time between treatments to ensure a safe and effective outcome. Dry or dehydrated skin can present difficulties because both short wave diathermy and direct current require moisture to work effectively. Dead skin cells may also block the follicle opening, causing difficulty with needle insertion. It is important to also consider the skin's reaction.

Moist skin

This skin type has high moisture content in both the epidermis and dermis. When there are varying degrees of moisture found on the facial area, there may be varying skin reactions to the treatment. These should all be noted and acted upon by adjustment to the intensity, timing and method in the various areas and, if appropriate, even changing the needle. Blend is the more suitable current because of the lower intensity of short wave diathermy current. The use of short wave diathermy current on this skin type is not recommended as the current may rise too quickly to the surface of the skin before effective treatment of the lower follicle.

Mature skin

This skin type may react quickly to epilation with a pronounced erythema and the client's pain threshold may also be affected, so the current intensity should be as low as possible. Insertion spacing, length of and frequency of treatments will all have to be taken into consideration to ensure no undesirable reactions occur. The blend method may prove more suitable for this skin type because of the lower intensity of the short wave diathermy current. Skin sensitivity can appear, with allergy to products or treatment.

Global origins

A client's ethnic origin will directly affect the type of treatment chosen. Their follicle shape and depth will impact on all aspects of the treatment, including the treatment plan and needle choice.

There are a number of differences between the structures of white/Caucasian, black, Asian, Oriental and Mediterranean/ Latino skins, so each skin type should be treated differently when epilation is being carried out. People of different ethnic origins have differing amounts of hair. White-/Caucasian-skinned Northern Europeans (including people from Britain and Scandinavia) have less hair than those with darker skins in Asia. Black skins have relatively little hair, while Oriental skins have the least body hair.

Black skin
Characteristics:

- The stratum corneum of the epidermis is much thicker and skin desquamates more easily.
- Collagen fibres are more numerous, making it stronger.
- The ageing process is slower because the elasticity in the skin lasts longer.
- Sebaceous glands are more numerous and larger.
- A greater number of sebaceous glands open onto the skin's surface instead of into a hair follicle.
- Suderiferous glands are more numerous and larger.
- The suderiferous duct opens onto the surface of the skin — it is longer and more obvious.

Advice on epilation:

- Curly and distorted hair follicles are a consideration.
- Black skin tends to hyperpigmentate more than white skin (although this can rectify itself).
- When a hair regrows in a hair follicle that has been treated previously, it grows straight and very shallow. This hair can then be treated as for hair on white skin.
- It is difficult to detect erythema, so there is a risk of over-treating.
- The area can be prone to heat retention and swelling as the skin is extremely sensitive to heat.
- The skin is prone to keloid scarring — ensure a full and accurate consultation.
- Complete a short test treatment to assess healing rate.
- The preferred method of treatment should be blend, so that the lye produced reaches the curved hair follicles effectively. Consider a gold needle for less skin reaction. If using short wave diathermy, use an insulated needle so that the current is concentrated at the tip of the needle to reduce surface reaction, and ensure current is of a low intensity.
- Difficulty probing a curved hair follicle can be experienced as the hair shaft is usually flattened. Ensure firm but light stretch is used and positioning of body is correct.

- Use the correct diameter of needle, matching the diameter of hair treated.

- Space out the treatments and the probing area — one in five to prevent overheating of the skin tissue.

- Ensure aftercare is applied immediately — use a compress of witch hazel or aloe vera gel.

- Discuss homecare advice and give the client an aftercare leaflet.

- Book the next treatment after sufficient healing time has occurred.

Asian and Mediterranean/Latino skin

Characteristics:

- Normally a finer texture than black skin.

- The skin colour can vary from dark brown to light brown.

- The hair growth tends to be fine, dark and dense, although dark and coarse hairs are often found among the finer hairs.

- The fine hairs usually grow from follicles that are small, straight and superficial to the skin's surface.

- The coarse, terminal hairs are from follicles that are straight but deep.

- This skin type is prone to sensitivity and increased pigmentation.

- The pigmentation may not be evident for several days or weeks and can take many months to fade.

- Mediterranean/Latino skin is usually olive in colour, moist and oily which allows easy insertion due to the elastic nature of the skin.

Advice on epilation:

- The blend method is recommended, teamed with a gold needle to combat sensitivity and problematic reaction.

- If the short wave diathermy method is used, ensure a low intensity and use an insulated needle to keep the intensity in the lower half of the follicle.

- Space out the treatments and the probing area.

- Avoid over-treating the area and allow sufficient healing time.

Oriental skin

Characteristics:

- Oriental skin is prone to pigmentation, sensitivity, discoloration and pit marks if it is over-exposed to heat.

Advice on epilation:

- See the advice for Asian skin above.

- The pores will usually be small and tight, so a size 2 or 3 short needle may be required.

Sizes and types of needles

There are several needle manufacturers, with Sterex probably being the most well-known, as they developed the first sterilised needles. Types of needles include two-piece, one-piece, gold and insulated needles. Needles are made from the highest quality materials, with a polished tip for perfect insertion comfort. They are most commonly sterilised using gamma irradiation and are guaranteed for five years with a visible date mark.

Needle types

Two-piece needles: available in stainless steel, gold and insulated

Stainless steel: available in sizes 2, 3, 4, 5, 6 and 10 (size 10 for advanced techniques)

Gold: available in sizes 2, 3, 4 and 5

Insulated: available in sizes 2, 3, 4 and 5

One-piece needles: available in sizes 2, 3, 4 and 5

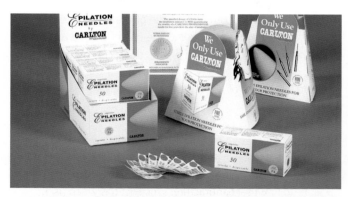

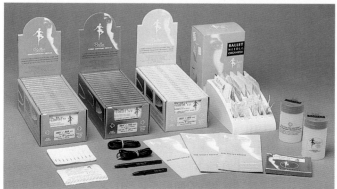

A selection of needles

Think about it

Think about it

The electrolysis needle fulfils two roles:

- to position the needle
- to conduct the current.

The smaller the size number, the thinner the needle. Therefore, when treating fine hair, a 2 or 3 needle which is 0.02 or 0.03 of a millimetre would be selected. To work on very coarse hair, a size 6 might be chosen; 4 and 5 are used for hairs of in-between thickness.

The choice of diameter of needle is essential to the effectiveness of the treatment. A smaller needle is easier to insert into a larger follicle. It is wrongly believed that by using a smaller needle than is suitable, less discomfort is caused. In reality, a greater discomfort is caused because the same current is released from a smaller surface area, thus causing a more concentrated expulsion of current.

Importance of using the correct diameter of needle

It is important to use the correct diameter of the needle:

- to ensure that the destructive agent (heat or chemical) is adequate to be effective
- to help prevent (diathermy) heat rising to the surface and damaging the surface of the skin
- to prevent skin damage and over-treatment if too large a needle is used
- to prevent needle movement within the follicle if the needle used is too small
- because the smaller the size of the needle, the smaller the surface area and the sharper it is, causing a more intense sensation for the client.

Think about it

Always follow the manufacturer's instructions when using needles.

Two-piece needles are also available in different shaft lengths (the part that goes in the follicle) — short is .48 centimetres long; regular is .63 centimetres long. Short is recommended for the face and regular for the body, but all clients are different and it really is a matter of the electrologist's personal preference and client requirements.

There are also different shank sizes (the part that fits into the needle holder) — F and K. F is the standard size for the UK. They are both the same length, but F has a larger diameter than K.

The difference between two-piece and one-piece needles

A two-piece needle is a strong yet flexible needle, offering the electrologist essential flexibility and 'feel'. This type of needle flexes when it meets resistance, indicating to the electrologist whether the insertion is correct or incorrect.

The one-piece needle is more rigid, and is ideal for advanced techniques and for the experienced electrologist.

Think about it

The client may be allergic to nickel, in which case gold needles should be used, or if allergic to gold, insulated needles may be used.

Gold needles

The benefits of using gold needles include the following:

- Smoother insertion — gold is a very smooth metal and glides into the follicle more easily than other needles, proving more comfortable for the client, with less erythema.
- A more comfortable treatment — it is an excellent conductor of electricity, which sometimes allows the current to be reduced, resulting in a more comfortable treatment for the client and less erythema.
- Gold is hypoallergenic and therefore suitable for those with allergic reactions to metal and those with sensitive skins.

Additional knowledge

The flash technique

The flash technique uses a very high current for a very short period of time. This method is popular in the US but is not widely used in the UK. The heating pattern is very different with a narrower field of current spread. Specialised equipment is required for this technique.

Insulated needles

These needles are coated with a medical-grade insulation material that is used in hospitals for the lining of catheters, heart bypass tubing and endoscopes. They are recommended for the client who has sensitive skin and are suitable for the flash technique.

They offer the electrologist more choice and freedom to treat even the most difficult skins. By insulating the needle all the way down its surface, leaving only the very tip exposed, they help prevent heat (diathermy) rising to the surface of the skin, concentrate the current at the hair root and offer a smooth insertion. Insulated needles are recommended for diathermy only, as there is evidence to suggest that the insulation material can be distorted by the lye produced when using blend or galvanic.

Loading and unloading the needle holder

A new sterile needle is required for each client. You must avoid contaminating the needle by ensuring fingers, tweezers etc. do not come into contact with it.

It is important to load the needle into the needle holder correctly. Manufacturers have produced many different needle holders and needles which all load differently, so whichever needle holder you use, follow the manufacturer's instructions to ensure **aseptic** loading. If the needle is contaminated in any way, cross-infection could take place and infections or diseases could be passed on. If the needle is damaged, for example upon removal of the plastic sleeve or knocking the magnification lamp, then it should be disposed of and a new one loaded. Not only could cross-infection occur but also once a needle is bent, the metal is weakened and current could build up or be discharged at the weakened section, resulting in skin damage.

Key terms

Aseptic – to be free of pathogenic micro-organisms, for example aseptic surgical instruments, or to use methods to protect against infection by pathogenic microorganisms, for example aseptic surgical techniques. The term is used in electrolysis to illustrate sterile needles and other equipment as well as needle-loading techniques.

Loading a two-piece needle

Two-piece needles are individually wrapped and come complete with a plastic protective sleeve protecting the needle.

1 With gloved hands load a sterilised chuck cap onto the needle holder but leave slack and do not tighten on the needle holder mechanism. If the chuck cap is tightened with no needle in the needle holder mechanism it is forced shut and future needle loading becomes difficult. Tear open the needle packet at the nicked opening and withdraw the sterile needle

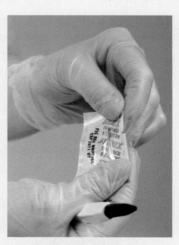

2 The needle, complete with protective sleeve, is fully inserted through the chuck cap opening down into the needle holder

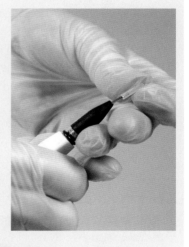

3 Once positioned gently start to tighten the chuck cap. Whilst this procedure is being undertaken carefully look through the plastic sleeve and manoeuvre the shank of the needle so that it very slightly protrudes from the chuck cap opening once the chuck is fully tightened. This position ensures maximum needle vision when inserting the needle and helps achieve the correct depth of insertion

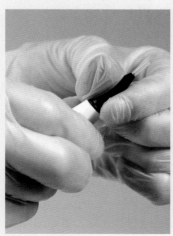

4 Firmly tighten the chuck cap and once it is tightly secure one quick 'twist and pull' movement ensures the protective sleeve covering the needle easily lifts off and a perfectly loaded needle is revealed

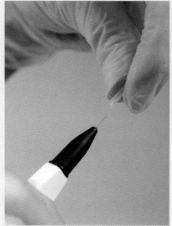

Loading a one-piece needle

One-piece needles are 'blister' packed in sleeves of 10 and have no plastic protective sleeve. The loading technique is very different to that of the two-piece needle.

1 With gloved hands load a sterilised chuck cap onto the needle holder but leave slack and untightened on the needle holder mechanism. Carefully and gently tear one needle from the 'sleeve' using the shank end (the part which fits into the needle holder). If the needle is torn from the sleeve using the needle-tip end the needle could easily become bent from the pressure

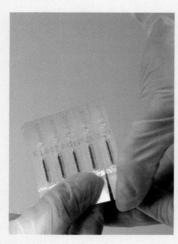

2 Peel the paper tab up away from the plastic container exposing the shank of the needle

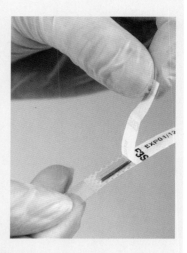

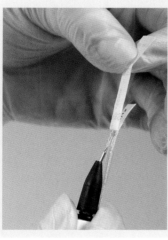

3 Approach the exposed shank of the needle with the loosened chuck cap on the needle holder and bring them together so that the shank of the needle enters into the chuck cap

4 Lift the angle of the hands so that the needle drops to the required depth and tighten the chuck cap. The result will be a perfectly loaded needle

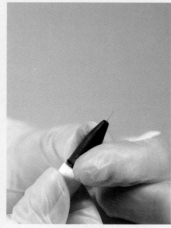

Unloading the needle

(This procedure should be undertaken with gloves still in situ from the treatment.)

- Unscrew the chuck cap loosening it from the needle holder.

- Position the needle holder facing downwards, over the sharps box, holding the loosened chuck cap. Gently tap the holder to allow the needle to fall into the box.

- If the needle does not move, slacken the chuck cap a little more and repeat the procedure.

- If the needle still does not move, gently grip and pull out the needle with tweezers while positioned facing downwards over the sharps box.

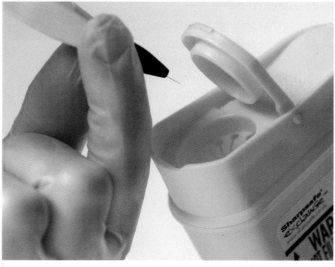

Correct needle disposal into a sharps box

Salon life

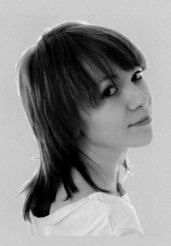

fiona's story

I was having an extremely busy day in the salon with back-to-back treatments. One of my regular clients arrived for her facial treatment but I did not have time to test the machine prior to treating her.

I began as usual, gradually increasing the current intensity, but at the normal setting she could feel nothing. I thought this was a little strange but turned up the current because the hairs were not coming out. Again the client felt nothing. Once more, I turned up the current — by this time it was quite high — but the hairs started releasing from the follicles, so I was just relieved the treatment was working.

I completed the treatment on one side of her upper lip, and gently moved the client's face towards me to work on the other side. I slightly moved the positioning of the needle holder and lead to make it easier to reach her and again started inserting. Suddenly, the skin blistered and the client jumped in pain. We were both shocked and I stopped the treatment immediately.

ASK THE EXPERTS

Q *What did Fiona forget to do?*

A Equipment should always be tested prior to use and the accessories cared for and stored correctly. Inside the needle holder lead are very fine copper fibres, and if the lead is damaged or incorrectly stored, some of these integral fibres may be damaged. The current flowing down the lead may then become impaired or intermittent. This, in turn, can lead to ineffective or even dangerous treatment as current levels are unpredictable.

Q *What should she do now?*

A Immediate action to cool the skin is required if the skin blisters, and aftercare lotion must be immediately applied to prevent any infection and promote healing. The client will also need careful and considered care and attention to reassure them and try to reduce the damage caused.

Effects for the therapist:

- Using untested and unsafe equipment could result in ineffective and potentially dangerous treatment
- The very ethos of being a therapist is to help people and make them feel better about themselves. Causing a client pain and possible permanent skin damage will knock a therapist's confidence and may affect her psychological wellbeing
- The therapist could potentially lose her job if her employer felt she behaved in an unsafe manner
- The therapist could potentially lose a client and word may spread to other customers
- The therapist's future job prospects could be affected
- The therapist could be sued by the client irrespective of whether the skin damage caused is temporary or permanent

Effects for the client:

- The skin damage caused could be permanent, but even if temporary it will cause embarrassment and affect the client's emotional and psychological wellbeing
- Causing the client to jump in pain may scare the client and prevent them from having another electrolysis treatment
- Causing blistering and sudden pain will certainly result in the client losing all confidence in the therapist's skills and they could go elsewhere for future treatments
- If any permanent skin damage occurs it could cause huge psychological scars affecting the client's confidence, self esteem and happiness

If the needle cannot be removed easily, check that the needle holder clamp mechanism, supporting the needle underneath the chuck cap, is of the correct grip. If necessary, gently ease the mechanism open with a redundant pair of tweezers to loosen them apart fractionally. However, if they are too loose, apply gentle pressure with gloved fingers or tweezers to tighten them. This should then ensure the correct disposal of the needle.

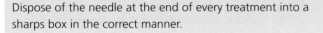

Think about it

Dispose of the needle at the end of every treatment into a sharps box in the correct manner.

Working safely to avoid contra-actions

There are many different types of epilator available, including:

- computerised units costing many thousands of pounds that will calculate the amount of hair that is removed and allow you to programme in the client's details
- units that will allow you to operate DC and AC separately (or together)
- modern digitalised units which offer three-in-one modalities
- simple straightforward diathermy or galvanic-only units.

Think about it

Always check that the electrical machinery you are about to use shows its electrical maintenance check date and that it is current. Ensure that the wires and leads are not frayed or loose and follow the manufacturer's recommended testing procedures to ensure that the leads are in good working order. Leads are made of very fine copper fibres, which if coiled too tightly can break. This can cause the current to become intermittent and unpredictable.

Methods of epilation

To refresh your memory about the types of electrical current, see Facial treatments — theory and consultation, page 272.

There are three different methods of epilation:

- galvanic (meaning 'direct current')
- alternating (often referred to as short wave diathermy or thermolysis)
- blend.

Galvanic electrolysis

This is the first form of electrical epilation and uses a direct current (a current that flows in one direction only) through a circuit consisting of one negative and one positive electrode. When a direct current passes through an electrolyte containing ions, the ions move in opposite directions.

The ions carry the current. When this is applied to tissue salts and moisture or a salt/water solution, 'electrolysis' takes place. The salt and water split into their chemical elements, which then rearrange themselves to form entirely new substances. In galvanic electrolysis, the client holds the anode connected to the positive outlet on the epilation machine and the needle holder electrode is connected to the negative outlet and therefore negatively charged. A needle is inserted into the hair follicle which contains water (H_2O) and salt (NaCl) which together act as a natural electrolyte. This increases the conductivity of the skin and allows the current to flow freely through the skin. The direct current causes a chemical reaction resulting in the atoms of the salt and water breaking down.

The atoms split into negatively and positively charged ions called cations and anions which rearrange themselves to form completely different chemical substances. Sodium hydroxide (NaOH), known as lye, a strong caustic alkali, provides the destructive force in galvanic electrolysis, and hydrogen gas (H_2) at the cathode and chlorine gas at the anode, which in turn change into hydrochloric acid.

Galvanic electrolysis is a very effective method of permanent hair removal and offers a wide field of tissue destruction which is useful for curved and distorted follicles. However, a minimum of ten seconds is required for each hair, making it an effective but slow treatment.

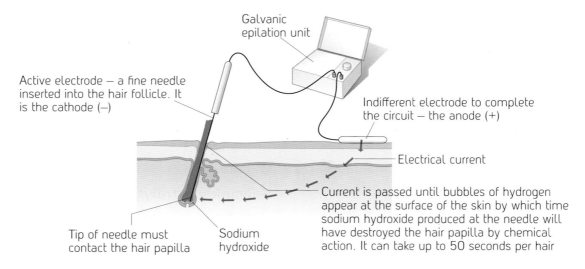

Active electrode — a fine needle inserted into the hair follicle. It is the cathode (–)

Galvanic epilation unit

Indifferent electrode to complete the circuit — the anode (+)

Electrical current

Current is passed until bubbles of hydrogen appear at the surface of the skin by which time sodium hydroxide produced at the needle will have destroyed the hair papilla by chemical action. It can take up to 50 seconds per hair

Tip of needle must contact the hair papilla

Sodium hydroxide

Destruction of the hair follicle by galvanic electrolysis

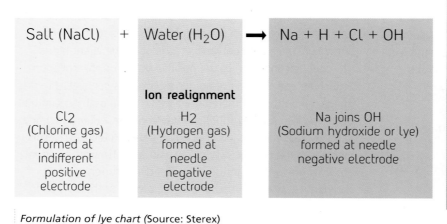

Salt (NaCl)	+	Water (H_2O)	→	Na + H + Cl + OH
		Ion realignment		
Cl_2 (Chlorine gas) formed at indifferent positive electrode		H_2 (Hydrogen gas) formed at needle negative electrode		Na joins OH (Sodium hydroxide or lye) formed at needle negative electrode

Formulation of lye chart (Source: Sterex)

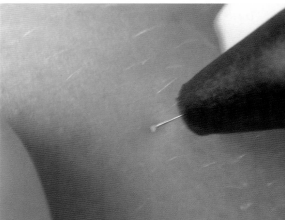

The current is discharged and a small amount of tissue fluid mixed with hydrogen gas bubbles up the follicle and appears at the follicle opening

Benefits of galvanic

- There is generally less discomfort than other methods.
- The chemical reaction has a wider field of destruction.
- It is a more effective (but much slower) method.
- It can treat distorted follicles.
- The current is attracted to the area of greatest moisture (the dermal papilla), therefore there is less risk of surface over-treatment, as the moisture gradient of the skin ensures the action is kept below the skin's surface.

Alternating current treatment

High frequency, radio frequency, thermolysis or short wave diathermy is an alternating (oscillating) current of very high frequency and low voltage ranging from 2–30 MHz or 3–30 million cycles per second. This method directs the radio frequency to the moist tissue at the base of the hair. The moisture in the cells resists the radiant energy and heats up only to be dehydrated and destroyed. These light waves heat the moist living tissue, and the dry keratinised tissue of the epidermal wall of the surrounding hair follicle is left unaffected. This is similar to placing meat in a paper bag into the microwave — the meat will be heated enough to be cooked, yet the bag will be unaffected.

By the 1930s, the alternating method began to replace the galvanic method because of its ability to destroy tissue in milliseconds rather than minutes. However, the disadvantage of short wave diathermy was its high percentage of regrowth coupled with its inability to treat curly or distorted follicles.

In short wave diathermy treatment, the molecules within the tissues are altered. The rapid agitation of atoms causes them to vibrate against each other resulting in friction which, in turn, causes heat to concentrate close to the needle tip, known as the high frequency field. Therefore, the friction that is produced by these oscillations (cycles) produces heat that builds up in the hair follicle and destroys tissue by either cauterisation or coagulation. Electrologists aim at coagulation (where the cellular structure in the tissue breaks down and protein is congealed) of the lower hair follicle in order to destroy it without damaging the surrounding tissue

Benefits of diathermy

- Short treatment time.
- Many hairs are removed in one sitting.
- Flash can be used.
- Some clients prefer the sensation of a short sharp sting.

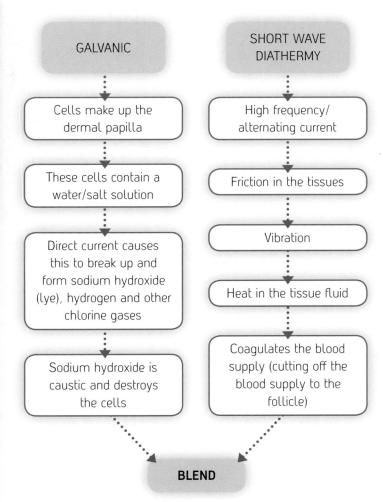

The three currents used in epilation – galvanic, short wave diathermy and blend

Blend

The thoroughness of galvanic electrolysis and the speed of short wave diathermy have been combined to produce a method of permanent hair removal known as the blend. It was introduced to the UK in 1987 and has been steadily growing in popularity because of its effectiveness. The principle of the blend is to enhance the chemical action of galvanic electrolysis with the application of high frequency simultaneously. Both currents retain their own individuality and work together to provide the most effective method in a versatile, efficient and comfortable treatment. It is suitable in treating any type of hair follicle including curly or distorted hairs because of its wide and deep field of destruction, and the regrowth experienced with shortwave diathermy is reduced.

Blend is primarily a galvanic treatment with minimal use of the short wave diathermy current. Short wave diathermy's only function (in blend treatments) is to produce warmth to speed up the chemical reaction brought about by the galvanic current. This warmth heats the lye as it is produced within the follicle by the galvanic current and makes it a more effective destructive pattern as well as creating more receptive skin tissues.

Benefits of blend

- Shorter treatment time than galvanic alone.
- There is less regrowth than with short wave diathermy.
- The chemical reaction when mixed with warmth provides the most effective destruction pattern and results.
- There is less discomfort than with short wave diathermy.
- It is effective on curved and distorted follicles.
- The current is attracted to the area of greatest moisture (the dermal papilla), therefore there is less risk of surface over-treatment, as the moisture gradient of the skin ensures the action is kept below the skin's surface.
- When blended, the lye becomes more turbulent, enabling it to invade all parts of the follicle.
- The warmth of the diathermy affects the tissues surrounding the dermal papilla, causing them to become more porous and allowing the caustic lye to diffuse into them, making the treatment more thorough.
- Research indicates that the wide field of effectiveness destroys any hair germ cells which may develop at a later date.
- Its effectiveness is ensured as research indicates the lye remains in the follicle for a period of time after treatment.

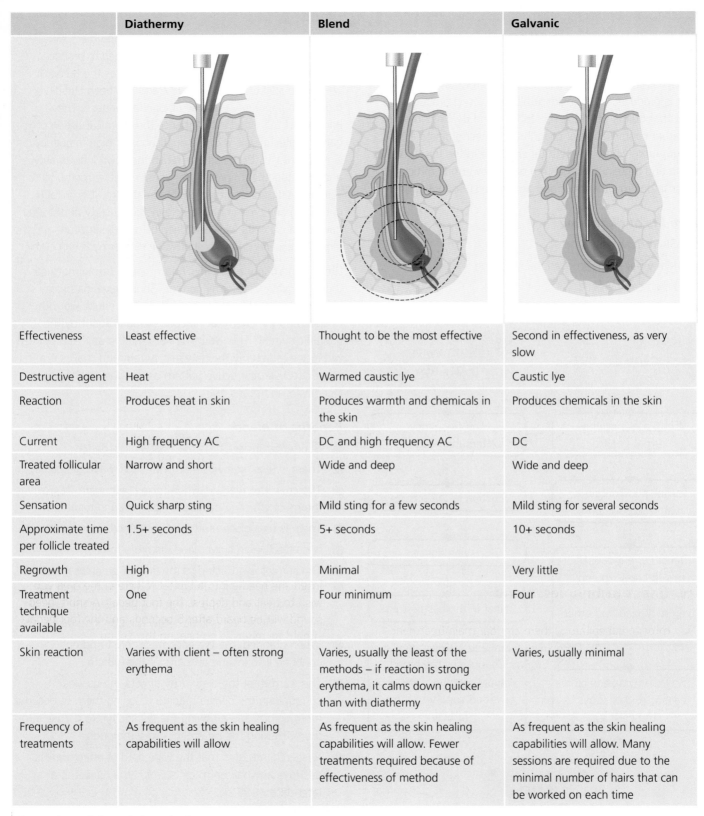

	Diathermy	Blend	Galvanic
Effectiveness	Least effective	Thought to be the most effective	Second in effectiveness, as very slow
Destructive agent	Heat	Warmed caustic lye	Caustic lye
Reaction	Produces heat in skin	Produces warmth and chemicals in the skin	Produces chemicals in the skin
Current	High frequency AC	DC and high frequency AC	DC
Treated follicular area	Narrow and short	Wide and deep	Wide and deep
Sensation	Quick sharp sting	Mild sting for a few seconds	Mild sting for several seconds
Approximate time per follicle treated	1.5+ seconds	5+ seconds	10+ seconds
Regrowth	High	Minimal	Very little
Treatment technique available	One	Four minimum	Four
Skin reaction	Varies with client – often strong erythema	Varies, usually the least of the methods – if reaction is strong erythema, it calms down quicker than with diathermy	Varies, usually minimal
Frequency of treatments	As frequent as the skin healing capabilities will allow	As frequent as the skin healing capabilities will allow. Fewer treatments required because of effectiveness of method	As frequent as the skin healing capabilities will allow. Many sessions are required due to the minimal number of hairs that can be worked on each time

Comparison of electrolysis methods

Mixing methods

The method chosen should be jointly agreed between the electrologist and the client. The severity of the hair growth will influence that decision. If the client has a large amount of superfluous hair, then short wave diathermy taking only one second or so per hair will clear the area in salon treatment time, allowing the psychological benefits this can bring. It may be that a section, for example just the upper lip, can be treated with blend. Once the blend area has been cleared, a further section can be set aside for blend treatments.

Think about it

Diathermy, galvanic and blend epilation units are very different in their use. Follow the manufacturer's instructions or attend a training course before operating. Settings vary with different machines.

With this method of working, the client gains the benefit of the most effective method teamed with the greatest number of hairs removed. For example, with an area of dense and scattered hair growth, it is important to work systematically and methodically. Use short wave diathermy in order to clear the area quickly with treatment duration of up to one hour per week, which will, over a period of time, change to treating a specific area (for example upper lip) with blend. Then as the hair weakens and starts to disappear, move to fortnightly sessions with blend on upper lip and chin. Eventually, blend treatments only will be used for the remaining hair. The length and frequency of treatments will be determined by the appearance of regrowth, and the needle size will reduce as treatment continues.

Treatment techniques: blend

With most blend epilators, there are four main treatment techniques available. Combining techniques allows the treatment to be tailored to the individual. Some epilators are digital, others use dials. Do not be concerned if the numbers fluctuate up or down by one digit when using a digital epilator as this is acceptable with digital readouts and simply means the current differentiation is so minimal the digital readout cannot register it.

Technique 1 (using the Sterex SXB Blend digital epilator)

Technique 1 is the main technique and generally used first, but if the client feels uncomfortable, one of the other three techniques (see pages 548–549) can be used. Check the wellbeing of the client after each increase. Do not inform the client that you have just increased the current, but rather that you are adjusting the current. Discuss the sensations felt by the client, as you can offer other techniques and combinations of techniques to suit each client to ensure acceptable comfort levels at all times.

- Prepare the client. It is recommended that the client's jewellery is removed.
- Give the client the indifferent electrode to hold – damp cotton wool pads or damp tissue can be wrapped around this if the client's hands are dry thereby assisting the conductivity (refer to manufacturer's instructions).
- Position yourself comfortably, with easy access to the footswitch.
- Choose a needle appropriate to the diameter of the hair and length of the follicle.
- Attach all accessories.
- Switch on the current at the back of the epilator, ensuring there is nothing blocking the fan situated beneath the unit, for example towels/couch roll.
- Switch on the diathermy, galvanic and timer sections – the digital readouts will register 01 or 00. Whenever pressure is released from the foot pedal, the current digital readouts will register back to 00 or 01.
- To alter the diathermy intensity, depress the foot pedal and set to 04. To alter the galvanic intensity, depress the foot pedal and increase to .20.
- Insert the needle into a typical follicle in the area you wish to treat and depress the foot pedal. A short 'beep' sound will be heard after 5 seconds and the foot pedal should be released on hearing this sound.
- Try releasing the treated hair. If it doesn't release, check the client's level of sensation and increase the galvanic current. If the client feels nothing, increase by 10 digits; if the client can feel something, increase by only 5 digits.
- Increase the galvanic in this way, one follicle at a time, until you have reached **the working point**. Record these data on the client's record card.

Key terms

The working point – the point when hairs remove without traction.

Provide electrical epilation treatments B29

- The level of galvanic current required will vary for every client. Check to ensure the client is comfortable and no adverse skin reaction is apparent.
- The level of galvanic current may vary dramatically between clients, whereas the level of diathermy will vary less. (It may be necessary to increase the diathermy a little but remember the diathermy only acts as a catalyst to increase the action of the more effective galvanic.)
- There may be more erythema and even oedema than associated with diathermy — this is a normal galvanic reaction that calms down very quickly.

Set digital readouts at short wave diathermy 04; timer 05.00; galvanic 0.20

⬇

Insert the needle and depress the footswitch

⬇

Wait for the 'beep' and then remove your foot

⬇

Try the hair to see if it will release

⬇

If not, increase the galvanic intensity by 5 digits. Insert into another follicle and depress the footswitch

⬇

Increase galvanic intensity 5 digits at a time until you reach the working point

Technique 1

Technique 2

This is known as the 'lower for longer' technique, as the galvanic intensity is lowered but the time is lengthened. This technique is used if the client feels uncomfortable with the higher current and shorter time of technique 1.

If, when using technique 1, the client says he or she is finding it too uncomfortable, then reduce the galvanic current by 5 digits and increase the time by 1 second, or reduce by 10 digits and increase by 2 seconds.

Technique 2 will not treat as many hairs as the main technique, as you will be in the follicle for longer, but the sensitive client may prefer it. If the treatment area is the face, however, the client may decide to have the main technique, even though she may prefer the sensation of the second, as it will remove more hairs.

Turn the galvanic intensity down 5 digits from the working point

⬇

Increase the time by 1 second (to 06.00 seconds)

Technique 2

Technique 3

This is known as the 'treat and leave' technique, as you treat a group of hairs but do not remove them immediately. If the client is sensitive but anxious to have as many hairs removed as possible, this technique is a useful and popular one to offer.

If the client says he or she is finding technique 2 too uncomfortable, then reduce the time back to 5 seconds. Treat a group of at least ten hairs, then treat a further group of at least ten hairs. After treating the second group, go back to the first group with your tweezers and remove the hairs, then go back to the second group and remove those hairs.

The action of the lye continues for a brief period of time, even though the current is switched off and the needle is withdrawn. In this technique the electrologist specifically uses the 'carry-on effect' of the lye.

The benefit of this technique is the use of lower levels of current but with a quick treatment time. The fact that many hairs are removed saves time, too.

From technique 2, decrease the time to 5 seconds; leave the galvanic intensity as set

Treat a group of approximately ten follicles but do not remove the hairs, thus allowing time for the lye to take effect

Treat another similar-sized group of hairs but do not remove them

Gently release the hairs from the first group of follicles with tweezers

Gently release the hairs from the second group of follicles

Technique 3

Technique 4

Galvanic-only is a technique that is rarely used as it takes so long. Some clients prefer the sensation of the galvanic-only technique but few are happy with the longer treatment time of 10 seconds, minimum, per follicle. It is an option, though, for the very sensitive client or those with just a few hairs. If the client finds all the blend techniques too uncomfortable, then turn off the diathermy and increase the time to 10 seconds.

With the fourth technique, if the client is not comfortable you can decrease the current and increase the time, thereby having a 'lower for longer' method, or offer 'treat and leave' as a method of increasing the number of follicles treated.

Treatment technique using a Sterex SXT diathermy-only unit:

- Attach the switched needle holder — *or* attach a Sterex unswitched needle holder and footswitch.
- Plug in and switch on the epilator.
- The mains light will come on and you will hear the internal fan.
- Switch on the on/off button.
- Using the up and down buttons, set the diathermy intensity to the level required. (If using a footswitch and unswitched needle holder, you will need to depress the footswitch when altering the current intensity.)
- If working on a new client, start at 10 and increase 5 digits at a time, working on a different follicle each time, until you reach the working point. (The working point is reached when the hairs remove without traction.)
- All clients have different tolerance levels and current intensity requirements, but as a rough guide the average working points are 20–40. Some clients will need lower levels, some higher.

From technique 3, increase the timer to 10 seconds

Switch off the diathermy but leave the galvanic intensity as set

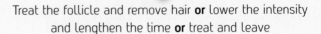

Treat the follicle and remove hair **or** lower the intensity and lengthen the time **or** treat and leave

Technique 4

Think about it

Technique 1 = higher for shorter
Technique 2 = lower for longer
Technique 3 = treat and leave
Technique 4 = galvanic only

Think about it

Whichever treatment technique is chosen is ultimately the client's choice.

Possible faults

With all techniques, if the occasional hair does not want to release, do not attempt to treat it again or force it; let the carry-on effect work, return and remove the hair at the end of the treatment.

Accurate probing is essential for a successful epilation treatment:

- The needle should enter the follicle easily with no 'bending' of the needle.
- The needle should gently slide into the follicle with no depression of the skin.
- A steady, supportive three-way stretch helps ensure an accurate insertion by clearly 'presenting' the hair and direction and angle of growth to the electrologist. When performed correctly, that is firmly but gently, it also assists with client comfort and confidence (see the diagram on page 534).
- The action should be smooth, rhythmic and unhurried, with no sign of traction when removing the hair from the follicle.

- Contact with the client at all times is most important. The 'supportive stretching hold' should never be removed from the client when passing over the tweezers to the needle holder hand to release the hair.
- A smooth, rhythmic change-over of tweezer to release the hair should be achieved.
- Slight resistance will be felt when the needle tip reaches the base of the follicle.
- The needle should remain stationary in the follicle, not be shaken or moved.
- The finger switch or footswitch should be depressed gently and smoothly.
- Double shots of current either by finger switch or foot pedal are not recommended. This can cause the needle to shake inside the follicle when the current is released, causing tissue damage and discomfort.
- The angle of insertion should mimic the direction of hair growth.
- The needle should not 'lean on' the surface of the skin nor the skin be used to rest and glide the needle into the follicle.

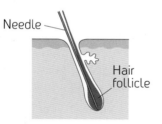

(a) Correct probing angle

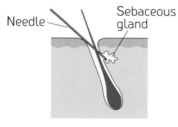

(b) Incorrect probing angle — sebaceous gland pierced

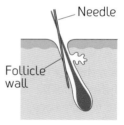

(c) Probing angle too steep follicle wall pierced

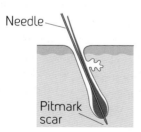

(d) Probe is too deep — base of follicle pierced. Tissue below follicle destroyed causing pitmark scar

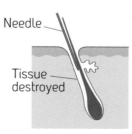

(e) Probe is too shallow — current application too close to surface. Tissue close to skin's surface destroyed

The effects of incorrect needle insertion

- Too deep an insertion may pierce through the follicle wall and cause discomfort, tissue damage and ineffective treatment. Repeated insertions of this type will cause pitting on the surface of the skin.
- Too shallow an insertion may cause surface skin damage, discomfort and ineffective treatment.
- A needle holder held lightly without tension ensures electrologist achieves sensitivity during probing.
- A steady, supportive three-way stretch helps ensure accurate insertions (see image on page 534).

Contra-actions

Possible contra-actions are shown in the table below.

Contra-action	Action required
Bending the needle	If the needle is bent in any way it should not be straightened, as distortion of the metal in the area will have taken place. This may cause a build-up of current in that section of the needle and therefore a possible burn to the client. Remove the needle safely, replace and continue treatment. (This is not to be confused with angling of the needle, when the needle is deliberately angled from the base in order to assist difficult insertions.)
Blanching or whitening	Blanching or whitening around the follicle during insertion and treatment may be the inappropriate use of short wave diathermy on a black or Asian skin or could indicate too high a current or too superficial an insertion. Treatment should immediately stop in the area and a cold compress should be applied. The reason for the whitening should be pinpointed and rectified. Hypopigmentation marks may fade over time and exfoliation of the area and a good skin regime will help; however, sometimes pigmentation can be permanent. A build-up of whiteness under the skin surrounding the follicle during blend or galvanic treatment can be the result of lye building up under the skin's surface during treatment – this is not to be confused with blanching and is not an uncommon phenomenon.

Contra-action	Action required
Blood spot or bleeding	If an incorrect insertion is made, a blood spot could appear on the surface of the skin. Immediately stem the blood with a fresh piece of cotton wool or cotton bud and depress gently but firmly for several seconds. This action is twofold – bruising is prevented by the pressure stopping the blood spreading under the surface of the skin; blood is prevented from spreading on to other items, e.g. gloves. The pressure and cotton wool can remain in place while the electrologist continues her work on other hairs in a nearby area.
Palpitations	If the client suffers palpitations, it could be because he or she is nervous or it could indicate that the individual's breathing is restricted by being in a supine position – that is, flat on the couch. Stop the treatment, loosen the client's clothing, and gently reassure the client. Fetch a glass of water to help the client calm down and raise him or her into a more seated position. Adjust your working angle to suit. It may be that the client is unsuitable for treatment.
Profuse sweating	The client may be nervous or ill, or have recently performed aerobic exercise, or it may be very hot. It is important to check the cause in order to know how to continue. Profuse sweating makes a treatment very difficult to perform. Because of the excess moisture in the skin, accuracy of insertion can be affected and also the moisture in the skin will exacerbate the current, so the current needs to be very low. Stop treatment and try to cool and calm the client as much as possible. Allow time for composure, and offer a cool glass of water. If the sweating can be calmed, continue the treatment.

Continued

Erythema and oedema	A certain amount of erythema and oedema (swelling) of the area are to be expected and is normal. Every client is different in his or her reactions to treatment. With sensitive skin, the area often becomes very red and swollen. Spacing of insertions can help, working to strict time limits and short treatments, covering perhaps two areas rather than one intensive area, and ensuring the skin has plenty of time to heal between treatments should all assist the problem. Cool water can be applied via a fresh cotton wool pad. Witch hazel is very cooling and this can be used on a fresh cotton wool pad. Some electrologists use ice (ensure this is not put directly on the skin) to take the heat out of the skin and to assist with the prevention of swelling. Good camouflage products are recommended.
Bruising	A blue or black bruise appearing during or after treatment could indicate inaccurate and too deep probing which pierces or damages the capillaries. It could also indicate too firm a stretch and handhold and too large a probe. Immediate pressure should be applied with dry sterile cotton wool or a cold compress.
Weeping follicles	These could indicate that too much galvanic current has been used, resulting in excessive chemical decomposition of the tissues of the skin. A cold compress and good aftercare are recommended if over-treatment has occurred.

Contra-actions to epilation

Other contra-actions can occur which may not directly involve the electrologist but may be linked to inaccurate or irresponsible aftercare by the client, or as a result of not following manufacturers' machine instructions and recommendations. For example, if the fan designed to keep an epilator cool for continuous use is blocked by a towel or couch roll it may overheat and this could affect the output of the machine and ultimately the client.

Provide aftercare advice

In this section you will learn about:

- Home care
- Giving accurate and constructive advice
- The cataphoresis procedure

Home care

Immediately after treatment show the client the removed hair and discuss the progress to date. Any photographs of the area(s) treated taken with the client's consent may be referred to as appropriate. Allow the client to view the area by giving the client a mirror and checking back to the treatment plan — ensure that the finished result is to the client's satisfaction. Follow this with full aftercare and homecare advice, product sales as appropriate and confirm the next treatment booking in the salon's diary and with the client.

There are many different aftercare products on the market specially designed for epilation. It must be impressed upon the client that a good programme of hygienic homecare will prevent any spots or minor infections occurring. It is important for the client to know that extra care of the treated area must be taken, especially within the first 36 hours, giving the skin a chance to settle and return to 'normal'.

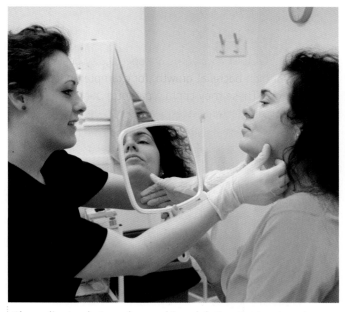

Show clients what you have achieved during the treatment

My story

Aya's story

I finished a treatment with a new client and, as she had never had epilation before, I spent an extra few minutes on my aftercare product advice. She listened carefully to what I said, including how to use the Sterex aloe vera gel I was recommending — it contained 95 per cent aloe whereas other similar products may contain only 2 per cent. However, the client chose not to purchase the gel.

Later that night, she cleansed her face with a product that had a high alcohol content. This stung a little, so in the absence of a specialised aftercare product, the client spread some petroleum jelly over the still slightly sore and raised treatment area, thinking that this would help calm it.

The next morning the area was moist, sore and swollen. The petroleum jelly had blocked the area (keeping the heat in) and encouraged bacterial growth. She rang me in distress, worried that something had gone wrong. I realised that...

What should Aya have done?

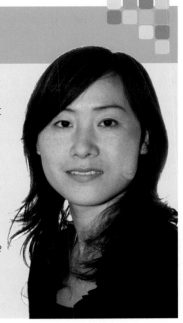

Giving accurate and constructive advice

- Aftercare products such as aloe vera or witch-hazel gel are designed to assist in the healing process of the area. They are specifically formulated to soothe the skin and help prevent any infection of the treated follicles, which will be more prone to infection after the hairs have been removed. Witch hazel, with its natural aseptic qualities, applied immediately following treatment helps prevent infection and so is generally used to soothe and cool the area for 24–48 hours (depending on skin type and area treated). Other creams are specifically designed for areas of high bacterial growth, for example underarms and groin. These may contain products such as Triclosan (a strong antibacterial agent) which, for these areas, is recommended instead of witch hazel for the first 24–48 hours to assist in preventing any infection occurring. Aloe vera with its renowned capabilities of cellular regeneration and renewal is ideal following this initial regime, for regular daily use right up to the next treatment.

- Once the skin has absorbed aftercare products, a specialised coloured cream to camouflage erythema can be used. The client's normal foundation may not be suitable as it may contain perfume or chemicals that could irritate the treated area.

- Any aftercare product should always be applied using fresh cotton wool, with the protection of gloved hands, and the manufacturer's instructions should always be followed.

- Advise the client not to touch the treated area for 12–24 hours to avoid contamination. After this time, gently cleanse with perfume/alcohol-free products, otherwise the skin may be sensitised. At home, the aftercare product should be applied using clean cotton wool. Rich creams will block the skin, preventing heat from escaping.

- Advise the client to avoid wearing tight restrictive garments on or around the treated area as these may block the area, trapping heat and causing greater irritation. They may also rub on the treated area, causing friction and therefore heat, both of which may ultimately result in an infection.

- Advise the client to avoid heat treatments such as sunbathing, sunbeds and saunas following epilation. This is because there is still heat remaining in the skin and it must be allowed to cool down and recover. Swimming is not recommended for a minimum of 24 hours as the skin is healing itself and must be given time to recover. Client participation in any of these may result in irritation, oedema, erythema, soreness or even infection.

● Advise the client on how to deal with regrowth between treatments (see the section on hair management techniques on page 522).

● An appointment should be made for the next treatment.

It is essential that the skin is allowed to heal completely between treatments. Some clients heal at a slower rate than others and this depends on several factors.

General wellbeing and self-care have a direct effect on the speed of healing. For example, vitamin C assists the body's healing process, with smokers requiring double the amount of vitamin C. Taking all these points into account, allow a healing period of one to two weeks for the majority of clients for each area of the face or body.

Think about it

Aftercare leaflets are available from the manufacturers and it is recommended to give clients one after the initial consultation and patch test and one following each subsequent treatment, to encourage them to maintain 'best practice'. Written aftercare advice to substantiate verbal advice is a pre-requisite in the small print of some insurance cover documents and if this were not carried out they may not validate a claim. Write the date and time of the client's next appointment on the back of the aftercare leaflet.

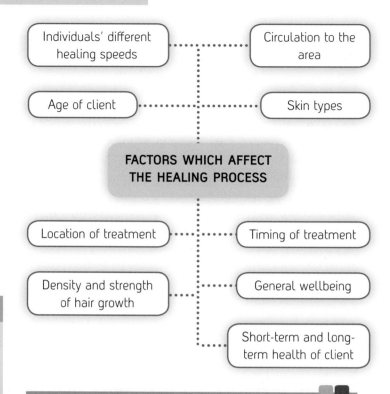

FACTORS WHICH AFFECT THE HEALING PROCESS

- Individuals' different healing speeds
- Circulation to the area
- Age of client
- Skin types
- Location of treatment
- Timing of treatment
- Density and strength of hair growth
- General wellbeing
- Short-term and long-term health of client

Key terms

Anaphoresis – opens pores, relaxes the tissues, increases erythema and aids insertions.

Cataphoresis – closes pores, calms the skin and soothes nerve endings.

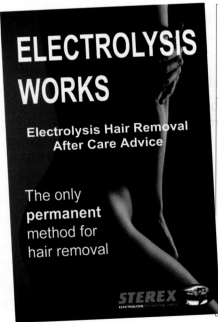

ELECTROLYSIS WORKS

Electrolysis Hair Removal After Care Advice

The only **permanent** method for hair removal

STEREX

Following electrolysis treatment a healing process takes place. Initially the skin may appear red and slightly swollen and sensitivity may also be experienced. This is normal during the healing process and these temporary reactions should reduce within 24-48 hours depending upon the area treated.

The healing process continues below the skin's surface and it is imperative to adhere to the verbal and written after-care advice recommended by your electrologist to ensure optimum results and help avoid any adverse reactions.

Please ensure you have read, understood and will comply with this after care advice. Please ask your local practitioner if you have any questions or concerns and return for further treatments as advised.

- The treatment area can be gently washed or cleansed using products recommended by the electrologist. The area should be patted dry with paper tissues (not towels) until healed. Use specialist recommended make-up and avoid perfumed products and soap. Ensure any make-up products are applied using sterile methods.
- Do not touch, pick or irritate the treated area
- Avoid UV exposure, sunbeds and fake tan. Wear sunscreen if directed to do so by your specialist
- Avoid wearing jewellery/accessories in the area or any tight restrictive clothing which could cause friction or irritation to the area
- Avoid electrical or heat treatments for 24-48 hours or until area is completely healed.
- Swimming, saunas, steam rooms, hot baths, facial scrubs and micro-dermabrasion should be avoided until the area has completely healed
- If you use a product to bleach the downy growth between treatments it should not be applied for at least 48 hours.
- Hair should not be plucked or removed with a wax or cream remover between treatments. It is safer to simply cut any noticeable hairs with scissors
- Remember to tell your electrologist about any unusual reactions immediately in order that she may modify your treatment and advise accordingly.

Appointments

Date	Time

An aftercare leaflet from Sterex (Source: Sterex Electrolysis International Ltd)

The cataphoresis procedure

During blend or galvanic electrolysis treatment, when the direct current is used, the needle acts as the negative electrode (cathode) which has an alkaline effect on the skin, producing the caustic chemical known as lye (sodium hydroxide). It is normal for the skin to become sensitised resulting in erythema and raised bumps and if this reaction is excessive it may be considered beneficial to follow with a cataphoresis procedure.

A cataphoresis procedure involves moving a small positively charged roller over the skin. The roller used in this procedure is the positive electrode (anode) and this has a balancing effect as the positive electrode produces a mild acid reaction on the skin, thereby neutralising the alkaline effect produced during treatment.

Note that the skin is naturally mildly acidic with a pH of 4.5–5.5. The skin's reaction from the electrolysis treatment will be reduced as the positive electrode neutralises the lye.

However, with sophisticated modern digital equipment and high quality medical-grade needles (in particular 24-carat-gold needles), as well as high quality aftercare products, clients' skin reactions are commonly far less severe and quite acceptable. Therefore, although cataphoresis is taught as part of the syllabus within colleges and centres, it is not often practised within industry due to constraints such as time, cost and client expectations.

Advantages

- It balances the skin's pH.
- It neutralises lye.
- The skin should appear and feel soothed/calmed.

Disadvantages

- It lengthens the treatment time.
- The cost of equipment.
- Client expectations – clients may want the time spent doing cataphoresis used to remove hairs instead.

Check your knowledge

1 What is the hormone that stimulates hair growth?
   a) Androgen
   b) Adrenaline
   c) Noradrenaline
   d) Testosterone

2 What current is mixed with the galvanic current to create the blend method?
   a) Direct current
   b) High frequency
   c) Microcurrent
   d) Macrocurrent

3 Which endocrine disorder affects hair growth?
   a) Myxoedema
   b) Grave's Disease
   c) Cushing's Syndrome
   d) Diabetes

4 Why is it is important not to treat a minor or an under-age client?
   a) The electrologist will be uninsured.
   b) Police checks are required prior to treatment.
   c) The parent or guardian have not given permission.
   d) An under-age client will be more nervous of the treatment.

5 What is Stein-Leventhal Syndrome better known as?
   a) Cretinism   c) Diabetes
   b) Dwarfism   d) Polycystic ovaries

6 How do you know how deep to introduce the probe into the follicle?
   a) Insert the full length of the probe
   b) Insert only half of the length of the probe
   c) Adjust insertions according to hair size
   d) Adjust insertions until a resistance is felt

7 How would abnormal swelling in the area following an epilation treatment be best avoided?
   a) Using a high current intensity
   b) Not overworking the area
   c) Ensuring your probing is closely spaced
   d) Ensuring your treatment is of a long duration

8 How do you select the needle size?
   a) The smaller the needle the easier the insertion
   b) Equal in diameter to match the hair
   c) All needle sizes are suitable for all hairs
   d) The larger the needle the larger the heating pattern

9 Which pole is held by the client during galvanic electrolysis?
   a) Negative – cathode   c) Negative – anode
   b) Positive – anode   d) Positive – cathode

10 What is the growing phase of the hair growth cycle called?
   a) Telogen   c) Melanin
   b) Catagen   d) Anagen

Getting ready for assessment

- Personal presentation is of vital importance, particularly for an electrologist who is dealing with clients on such a sensitive issue as unwanted hair growth. All the rules on personal hygiene must be even more closely adhered to, to ensure a hygienic, safe and effective treatment.

- The client should be in a relaxed position, their comfort levels regularly checked. It is important to treat them with respect and to ensure that their modesty and privacy levels are upheld at all times.

- You should perform all treatments in a cost-effective manner and within a commercially viable time. Efficiency and organisation in all aspects of working practice are required to achieve this, including equipment maintenance, set-up and preparation of treatment area, prepared sterilisation, adequate supplies to hand, timed consultation and efficiently carrying out verbal and written aftercare etc. Some electrologists have a small timer which, once the client is prepared and ready for treatment, they set for the required and paid time. Once this timer 'beeps', the treatment finishes and the aftercare is performed.

- Your assessor will be looking for you to demonstrate clear explanation and agreement in writing on the projected cost, likely duration, frequency, type of treatment and client commitment needed, as well as identification and agreement in writing of the area to be treated to meet with client expectation and attain realistic and achievable treatment objectives.

- You will also be expected to show a polite, sensitive and supportive manner to determine the client's treatment needs and the firm foundation for the start of a developing bond and good professional working relationship between the client and electrologist.

- Your assessor will want to see that the area to be treated is kept clean, oil-free and dry prior to treatment and that you select the size and type of needle appropriate for the client's follicle size, hair and skin type and the method of epilation chosen.

- Each manufacturer of epilation machines will have a manual for that machine which will detail instructions of how to perform a testing procedure prior to treatment. This allows you to check the machine is performing as it should and thus avoids the potential of contra-actions occurring.

- You must demonstrate that you are working systematically, removing hair within the desired treatment area(s) and within the boundaries of the skin's tolerance.

- Your assessor will be looking for aftercare advice and recommendations given accurately and constructively, with individual advice given that is specific to the client's needs.

Index